McAlpine's Multiple Sclerosis

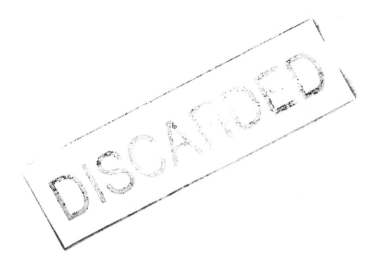

Volume Editor:

W. B. Matthews

Professor Emeritus of Clinical Neurology, University of
Oxford, Oxford, UK

McAlpine's Multiple Sclerosis

W. B. Matthews
Professor Emeritus of Clinical Neurology, University of Oxford,
Oxford, UK

A. Compston PhD MB BS FRCP
Professor of Neurology, Addenbrooke's Hospital Medical School,
Cambridge, UK

Ingrid V. Allen DSc MD MB BCh BAO FRCPath
Professor of Neuropathology, Institute of Pathology, Queen's
University, Belfast, UK

Christopher N. Martyn MA DPhil MRCP
Epidemiologist, MRC Environmental Epidemiology Unit, Southampton
General Hospital, Southampton, UK; Honorary Senior Registrar in
Neurology, Wessex Neurological Centre, Southampton General Hospital,
Southampton, UK

SECOND EDITION

CHURCHILL LIVINGSTONE
EDINBURGH LONDON MELBOURNE AND NEW YORK 1991

CHURCHILL LIVINGSTONE
Medical Division of Longman Group UK Limited

Distributed in the United States of America by
Churchill Livingstone Inc., 650 Avenue of the Americas,
New York, 10011, and by associated companies, branches and
representatives throughout the world.

First edition 1985
Second edition 1991
    Reprinted 1992 (twice)

ISBN 0-443-04047-8

British Library Cataloguing in Publication Data
McAlpine, Douglas 1890–
    McAlpine multiple sclerosis. – 2nd. ed.
    1. Man. Multiple sclerosis
    I. Title II. Matthews, W. B. (Walter Bryan)
    616.834

Library of Congress Cataloging in Publication Data
    McAlpine's multiple sclerosis / W. B. Matthews . . .
    [et al.].—2nd ed.
        p. cm.
    Includes bibliographical references.
    Includes index.
    ISBN 0-443-04047-8
    1. Multiple sclerosis. I. McAlpine, Douglas.
II. Matthews, W. B. (Walter Bryan) III. Title: Multiple
sclerosis.
    [DNLM: 1. Multiple Sclerosis. WL 360 M478]
RC377.M43 1991
616.8'34—dc20
DLC   90–1947
for Library of Congress   CIP

The
publisher's
policy is to use
**paper manufactured
from sustainable forests**

Produced by Longman Singapore Publishers (Pte) Ltd
Printed in Singapore

Preface to the First Edition

This book is in some sense a fourth edition of the original *Multiple Sclerosis* of 1955 by McAlpine, Compston and Lumsden. This was succeeded by two editions of *Multiple Sclerosis: A Reappraisal* by McAlpine, Lumsden and Acheson. Each edition owed much to the enthusiasm and original observations of the late Douglas McAlpine, and it seemed appropriate to continue to use his name, even though the present volume contains very few words written by him, and perhaps a number of which he would not have approved.

It is no longer possible even to attempt a comprehensive work on multiple sclerosis and we have had to be selective. The absence of a virologist, a biochemist and an expert on experimental allergic encephalomyelitis may be regretted. The virologist could, however, only have written on the continuing failure to demonstrate a virus as the cause or even the precipitating factor of multiple sclerosis, despite the most intensive search. The biochemist could have described the composition of myelin but not the reason or mechanism of its breakdown in multiple sclerosis. The expert in EAE would have had to confess that despite remarkable similarities the disease is not identical with multiple sclerosis.

Considerable emphasis has again been laid on clinical aspects of the disease and surprise might therefore be felt at the omission of the chapter in earlier editions on medico-social aspects. This omission is not because the often literally vital significance of this topic to the patient has been ought unimportant. The provision of help and the means of obtaining it vary greatly with the economic climate and from one country to another. The ideal requirements might have been discussed but their fulfilment is a political decision that may be influenced but seldom implemented by doctors or patients.

The pathology section concentrates upon the basic neuropathology of the different phases of multiple sclerosis, where possible relating it both to the clinical aspects of the disease and to the result of immunological and experimental studies.

At a time when *Current Contents* averages six references to multiple sclerosis every week, the problems of preparing an up-to-date manuscript are severe and have almost certainly not been fully overcome. This is not always disadvantageous, however, as advancing knowledge of multiple sclerosis is apt to follow a somewhat halting course, the latest contribution all too often not being confirmed by the next investigator.

1985

W. B. M.
E. D. A.
J. R. B.
R. O. W.

Preface to the Second Edition

In the previous edition of this book, knowledge of selected topics in multiple sclerosis was surveyed up to 1983. Succeeding years have seen notable advances in means of diagnosis and increasing sophistication in the collection of epidemiological data and in the organisation and assessment of therapeutic trials. In the laboratory, the nature of the disease process has been tenaciously pursued and imaging techniques have thrown unexpected light on the natural history and pathophysiology of multiple sclerosis. Despite this continuously increasing endeavour, the goal of revealing the cause of the disease has not yet been achieved.

In this edition, the plan previously adopted has been followed, but with a new cast. Sir Donald Acheson, a contributor to *Multiple Sclerosis, a Reappraisal* and to the last edition, now has exacting tasks that have prevented his continued association with this book and has been succeeded by Dr Christopher Martyn from the same University Department. Professor Ingrid Allen needs no introduction as a major authority in her field. It is a pleasure to welcome Professor Alastair Compston, the son of the late Dr Nigel Compston, a contributor to the original 1955 edition.

As before, emphasis has been placed on clinical aspects, but even here the topic is so vast that important areas have had to be neglected, in particular the social implications of the disease, the management of day-to-day problems in the home and the extent of practical help available. These are covered by many admirable publications, written with the necessary involvement of people with multiple sclerosis. In the scientific field, subdivision between topics is not always clear cut. Heredity, for example, has important implications for epidemiology, for immunology and for clinical practice, and some overlap between chapters has proved necessary and helpful in permitting contributors to express their ideas fully.

The major disappointment of the years since the last edition is that, despite great expansion of the chapter on treatment, it is not possible to claim for any regime that it will consistently ameliorate the course of the disease.

Oxford, 1990   W.B.M.

Contents

Epidemiology

Christopher Martyn

1. The epidemiology of multiple sclerosis

Epidemiologists are concerned with the patterns of disease within populations, with the geographical distribution of disease and with the way in which the occurrence of disease varies over time. To put it in the most straightforward terms, they are trying to answer three questions: Where does the disease occur? When does it occur? And who gets it? The purpose of this endeavour is to identify causes and to provide a description of the natural history of the disease.

THE EPIDEMIOLOGICAL APPROACH TO MULTIPLE SCLEROSIS

Clinicians, accustomed to focusing on the unique diagnostic and therapeutic problems of individual patients, sometimes find difficulty in adjusting to the wider angle view needed when patterns of disease are being considered in populations. A general explanation of the methods of epidemiology would be out of place here (the interested reader is referred to one of the several excellent textbooks on the subject)[1,2] but a brief discussion of some of the techniques used and difficulties faced by epidemiologists studying multiple sclerosis may be helpful.

Measurement of rates of disease

Several different indices are used to describe the frequency of disease in a population. The most informative of these, particularly where the intention is to identify aetiological factors or determine whether the risk of disease has changed over time, is **incidence** or the rate of occurrence of new cases.

Incidence is calculated as a simple ratio in which the numerator is the number of people who develop a disease during a fixed period of time, usually a year, and the denominator is the total number of people who are at risk of developing the disease during the same period. It can be defined as:

$$\frac{\text{number of new cases of}}{\text{disease in a period of time}}$$
$$\text{number of people at risk}$$
$$\text{of developing disease}$$
$$\text{in the same period}$$

In practice, unfortunately, there are two reasons why a satisfactory estimate of incidence of multiple sclerosis in a population is hard to obtain. Multiple sclerosis is an uncommon disease so that, unless the population being investigated is very large or studied for a long period of time, only a small number of new cases will occur. Estimates of incidence based on small numbers are too easily influenced by random variation to be of much value. The second reason concerns the difficulty in making a definite diagnosis in the early stages of the disease. Cases which should have been included in the numerator of the ratio defined above may be lost because a firm diagnosis could not be made during the period of the study.

These problems in measuring incidence have led most investigators to rely upon **prevalence** as the index of disease frequency. Prevalence is the ratio of the number of cases alive at a given time (prevalence day) to the size of the population at risk at the same time. It can be defined as:

$$\frac{\text{number of cases of disease alive on a particular day}}{\text{number of people at risk of having the disease on the same day}}$$

All cases of the disease alive on prevalence day are included, regardless of how long they have suffered from the disease. Only those cases who have died or who have left the area before prevalence day are excluded. For chronic diseases such as multiple sclerosis, the prevalence may be 20 or 30 times higher than the incidence. This is why prevalence has a great advantage over incidence as an index of disease frequency. Because the numerator includes all living cases, it is large enough, in relation to the denominator of people at risk, to allow stable estimates to be calculated for quite small populations.

There are, however, a number of disadvantages associated with its use as a summary measure of disease frequency. Prevalence is arithmetically related to incidence by duration of disease:

$$\text{prevalence} = \text{incidence} \times \frac{\text{mean duration}}{\text{of disease}}$$

Because of this dependence on duration of disease, differences in survival of cases due to variation in the severity of the disease or in the efficacy of treatment of its complications have a major influence on estimates of prevalence. This must be taken into account when comparing prevalence of disease in different places. For example, in communities where the standard of living is low and quality of medical care poor, the development of disability often quickly leads to under-nutrition, inter-current infection and death. The prevalence of chronic disease will inevitably be lower than in a community where the incidence of disease is the same, but where living conditions and access to medical care are better.

Nor does a change in prevalence over time necessarily indicate a change in the underlying in-cidence of disease. It might also be caused by: a change in the duration of disease; a difference in the ascertainment of cases; a change in the age structure of the population; differential migration of people with the disease compared with the general population. A clear example of how these factors may operate is found in reports of studies in the Orkneys. In repeated surveys of these islands, the prevalence of probable multiple sclerosis increased from 82 per 100 000 population in 1954 to 258 per 100 000 population in 1974.[3] Incidence rates remained fairly constant over this period. Indeed, there is evidence that the incidence of multiple sclerosis in the Orkneys has been falling in recent years.[4] The apparent paradox of rising prevalence and falling incidence is mainly explained by more complete ascertainment of cases in later surveys and by an increase in the average duration of disease. Changes in the age structure of the population and differential emigration of healthy individuals probably made a minor contribution to the rise in prevalence too.

Other indices of disease frequency based on hospital admission or discharge rates, or on mortality data, are sometimes used to study patterns of multiple sclerosis. The information needed to calculate these indices is usually collected routinely by a country's Central Office of Health Statistics and investigators may be allowed access to it. Studies that utilise this source of data often seem attractive because they can be carried out more cheaply and with less effort than a population-based survey of prevalence. However, hidden biases exist in the way the data are collected, and indices of disease frequency based upon them may be unreliable. Hospital admission and discharge rates are strongly influenced by quality and availability of medical care, as well as by rates of disease. They are not usually helpful when comparing frequency of disease in different communities. Mortality data ultimately depend on what was written on the death certificate by the medical practitioner certifying death. The Central Office of Health Statistics uses this information to identify and code the underlying cause of death. Because the terminal event for many patients with multiple sclerosis is a respiratory or urinary tract infection, multiple sclerosis often appears on the death certificate only as a contributory cause or an associated condition. Of course, some patients die because of an unrelated illness and multiple sclerosis may not be recorded at all. In these circumstances, the underlying cause of death will not be attributed to multiple sclerosis. Studies in the USA, England and Norway have shown that as many as 40% of patients diagnosed during life as having multiple sclerosis do not have this diagnosis coded as the underlying cause of death.[5-7] Rates of multiple sclerosis derived from mortality data are certain to underestimate the true frequency of disease.

There are other disadvantages in using mortality data to study multiple sclerosis. Because the disease is chronic, death rates give no indication of the current pattern of incidence of the disease. Instead, they reflect what was happening 20 or 30 years earlier. They are also influenced by improvements in the treatment that lead to longer survival of cases. In many places mortality from multiple sclerosis has declined, not because the disease is occurring less frequently, but because its duration has increased.

Sufficient information to obtain a fairly complete picture of the distribution of multiple sclerosis is now available from surveys carried out with the specific aim of establishing the prevalence of the disease. The value of mortality and hospital admission and discharge rates has therefore diminished, although these indices may still be useful in circumstances where prevalence data are scanty. They can also provide independent corroboration of estimates of rates of disease based on other data.

Case ascertainment in surveys of prevalence and incidence

Accurate estimates of rates of multiple sclerosis in a population depend absolutely on completeness of case ascertainment. Since the prevalence is usually less than 1 case per 1000 population, it has only been practicable in very few studies to employ trained field workers to carry out a door to door survey to identify cases. Most surveys have used less direct methods; usually the primary source of information has been the records of hospitals, neurologists and other medical practitioners serving the population in which the survey is carried out. Sometimes, additional sources of information, such as the membership records of patient societies for multiple sclerosis, records of community nursing services and diagnostic indices of departments of neurophysiology, where patients with suspected multiple sclerosis might have been referred for examination of visual and other evoked responses, are used to supplement the primary source and increase completeness of case ascertainment.

It is obvious that these indirect methods of case finding rely heavily on the standards of medical care and record keeping that prevail in the community studied. The attitudes that patients have towards seeking medical advice about neurological disability, whether such advice is free, and the ease of access to physicians with special training in diseases of the nervous system, are all likely to be important determinants of the number of diagnosed cases of multiple sclerosis. The results of two recent surveys emphasise how, even in areas with excellent medical resources, a considerable proportion of cases of multiple sclerosis remain unknown to local medical services. In a south London borough, only 79% of cases could be identified from hospital and general practitioner records.[8] In another survey, of the health district of Southampton and south west Hampshire, 38% of cases were unknown to the general practitioners working in the area.[9] There is no reason to believe that these figures are atypical and in many areas of the world the proportion of cases that can be identified from medical records alone is probably much smaller.

In areas that have been studied on more than one occasion, the prevalence of multiple sclerosis in later surveys is almost always higher than that found in the first. Part of the explanation is likely to be that the first study raised the level of awareness of the disease amongst medical practitioners working in the survey area. In the years following the survey, missed cases become identified and diagnosis of new cases is earlier and more complete. If the area is surveyed a second time, prevalence appears to have increased.

A further factor that affects case ascertainment is the size of the population being surveyed. Dean's work in Sicily shows how case-finding is improved by concentrating on a small and well-defined population instead of trying to cover a large region. Multiple sclerosis was thought to be a rare disease in southern Italy until his intensive studies of small communities revealed that the prevalence in some places exceeded 50 per 100 000 population.[10–14]

The factors that influence completeness of case ascertainment operate so consistently that it is possible to formulate four rules that should be borne in mind when judging the significance of differences in reported prevalence. Estimates of the prevalence of multiple sclerosis are almost invariably higher:

1. in recent surveys compared with earlier surveys
2. in second and subsequent surveys (compared with the first) when an area has been studied more than once
3. in surveys that have used many sources of information to identify cases compared with surveys that have relied on a single source
4. in surveys of small populations compared with surveys of large populations.

Accuracy of diagnosis

A major problem in the past for epidemiologists trying to identify cases of multiple sclerosis arose because of the lack of any satisfactory diagnostic test for the disease. Sets of standard clinical criteria for the diagnosis have been proposed in an attempt to get around this difficulty.[15–21] Many carefully carried out surveys have included an independent clinical assessment of cases to ensure that they fulfilled these criteria. Some difficulties remain because the diagnostic criteria for multiple sclerosis have undergone modification to improve their sensitivity and specificity and to include information derived from laboratory tests. Different investigators have used different sets of criteria for diagnosis and classification and the details of whose criteria have been used are not always given in published work. An assessment of variation between neurologists in the application of one set of these criteria showed that there was a considerable amount of disagreement over the diagnosis in individual patients,[22] but few investigators engaged in surveys have checked on the reproducibility of their diagnostic classification.

Frequently, of course, a gap of several years intervenes between the onset of symptoms and the point when a definite diagnosis of multiple sclerosis is established. This may occur because the patient delays seeking medical advice, or because the clinical features at presentation are not sufficiently characteristic of multiple sclerosis for the diagnosis to be made at the time.

The effect of these diagnostic difficulties is twofold. First, the lack of a test to confirm the diagnosis means that, even in the best conducted surveys, a proportion of cases will be misclassified. The number on which the estimate of prevalence is based will inevitably include some people who do not have the disease. Second, delay between the onset of symptoms and diagnosis will cause the numbers of patients with multiple sclerosis to be underestimated. There is a fortunate tendency for these effects to operate in opposite directions; the overestimate caused by inclusion of people with other diseases is, to some extent, balanced by the underestimate caused by delay in diagnosis.

In the past few years, the wider use of evoked potential studies and laboratory analysis of CSF has almost certainly led to earlier and more accurate diagnosis. As magnetic resonance imaging techniques become available, further improvement can be expected and the proportion of cases that must be excluded from surveys because of doubt about the diagnosis will decline. Unfortunately, these advances are only likely to be of benefit to epidemiologists working in developed countries.

The age structure of the population

When comparing rates of disease between different places or in the same place at different times, it is essential to avoid the distorting effects of differences in the age structure of the population. Rothman has given a clear example of how failure to do this may give a misleading impression.[1] He compared the annual death rates from all causes in Sweden and Panama. In 1962 the death rate in Sweden was 98 per 10 000, whereas in Panama it was nearly 30% lower, at 73 per 10 000. At first sight this is a surprising finding, but an explanation can be found by examining the age structure of the population of the two countries. In Panama, 69% of the population were under the age of 30, while in Sweden, the corresponding figure was only 42%. The apparently lower mortality in Panama can be entirely accounted for by the fact that the Panamanians were younger than the Swedes.

Differences in age structure of populations tend to have their most profound effects on estimates of rates of diseases that affect the very young or very old. Rates of diseases like multiple sclerosis that strike young or middle-aged adults are less subject to distortion. Adjustment of estimates of crude prevalence for age differences is unlikely to change the interpretation placed upon large differences between countries whose population structure is fairly similar. However, where areas with populations of very different age are being compared, for instance a third world country with an industrialised nation, adjustment for age becomes important. In a survey in Bombay, the estimate of the crude prevalence rate fell by more than 25% when adjusted to the population of the USA.[23] Another situation in which adjustment for age becomes necessary is when comparing rates of disease in immigrants with the native-born population of a country. In Australia, crude prevalence rates of multiple sclerosis in people born overseas were found to be significantly higher than in people who had been born there. Because the age distribution of the immigrant population was weighted towards the older age groups, much of the difference was removed by age-standardisation.[24]

Provided that the age structure of the populations being compared is known, simple mathematical techniques can be applied to adjust for differences. No firm conclusions should be drawn from estimates of crude prevalence until this has been done.

Case-control studies

The discussion so far has concerned the application of the techniques of descriptive epidemiology to multiple sclerosis — the gathering of quantitative information about the occurrence of the disease in populations. Another approach has been to use case-control methodology. In a case-control study, patients with a disease are compared with controls who do not have the disease. Rates of past exposure to known or suspected risk factors are measured in each group and from this, the relative risk associated with each factor is estimated.

Case-control studies are an efficient way in which to test specific aetiological hypotheses. But the apparent simplicity of the method disguises the difficulties that can arise both in the choice of cases and an appropriate control group, and in the unbiased measurement of exposure to the risk factors of interest.

Selection of cases

Investigators in case-control studies of multiple sclerosis usually recruit prevalent, i.e. existing, cases of disease rather than incident, i.e. new, cases. The reason for choosing prevalent cases is fairly obvious. An investigator who restricted himself to new cases would find it hard to recruit enough people to achieve adequate statistical power for his study. But the use of prevalent cases may cause problems in interpretation. If an association between disease and exposure is found it may reflect an effect, not on the occurrence of disease, but on survival. For example, the finding that cases of multiple sclerosis experience lower rates of respiratory infection than controls[25] may not mean that people with multiple sclerosis have superior immune defences against common viruses, but merely that cases who do not get these infections survive longer than those that do and so have a greater chance of being recruited into the study.

Another serious problem in using prevalent cases in investigations of chronic disabling disease arises because the presence of disease modifies the way in which patients lead their lives. If differences are found between cases and controls, they may be a result of having the disease rather than a cause of the disease.

Even if it proves possible to use incident cases of disease, there may be uncertainties about the correct interpretation of the results. No case can be entered into the study until the diagnosis has been made and because of the variability of the initial presentation of multiple sclerosis, time of diagnosis in relation to the onset of disease is unlikely to be uniform throughout the study population. If the influences that determine the time of diagnosis are related in some way to the exposure being investigated, spurious associations might arise. For example, in a case-control study designed to find out whether urban dwellers are at greater risk of multiple sclerosis that those living in a rural environment, a positive result might be found because people living in towns have easier access to neurological centres and, as a result, a greater chance of being diagnosed at an earlier stage of the disease.

Selection of controls

Choice of an appropriate control group is a crucial part of the design of a case-control study. Two requirements must be fulfilled: (i) the exposure of controls to the risk factors under investigation must be representative of the study population at risk of becoming cases, and (ii) it must be possible to measure the exposure of controls to these risk factors with the same degree of accuracy as for cases.

In hospital-based studies, patients with other neurological diseases are frequently used as a convenient source of controls. This has the advantage that measurement of exposure can often be made comparable to that for cases. A danger in studies that rely on recall to assess exposure is that, because of a natural interest in trying to understand why they have become ill, cases are more motivated to search their memories than controls. If the controls are also ill, they too will be seeking an explanation for their disease. There is the further advantage that the diagnoses of controls can be chosen so that their catchment population is similar to that of cases.

The main weakness of using patients with other diseases as controls is that their exposure may not be representative of that of members of the study population who are at risk of becoming cases. For example, if patients with epilepsy are included in the control group, restrictions on driving are likely to affect both the jobs in which they can be employed and their leisure activities. This will make them unrepresentative of the study population for a whole range of occupational and leisure-time exposures.

An alternative to using other patients as controls is to select controls from the general population. Population registers derived from censuses or, in countries with a nationalised health service, health service records can be taken as the sampling frame, or a predetermined algorithm can be used. to select controls living in the same neighbourhood as cases. The exposures of controls selected in one of these ways from the general population are likely to be more representative of those in the population at risk than if controls with other neurological diseases are used. However, biases may occur if there is a poor response rate from controls, because the exposure patterns of non-responders are often different from those of people who agree to take part in the study.

The hardest problem to overcome when using controls selected from the general population is in the unbiased ascertainment of exposure. Subjects selected from the community will usually be less inclined than cases to put time and effort into helping with a study. Some investigators have resorted to using two control groups, one derived from the community and the second from patients with other diseases, to try to overcome these difficulties.

When weighing up the validity of a case-control study, three questions should be asked about the control group(s) used:

1. Did the controls come from the same population as the cases? That is to say, would a subject recruited as a control have been recruited as a case if he had developed the disease being studied?
2. Was the method used to ascertain exposure similar in cases and controls? For example, if information was obtained from cases by an interviewer while they were in hospital, comparison with information obtained from controls by a postal questionnaire would be suspect.
3. Were those involved in collecting data blind to the case/control status of the subject? In order to avoid subconscious biases, the person collecting information, whether he is administering a questionnaire, carrying out a physical examination or performing an analysis in a laboratory, should not know whether he is dealing with a case or a control.

This account of the methods used and problems encountered in carrying out epidemiological studies of multiple sclerosis is intended to encourage caution in the interpretation of results. Examples like that of the Orkneys, where prevalence increased threefold over a period of 30 years despite stable or declining incidence rates, or Southern Italy and Sicily, where multiple sclerosis was considered rare until intensive surveys of small communities were carried out, should be borne in mind by anyone tempted to put much weight on the results of a single study. But there is no need to take too negative a view; many of the features of the epidemiology of multiple sclerosis have now been confirmed by different investigators, using a variety of methods. One may be confident that the unusual pattern of the disease contains important clues about its cause.

THE PATTERN OF MULTIPLE SCLEROSIS IN POPULATIONS

Sex

Population surveys consistently show that multiple sclerosis is more common in women than in men. By averaging data from 14 well-conducted prevalence surveys carried out before 1977, Acheson calculated that the risk for women was 1.4 times greater than that for men.[26] The results of several investigations carried out since suggest that this may be an underestimate; recently reported values for the sex ratio range between 1.9 and 3.1.[24,27–29]

Because these ratios are based on prevalence data, the possibility exists, at least in theory, that they may have been affected by differential survival between the sexes. Known differences in duration of disease or mortality between men and women are not great enough to account for a sex ratio of this magnitude and the surveys of incidence that give rates for the sexes separately confirm that incidence in women is consistently higher than in men. It is reasonable to conclude that women are about twice as likely to develop the disease as men.

Differences between the sexes in the incidence of disease occur very commonly and, even when the differences are large, they often fail to provide any strong clues about aetiology. It is possible that the higher incidence of multiple sclerosis in women reflects a hormonal factor that increases susceptibility, but there are many other, equally probable, explanations.

Age

The pattern of age of onset of multiple sclerosis established in early studies remains unchallenged by recent work. Onset of the disease is rare before puberty, but subsequently the incidence increases rapidly to reach a peak around the age of 30 years. It remains high in the fourth decade but then declines steeply. After the age of 60 years, the incidence is negligible. In the majority of surveys, the average age of onset of multiple sclerosis is slightly lower in women than in men. The difference is rarely more than 2 years and often much less. A difference of this magnitude could easily be the result of a systematic bias as might arise, for instance, if women tended to seek medical advice earlier in the course of an illness than men or if neurologists, aware that multiple sclerosis is more common in women than men, were inclined to make the diagnosis more readily in women.

A remarkable feature of the age-specific incidence curve for multiple sclerosis is that its shape does not vary with the underlying frequency of disease. In an American study, identical methods were used to survey populations in Seattle and Los Angeles.[30,31] The prevalence of multiple sclerosis in Seattle was more than twice that in Los Angeles, but the average age of onset of the disease and shape of the age-specific incidence curve showed little difference between the cities. The same phenomenon has been found in a recent survey of three towns in Australia.[24] The incidence of multiple sclerosis in Perth, W A; Newcastle, Queensland; and Hobart, Tasmania was measured over the period 1971–1981. There was a nearly threefold difference in incidence rates, but again, the shape of the age-specific incidence curves of the individual towns was similar. The observation holds true in the most extreme cases; the age-specific incidence curve for multiple sclerosis in Japan, where the overall prevalence is only about 2 per 100 000 population, can be made to coincide with that of Denmark, where the prevalence is

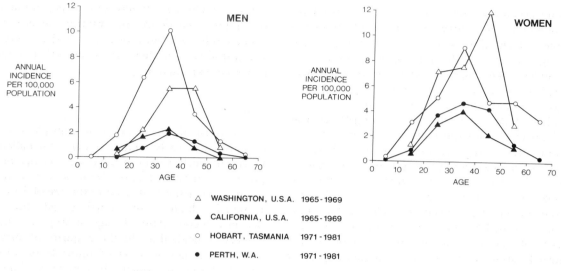

Fig. 1.1 Age-specific incidence rates for multiple sclerosis.

nearly 50 times higher, simply by adjusting the scale of the vertical axis of the graph.[32] These examples are illustrated in Figure 1.1.

The age-specific incidence curve for multiple sclerosis is unusual and some tentative inferences may be drawn from it. The unimodal shape and lack of variation with underlying frequency of disease are consistent with the view that multiple sclerosis is a single disease and that its aetiology does not differ between places. The way in which the curve rises steeply to a maximum around the age of 30 years before rapidly falling away again suggests either that the chances of exposure to the causal agent increase to a peak with age and then decline, or that some factor that determines susceptibility behaves in the same way. The shape of the curve is hardly compatible with the idea that multiple sclerosis is caused by cumulative exposure to an environmental factor. In diseases for which cumulative exposure to a noxious agent is aetiologically important, e.g. many cancers, the usual pattern of incidence is an exponential increase with age.

Except that the peak occurs 20 years later, the age-specific incidence curve for multiple sclerosis resembles that of many of the acute infections of childhood. The incidence of these acute infections rises rapidly in the first few years of life to reach

a peak sometime in the first decade. Because the first attack confers lifelong immunity, incidence then quickly declines as the proportion of the population that are immune increases. The age at which the peak in incidence occurs varies with the pattern of exposure to the infectious agent. Where the infection is most common, first exposure to the infective agent occurs early and the highest incidence is in the very young. In places where the infection is less common, first exposure is relatively delayed and the peak in incidence occurs at an older age. In parts of Africa, for example, the highest incidence of measles is found in children under the age of 2 years, whereas in the developed countries of the world, the peak in incidence occurs in children in the 5–10-year-old age group.[33,34] It has been suggested that multiple sclerosis may be a rare sequel to a childhood infection that only becomes manifest after a long latent period. If this were so, one would expect that the age-specific incidence curve would be shifted to the right (i.e. the average age of onset of disease would be later) in places where multiple sclerosis is rare and, as we have seen, the evidence is against this.

A few other diseases, for example, schizophrenia, thyrotoxicosis, migraine and chronic sinusitis, have been noted to have an age-specific incidence curve like that of multiple sclerosis.[35] But these conditions are likely to be diverse in their aetiology, and the parallels in age of onset do not suggest any useful hypotheses about the cause of multiple sclerosis.

World distribution

The striking differences in the frequency of multiple sclerosis between different parts of the world have been written about and discussed for more than 40 years. In 1975, Kurtzke undertook an encyclopaedic review of nearly 200 surveys in which an attempt had been made to establish the prevalence of multiple sclerosis.[36,37] He critically evaluated the methodology used in each of these surveys and graded them into three categories. Class A studies represented surveys of a delineated population carried out using well-defined and reasonably comparable methodology and diagnostic standards. Studies contained in Class B were considered satisfactory in methodology, but there was some reason why they were not fully comparable to those in Class A — most commonly because the survey had been carried out to investigate an area where there was a prior reason to suspect that the frequency of disease was unusual. Class C surveys contained obvious methodological flaws. An additional group, Class E, represented an estimate of prevalence obtained by taking the ratio of cases of multiple sclerosis to cases of amyotrophic lateral sclerosis in series from hospitals and clinics. When calculating this estimate, amyotrophic lateral sclerosis was assumed to have a prevalence of 5 per 100 000 population worldwide. Kurtzke also recalculated prevalence rates for these surveys using only cases which fell into the diagnostic categories: probable; early probable or latent; and definite, and excluded cases where the diagnosis was possible multiple sclerosis using, as far as possible, the criteria of Allison & Millar.[15] He also gave 95% confidence intervals for each rate.

It is impossible to describe each of these surveys here; in any case, Kurtzke's review makes the task unnecessary. Instead, his invaluable work has been taken as a starting point and in the description of the world distribution of multiple sclerosis that

follows, emphasis has been given to surveys carried out since 1975.

Recently, it has been shown that mortality from amyotrophic lateral sclerosis has increased considerably in several countries over the past 25 years.[38–42] There is also evidence that the geographical distribution of the disease may be less uniform than was previously supposed. Estimates of the prevalence of multiple sclerosis based on ratios with amyotrophic lateral sclerosis may therefore be misleading and studies that fall into Class E have largely been ignored. Nor has much weight been given to surveys that fall into Class C.

Geographical regions are sometimes grouped into high, medium and low risk zones according to their prevalence of multiple sclerosis. The exact prevalence that is used to determine the cut-off points between zones of risk varies between authors. The most widely used grouping follows Kurtzke's definitions: areas having a prevalence equal to or greater than 30 cases per 100 000 population are high risk; areas where the prevalence falls between 5 and 25 cases per 100 000 population are medium risk, and areas with fewer than 5 cases per 100 000 population are low risk. This convention may be helpful, particularly when displaying information graphically, but it has several disadvantages. The first is that important differences within zones may be masked. In northern Europe, for example, there are five or sixfold variations in the prevalence of multiple sclerosis within the high risk category. The second disadvantage is that undue significance is given to the rates that define cut-off points between categories. It is not unusual to find statements in the literature to the effect that the most recent survey has revealed that prevalence in such and such a place is greater than 30 per 100 000 population and that it should now be considered a high risk zone for multiple sclerosis. As we have seen, large increases in prevalence may occur independently of any change in the incidence of the disease. The implication associated with the re-definition of an area as a high risk zone is that the aetiological factors that determine disease frequency have changed; this view is often unjustified. Lastly, the reader should note that the rates of disease used to define the cut-off points between categories are arbitrary. The boundaries

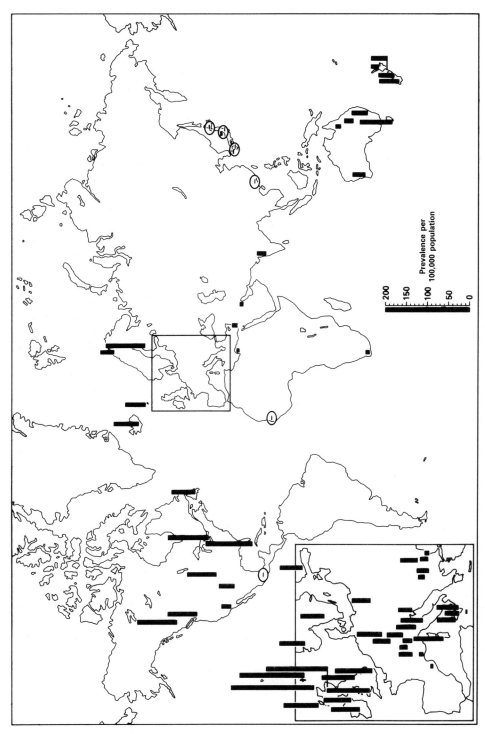

Fig. 1.2   Prevalence of multiple sclerosis throughout the world. (Bars represent estimates of prevalence obtained from population based surveys. Where areas have been studied repeatedly, only estimates from surveys in which case-ascertainment was judged to be most complete and which were carried out most recently have been shown.)

between the zones have no special significance and there is no reason to suppose any sudden discontinuity in the risk of multiple sclerosis between zones

Europe

The prevalence of multiple sclerosis is high over the whole of the northern part of Europe. The highest rates of all have been reported from the Orkneys, a group of small islands situated to the north of the Scottish mainland, where the prevalence in 1974 exceeded 250 per 100 000 population.[3] The prevalence is also very high in other parts of the United Kingdom. The frequency of the disease exceeds 100 per 100 000 population in the Shetland Islands,[43] in north east Scotland[29] and south east Wales.[44] In all of the five other regions of the United Kingdom that have been surveyed in the last 25 years or so, the prevalence is at least 80 per 100 000 population.[45–50]

Most reports indicate that rates of the disease are generally slightly lower in Scandinavian countries than in the United Kingdom. Surveys in Norway and Finland in the 1950s and 1960s found rates of less than 30 per 100 000 population, but recent work shows that the prevalence is now considerably higher. Conclusive evidence that the increase in prevalence indicates a rising incidence of disease is lacking and the rise may be partly or even wholly explained by improvements in case ascertainment and in the longer survival of cases. Within the countries of Scandinavia there are significant differences in the prevalence of multiple sclerosis. The methodology of the two most recent studies from Norway is comparable and the results show that the rate of disease is lower in the far north of the country (32 per 100 000 pop.) than it is in the south west (60 per 100 000 pop.).[51,52] In Finland, the prevalence is significantly higher in the rural western part of the country (93 per 100 000 pop.) than in the industrial south (53 per 100 000 pop.)[53] A recent study examined the incidence of disease in these two areas and confirmed that this is a genuine difference in the rate of occurrence of disease.[54]

The prevalence of multiple sclerosis in Germany and the Netherlands is similar to that found in Scandinavian countries. The most recent survey was carried out in the state of Hesse in West Germany where an overall prevalence of 58 per 100 000 for clinically definite and probable cases was reported.[55]

Reliable information about the frequency of multiple sclerosis in the countries of Eastern Europe is meagre and no new data have emerged from Czechoslovakia, Romania, Hungary or Turkey since Kurtzke's review. Only four surveys, from Poland, Czechoslovakia, Romania and Estonia in the USSR were graded Class A and these gave estimates of prevalence ranging between 22 and 52 per 100 000 population. The fact that the surveys which employed the best methodology gave the highest estimates of prevalence suggests that the true frequency of the disease in eastern Europe may not be much lower than in the countries of north west Europe.

The results from a recent study in Poland provide a rare counter-example to the general rule that prevalence estimates are higher in second surveys.[56] These investigators reported a fall in prevalence, from 51 to 43 per 100 000 population between 1965 and 1981. The probable reason for the decrease was a marked change in the age structure of the population because of a very high birth rate, rather than any underlying change in the incidence of disease.

In a study of 5 districts in Bulgaria in 1987, the prevalence varied between 10 and 28 per 100 000 population.[57] Both the low rate of disease and the differences between districts may have been the result of under-ascertainment of cases.

No recent data are available for France and Spain. Some of the estimates of prevalence based on earlier work are questionable, either because they depend on small numbers of cases, or because of doubts about the completeness of case ascertainment. For France, estimates of prevalence range between 14 and 63 per 100 000 population. In the single available survey for Spain, in the province of Cataluna, prevalence was estimated at 6 per 100 000 population.

Several studies carried out in Italy before 1975 suggested that multiple sclerosis was uncommon, particularly in the south of the country.[58] This view must now be reconsidered in the light of a series of surveys of small communities on the mainland of Italy[14,59] and in Sicily [10–13] and Sardinia,[60] all of which have reported prevalences of more than 45 per 100 000 population.

Malta, an island less than 100 miles from Sicily, provides an interesting contrast. Here, the prevalence of multiple sclerosis is only 4 per 100 000 population.[61] The population of Malta is about 280 000, which is much larger than that of the towns surveyed in Sicily, but the methods used to identify cases in the two islands were identical and the investigators found that, in Malta, patients with suspected disease of the nervous system were generally fully investigated. It does not seem likely that a difference in prevalence of this magnitude can be explained simply by less complete case ascertainment in the larger Maltese community.

In 1975, Kurtzke suggested that the geographical distribution of multiple sclerosis in Europe could be summarised by considering areas north of the 45° parallel of latitude as a high risk zone and areas to the south as being of distinctly lower risk. Almost all surveys since then have shown a rise in the prevalence of multiple sclerosis, but the size of the increase has been much greater in Italy than elsewhere. A pattern of decreasing risk of multiple sclerosis from north to south is still apparent, especially if allowance is made for the fact that surveys in Italy were carried out in smaller populations than most of the studies in the countries of northern Europe. But no discontinuity in the gradient of risk can be discerned and the notion of a dividing line between zones of risk is no longer tenable.

North America and Canada

The prevalence of multiple sclerosis in Canada and in the northern states of the USA is similar to rates in European countries at the same latitude. A recent study in Ontario, in which multiple sources of information were used to ensure nearly complete case ascertainment, found a prevalence of clinically definite cases of over 80 per 100 000 population.[27] In British Columbia, another study of high quality found a prevalence of 93 per 100 000 population, although this estimate included probable as well as definite cases.[62] In Newfoundland and Labrador, the prevalence of clinically definite and probable cases was 55 per 100 000.[63] A nationwide survey carried out in the USA reported an overall prevalence of 69 per 100 000 population in areas north of the 37° parallel of latitude.[64,65]

Further south, in the North American continent, the prevalence of multiple sclerosis declines. In the nationwide survey, areas south of 37°N were found to have a prevalence of 36 per 100 000 population. These recent data confirm the findings of many earlier studies that demonstrated a decreasing risk of multiple sclerosis from north to south in North America. Several of these surveys were carried out with the express intention of comparing the prevalence at different latitudes using identical methods in two or more places.[30,31,66–69]

Special mention must be made of a series of case-control studies of US ex-servicemen (veterans) from World War II and the Korean conflict.[69] Because these people, whatever their place of origin, had the benefit of similarly high standards of medical care both during and after their period of military service, geographical bias in diagnosis is eliminated. The studies recruited patients from all states in the USA and were able to exploit military records to obtain a control group matched for age, date of entry and branch of service and survival of the war. Table 1.1 shows case-control ratios for the USA for white male ex-servicemen according to place of residence before enlistment. A clear pattern of decrease in risk can be seen from north to south.

The same source of data shows that the risk of multiple sclerosis is considerably lower in the black population of the USA. Overall, the relative risk for blacks as compared with whites was 0.4. The gradient in risk from north to south by place of residence before entry into the Armed Services was also present in blacks.

Table 1.1 The risk of multiple sclerosis in US veterans by tier of latitude of residence at entry to military service. Numbers are case/control ratios

Sex and race	Tier of latitude		
	North	Middle	South
White males	1.41	1.02	0.58
White females	2.77	1.71	0.80
Black males	0.61	0.59	0.31
Total	1.41	1.00	0.53

Central and South America

Apart from a survey of government employees and their dependents in Mexico that showed an extremely low prevalence of the disease (1.5 per 100 000 pop.),[70] no reliable population-based studies of this area have been performed.

Australia and New Zealand

Australia and New Zealand are both countries with evenly high standards of medical care and populations of predominantly European origin. They provide an opportunity to observe whether the gradient of prevalence of multiple sclerosis, which exists in Europe and North America from north to south, is also present in a population of similar racial origins in a different location.

Surveys carried out in Australia in the 1960s suggested that a gradient of risk with increasing latitude did, indeed, exist.[71–73] The direction of the gradient is, of course, reversed in the southern hemisphere, with higher rates being found in more southerly latitudes. Multiple sclerosis was uncommon in Queensland, significantly more frequent in Perth, Western Australia and Newcastle, New South Wales, and commonest of all in Hobart, Tasmania. Any questions about completeness of case ascertainment and the diagnostic criteria that were employed in these studies have been answered by a second series of surveys published recently.[24,74] Following the pattern seen so frequently elsewhere, the prevalence of multiple sclerosis had risen in each of these places, but a gradient of increasing risk from north to south was still clearly present. Current prevalence rates for Australia are given in Table 1.2. Mortality data for multiple sclerosis in Australia have recently been analysed.[75] They confirm the relation between increasing frequency of the disease and increasing southerly latitude. They also show that mortality from multiple sclerosis has fallen in all areas of the country over the past decade. This provides at least a partial explanation for the observed increase in prevalence.

A difference in the risk of multiple sclerosis was also found when areas in the north and south of New Zealand were compared. The prevalence of the disease in Otago and Southland in the most

Table 1.2 Prevalence of multiple sclerosis by latitude in Australia and New Zealand

Location	Latitude	Prevalence (per 100 000 pop.)
Australia		
N Queensland	<23°28'S	12
S Queensland	>23°28'S	21
Perth, WA	32°S	30
Newcastle, NSW	33°S	37
Hobart, Tasmania	43°S	76
New Zealand		
Waikato	38°S	30
Otago and Southland	46°S	79

southerly part of the country was more than twice that in the Waikato Hospital Board area in the North Island[28,76] (see Table 1.2).

South Africa

South Africa is the only other area in the southern hemisphere in which the prevalence of multiple sclerosis has been investigated by population-based surveys. The prevalence is low in all four provinces of the country. There are important differences in the prevalence between different racial groups. Only one case has ever been reported from the black population.[77] Amongst whites, the prevalence is higher (11 per 100 000 pop.) in the English speaking population than in the Afrikaans-speaking population (3 per 100 000 pop.).[78]

Japan

Several, well-performed studies have demonstrated that multiple sclerosis is rare in Japan. Prevalences of less than 5 per 100 000 population have been found in regions situated both in the north and south of the archipelago.[79–81] This low figure is not the result of using different diagnostic criteria or of failure of Japanese neurologists to recognise multiple sclerosis. Neurologists from countries where multiple sclerosis is common (including McAlpine himself) have been involved in some of the surveys. Although higher rates of visual impairment at onset and a higher rate of optic nerve involvement during the course of the disease have been observed in Japanese patients with multiple sclerosis compared with patients in Western countries, the natural history of the disease is essentially the same.[82] Recently published work gives no indication that the prevalence is increasing.[83]

China and the far East

In Hong Kong prevalence in the Chinese is less than 1 per 100 000.[83a] Information from case-series from hospitals providing a neurological service suggests that the disease is also rare in Korea[84] and mainland China.[85]

India

Multiple sclerosis has traditionally been considered extremely uncommon in India. Jain and Maheshwari,[86] who reviewed all work on multiple sclerosis in the sub-continent published before 1985, were able to find only 354 cases collected over a period of 30 years. But a meticulous study of Parsees living in Bombay,[23] where a community of some 14 000 people were screened in a door-to-door survey, suggests that this view may be mistaken. This study found a crude prevalence of 21 per 100 000 population. When age-adjusted to the 1960 population of the USA, the rate was 15 per 100 000. These rates, however, are based on only three cases and their precision is low; the 95% confidence interval surrounding the estimate of prevalence (3.1 to 43.8 per 100 000 pop.) extends from highest to lowest of Kurtzke's zones of risk. There are also indications from case-series that multiple sclerosis may be commoner in Parsees than in other ethnic groups.[87,88] No definite conclusion about the prevalence of multiple sclerosis in India can be reached at present.

The near and middle East

Israel is the only country in this area that has been subject to intensive study with regard to multiple sclerosis. The prevalence in 1960 was 15 per 100 000 population, but the population contains immigrants from more than 70 countries and the rates of disease among them differ considerably according to country of birth.[89,90] The significance of this variation is discussed later.

Estimates of prevalence are available for Arab populations from Kuwait (8 per 100 000 pop.)[91] and Libya (6 per 100 000 pop.).[92] A case-series from Saudi Arabia indicates that the disease is uncommon there.[93]

Race

The first question to be answered when trying to interpret the global pattern of multiple sclerosis concerns differences in susceptibility to the disease between different races. To what extent can the variation in prevalence of multiple sclerosis throughout the world be attributed to genetically determined ethnic factors?

Whites of European origin

There can be no disagreement about the fact that white people of European stock are susceptible to multiple sclerosis. The highest prevalence of the disease is found in areas of northern Europe and in those countries now populated with people of European descent — North America, Canada, Australia and New Zealand. However, the rarity of multiple sclerosis amongst the white population of South Africa and, to a lesser extent, Queensland and the southern states of the USA, shows that susceptibility alone does not inevitably lead to high rates of disease in white populations.

Blacks of African origin

Multiple sclerosis is almost unknown in the black population of South Africa and what data are available suggest that it is rare over the whole of the African continent. Other black populations manifest higher rates of the disease. The US veterans study provides reliable information about the incidence of the disease in black males in the USA. For all practical purposes, any bias towards underdiagnosis of the disease in blacks is eliminated in this study. The disease is less common in blacks than whites (the relative risk for black males compared with white males = 0.4) but the incidence is far higher than it is in Africa. The declining gradient in risk from north to south observed for whites, also exists for American blacks. This is strong evidence that, even if blacks are relatively protected from the disease by their genetic constitution, the environmental factors causing the disease are similar to those that operate in whites.

Evidence from Jamaica indicates that multiple sclerosis is probably rare in the West Indies[94] and hospital admission rates for multiple sclerosis in first generation West Indian immigrants in Britain are very low.[95,96] This must be set against the findings of a recent study of second generation black immigrants in London (i.e. blacks of West Indian origin born in the UK) which suggests that the incidence of multiple sclerosis is as high in this group as it is in the native white population.[97]

A possible reason for the higher rates of multiple sclerosis observed in blacks of the USA when compared with rates in Africa is that, as a result of interbreeding with the white population, they have become more susceptible to the disease. But this explanation cannot account for the very rapid increase in the frequency of multiple sclerosis, within one generation, that has occurred in West Indians in London. The evidence that black people have an innately low susceptibility to multiple sclerosis is far from conclusive; the low rates of the disease observed in some black populations may be explicable in terms of different exposure to environmental factors.

Orientals

Rates of multiple sclerosis are very low in Japan and evidence from Hong Kong, China and Korea suggests that the disease is rare in other oriental populations. Death rates from multiple sclerosis in Japanese and Chinese immigrants in California and Washington are about 4 times lower than for the white population. The numbers of deaths on which these rates are based are very small,[98] but subsequent prevalence surveys of the same areas identified only 8 cases of multiple sclerosis out of a total population of 120 066 Japanese-Americans.[99] An intensive search was made amongst the Japanese communities living in these areas and it is not likely that the low prevalence of the disease is due to under-ascertainment of cases. Nor can the deficiency of cases be explained by a shorter duration of disease in the Japanese than in the whites. The Japanese living in these American cities do not tend to cluster into tight ethnic communities and, with the possible exception of diet, the investigators could not identify any environmental factors that might operate

among the Japanese but not amongst the white population. A low prevalence of multiple sclerosis has also been found in Japanese, Chinese and Filipino immigrants in Hawaii.[100]

The data are highly suggestive that the Japanese and probably other oriental groups too, possess low susceptibility for multiple sclerosis and that this has a genetic basis. However, the effect of migration on risk of disease is sometimes delayed. The incidence of gastric cancer, for example, is lower in the second generation of Japanese immigrants to the USA than in the first, but still higher than in American whites.[101] Final confirmation of low inherent susceptibility must await studies of occurrence of multiple sclerosis in third generation American Japanese who have fully adopted the way of life of their host country.

Arabic peoples

Unfortunately, there are no data which allow the possible contribution of protective genetic factors to the low rates of multiple sclerosis in arabic countries to be assessed.

People from the Indian sub-continent

Evidence from hospital discharge rates in the United Kingdom suggests that immigrants from India and Pakistan retain the (probably) low risk of multiple sclerosis of their countries of origin.[95,96] The population in this study however, consisted mainly of first-generation immigrants and their period of residence in the United Kingdom may have been too short for any change in risk of the disease to become apparent. For this group the question of racial susceptibility, or lack of it, remains open.

Maoris

A recent survey in New Zealand failed to identify any cases of multiple sclerosis in the Maori population.[28] Ethnic differences in access to specialist medical services were not considered great enough to explain this finding. The current way of life of Maoris was said by the investigators to be similar to that of the European population and, if this is correct, it may indicate a genetic basis for the low risk. However, it is known that Maori families are generally larger than those of the European population and that Maori households often contain more than one family.[102] Further, the overall prevalence of hepatitis B surface antigen in the non-European population is more than 4 times greater than in the European population and it is particularly high in the 15–29-year-old age group (16% HBsAg +ve).[103] The patterns of childhood infection in the two populations are therefore rather different and this may be relevant to their different experience of multiple sclerosis.

Eskimos

There are no reports of multiple sclerosis in the native born people of Alaska and Greenland but, in the absence of proper surveys, these data should only be considered anecdotal. In a prevalence survey in the northern part of Norway, no cases were found in a population of 26 000 Lapps;[52] the expected number of cases, calculated from local population rates, was between 7 and 8.

The ethnic aspects of the geographical distribution of multiple sclerosis have recently been reviewed by Lowis[104] and parts of the following summary are adapted from his useful discussion of the subject. The evidence showing that multiple sclerosis occurs in all three of the main racial groups in the world — white, oriental and black — is beyond doubt. However, it seems that, regardless of the country in which they are living, orientals manifest low rates of the disease. There is fragmentary evidence that Eskimos and North American indians, who, by origin, are oriental, also have very low rates of multiple sclerosis. The most likely explanation for the low rates in orientals is that they are protected against the disease by some racially determined genetic factor.

The highest frequency of multiple sclerosis is found in areas of the world largely inhabited by white people and the lowest frequency in areas inhabited by non-whites, but large geographical variations in the frequency of multiple sclerosis are present in both white and black populations. White populations exist in which the disease is rare, and the recent study of second generation West Indian immigrants in Britain provides an example of a black population in which the disease is common.

Different ethnic groups living in the same area may experience different rates of the disease. Although this may be partly due to differences in susceptibility, it is clear that racial differences alone cannot account for the global distribution of multiple sclerosis.

The relationship with latitude

The difference in prevalence of multiple sclerosis between the north and south of the USA was first described in 1922,[105] but it was not until 1950 that Limburg first put forward the idea that the frequency of multiple sclerosis could be described by its relation to latitude.[106] His hypothesis, based mainly on crude mortality rates for individual states in the USA and for the provinces of Canada, suggested that rates of multiple sclerosis rise with increasing distance from the equator. Since then, numerous prevalence surveys have greatly improved the quality of our information about the geography of the disease. As we have seen, within the tropics (about 23°N to 23°S) the disease is very rare. As latitude increases, multiple sclerosis becomes more common, with the highest rates being found in areas above 50°N and below 50°S. Data are patchy for latitudes greater than 60°N and S but there is some suggestion from surveys in Scandinavia that rates begin to decline again. The obvious exception to this general pattern is Japan (30°–45°N), where rates of multiple sclerosis are very low. There are some areas of the world, notably South America and the USSR, for which no reliable data are available.

Even after allowance has been made for all the difficulties that must be taken into account in making comparisons between the results of prevalence surveys, the evidence for a genuine relationship between the frequency of multiple sclerosis in peoples of north and central European stock and latitude of place of residence seems overwhelming. A gradient in risk of the disease from north to south has now been well-documented in three continents. There is evidence that the relationship also holds good for the black population of the USA.

The possibility that the relationship represents

an artefact caused by different standards of medical care has effectively been refuted by the results of the US veterans survey which, for all practical purposes, elimated geographically-based diagnostic bias, and by the recent surveys in Australia and New Zealand, where the provision of medical services is uniformly good.

The importance of the relationship, as Acheson has pointed out, lies in what it can suggest about the existence of a relationship between the occurrence of the disease and other variables which are themselves correlated with latitude. Attempts have been made to explain the relationship in terms of the distribution of people with a high degree of genetically-determined susceptibility to the disease. In the United Kingdom, the gradient in prevalence of multiple sclerosis from north to south was found to correlate with regional differences in the frequency of the HLA subtype DR2 in the population.[107] But this explanation is unsatisfactory because, in regions where the prevalence of multiple sclerosis is highest, no association between HLA DR2 and multiple sclerosis was found.[108] It is unlikely that if HLA DR2 is an important determinant of the rate of multiple sclerosis in a population, there will be no association between this phenotype and disease in individuals. The authors have tried to account for the inconsistency by suggesting that the association in individuals might disappear in areas where a high proportion of the general population possessed HLA DR2. But the assertion that the strength of an association between a risk factor and disease depends on the prevalence of the risk factor in the population is incorrect. In any case, even in areas where HLA DR2 is most common, the proportion of the population with this phenotype does not exceed 50%. When the frequency of a risk factor in a study population is around this level, the power of case-control studies to detect an association is at its maximum.

In the USA, a correlation has been reported between the prevalence of multiple sclerosis in each state and the proportion of the population who are of Scandinavian descent.[109] Because Scandinavia is an area where the prevalence of multiple sclerosis is high, it is suggested that this correlation indicates the distribution of genetic susceptibility. At best, this can only be a partial explanation; it is unable to account for the gradient in prevalence of the disease from north to south found in the US veterans study in American blacks, nor can it explain the gradient of prevalence of the disease seen in immigrants to Australia, where the countries of origin of immigrants to Perth and Hobart were similar, yet the experience of multiple sclerosis very different.

Climate

An obvious possibility for a disease whose frequency varies with latitude in three continents and both hemispheres is that the occurrence of the disease may be directly or indirectly related to climate. There have been several attempts to identify specific meteorological and climatic variables that correlate with the risk of multiple sclerosis. Using data from the US veterans study, a closer correlation was found between rates of multiple sclerosis and indices of annual and winter sunshine than with latitude, temperatures in summer and winter, or precipitation. The strongest correlation was with December solar radiation.[110] A second, larger case-control study of a different sample of veterans investigated 10 climatic variables including an air pollution index, concentrations of minerals in ground water, measures of annual solar radiation, both in energy per unit area and in hours of sunshine, mean annual periods of high and low temperatures, and measures of annual rainfall and humidity as well as altitude.[111] All these variables significantly influenced the risk of multiple sclerosis when considered separately, but when the data were analysed in a multiple regression model, the effect was found to be due to the correlation of these variables with latitude. The authors concluded that the explanation for the influence of latitude must be sought outside the realm of conventional meteorological variables. But this conclusion may be mistaken, because when many variables are highly correlated, multiple regression may not be a satisfactory way of determining which of them is biologically most important.

Nonetheless, with the exception of rickets, cataracts of the crystalline lens and malignant melanoma, rather few diseases are known in which climatic variables act directly in their causation. A more plausible suggestion, if the link between the frequency of multiple sclerosis and latitude involves climate, is that the effect is mediated indirectly. Climate influences diet, design of housing, means of sanitation, social customs and many other aspects of the way of life of a population. Differences in one or more of these factors might provide a mechanism by which environmental factors could influence the incidence of the disease.

Studies of migrants

Brief mention has already been made of observations of the occurrence of multiple sclerosis in migrant populations. The subject deserves further consideration because of the potential value of migrant studies in indicating the sort of aetiological factors that might be operating. It is obvious that the incidence of diseases whose cause is entirely genetic is unaffected by migration. Nor will migration have any effect on incidence if the disease is transmitted vertically or caused by events occurring in the perinatal period. For diseases with one of these aetiologies, the incidence in a migrant population is determined by place of birth and not by the country to which they move. On the other hand, if the risk of disease alters after migration, this is compelling evidence implicating an environmental factor working some time after birth in the aetiology. Where details of age at migration are available and the migrant population sufficiently large, it may be possible to examine the risk of disease in groups of people who migrated at different ages and so gain information about the age at which the disease was acquired.

There are, however, several possible confounding factors that have to be taken into account when comparing rates of disease in a migrant population with the rates of disease in their country of origin. First, people who migrate are unlikely to be typical of the general population in the country which they have left either in age, social class or general health. If, as seems probable, people with chronic disease are less likely to move than people who are well, it is only to be expected that rates of disease in a migrant population will be lower than that of the general population of the country that they left. Second, the country to which they emigrate may impose restrictions on the race, age, edu-

cational attainments, and health of the people they will accept. The migrant population may not therefore be directly comparable to the native-born population of the host country. Additional difficulties in interpretation arise because it may be some time before migrants fully adopt the way of life of the inhabitants of the country to which they emigrate. The environmental factors to which they are exposed cannot always be assumed to be the same as the general population of the host country.

Epidemiologists investigating rates of disease in migrants have to contend with a number of practical problems. The numbers of people who migrate must be sufficiently large for adequate statistical analysis. Enough information about the migrants must be available to allow the size of the population at risk of the disease to be estimated, and adjustment must be made to estimates of rates of disease to allow for differences in the age structure between the migrant and native-born populations.

Migration from areas of high risk to areas of lower risk

If rates of disease are considered without regard to age at migration, studies of people from northern Europe who moved to South Africa, Australia and Israel suggest that their risk of multiple sclerosis is intermediate between that of their country of origin and that of the host country.

In South Africa, the prevalence of multiple sclerosis in immigrants from the United Kingdom and other European countries is about 36 per 100 000 population.[78] This rate should be contrasted with rates of 50 to 100 per 100 000 population in the countries from which these people originated and rates of 11 per 100 000 population for native-born South Africans.

The most recent data for Australia, after age-standardisation to the local population, shows that the prevalence of multiple sclerosis in immigrants is similar to the prevalence in Australian born people, except in the areas of highest risk. Furthermore, the north to south gradient in risk of multiple sclerosis present in the Australian born population is also apparent in the immigrant population.[24] Immigrants to Perth and Newcastle have a prevalence of 30–40 per 100 000 population, which is not significantly different from the rate for the native born population, but considerably lower than the current rate of disease in northern Europe. In the higher risk area of Hobart, Tasmania, the prevalence in immigrants was 103 per 100 000 population. This is significantly higher than the prevalence in the local population, but very similar to the prevalence in the UK and Ireland, from which the majority of the immigrants came. Comparison of immigrants to Perth and Hobart showed no differences in age at migration, duration of residence in Australia or in their countries of origin.

Interpretation of data from Israel is particularly difficult because of the unusual and rapidly changing age structure of the population. However, comparison of age-specific prevalence rates makes it clear that, at all ages, the disease is less common in European immigrants to Israel than it is in countries in Northern Europe.[112]

The effect of migration on the risk of multiple sclerosis has been examined in the US veterans study.[113] This gives information about changes in risk of disease in those who moved between three tiers of latitude (north, middle and south) within the USA in the period between birth and entry into the Armed Forces. Interpretation of the results of this study is simplified because recorded migration preceded diagnosis. The observations cannot therefore be accounted for by differential migration of healthy people. The results are summarised in Table 1.3. Looking first at the margins, it can be seen that case/control ratios are highest in the most northerly tier and lowest in the most southerly, both for place of residence at birth and at enlistment. This relationship between risk of multiple sclerosis and latitude has already been discussed. Comparing now the case/control ratios for those who entered the Armed Forces from a place of residence in a more southerly tier of latitude than that in which they were born with the ratios for those who remained in the same tier, a consistent fall in risk is seen; a move south in the first two decades of life is associated with a decrease in the risk of multiple sclerosis.

A decrease in risk of multiple sclerosis was also observed in a study of people who had migrated internally within the USA from northern states to California.[30]

Migration from areas of low risk to areas of high risk

Studies of first generation immigrants to Greater London from the West Indies, where multiple sclerosis is probably rare,[94] showed that, during the years 1960–1972, their risk of being hospitalised with a first diagnosis of multiple sclerosis was only one-eighth of that of people born in the United Kingdom.[95,96] Although this work has been criticised because the period of residence of these immigrants within the UK may have been very short and because an inappropriate population denominator may have been used,[114] it does suggest that emigration from a low-risk area to a high-risk area has no immediate effect on the risk of disease. This work was later followed up by a study of incidence of multiple sclerosis in the children of these immigrants.[97] The rate in the second generation was strikingly higher than that in the first, and comparable to the incidence of multiple sclerosis reported from Northern Ireland and the Irish republic. At the time the study was published, no recent data for the Greater London area was available for direct comparison. Since then, a prevalence survey of a South London borough has shown the prevalence of probable multiple sclerosis to be 87 per 100 000 population.[8] This rate is very similar to that in Northern Ireland and the Irish republic, with which the original comparison was made. Given that the methods of case ascertainment used probably underestimated the rate in the children of immigrants, it is likely that the risk of multiple sclerosis in this population is at least as high as that of the white UK-born population.

The US veterans study was also able to compare the risk of multiple sclerosis in men who moved from south to north within the USA between birth and entry to the Armed Forces with the risk in those who remained at the same latitude. An increase in risk was present in those who moved north, but the magnitude of this increase was less than the corresponding decrease found in those who moved from north to south (see Table 1.3).

Table 1.3 The effect of migration in the time between birth and entry to military service on the risk of multiple sclerosis in US veterans. Numbers are case/control ratios

Residence at birth (by tier of latitude)	Residence at entry to military service (by tier of latitude)			
	North	Middle	South	Total
North	1.41	1.26	0.70	1.38
Middle	1.30	1.04	0.72	1.04
South	0.73	0.62	0.56	0.57
Total	1.39	1.04	0.58	1.04

Another study of migration within the USA failed to confirm these findings. The prevalence of multiple sclerosis among people who had migrated from southern states to Seattle was not significantly different from the prevalence among migrants to Los Angeles.[30] However, as the authors pointed out, the number of migrants from southern states to Seattle was small and the power of the study was insufficient to detect small changes in risk.

A study of rates of multiple sclerosis in a group of half-oriental (offspring of Vietnamese mothers and French fathers) born in Vietnam and brought to France suggested that the cumulative risk of multiple sclerosis in this group was similar to that of north European populations of the same age. This, of course, is much higher than the expected risk of the native Vietnamese population.[115] The estimate though, is based on very small numbers — 3 cases of probable or definite multiple sclerosis and 3 cases in whom the disease was suspected. Also, because of the mixed parentage of these cases, it is not possible to separate genetic from environmental factors.

In Israel, the disease was only one fifth as prevalent among immigrants from African and Asian countries compared to immigrants from Europe. In contrast, native Israelis of either European or Afro-asian origin have the same prevalence rates.[112]

Age at migration

A further study by Dean & Kurtzke[116] of Europeans migrating to South Africa, showed that the risk of multiple sclerosis was dependent on the age at which migration took place. In the group who had migrated before the age of 15 years, the number of people developing the disease was only one third of the number expected from rates in the European population generally. Surveys in Israel also suggest that the age of 15 years is an important dividing line between those who retain the risk of multiple sclerosis of the country in which they were born and those who acquire the lower risk of the country to which they emigrate.[117,118] However, these findings are based on rather small numbers and in the analyses, immigrants were combined into age groups of 5 years or more for age at immigration. The impression that the change in risk occurs sharply at the age of 15 years may be false. In a study of migrants within the USA, the results suggested that the reduction in risk of multiple sclerosis associated with a move from north to south was greater the earlier in life the move took place, without any sharp dividing line at a particular age.[119] The reduction in risk was greatest in those moving before the age of 9 years, but an effect was still apparent in those who moved at ages 15–19 years. In the recent Australian surveys, differences in risk between those moving to Perth and Newcastle compared with those moving to Hobart were seen, despite the fact that about 70% of immigrants were over 15 years of age at the time of migration.[24] However, the fact that risk of multiple sclerosis in US veterans was not affected by the place where they were stationed during their period of military service,[120] points to environmental exposures in the first two decades of life as being more important than later exposures in determining risk.

In summary, the evidence that migration from

a high to a low risk area in early life results in a reduction in the risk of multiple sclerosis is clear and consistent. The evidence that migration in the opposite direction — from a low to a high risk area — increases the risk of multiple sclerosis is less consistent, and there is a suggestion that the increase in risk may be less than the corresponding decrease in risk associated with a move in the other direction. If this asymmetry in the change of risk associated with migration is real, it suggests that the obvious hypothesis that the causative factors are common where the disease is common and rare where the disease is rare, is wrong. If this were the case, one would expect a move from an area of low frequency of disease to an area of high frequency to be associated with an increase in risk of disease of a similar magnitude to the reduction in risk associated with a move in the opposite direction. One interpretation of the asymmetry in change of risk is that in low risk areas, there is some protective mechanism which operates during early life to confer a degree of life-long protection from the disease.

The evidence also suggests that migration from a high to low-risk area has a greater effect on modifying the probability of developing multiple sclerosis if the move takes place in early life, than if the move is delayed to adulthood. Nonetheless, several studies indicate that a move in adult life can still alter the chances of developing the disease.

An interesting recent observation from case-control studies in the USA complicates the interpretation of migrant data still further by suggesting that multiple moves during childhood might themselves be associated with an increased risk of multiple sclerosis, independently of the origin or destination of the move.[121,122]

Clusters and epidemics

A search of the literature on multiple sclerosis reveals many reports of apparent clusters of the disease.[123–127] Two recent examples are the occurrence of 29 cases of clinically definite or probable multiple sclerosis on the small island of Key West, off the coast of Florida,[128] and of 4 cases, all developing first symptoms of disease within a short period of time, who had previously lived in the same tenement building in Glasgow.[129] While these observations are superficially attractive to those seeking clues about causation, biases in reporting usually make it impossible to evaluate whether such clusters occur significantly more often than could be expected. Poskanser and colleagues demonstrated more than 25 years ago that, in small populations, large variations in the frequency of uncommon diseases may be accounted for by chance alone.[130] In their investigation of multiple sclerosis in Northumberland and Durham, they found a striking variation in the prevalence among the 53 smaller administrative districts within the two counties. Rates ranged from 19–85 per 100 000 population. But when the Poisson distribution was used to model the frequency distribution of rates that could be expected if the variation were due to chance, they discovered that the observed rates could be accounted for by random variation.

In other places where rigorous statistical techniques have been used to explore data collected by systematic surveys, no positive evidence for geographical or temporal clustering has been found.[131–134]

The only exception to this is the finding of geographical clustering of cases at the onset of symptoms and 23 years previously in the Orkneys.[135] It was suggested that this indicates that two environmental exposures at different times are required for the development of disease. The failure of the same workers to find evidence of clustering in the Shetland Islands, and of other workers to find evidence of clustering elsewhere, makes one hesitant in accepting this interpretation.

Reports of clusters are more valuable if they can suggest a hypothesis about the cause of the disease. A higher than expected incidence of multiple sclerosis in workers at a zinc manufacturing plant led to a case-control study of indicators of exposure to zinc.[136] The control group selected from workers in the plant had higher plasma concentrations of zinc than controls from the local community, but no differences were found between cases and controls.

The Faroes epidemic

The most famous cluster of cases of multiple

sclerosis, which some have interpreted as representing a point-source epidemic, occurred in the Faroes, a group of small islands lying between Norway and Iceland. In a series of papers, Kurtzke & Hyllested have now reported 46 cases of probable multiple sclerosis in Faroese people, all with the onset of disease between 1943 and 1973.[137-139] Their first paper concerned the 34 cases that had been identified by 1977. After exclusion of 5 cases born in Denmark, 4 who had been resident abroad for long periods and 1 with onset of disease in 1970, a cluster of 24 cases was found, all of whom experienced the first symptoms of disease between the beginning of 1943 and the end of 1960. This was interpreted as representing an epidemic with a common source of exposure.

A remarkable event took place in the Faroes just before the onset of this putative epidemic of multiple sclerosis. Following the invasion of Denmark by Germany in April 1940, the Faroe islands were occupied by the British Armed Forces. The size of the British garrison varied between 1500 and 7000 men and they were present on the islands during the period 1940–1945. The population of native Faroese at the time was about 26 000. When the place of residence of the cases was compared with the location of the British troops, 21 out of the 24 cases were found to have lived in places where the troops had been stationed. The remaining 3 cases were said to have had extensive contact with the troops in the Faroese ports.

In later reports, 12 additional cases in native-born Faroese were described. The analyses in these papers concern 32 cases, all born on the Faroes and with periods of residence abroad totalling less than 2 years. Three of these cases were born after the occupation of the islands had ended. Kurtzke & Hyllested now interpret the occurrence of multiple sclerosis on the islands as three separate epidemics beginning in 1943 and ending in 1973. They believe that asymptomatic British troops introduced the first epidemic during 1941–1942 and that subsequent epidemics resulted from transmission by affected but asymptomatic Faroese.

This conclusion has been widely discussed and criticised.[140-143] The central pillars of the argument are that the occurrence of cases fits a log normal frequency distribution — a phenomenon

typical of an epidemic caused by a short period of exposure[144] — and that there was close contact between cases and British troops who occupied the islands. Neither of these has a completely solid base. Although no cases of multiple sclerosis with onset of disease before 1943 have been found, in view of the remoteness of the islands and their very scattered population, it is impossible to be certain that none existed. In order to accommodate cases of multiple sclerosis which occurred after 1960, it has been necessary to elaborate the original hypothesis of a single epidemic. It is now proposed that there were three separate epidemics and also that the period of exposure to the putative infectious agent necessary for the development of the disease has become longer. Numbers of cases in the later epidemics are very small — only three cases in the last — and no convincing explanation is offered as to why longer exposure is necessary after the disease has become endemic.

Information from official War Diaries and Order of Battle reports, as well as from an investigation carried out in the islands themselves, confirms evidence obtained from patients that contact between cases and British troops was close. There can no longer be any doubt that a real geographical association exists between the location of the troops and the occurrence of multiple sclerosis. However, there has been no comparison between cases and controls which indicates that contact of individual cases with the troops was any more frequent or prolonged than that of others living in the same locations. Many changes in the way of life of the islanders have taken place in the last 50 years and it is not impossible that these may have affected both the risk of multiple sclerosis and the chances of the disease being diagnosed.

The occurrence of multiple sclerosis has also been investigated in Iceland.[145] This island too, was occupied by troops from Britain, and also from the USA and Canada, during World War II. A rise in incidence of multiple sclerosis was found, starting in 1945 and declining in 1954. However, unlike the Faroes, multiple sclerosis is known to have been prevalent in Iceland in the years before the war and there is, as yet, no evidence pointing to especially close contact between cases and the occupying forces. A possible confounding factor is that the first neurologist in Iceland was appointed in 1942. This, in itself, may have lead to an increase in the number of cases that were diagnosed in the following decade.

Another possible outbreak of multiple sclerosis associated with British troops has been reported in the Orkney and Shetland Islands.[146] Here, the incidence of the disease began to increase within 18 months of the arrival of the troops.

A further intriguing 'epidemic' has recently been described in the small, previously inaccessible community of Macomer in Sardinia.[147] In 1945, a large influx into the local population took place when an army training camp was established there. No cases of multiple sclerosis had ever been recorded in Macomer until 1952. In the years 1952–1960, 6 cases were diagnosed. A further 7 cases occurred between 1964 and 1980. The period between first contact with outsiders and the occurrence of the first cases of multiple sclerosis in Macomer is much longer than in the Faroes. The mean time between arrival of the newcomers and onset of disease for the original 6 cases is more than 12 years.

The authors of the reports of these four instances of increasing incidence of multiple sclerosis in isolated communities following contact with large numbers of people from outside have all inclined towards interpreting them as evidence that multiple sclerosis is a transmissible disease. But more prosaic explanations are also possible. None of these communities had easy access to specialist neurological services before the observed increase in incidence and none had previously been studied with regard to the frequency of multiple sclerosis. Other events occurring in parallel with the influx of people into the local population may have led to improved recognition of the disease and hence to an increase in recorded incidence.

Several epidemiologists who have independently studied the data collected by Kurtzke & Hyllested from the Faroes have concluded that the epidemic there remains unproven.[140–143] The same conclusion applies, with at least equal force, to the epidemics reported in Iceland, the Orkney and Shetland Islands and Macomer.

Swayback

The cluster of 4 cases of multiple sclerosis that occurred in a group of 8 research workers investigating swayback, a demyelinating disease affecting new-born lambs, also deserves special mention.[148,149] Three of these workers developed their first symptoms of disease within a few months of each other and the fourth 6 years later. All of the group have now died; in 2 of the affected people, autopsy was performed and the clinical diagnosis was confirmed by the presence of multiple areas of demyelination within the central nervous system. The likelihood that 4 people out of a group of 8 chosen at random will develop multiple sclerosis has been put at one in a thousand million. But this is not a fair yardstick to use. By no stretch of the imagination can these 8 people be thought of as being chosen at random. Indeed, 2 of them had been at school and university together and other similarities in the background, education and interests of members of the group make it likely that they shared many environmental exposures other than contact with pathological material from the brains of sheep with swayback. It is now established that the disease of swayback is a nutritional disease resulting from copper deficiency and there is no evidence that it is infectious or transmissible. Furthermore, multiple sclerosis is uncommon in areas where copper deficiency in pasture and swayback have been a serious veterinary problem. Systematic enquiries have revealed no further cases of multiple sclerosis in other scientists and laboratory workers investigating the disease of swayback.

Clusters in families

Familial clustering of cases has been shown for a very large number of diseases and multiple sclerosis is no exception. A significantly increased prevalence of multiple sclerosis in other members of the families of patients suffering from the disease has been observed many times.[150] The risk is higher in the siblings of an affected person than it is in the parents or children.[151] An interesting observation made recently is that there is a significantly increased sex concordance in non-twin sibling pairs with the disease.[152]

Familial aggregation can, of course, be the result of shared genes, shared environment or a combination of both of these. A systematic study of population genetics in the Orkney Islands, where inbreeding is high compared with the rest of the United Kingdom, did not find that the number of inbred people amongst patients with multiple sclerosis was higher than amongst controls.[150] Analysis of kinship coefficients and family histories suggested that single locus inheritance was very unlikely. The authors concluded that genetic involvement was probably multifactorial and possibly subordinate to an environmental aetiology. Other data, including twin studies (discussed later in this chapter), also indicate that the increased risk of disease in other members of the family of cases is due to interaction between shared environmental risk factors and genetic susceptibility.

Socio-economic factors

Factors associated with socio-economic status are powerful determinants of risk for many diseases. Several studies suggest that multiple sclerosis is unusual in that it tends to be more common in members of higher socio-economic groups. In two adjacent counties in the North of England, Northumberland and Durham, there was a significant excess of men of social classes 1 and 2 with multiple sclerosis.[153] Similar findings have been reported from Oxford[154] and north-east Scotland.[29] Mortality data for England and Wales shows that deaths from multiple sclerosis are commonest in social class 3 (non-manual).[155] In view of the inevitable downward drift in social class in people with chronic disease because of the effect of disability on occupation, this should probably be interpreted as further evidence that the disease is more frequent in higher social classes.

In the US veterans study, high socio-economic status at enlistment was associated with increased risk of multiple sclerosis,[120] but other studies in North America have failed to support this finding.[65,156] No association with socio-economic status has been found in Israel.[90]

Multiple sclerosis was more common amongst higher social classes in the Shetlands, but not in the Orkneys.[157] Unfortunately, these communities are unsatisfactory for this sort of analysis because the range of occupations amongst the islanders is small and because there is little difference in wealth between the poorest and richest inhabitants.

The balance of the evidence seems to suggest that members of higher socio-economic groups are at higher risk of multiple sclerosis. There is certainly no indication that the disease is positively related to poverty, overcrowding or other indices of low socio-economic status.

Urban-rural differences

The evidence concerning differences in risk of multiple sclerosis for people born or living in rural or urban areas is conflicting. In Israel, a significantly higher percentage of cases compared with controls lived in communities where the population was greater than 500 000 before the onset of disease, but no difference was found when the comparison was made between residence in communities where the size of the population was under and over 25 000.[90] Residence in large centres of population at birth and at the time of entry into the Armed Forces was associated with a four-fold increase in risk of multiple sclerosis in the US veterans study.[120] The most recent descriptive study of multiple sclerosis in the north east of Scotland noted an excess of prevalent cases living in urban areas, but this might have reflected migration of disabled patients into towns. A similar explanation is thought to account for the deficiency of rural dwellers among patients with multiple sclerosis in Western Australia. In the Orkneys, significantly more cases lived in towns rather than in rural areas at the time of onset of the disease, but no differences were found for place of residence at birth. In the Shetland Islands, the pattern was reversed, with cases being more likely to live in rural areas at onset of disease, although this difference was not statistically significant. It should be noted that towns in the Orkneys and Shetlands have populations of only a few thousand and the environmental factors associated with urban residence in these islands are likely to be very different from those associated with urban living in the USA and Israel.

Data from several other countries including Norway,[158] Denmark,[159] Germany,[160] Canada,[27] England[135] and Northern Ireland[48] either fail to demonstrate any differences in prevalence between town and country, or show an excess of cases in the rural population.

No simple resolution of these divergent findings is possible. In most studies, there is probably a bias towards identifying cases in urban areas, which leads one to place more reliance on data which point to an increased risk for those living in rural areas. Against this is the strong association of urban dwelling with risk of multiple sclerosis found in the US veterans study in which the design of the investigation elimated these sources of bias.

Time trends

Reliable data concerning changes in the incidence of multiple sclerosis over time can only be obtained prospectively and therefore require sustained epidemiological investigation of a population over many years. It is not surprising that such data are sparse. The Orkney and Shetland Islands have been surveyed on four occasions between 1954 and 1974, allowing annual incidence to be estimated over a period of 42 years. The total population of the Orkneys is about 20 000 and there is considerable variation in incidence from year to year. Nonetheless, there has been a slow but convincing downward trend in the incidence of multiple sclerosis since 1965 and a suggestion that rates may have been falling since 1941.[4]

In contrast, long-term studies of larger populations in Northern Ireland and Rochester, Minnesota suggest that incidence rates have remained stable over long periods of time, despite a nearly two-fold increase in the prevalence of the disease.[48,161]

An apparent increase in incidence in Hobart, Tasmania and in Newcastle, New South Wales between 1961 and 1981 is thought to be a result of immigration of a population at higher risk of multiple sclerosis than the Australian-born population.[24]

The constancy of the low prevalence rates of multiple sclerosis in Japan over the past quarter of a century has already been noted.

Rosati and colleagues have suggested that incidence of multiple sclerosis more than doubled in the town of Sassari in Sardinia over the period 1965–1985.[162] They point out that the discovery of

Sardinia as a tourist attraction has brought native Sardinians in contact with large numbers of people from high-risk areas for multiple sclerosis and favour, as an explanation for the increase in incidence, transmission of the disease by contact with sub-clinical cases. Their estimates of incidence were however, obtained retrospectively. In 1984, an intensive search was made for all living patients. The date of onset of disease was established after interview and examination by a neurologist. This method would have missed cases who had died or left the study area since disease onset and so would have underestimated incidence for all but the most recent years. If the mean duration of disease is 20 years, half the cases with disease onset in 1965 would have died by 1985 and the estimate of incidence for 1965 would be only half the true rate. The apparent increase in incidence between 1965 and 1985 may therefore be entirely accounted for by the expected mortality.

This methodological problem was avoided in estimating incidence in north east Scotland.[29] Here, there does seem to have been a genuine increase in the annual incidence of multiple sclerosis, from 4.2 per 100 000 population in 1959–1961 to 7.2 per 100 000 population in 1977–1980, though, as the authors admit, this may be partly due to increased local awareness of the disease following a survey in 1970, and to the increasing use of evoked responses, analysis of CSF and CT scanning in diagnosis.

Overall, the impression is of remarkable stability in the incidence of multiple sclerosis. The point has been made that, in view of the general improvement in both knowledge of the disease and in methods of diagnosis, this is surprising.[144] It might have been expected that better diagnosis would by itself lead to an increase in reported incidence of the disease. Perhaps the correct interpretation of the apparent stability in incidence is that the rate of occurrence of the disease is actually declining, at least in parts of the UK, Europe and the USA.

Genetic factors

For most diseases, argument about whether the cause is genetic or environmental is unproductive. It is true that the causation of a few diseases, for example, measles or rabies, can be accounted for by exposure to a single environmental agent. Regardless of genetic constitution, an individual is almost certain to develop the disease on first contact with the infective agent. For a few other diseases, the cause is entirely genetic. A male who inherits the gene for Duchenne muscular dystrophy inevitably develops the disease. In the vast majority of diseases however, causation is more complex. Neither genes nor environmental agents are sufficient cause by themselves.

Epidemiologists seeking environmental causes for disease rarely find themselves in conflict with those investigating its genetic basis. On the contrary, knowledge of the genetics of a disease allows the search for environmental causes to be carried out more efficiently. An epidemiologist designing a case-control study to investigate the environmental factors involved in the causation of ankylosing spondylosis might well decide to include only cases and controls who were HLA B27 positive in order to avoid diluting his sample with subjects whose risk of disease is low.

Sometimes, attempts are made to estimate the relative importance of genetic and environmental factors in the causation of a disease. Heritability may be used as a measure of the genetic contribution. This is defined as the proportion of the variance in risk of developing the disease that can be attributed to genetic factors. It is not always appreciated that an estimate of heritability applies only to the population in which it was made. It cannot be extended to other groups. An example may make the reason for this clear. Suppose a disease is caused by the simultaneous presence of a genetic factor and an environmental factor. In a population where the genetic factor is very common and the environmental factor is rare, who gets the disease will mainly be determined by the pattern of exposure to the environmental factor. If the circumstances are reversed, so that most of the population is exposed to the environmental factor but only a few possess the genetic factor, who gets the disease will be mainly determined by the distribution of the necessary gene. In both these situations, the environmental factor and the genetic factor are essential for the disease to develop and therefore, in biological terms, they can be considered equally important causes. But

an investigator might easily come to the conclusion that the disease was primarily environmentally determined if he studied the first population, or mainly genetically determined if he studied the second.

Where multiple sclerosis is concerned, three lines of evidence point to the involvement of a genetic factor. The first is the differences in racial susceptibility. Low rates of disease in Japanese and other oriental people persist even after migration to countries where multiple sclerosis is common in the native-born population. As has been previously discussed, this is a strong indication that racially-determined genetic factors influence risk of disease.

The second line of evidence is that particular HLA antigens are found more frequently in cases of multiple sclerosis than in controls. The relationship between histocompatibility antigens and multiple sclerosis is reviewed in detail in Chapter 10, but it is worth mentioning in this context that the increase in risk of disease associated with these antigens is not great. For example, the association between HLA DQw1 and multiple sclerosis in north east Scotland, although highly statistically significant, has a relative risk of only 2.1 (95% confidence interval, 1.2–3.4); these figures were calculated from published data.[163] In south east Wales, the relative risk associated with HLA DR2 is 2.9 (95% confidence interval, 1.7–5.0).[164] Futhermore, the HLA haplotypes that are linked to increased risk of disease differ between populations.

The third line of evidence comes from studies of the occurrence of the disease in twins. This is an approach that has been used in a number of diseases to determine whether genetic factors are operating: the principle is simply to compare concordance rates for the disease in monozygotic and dizygotic twins. To obtain an unbiased estimate of the genetic contribution, it is important that twin pairs are recruited independently of their disease status. Unfortunately, many twin studies of multiple sclerosis are flawed by the way in which twin pairs have been selected. When investigators advertise for twins, either in magazines and newsletters of patient societies or in the national press or by making inquiries amongst neurologists, there is a danger that concordant twin pairs will be over-represented. Three studies have managed to avoid this source of bias by using a national twin registry as a starting point and determining the presence or absence of multiple sclerosis prospectively.[165–167] A fourth study used a national register of cases of multiple sclerosis to identify cases of disease and then asked the cases whether they had a twin.[168] The latter method is less satisfactory because it relies on the testimony of patients to identify twin pairs and because there may be a bias towards identifying concordant pairs. Clearly, if both members of a twin pair suffer from the disease, the chances that at least one of them will be included on the register are greater than if only one member has the disease. Nonetheless, any bias is likely to operate equally for both mono- and dizygotic twin pairs. The results of these four studies are summarised in Table 1.4.

Concordance rates among monozygotic twin pairs are consistently higher than amongst dizygotic pairs but, assuming aetiological homogeneity, it is apparent that there is no genotype that, irrespective of environment, always leads to the development of multiple sclerosis. There are certain genotypes that are associated with increased susceptibility, but multiple sclerosis cannot be due only to the action of a single gene. Non-genetic differences are decisive in determining who gets the disease.

One interesting feature to emerge from twin studies is that concordance rates for dizygotic twins seem to be higher than would be expected from the rates calculated from sibship risk, even after allowance has been made for bias present in many studies towards identification of concordant twin pairs.[169] Dizygotic twins are, of course, no different from other siblings in the amount of genetic material that they share. However, environmental exposures for dizygotic twins in the first years of life are likely to be more similar than for brothers and sisters who are not twins. The raised concordance rate in dizygotic twins is compatible with the hypothesis that events in the early part of life are important in determining the subsequent risk of multiple sclerosis.

Multiple sclerosis and infection

The suggestion that multiple sclerosis is caused by infection, particularly viral infection, recurs throughout the literature on the disease. Part of its appeal derives from the fact that viruses are known to provoke demyelination in animals and, in some circumstances, man too. Many microorganisms have been pursued as likely culprits but none, so far, has been unequivocally incriminated.

Measles

A generally consistent finding in serological investigations of viral infection in multiple sclerosis has been that serum antibody levels to measles are elevated in cases compared with controls. Norrby, reviewing studies which addressed this question in 1978, found that 31 out of 35 of them demonstrated a significantly higher titre of measles antibody,[170] and there have been further positive reports since.[171] Titres of antibodies to measles are also raised in siblings of cases of multiple sclerosis,[172] particularly if they share the same HLA haplotype.[173]

There are, however, some important exceptions to this pattern. In the Orkneys and Shetlands, where, because of the isolated nature of the communities, childhood infections generally occur at a later age than on the mainland of Britain, no differences in levels of antibodies to measles or in the age of measles infection between cases and controls were found.[174] An important additional finding was that 6 cases of multiple sclerosis had measles between 2–14 years after the onset of the first symptoms of multiple sclerosis. The extensive inquiries made about these patients makes it very unlikely either that the diagnosis of measles was incorrect or that it was a second attack of the infection.

Table 1.4 Concordance rates for multiple sclerosis in monozygotic and dizygotic twin pairs

	Concordance rate		
	Monozygotic	Dizygotic	Unknown
Bobowick et al 1978[165]	1/6	0/8	0/1
Ebers et al 1986[168]	7/27	1/43	–
Heteberg 1987[167]	4/19	1/31	–
Kinnunen et al 1987[166]	2/11*	1/10*	–

* Includes one member of a twin pair with optic neuritis only.

Raised titres of antibodies to many other viruses have been reported in cases of multiple sclerosis. These include vaccinia, rubella, herpes zoster, herpes simplex, mumps and Epstein–Barr virus. Unlike measles, the findings are not consistent.

Canine distemper

Infection with canine distemper virus as a factor in the causation of multiple sclerosis first received attention following a remarkable report of three sisters whose first symptoms of multiple sclerosis occurred shortly after their pet dog developed an acute encephalopathy.[175] Since then, outbreaks of canine distemper have been linked to clusters of multiple sclerosis in Alaska,[176] Iceland,[177] the Faroe Islands[178] and Key West, Florida.[179] Whether this link is any more than coincidence is doubtful. A series of case-control studies has failed to demonstrate a consistent pattern of increased exposure to animals and household pets in cases of the disease.[180–184] The epidemic of canine distemper in the Faroe Islands is particularly interesting because there is little doubt that the disease was introduced by the British troops occupying the islands in World War II. Kurtzke and colleagues have investigated the possible connection of canine distemper with the epidemic of multiple sclerosis which they believe to have occurred in the islands. They found no geographical correlation between the villages in which canine distemper was reported and the residence of cases of multiple sclerosis. In a case-control comparison, cases had no excess contact with sick dogs and there were no differences between cases and controls in antibody titres for canine distemper.[185]

Enteric infection

Poskanser and colleagues have drawn attention to a possible parallel between multiple sclerosis and poliomyelitis.[186] The epidemiology of poliomyelitis is unusual: unlike almost all other infectious diseases, poliomyelitis responds to improved sanitation and hygiene by becoming more common. Over the first half of this century, all countries of the developed world experienced a steep decline in incidence and mortality from almost all infectious diseases. The only exception

was acute paralytic poliomyelitis, whose incidence gradually increased to reach a peak in the late 1940s and early 1950s. Rates of poliomyelitis declined only after the development of vaccines and the widespread introduction of immunisation policies. The explanation of this paradox lies in the increasing vulnerability of the central nervous system to poliovirus infection with increasing age. Poliovirus infection during infancy is very much less likely to involve the nervous system and produce paralysis than infection at a later age. As hygiene and sanitation improved, the proportion of children who escaped poliovirus infection in the relatively safe period of infancy increased and paralytic poliomyelitis became more frequent.[187]

If multiple sclerosis were the result of an enteric infection that behaved in a similar way to poliomyelitis, a plausible explanation could be given for much of its epidemiological pattern. It would account for the rarity of the disease in tropical and sub-tropical countries where sanitation is poor and the towns densely populated, and the higher incidence in developed countries in the temperate zone in Northern Europe, North America and New Zealand. Dean has pointed out that the hypothesis can also explain the rarity of multiple sclerosis in white native-born South Africans despite their generally excellent sanitation.[116] He suggests that these people are exposed to enteric infection at an early age because of their intimate contact in infancy and childhood with African servants. The very low rate of poliomyelitis observed in white South Africans supports his view.[188]

However, the hypothesis is deficient in several respects. If multiple sclerosis were the result of delayed exposure to enteric infection, large changes in the incidence of the disease would have been expected to occur in parallel with the improvements in sanitation that have taken place in the countries of Europe and North America over the last 80 years. Although reliable data concerning the time trends of the incidence of multiple sclerosis are scanty, they contain no hint of such an increase. The hypothesis is hard to reconcile with the gradient in risk of multiple sclerosis from north to south in Australia and New Zealand. The living conditions of the population are similar throughout these countries. The hypothesis has been tested specifically in case-control studies in the Orkney and Shetland Islands[157] and in Israel.[189] There is no suggestion that cases tended to come from homes with better sanitation than controls.

Although the hypothesis cannot be sustained, the analogy with poliomyelitis contains ideas that may yet prove to be right. Poliomyelitis provides an example of a disease whose causative agent is less commonly encountered in places where the disease is frequent than in places where it is rare. It also shows how the same agent may be protective in one set of circumstances and inimical in another.

Slow viruses

As for many degenerative neurological diseases whose aetiology is obscure, the suggestion has been made that multiple sclerosis may be caused by a slow virus. There is no evidence indicating that this is likely. None of the neurological conditions in man that are thought to be caused by infection with a slow or persisting virus or virus-like agent — kuru, Creutzfeldt–Jakob disease, sub-acute sclerosing panencephalitis, progressive multifocal leukoencephalopathy, Gerstmann–Sträussler syndrome — show epidemiological patterns remotely like that of multiple sclerosis. The single observation that sheep inoculated with brain tissue from a case of multiple sclerosis developed scrapie has never been confirmed.[190]

Sinusitis

Evidence for an association between multiple sclerosis and chronic sinusitis has recently been put forward.[191] This association is of particular interest because of the similarities between the two diseases in their changing incidence with age. The study was carried out in 10 general practices in southern England. Significantly higher rates of chronic sinusitis were found in cases of multiple sclerosis than in controls and it was also reported that attacks of sinus infection were associated with the timing of first attacks of multiple sclerosis and with subsequent relapses. The authors ingeniously suggested a mechanism of pathogenesis, albeit with little supporting evidence, that involved

direct infection of the central nervous system by migration of motile spirochaetal organisms through defects in the bony walls of the paranasal air sinuses.[192] The study was widely criticised because of the difficulty of making a reliable diagnosis of sinusitis on clinical grounds alone, and because of doubts about the unbiased selection of the control groups.

An attempt was made to confirm the association, by comparing the prevalence of radiological signs of chronic sinus infection in cases of multiple sclerosis and controls with other neurological diseases.[193] Cases of clinically definite multiple sclerosis were identified from the diagnostic index of a regional neurological centre. Forty three cases were found who had both an antero-posterior and lateral skull X-ray taken at the time of first diagnosis. Each case was matched to 2 controls of the same sex within the same 5 year age group. Controls were selected from the index of patients examined in the neuroradiology department. Starting at the entry for the case, the index was searched for the next 2 patients of the same sex and age group who had also had antero-posterior and lateral skull X-rays taken. Controls were excluded if they had been referred because of headache or if their skull X-rays showed evidence of a neurosurgical procedure. Radiological signs of sinusitis were evaluated by one neuroradiologist, who was blind to the disease status of the patient. Repeat assessment of a random sample of X-rays showed that 76% of the neuroradiologist's evaluations were the same. No excess of radiological signs of sinusitis was present in cases. The relative risk of radiologically-diagnosed sinusitis was 0.95, with a 95% confidence interval of 0.42–2.12. Analysis of signs of infection in maxillary, frontal, ethmoid and sphenoid air sinuses separately, showed no differences between cases and controls. As can be seen from the confidence interval, the study was too small to exclude a small excess of sinusitis in cases of multiple sclerosis, but it provides no support for the original observation of a strong association between the conditions.

Borrelia burgdorferi

Apparent similarities between the clinical features of multiple sclerosis and some of the neurological sequelae of Lyme disease and a report of a cluster of cases of multiple sclerosis in a single general practice in the New Forest area of Hampshire in the south of England, where exposure to Borrelia-carrying ticks is thought to be high, has led some authors to speculate that *Borrelia* spp. may be a cause of multiple sclerosis.[194] Two studies have been reported in which the possible link has been investigated systematically. In Austria, the prevalence of antibodies to *Borrelia burgdorferi* was lower in a group of 106 patients with multiple sclerosis than in controls.[195] In a study in an area endemic for Lyme disease in the USA, only one patient out of a series of 89 cases with multiple sclerosis was serologically positive for Borrelia infection.[196] Unfortunately, there was no control group with which to compare this observation, but the very low prevalence of seropositivity does not suggest that exposure to *Borrelia* spp. is important in the aetiology of multiple sclerosis. Most neurologists now agree that the neurological features of neuroborreliosis and multiple sclerosis do not resemble each other very closely and the geographical distribution of Lyme disease is very different from that of multiple sclerosis.

Herpes zoster

A small study in Scotland reported that the incidence of Herpes zoster was significantly increased in patients with multiple sclerosis.[197] A higher incidence was also claimed in a later study in an adjacent region, although the choice of control group was questionable and an error was made in calculating the statistical significance of the odds ratio.[29]

An investigation of the possible association was undertaken in a community based study in Rochester, Minnesota.[198] A cohort of 590 people diagnosed with Herpes zoster between 1945 and 1959 was assembled retrospectively. No cases of multiple sclerosis had occurred in this group at the time the study was carried out, whereas the expected number, calculated from incidence data for multiple sclerosis in Rochester, was 0.2. In the complementary investigation, in which 48 cases of multiple sclerosis were followed up to determine the incidence of Herpes zoster, 3 cases were observed where the expected number was 1.8.

The statistical power of these studies is not great enough to detect a weak association between the two conditions, but the results do not suggest that it is worth pursuing further.

Herpes simplex

The hypothesis that multiple sclerosis was caused by infection with Herpes simplex type 2 in people lacking Herpes simplex type 1 immunity was suggested as being compatible with some of the features of the epidemiology of the disease.[199] It did not survive testing in a case-control study; mean titres of antibody to Herpes simplex of both types were not significantly different between cases and controls and 22% of cases showed no serological evidence of infection with Herpes simplex type 2.[200] The same study demonstrated significantly higher titres to measles virus measured by both complement fixation and haemagglutination inhibition assays in cases.

Retrovirus infection

The recent evidence concerning retrovirus infection in cases of multiple sclerosis is not based on epidemiological studies and is considered elsewhere in this book. Much of the controversy has centred around technical aspects of the work, but it may be worth pointing out that other difficulties in interpretation stem from the lack of knowledge about the prevalence of nucleic acid retrovirus sequences and antibodies to human retroviruses in the general population and the unsatisfactory way in which the control groups of some of the studies were selected.

Multiple sclerosis as an age-dependent response to infection

The host response to many infections varies with the age at which the infection occurs. An obvious example is hepatitis B; infection with this virus during early childhood commonly results in a chronic antigen carrier state, but rarely causes an overt hepatitic illness; in contrast, when infection is delayed until adult life, the chronic carrier state is rare but hepatitis common. By a loose analogy, it has been suggested that the aetiology of multiple sclerosis might involve an age-dependent response to a common infection.

There are several studies that suggest that age of infection with some of the common communicable diseases of childhood tends to be older in cases of multiple sclerosis than in controls.[29,171,201–204] Most of these reports concern measles, but there is some evidence that age at infection may also be higher with mumps and rubella.

Infection with Epstein–Barr virus in early childhood is not associated with the typical symptoms of infectious mononucleosis whereas if infection is delayed until late adolescence or young adult life, about 50% of cases develop the condition. In the third world there is a high rate of seroconversion to Epstein–Barr virus before adolescence and consequently a low incidence of classical infectious mononucleosis.[205] The results of a recent case-control study of multiple sclerosis, in which an association with infectious mononucleosis was reported,[122] therefore provide further evidence that common infections are acquired late in cases of the disease. Although the numbers were small, the estimate of relative risk associated with infectious mononucleosis was very high (17) and it is to be hoped that this finding will be pursued.

Alter and colleagues have used existing data from 37 countries to explore global patterns of viral diseases and their relationship to frequency of multiple sclerosis.[206] Alter made the assumption, which is almost certainly justified, that if mortality from a particular infection in a country is high, it indicates that the infection was generally acquired early in life. There were significant negative correlations between mortality from dysentery, measles, typhoid fever, gastritis/colitis and tuberculosis, and mortality from multiple sclerosis. No correlation was present with infectious hepatitis, acute upper respiratory illness or influenza. Using data from published reports, Alter found that, in areas where multiple sclerosis is rare, the prevalence of seropositivity to a range of common viruses in early childhood tended to be much higher than in countries where multiple sclerosis is common.

These observations indicate that the hypothesis which links multiple sclerosis to delayed exposure to common viral infections is compatible with the broad geographical pattern of the disease. But it does not constitute strong evidence of a causal connection. Any disease that is more common in the countries of the developed world would be almost certain to show a negative correlation with infectious disease mortality when examined in this way. A much more stringent test would be to compare the age at which childhood infections were acquired in places which differed with regard to the prevalence of multiple sclerosis, but which were comparable in terms of ethnicity and general standard of living. Such places might be found, for example, in Australia and New Zealand.

Indirect evidence for delayed exposure to infection in cases of multiple sclerosis comes from studies of the effect of position in the birth order on risk of disease. James recently identified a subtle bias in several of the published studies that arises because of the trend towards decreasing family size.[207] Only two studies are free of this bias, but both suggest that, in multiple sibships, children higher in the birth order are at greater risk.[208, 209] Infections tend to be introduced into families by older children so that younger members of the family are first exposed at an earlier age.

Diet

The countries of the world in which multiple sclerosis is commonest are among the most affluent and there is no suggestion that the disease has a predilection for people in low socio-economic groups. The diet of people who enjoy a high standard of living is generally much more varied than the diet of people in poorer places and it is hard to imagine that multiple sclerosis could be the result of a specific dietary deficiency.

A well-known characteristic of the diet of people in affluent countries is that it contains a high proportion of animal fat. The idea that a high dietary intake of animal fat or an imbalance in the proportion of saturated to mono-unsaturated and poly-unsaturated fats might be associated with an increased risk of multiple sclerosis was proposed in 1950.[210] A suggested mechanism is that changes in the proportion of saturated to unsaturated fatty acids in cerebral lipids affect susceptibility to a demyelinating agent.[211] A survey in Norway, carried out to test the hypothesis, demonstrated lower rates of disease amongst coastal fishing communities than inland communities in agricultural areas. Actual measurements of dietary fat showed that there was a positive correlation between animal fat intake and risk of multiple sclerosis.[158] Evidence from this sort of ecological survey is far from conclusive because of the large number of possible confounding variables; many factors other than animal fat, both dietary and non-dietary, are likely to vary between the areas. No study demonstrating an increased risk of multiple sclerosis in individuals, as opposed to populations, with high intakes of animal fat has been published.

A survey of the usual dietary intake of 142 people with established multiple sclerosis who denied having changed their diet since diagnosis showed a reduction in total energy intake compared with the general population, but no differences in other nutrients.[212] In a study of consumption of unusual items of food in the Orkney and Shetland Islands, the only positive finding was that pig's brain had been eaten more frequently in childhood by cases resident in the Shetlands.[157]

CONCLUSION

Over the last 20 years, epidemiological investigation of multiple sclerosis has been dominated by prevalence surveys. In spite of the limitations on comparability imposed by differences in methodology, they have given us a fairly clear picture of the geography of the disease over much of the world. The results of the US veterans study and the recent surveys in Australia and New Zealand have confirmed beyond all reasonable doubt the general relationship, for populations of European origin, between the frequency of multiple sclerosis and latitude. There is good evidence too, in the USA at least, of a similar relationship in the black population.

The fact that this relationship holds good in Europe and North America and, in the southern hemisphere, in South Africa, Australia and New Zealand strongly suggests that the causation of the disease is the same worldwide. This view is reinforced by the similarity of the clinical features of the disease wherever it occurs, and by the way in which the shape of the age-specific incidence curve remains constant, regardless of whether the disease is common or rare.

Without underestimating the importance of genetic factors in influencing susceptibility both in populations and individuals, the results of migrant studies alone establish that environmental factors are decisive in determining risk of disease. But the nature of these environmental factors remains unclear. If we insist that aetiological hypotheses must be reconcilable with the epidemiology of the disease, the global scale over which the relationship with latitude applies allows us to eliminate geological factors associated, for example, with the type of soil or the water supply. Similar considerations relegate diet and contact with animals to a low position in the list of possible causes.

Evidence is beginning to accumulate to indicate that patients with multiple sclerosis have an unusual experience of infectious diseases. If multiple sclerosis is a rare sequel to delayed exposure to a common infectious agent, many of the epidemiological features of the disease can be understood. This hypothesis can account for the rarity of the disease in the tropics, where exposure to infection in early childhood is invariable. It can explain why migrants from areas where multiple sclerosis is uncommon tend to retain a low risk of disease and why migration in early life from an area where multiple sclerosis is common reduces the risk. Because of the role of the HLA system in modifying the immune response to foreign antigens, it also has the potential to provide a mechanism for the association of the disease with particular HLA haplotypes.

Many aspects of the idea remain to be explored. Although there is evidence that infection with measles, rubella, mumps and Epstein–Barr virus tends to be later in cases of multiple sclerosis than in controls, it is not known whether any one of these infections is especially important. Delay in acquiring these infections may be no more than a marker for delayed infection generally. Although multiple sclerosis might be the result of delayed exposure to a particular micro-organism, there is also a possibility that several different infections could be responsible. We have seen that the time trends and geographical patterns of enteric infections, transmitted primarily by the faecal-oral route, are incompatible with the epidemiological features of multiple sclerosis. The factors which determine age of infection by organisms that depend on other routes of transmission need to be investigated.

Another suggestion is that multiple sclerosis is caused by an infectious agent that is, as yet, unknown or poorly understood. The established connection between tropical spastic paraparesis and HTLV-I and the known neurotropism of other retroviruses make this group of agents possible candidates. The virus would, however, have to behave very differently from any known member of the group to produce the geographical distribution seen in multiple sclerosis.

The contribution that further studies of prevalence can make to the unravelling of the aetiology of multiple sclerosis is diminishing. They might contribute a detail to our knowledge of the pattern of the disease, but they are unlikely to change our view of it in any fundamental way. Epidemiologists now need to formulate specific hypotheses about causal environmental factors and find ways of testing them.

ACKNOWLEDGEMENTS

C.N.M. would like to thank the many people who helped with the preparation of this chapter. He is particularly grateful to Sir Donald Acheson who lent his large collection of reprints on the epidemiology of multiple sclerosis and to Dr David Coggon for advice about the design of case-control studies.

REFERENCES

1. Rothman K J 1986 Modern epidemiology. Little, Brown, Boston
2. Barker D J P, Rose G 1984 Epidemiology for clinicians, 3rd edn. Churchill Livingstone, Edinburgh
3. Poskanzer D C, Prenney L B, Sheridan J L, Kondy J Y 1980 Multiple sclerosis in the Orkney and Shetland Islands I: Epidemiology, clinical factors, and methodology. Journal of Epidemiology and Community Health 34: 229–239
4. Cook S D, Cromarty J L, Tapp W, Poskanser D, Walker J D 1985 Declining incidence of multiple sclerosis in the Orkney islands. Neurology 35: 545–551
5. Malmgren R M, Valdiviezo N L, Visscher B R 1983 Underlying cause of death as recorded for multiple sclerosis patients: associated factors. Journal of Chronic Diseases 36: 699–705
6. Larsen J P, Kvale G, Aarli J A 1985 Multiple sclerosis and mortality statistics. Acta Neurologica Scandinavica 71: 237–241
7. O'Malley F, Dean G, Elian M 1987 multiple sclerosis and motor neuron disease: survival and how certified after death. Journal of Epidemiology and Community Health 41: 14–17
8. Williams E S, McKeran R O 1986 Prevalence of multiple sclerosis in a south London borough. British Medical Journal 293: 237–239
9. McLellan D L, Roberts M H W 1986 Prevalence of multiple sclerosis in a south london Borough. British Medical Journal 293: 506–507
10. Dean G, Grimaldi G, Kelly R, Karhausen L 1979 Multiple sclerosis in southern Europe I. Prevalence in Sicily in 1975. Journal of Epidemiology and Community Health 33: 107–110
11. Savettieri G, Daricello B, Giordano D, Karhausen L, Dean G 1981 The prevalence of multiple sclerosis in Sicily I. Monreale city. Journal of Epidemiology and Community Health 35: 114–117
12. Dean G, Savettieri G, Giordano D et al 1981 The prevalence of multiple sclerosis in Sicily II. Agrigento city. Journal of Epidemiology and Community Health 35: 118–122
13. Savettieri, Elian M, Giordano D, Grimaldi G, Ventura A, Dean G 1986 A further study on the prevalence of multiple sclerosis in Sicily: Caltanissetta city. Acta Neurologica Scandinavica 73: 71–75
14. Morganti G, Naccarato S, Elian M et al 1984 Multiple sclerosis in the republic of San Marino. Journal of Epidemiology and Community Health 38: 23–28
15. Allison R S, Millar J H D 1954 Prevalence and familial incidence of disseminated sclerosis (A report to the Northern Ireland Hospitals Authority on the results of a three-year survey). Prevalence of disseminated sclerosis in Northern Ireland. Ulster Medical Journal 23 (suppl 2): 5–27
16. Alter M, Allison R S, Talbert O R, Kurland L T 1960 Geographic distribution of multiple sclerosis. World Neurology 1: 55–66
17. Schumacher G A, Beebe G, Kibler R F et al 1965 Problems of experimental trials of therapy in multiple sclerosis: Report by the panel on the evaluation of experimental trials of therapy in multiple sclerosis. Annals of the New York Academy of Science 122: 552–568
18. Liebowitz U, Alter M 1973 Multiple sclerosis: clues to its cause. Elsevier, New York
19. McAlpine D 1972 In: McAlpine D, Lumsden C E, Acheson E D (eds) Multiple sclerosis: a re-appraisal. Churchill Livingstone, Edinburgh
20. Rose A S, Ellison G W, Myers L W, Tourtellotte W W 1976 Criteria for the clinical diagnosis of multiple sclerosis. Neurology 26: 20–22
21. McDonald W I, Halliday A M 1977 Diagnosis and classification of multiple sclerosis. British Medical Bulletin 33: 4–8
22. Poser C M 1965 Clinical diagnostic criteria in epidemiological studies of multiple sclerosis. Annals of the New York Academy of Sciences 122: 506–519
23. Bharucha N E, Bharucha E P, Wadia N H et al 1988

Prevalence of multiple sclerosis in the Parsis of Bombay. Neurology 38: 727–729

24. Hammond S R, McLeod J G, Millingen K S et al. The epidemiology of multiple sclerosis in three Australian cities: Perth, Newcastle and Hobart. Brain 111: 1–25

25. Sibley W A, Bamford C R, Clark K 1985 Clinical viral infections and multiple sclerosis. Lancet 1: 1313–1315

26. Acheson E D 1977 Epidemiology of multiple sclerosis. British Medical Bulletin 33: 9–14

27. Hader W J, Elliot M, Ebers G C 1988 Epidemiology of multiple sclerosis in London and Middlesex county, Ontario, Canada. Neurology 38: 617–621

28. Skegg D C G, Corwin P A, Craven R S, Malloch J A, Pollock M 1987 Occurrence of multiple sclerosis in the north and south of New Zealand. Journal of Neurology, Neurosurgery and Psychiatry 50: 134–139

29. Phadke J G, Downie A W 1987 Epidemiology of multiple sclerosis in the north-east (Grampian region) of Scotland — an update. Journal of Epidemiology and Community Health 41: 5–13

30. Visscher B R, Detels R, Coulson A H, Malmgren R M, Dudley J P 1977 Latitude, migration, and the prevalence of multiple sclerosis. American Journal of Epidemiology 106: 470–475

31. Visscher B R, Clark V A, Detels R, Malmgren R A, Valdiviezo N L, Dudley J P 1981 Two populations with multiple sclerosis. Journal of Neurology 225: 237–249

32. Kurtzke J F 1983 Epidemiology of multiple sclerosis. In: Hallpike J F, Adams C W M, Tourtellotte W W (eds) Multiple sclerosis, pathology, diagnosis and management. Chapman and Hall, London, Ch 3, pp 47–95

33. Morley D, Woodland M, Martin W J 1963 Measles in Nigerian children. Journal of Hygiene 61: 115–134

34. The Registrar General's statistical review of England and Wales for the year 1960. Part I. Tables, medical. 1962 HMSO, London

35. Acheson E D 1965 The epidemiology of multiple sclerosis. In: McAlpine D, Lumsden C E, Acheson E D (eds) Multiple sclerosis — a re-appraisal. Churchill Livingstone, Edinburgh, Ch 1, p 20

36. Kurtzke J F 1975 A reassessment of the distribution of multiple sclerosis. Part one. Acta Neurological Scandinavica 51: 110–136

37. Kurtzke J F 1975 A reassessment of the distribution of multiple sclerosis. Part two. Acta Neurological Scandinavica 51: 137–157

38. Lilienfeld D E, Chan E, Ehland J, Godbold J, Landrigan P J, Marsh G, Perl D P 1989 Rising mortality from motoneuron disease in the USA. Lancet 1: 710–713

39. Kondo K 1978 Motorneuron disease: changing population patterns and clues for etiology. Advances in Neurology 19: 509–543

40. Flaten T P 1989 Rising mortality from motoneuron disease. Lancet 1: 1018–1019

41. Martyn C N, Barker D J P, Osmond C 1988 Motoneuron disease and past poliomyelitis in England and Wales. Lancet 1: 1319–1322

42. Durrleman S, Alperovitch A 1989 Increasing trend of ALS in France and elsewhere: are the changes real? Neurology 39: 768–773

43. Cook S D, MacDonald J, Tapp W, Poskanser D,

Dowling P C 1988 Multiple sclerosis in the Shetland islands: an update. Acta Neurologica Scandinavica 77: 148–151

44. Hennessy A, Swingler R J, Compston D A S 1989 The incidence and mortality of multiple sclerosis in south east Wales. In press

45. Dean G, Goodall J, Downie A 1981 The prevalence of multiple sclerosis in the Outer Hebrides compared with north-east Scotland and the Orkney and Shetland islands. Journal of Epidemiology and Community Health 35: 110–113

46. McCoubrie M, Shuttleworth D 1978 Prevalence of multiple sclerosis in west Yorkshire. British Medical Journal 2: 570

47. Brewis M, Poskanser D C, Rolland C, Miller H 1966 Neurological disease in an English city. Acta Neurologica Scandinavica 42 (suppl 24): 1–89

48. Millar J H D 1971 Multiple sclerosis, a disease acquired in childhood. Charles Thomas, Springfield

49. Millar J H D 1980 Multiple sclerosis in Northern Ireland. In: Rose F C (ed) Clinical Neuroepidemiology. Pitman Medical, Tunbridge Wells, Ch 15, pp 222–227

50. Brady R, Dean G, Secerbegovic S, Secerbegovic A-M 1977 Multiple sclerosis in the Republic of Ireland. Journal of the Irish Medical Association 70: 500–506

51. Larsen J P, Aarli J A, Nyland H, Riise T 1984 Western Norway, a high-risk area for multiple sclerosis: a prevalence/incidence study in the county of Hordaland. Neurology 34: 1202–1207

52. Gronning M, Mellgren S I 1985 Multiple sclerosis in the two northern most counties of Norway. Acta Neurologica Scandinavica 72: 321–327

53. Kinnunen E, Wikstrom J, Porras J, Palo J 1983 The epidemiology of multiple sclerosis in Finland: increase of prevalence and stability of foci in high-risk areas. Acta Neurologica Scandinavica 67: 255–262

54. Kinnunen E 1984 Multiple sclerosis in Finland: evidence of increasing frequency and uneven geographical distribution. Neurology 34: 457–461

55. Lauer K, Firnhaber W, Reining R, Leuchtweis B 1984 Epidemiological investigations into multiple sclerosis in southern Hesse. I. Methodological problems and basic epidemiologic characteristics. Acta Neurologica Scandinavica 70: 257–267

56. Wender M, Pruchnik–Grabowska D, Hertmanowska H et al 1985 Epidemiology of multiple sclerosis in western Poland — a comparison between prevalence rates in 1965–1981. Acta Neurologica Scandinavica 72: 210–217

57. Kalafatova O I 1987 Epidemiology of multiple sclerosis in Bulgaria. Acta Neurologica Scandinavica 75: 118–189

58. Societa Italiana di Neurologia 1975 XIX Congreso Nationale Genova, 3 December 1975

59. Granieri E, Tola R, Paolino E, Rosati G, Carreras M, Monetti V C 1985 The frequency of multiple sclerosis in Italy: a descriptive study in Ferrara. Annals of Neurology 17: 80–84

60. Rosati G, Aiello I, Pirastru M I et al 1987 Sardinia, a high risk area for multiple sclerosis: a prevalence and incidence study in the district of Alghero. Annals of Neurology 21: 190–194

61. Vassallo L, Elian M, Dean G 1979 Multiple sclerosis in southern Europe II. Prevalence in Malta 1978. Journal of Epidemiology and Community Health 33: 110–13

62. Sweeney V P, Sadovnich A D, Brandejs V 1986 Prevalence of multiple sclerosis in British Columbia. Canadian Journal of Neurological Science 13: 47–51

63. Pryse Phillips W E 1986 The incidence and prevalence of multiple sclerosis in Newfoundland and Labrador 1960–1984. Annals of Neurology 20: 323–328

64. Baum H B, Rothschild B B 1981 The incidence and prevalence of reported multiple sclerosis. Annals of Neurology 10: 420–428

65. Kurland L T 1952 The frequency and geographic distribution of multiple sclerosis as indicated by mortality statistics and morbidity surveys in the United States and Canada. American Journal of Hygiene 55: 457–476

66. Westlund K B, Kurland L T 1953 Studies on multiple sclerosis in Winnipeg, Manitoba, and New Orleans, Louisiana 1. Prevalence. Comparison between the patients groups in Winnipeg and New Orleans. American Journal of Hygiene 57: 380–407

67. Stazio A, Kurland L T, Bell L G, Saunders M G, Rogot E 1964 Multiple sclerosis in Winnipeg, Manitoba: methodological considerations of epidemiological survey. Ten year follow-up of a community wide study, and population re-survey. Journal of Chronic Diseases 17: 415–438

68. Stazio A, Paddison R M, Kurland L T 1967 Multiple sclerosis in New Orleans, Louisiana, and Winnipeg, Manitoba, Canada: follow-up of a previous survey in New Orleans and comparison between the patient populations in the two communities. Journal of Chronic Diseases 20: 311–332

69. Kurtzke J F, Beebe G W, Norman J E 1979 Epidemiology of multiple sclerosis in US veterans 1. Race, sex, and geographic distribution. Neurology 29: 1228–1235

70. Alter M, Olivares L 1970 Multiple sclerosis in Mexico. Arch Neurol 23: 451–459

71. Sutherland J M , Tyrer J H, Eadie M J 1962 The prevalence of multiple sclerosis in Australia. Brain 85: 149–164

72. Sutherland J M , Tyrer J H, Eadie M J, Casey J H, Kurland L T 1966 The prevalence of multiple sclerosis in Queensland, Australia: a field survey. Acta Neurologica Scandinavica 42 (suppl 19): 57–67

73. McCall M G, Brereton T Le G, Dawson A, Millingen K, Sutherland J M, Acheson E D 1968 Frequency of multiple sclerosis in three Australian cities — Perth, Newcastle, and Hobart. Journal of Neurology, Neurosurgery and Psychiatry 31: 1–9

74. Hammond S R, De Wytt C, Maxwell I C, Landy P J, English D, McLeod J G McCall M G 1987 The epidemiology of multiple sclerosis in Queensland, Australia. Journal of the Neurological Sciences 80: 185–204

75. Hammond S R, English D R, de Wytt C, Hallpike J F, Millingen K S, Stewart-Wynne E G, McLeod J G, McCall M G 1989 The contribution of mortality statistics to the study of multiple sclerosis in Australia. Journal of Neurology, Neurosurgery and Psychiatry 52: 1–7

76. Fawcett J, Skegg D C 1988 Geographic distribution of multiple sclerosis in New Zealand: evidence from hospital admissions and deaths. Neurology 38: 416–418

77. Bhigjee A I 1987 Multiple sclerosis in a black patient: a case report. South African Medical Journal 72: 873–875

78. Dean G 1967 Annual incidence, prevalence and mortality of multiple sclerosis in white South-African born and in white immigrants to South Africa. British Medical Journal 2: 724–730

79. Kuroiwa Y, Igata A, Itahara K, Shinzaburo K, Tsubaki T, Toyokura Y, Shibasaki H 1975 Nationwide survey of multiple sclerosis in Japan. Neurology 25: 845–851

80. Okinaka S, McAlpine D, Miyagawa K et al 1960 Multiple sclerosis in northern and southern Japan. World Neurology 1: 22–42

81. Okinaka S, Kuroiwa Y 1966 Multiple sclerosis and allied diseases in Japan: epidemiology and clinical aspects. Progress in Brain Research 21: 183–191

82. Shikasaki H, Okihiro M M, Kuroiwa Y 1978 Multiple sclerosis among orientals and caucasians in Hawaii: a reappraisal. Neurology 28: 113–118

83. Araki S, Urchino M, Kumamoto T 1987 Prevalence studies of multiple sclerosis, myasthenia gravis and myopathies in Kumamoto district, Japan. Neuroepidemiology 6:120–129

83a. Yu Y L, Woo E, Hawkins B R, Ho H C, Huang C Y 1989 Multiple sclerosis among Chinese in Hong Kong. Brain 112: 1445–1467

84. Kurtzke J F, Park C S, Oh S J 1968 Multiple sclerosis in Korea. Clinical features and prevalence. Journal of the Neurological Sciences 6: 463–481

85. Zhao B, Liu X, Guo Y, Yang Y, Huang H 1981 Multiple sclerosis — a clinical study of 70 cases. European Neurology 20: 394–400

86. Jain S, Maheshwari M C 1985 Multiple sclerosis: Indian experience in the last 30 years. Neuroepidemiology 4: 96–107

87. Singhal B S, Wadia N H 1975 Profile of multiple sclerosis in the Bombay region. On the basis of critical clinical appraisal. Journal of the Neurological Sciences 26: 259–270

88. Wadia N H, Trikannad V S, Krishnaswamy P R 1981 HLA antigens in multiple sclerosis amongst Indians. Journal of Neurology, Neurosurgery and Psychiatry 44: 849–851

89. Alter M, Halpern L, Kurland L T et al 1962 Multiple sclerosis in Israel. Archives of Neurology 7: 253–263

90. Antonovsky A, Liebowitz U, Smith H A et al 1965 Epidemiologic study of multiple sclerosis in Israel 1. An overall review of methods and findings. Archives of Neurology 13: 183–193

91. Al-Din A S N 1986 Multiple sclerosis in Kuwait: clinical and epidemiological study. Journal of Neurology, Neurosurgery and Psychiatry 49: 928–931

92. Radhakrishnan K, Ashok P P, Sridharan R, Mousa M E 1985 Prevalence and pattern of multiple sclerosis in Benghazi, north eastern Libya. Journal of the Neurological Sciences 70: 39–46

93. Yaqub B A, Daif A K 1988 Multiple sclerosis in Saudi Arabia. Neurology 38: 621–623

94. Cruickshank E K, Montgomery R D 1961 Multiple sclerosis in Jamaica. West Indian Medical Journal 10: 211

95. Dean G, McLoughlin H, Brady R, Adelstein A N, Tallett–Williams J 1976 Multiple sclerosis among immigrants in Greater London. British Medical Journal 2: 861–864

96. Dean G, Brady R, McLoughlin H, Elian M, Adelstein A M 1977 Motor neurone disease and multiple sclerosis

among immigrants to Britain. British Journal of Preventive and Social Medicine 31 (3): 141–147

97. Elian M, Dean G 1987 Multiple sclerosis among the United Kingdom-born children of immigrants from the West Indies. Journal of Neurology, Neurosurgery and Psychiatry 50: 327–332

98. Detels R, Brody J A, Edgar A H 1972 Multiple sclerosis among American, Japanese and Chinese migrants to California and Washington. Journal of Chronic Diseases 25: 3–10

99. Detels R, Visscher B R, Malmgren R M, Coulson A H, Lucia M V, Dudley J P 1977 Evidence for lower susceptibility to multiple sclerosis in Japanese-Americans. American Journal of Epidemiology 105: 303–310

100. Alter M, Okihiro M, Rowley R, Morris T 1971 Multiple sclerosis among Orientals and Caucasians in Hawaii. Neurology 21: 122–130

101. Haenszel W, Kurihara M 1968 Studies of Japanese migrants. 1. Mortality from cancer and other diseases among Japanese in the United States. Journal of the National Cancer Institute 49: 969–988

102. Milne A, Allwood G K, Moyes C D, Pearce N E, Lucas C R 1985 Prevalence of hepatitis B infection in a multi-racial New Zealand community. New Zealand Medical Journal 98: 529–532

103. Milne A, Allwood G K, Moyes C D, Pearce N E, Newell K 1987 A seroepidemiological study of the prevalence of hepatitis B infections in a hyperendemic New Zealand community. International Journal of Epidemiology 16: 84–90

104. Lowis G W 1988 Ethnic factors in multiple sclerosis: A review and critique of the epidemiological literature. International Journal of Epidemiology 17: 14–20

105. Davenport C B 1922 Multiple sclerosis from the standpoint of geographic distribution and race. Archives of Neurology and Psychiatry 8: 51–60

106. Limberg C C 1950 The geographic distribution of multiple sclerosis and its estimated prevalence in the United States. Proceedings of the Association for Research into Nervous and Mental Diseases 28: 15–24

107. Swingler R J, Compston D A S 1986 The distribution of multiple sclerosis in the United Kingdom. Journal of Neurology, Neurosurgery and Psychiatry 49: 1115–1124

108. Francis D A, Bachelor J R, McDonald W I et al 1987 Multiple sclerosis in north-east Scotland. An association with HLA-DQw1. Brain 110: 181–196

109. Ebers G C, Bulman D 1986 The geography of MS reflects genetic susceptibility. Neurology 36 (suppl 1): 108

110. Acheson E D, Bachrach C A, Wright F M 1960 Some comments on the relationship of the distribution of multiple sclerosis to latitude, solar radiation and other variables. Acta Psychiatrica Scandinavica 35 (suppl 147): 132–147

111. Norman J E, Kurtzke J F, Beebe G W 1983 Epidemiology of multiple sclerosis in US veterans: 2. Latitude, climate and the risk of multiple sclerosis. Journal of Chronic Diseases 36: 551–559

112. Liebowitz U, Kahana E, Alter M 1969 Multiple sclerosis in immigrant and native populations of Israel. Lancet 2: 1323–1325

113. Kurtzke J F, Beebe G W, Norman J E 1985 Epidemiology of multiple sclerosis in US veterans: 3

Migration and the risk of MS. Neurology 35: 672–678

114. Kurtzke J F 1976 Multiple sclerosis in immigrants. British Medical Journal 1: 1527–1528

115. Kurtzke J F, Bui Q H 1980 Multiple sclerosis in a migrant population. 2. Half-orientals immigrating in childhood. Annals of Neurology 8: 256–260

116. Dean G, Kurtzke J F 1971 On the risk of multiple sclerosis according to age at immigration to South Africa. British Medical Journal 3: 725–729

117. Alter M, Liebowitz U, Speer J 1966 Risk of multiple sclerosis related to age at immigration to Israel. Archives of Neurology 15: 234–237

118. Alter M, Kahana E, Loewenson R 1978 Migration and risk of multiple sclerosis. Neurology 28: 1089–1093

119. Detels R, Visscher B R, Haile R W, Malmgren R M, Dudley J P, Coulson A H 1978 Multiple sclerosis and age at migration. American Journal of Epidemiology 108: 386–393

120. Beebe G W, Kurtzke J F, Kurland L T, Auth T L, Nagler B 1967 Studies on the natural history of multiple sclerosis 3. Epidemiologic analysis of the Army experience in World War II. Neurology 17: 1–17

121. Visscher B A, Bunnell D H, Detels R 1981 Multiple sclerosis and multiple moves: an etiologic hypothesis. American Journal of Epidemiology 113: 140–143

122. Operskalski E A, Visscher B, Malmgren R M, Detels R 1989 A case-control study of multiple sclerosis. Neurology 39: 825–829

123. Deacon W E, Alexander L, Siedler H D, Kurland L T 1959 Multiple sclerosis in a small New England community. New England Journal of Medicine 261: 1059–1061

124. Eastman R, Sheridan J, Poskanser D C 1973 Multiple sclerosis clustering in a small Massachusetts community with possible common exposure 23 years before onset. New England Journal of Medicine 289: 793–794

125. Koch M J, Reed D, Stern R, Brody J A 1974 Multiple sclerosis: a cluster in a small north western United States community. Journal of the American Medical Association 288: 1555–1557

126. Murray T J 1976 An unusual occurrence of multiple sclerosis in a small rural community. Canadian Journal of Neurological Sciences 3: 163–166

127. Hoffman R E, Zack M M, Davis L E, Burchfiel C M 1981 Increased incidence and prevalence of multiple sclerosis in Los Alamos County, New Mexico. Neurology 31: 1489–1492

128. Sheremata W A, Poskanser D C, Withum D G, MacLeod C L, Whiteside M E 1985 Unusual occurrence on a tropical island of multiple sclerosis. Lancet 2: 618

129. Thomas M, Robertson M 1984 Multiple sclerosis in a Glasgow tenement. Scottish Medical Journal 29: 244–246

130. Poskanser D C, Shapira K, Miller H 1963 Epidemiology of multiple sclerosis in the counties of Northumberland and Durham. Journal of Neurology, Neurosurgery and Psychiatry 26: 368–376

131. Ashitey G A, Mackenzie G 1970 'Clustering' of multiple sclerosis cases by date and place of birth. British Journal of Preventive and Social Medicine 24: 163–168

132. Hargreaves E R, Merrington M 1973 A note on the absence of 'clustering' in multiple sclerosis. Journal of Chronic Diseases 26: 47–50

133. Neutel C I, Walter S D, Mousseau G 1977 Clustering during childhood of multiple sclerosis patients. Journal of Chronic Diseases 30: 217–224
134. Larsen J P, Riise T, Nyland H, Kvale G, Aarli J A 1985 Clustering of multiple sclerosis in the county of Hordaland, Western Norway. Acta Neurologica Scandinavica 71: 390–395
135. Poskanser D C, Walker A M, Prenney L B, Sheridan J L 1981 The aetiology of multiple sclerosis: temporal-spatial clustering indicating two environmental exposures before onset. Neurology 31: 708–713
136. Stein E C, Schiffer R B, Hall W J, Young N 1987 Multiple sclerosis and the workplace: report of an industry-based cluster. Neurology 37: 1672–1677
137. Kurtzke J F, Hyllested K 1979 Multiple sclerosis in the Faroe Islands. I: Clinical and epidemiological features. Annals of Neurology 5: 6–21
138. Kurtzke J F, Hyllested K 1986 Multiple sclerosis in the Faroe Islands. II: Clinical update, transmission, and the nature of MS. Neurology-36: 307–328
139. Kurtzke J F, Hullested K 1987 Multiple sclerosis in the Faroe Islands. III: An alternative assessment of the three epidemics. Acta Neurologica Scandinavica 76: 317–339
140. Sartwell P E 1966 The incubation period and the dynamics of infectious disease. American Journal of Epidemiology 83: 204–215
141. Poser C M, Hibberd P L, Benedikz J, Gudmundsson G 1988 Analysis of the 'epidemic' of multiple sclerosis in the Faroe Islands. I. Clinical and epidemiological aspects. Neuroepidemiology 7: 168–180
142. Poser C M, Hibberd P L 1988 Analysis of the 'epidemic' of multiple sclerosis in the Faroe Islands. II: Biostatistical aspects. Neuroepidemiology 7: 181–189
143. Dean G 1988 Was there an epidemic of multiple sclerosis in the Faroe Islands? Neuroepidemiology 7: 165–167
144. Acheson E D 1985 The epidemiology of multiple sclerosis. In: Matthews W B, Acheson E D, Batchelor J R, Weller R (eds) McAlpine's multiple sclerosis. Churchill Livingstone, Edinburgh, Ch 1, pp 22–25
145. Kurtzke J F, Gudmundsson K R, Bergmann S 1982 Multiple sclerosis in Iceland: 1. Evidence of a postwar epidemic. Neurology 32: 143–150
146. Martin J R 1987 Troop-related multiple sclerosis outbreak in the Orkneys. Journal of Epidemiology and Community Health 41: 183–184
147. Rosati G, Aiello I, Granieri E et al 1986 Incidence of multiple sclerosis in Macomer, Sardinia 1912–1981: onset of the disease after 1950. Neurology 36: 14–19
148. Campbell A M G, Daniel P, Porter R J, Ritchie–Russell W, Smith H V, Innes T R M 1947 Disease of the nervous system occurring among research workers on swayback in lambs. Brain 70: 50–58
149. Dean G, McDougall E I, Elian M 1985 Multiple sclerosis in research workers studying swayback in lambs: an updated report. Journal of Neurology, Neurosurgery and Psychiatry 48: 859–865
150. Roberts D F, Roberts M J, Poskanser D C 1979 Genetic analysis of multiple sclerosis in Orkney. Journal of Epidemiology and Community Health 33: 229–235
151. Schapira K, Poskanser D C, Miller H 1963 Familial and conjugal multiple sclerosis. Brain 86: 315–332
152. Grufferman S, Barton J W, Eby N L 1987 Increased sex concordance of sibling pairs with Bechet's disease, Hodgkin's disease, multiple sclerosis and sarcoidosis. American Journal of Epidemiology 126: 365–369
153. Miller H, Ridley A, Shapira K 1960 Multiple sclerosis. A note on social incidence. British Medical Journal ii: 343–345
154. Russell W R 1971 Multiple sclerosis: occupation and social group at onset. Lancet 2: 832–834
155. Occupational mortality. The Registrar General's decennial supplement for England and Wales 1970–1972. Office of Population Censuses and Surveys Series DS No 1. HMSO, London
156. Alter M, Speer J 1968 Clinical evaluation of possible etiological factors in multiple sclerosis. Neurology 18: 109–116
157. Poskanser D C, Sheridan J L, Prenney L B, Walker A M 1980 Multiple sclerosis in the Orkney and Shetland islands II: The search for an exogenous aetiology. Journal of Epidemiology and Community Health 34: 240–252
158. Swank R L, Lersted O, Strom A, Backer J 1952 Multiple sclerosis in rural Norway. New England Journal of Medicine 246: 721–728
159. Hyllested K 1956 Disseminated sclerosis in Denmark. Prevalence and geographic distribution. J Jorgensen, Copenhagen.
160. Lauer K, Firnhaber W 1985 Epidemiological investigation into multiple sclerosis in southern Hesse. IV. The influence of urban and rural environment on disease risk. Acta Neurologica Scandinavica 72: 403
161. Percy A K, Nobrega F T, Okazaki H, Glattre E, Kurland L T 1971 Multiple sclerosis in Rochester, Minn. Archives of Neurology 25: 105–111
162. Rosati G, Aiello I, Mannu L, Pirastru M I, Agretti V, Sau G, Garau M, Gioia R, Sanna G 1988 Incidence of multiple sclerosis in the town of Sassari, Sardinia. Evidence for increasing occurrence of the disease. Neurology 38: 384–388
163. Francis D A, Batchelor J R, McDonald W I et al 1987 Multiple sclerosis in north-east Scotland. Brain 110: 181–196
164. Swingler R J, Kirk P F, Darke C, Compston D A S 1987 HLA and multiple sclerosis in south east Wales. Journal of Neurology, Neurosurgery and Psychiatry 50: 1153–1155
165. Bobowick A R, Kurtzke J F, Brody J A, Hrubec Z, Gillespie M 1978 Twin study of multiple sclerosis: an epidemiologic inquiry. Neurology 28: 978–987
166. Kinnunen E, Koskenvus M, Kaprio J, Ano K 1987 Multiple sclerosis in a nationwide series of twins. Neurology 37: 1627–1629
167. Heltberg A 1987 Twin studies in multiple sclerosis. Italian Journal of Neurological Science (suppl 6): 35–40
168. Ebers G C, Bulman D E, Sadornick A D et al 1986 A population based study of multiple sclerosis in twins. New England Journal of Medicine 315: 1638–1642
169. James W H 1985 Sib risk and the dizygotic twin concordance rate for multiple sclerosis. Journal of Epidemiology and Community Health 39: 39–43
170. Norrby E 1978 Viral antibodies in multiple sclerosis. Progress in Medicine and Virology 24: 1–39
171. Compston D A S, Vakarelis B N, Paul E, McDonald W I, Batchelor J R, Mims C A 1986 Viral infection in patients with multiple sclerosis and HLA-DR matched

controls. Brain 109: 325–344

172. Ammitzboll T, Clausen J 1972 Measles antibody in serum of multiple sclerosis patients, their children, siblings and parents. Acta Neurologica Scandinavica 48: 47–56

173. Visscher B R, Sullivan C B, Detels R et al 1981 Measles antibody titres in multiple sclerosis patients and HLA-matched and unmatched siblings. Neurology 31: 1142–1145

174. Poskanser D C, Sever J L, Sheridan J L, Prenney L B 1980 Multiple sclerosis in the Orkney and Shetland Islands. Journal of Epidemiology and Community Health 34: 258–264

175. Cook S D, Dowling P C 1977 A possible association between house pets and multiple sclerosis. Lancet 1: 980–982

176. Cook S D, Dowling P C 1981 Distemper and multiple sclerosis in Sitka, Alaska. Annals of Neurology 11: 192–194

177. Cook S D, Dowling P C, Norman J, Jablon S 1979 Multiple sclerosis and distemper in Iceland. Lancet 1: 380–381

178. Cook S D, Dowling P C, Russell W C 1978 Multiple sclerosis and canine distemper. Lancet 1: 605–606

179. Cook S D, Blumberg B, Dowling P C, Deans W, Cross R 1987 Multiple sclerosis and canine distemper on Key West, Florida. Lancet 1: 1426–1427

180. Bunnell D H, Visscher B R, Detels R 1979 Multiple sclerosis and house dogs — a case-control study. Neurology 29: 1027–1029

181. Poskanser D C, Prenney L B, Sheridan J L 1977 House pets and multiple sclerosis. Lancet 1: 1204

182. Sylwester D L, Poser C M 1979 The association of multiple sclerosis with domestic animals and house pets. Annals of Neurology 5: 207–208

183. Hughes R A C, Russell W C, Froude J R L, Janett R J 1980 Pet ownership, distemper antibodies and multiple sclerosis. Journal of the Neurological Sciences 47: 429–432

184. Read D, Nassim D, Smith P, Patterson C, Warlow C 1982 Multiple sclerosis and dog ownership — a case-control investigation. Journal of the Neurological Sciences 55: 359–367

185. Kurtzke J F, Hyllested K, Arbuckle J D et al 1988 Multiple sclerosis in the Faroe Islands. IV. The lack of a relationship between canine distemper and the epidemics of multiple sclerosis. Acta Neurologica Scandinavica 78: 484–500

186. Poskanser D C, Shapira K, Miller H 1963 Multiple sclerosis and poliomyelitis. Lancet 2: 917–921

187. Burnet M, White D O 1972 Natural history of infectious disease. Cambridge University Press, Cambridge, Ch 7, pp 91–96

188. Dean G 1967 Poliomyelitis among white immigrants to South Africa. South African Medical Journal 41: 294–297

189. Liebowitz U, Antonovsky A, Medalie J M, Smith H, Halpern L, Alter M 1966 Epidemiological study of multiple sclerosis in Israel Part II. Multiple sclerosis and level of sanitation. Journal of Neurology, Neurosurgery and Psychiatry 29: 60–68

190. Field E J, Miller H, Russell H 1962 Observations on glial inclusion bodies in a case of acute disseminated sclerosis. Journal of Clinical Pathology 15: 278–284

191. Gay D, Dick G, Upton G 1986 Multiple sclerosis associated with sinusitis: case-controlled study in general practice. Lancet 1: 815–819

192. Gay D, Dick G 1986 Is multiple sclerosis caused by an oral spirochaete? Lancet 2: 75–77

193. Martyn C N, Colquhoun I. Unpublished data

194. Markby D P 1987 Distribution of multiple sclerosis in the United Kingdom. Journal of Neurology, Neurosurgery and Psychiatry 50: 505–506

195. Schmutzhard E, Pohl P, Stanek G 1988 Borrelia burgdorferi antibodies in patients with relapsing/remitting form and chronic progressive form of multiple sclerosis. Journal of Neurology, Neurosurgery and Psychiatry 51: 1215–1218

196. Coyle P K 1989 Borrelia burgdorferi antibodies in multiple sclerosis patients. Neurology 39: 760–761

197. Lenman J A R, Peters T J 1969 Herpes zoster and multiple sclerosis. British Medical Journal 2: 218–220

198. Ragozzino M W, Kurland L T 1983 Epidemiologic investigation of the association between herpes zoster and multiple sclerosis. Neurology 33: 648–649

199. Martin J R 1981 Herpes simplex virus types 1 and 2 and multiple sclerosis. Lancet 2: 777–781

200. Alter M 1981 Multiple sclerosis, herpes viruses, and immunity. Lancet 2: 1224–1225

201. Panelius M, Salmi A, Halones P E, Kivolo E, Rinne U K 1973 Virus antibodies in serum specimens from patients with multiple sclerosis, from siblings and matched controls. A final report. Acta Neurologica Scandinavica 49: 85–107

202. Alter M, Cendrowski W 1976 Multiple sclerosis and childhood infections. Neurology 26: 201–204

203. Andersen E, Isager H, Hyllested K 1981 Risk factors in multiple sclerosis: Tuberculin reactivity, age of measles infection, tonsillectomy and appendectomy. Acta Neurologica Scandinavica 63: 131–134

204. Sullivan C B, Visscher B R, Detels R 1984 Multiple sclerosis and age at exposure to childhood diseases and animals: cases and their friends. Neurology 34: 1144–1148

205. Warner H B, Carp R I 1981 Multiple sclerosis and Epstein–Barr virus. Lancet 1: 1290

206. Alter M, Zhen-Xin Z, Davanipour Z, Sobel E, Zibulewski J, Schwartz G, Friday G 1986 Multiple sclerosis and childhood infections. Neurology 36: 1386–1389

207. James W H 1984 Multiple sclerosis and birth order. Journal of Epidemiology and Community Health 38: 21–22

208. Visscher B, Liu K-S, Sullivan C, Valdiviezo N, Detels R 1982 Birth order and multiple sclerosis. Acta Neurologica Scandinavica 66: 209–215

209. Isager H, Anderson E, Hyllested K 1980 Risk of multiple sclerosis inversely associated with birth order. Acta Neurologica Scandinavica 61: 393–396

210. Swank R L 1950 Multiple sclerosis: a correlation of its incidence with dietary fat. American Journal of the Medical Sciences 220: 421–430

211. Dick G 1976 The aetiology of multiple sclerosis. Proceedings of the Royal Society of Medicine 69: 611–615

212. Hewson D C, Phillips M A, Simpson K E, Drury P, Crawford M A 1984 Food intake in multiple sclerosis. Human Nutrition: Applied Nutrition 38: 355–367

Clinical aspects
W. B. Matthews

2. Symptoms and signs

An entirely accurate account of the symptoms and signs of multiple sclerosis could only be compiled from a series of geographically diverse population studies of clinically definite and laboratory proven cases, minutely observed over the whole course of the disease to pathological confirmation. Such data are not available, nor are to be reasonably expected and, in any case, would be defective in the resolution of the problems of the doubtful case and of the delay in diagnosis. In default of such unattainable data, the mass of published material on the clinical features of multiple sclerosis consists largely either of lists of symptoms and signs encountered at the onset or during the course of the disease, or of accounts of small numbers of patients with symptoms of particular interest or rarity. In the former, diagnostic criteria are usually stated but detailed description of symptoms is obviously impossible. The reader is therefore inevitably left without useful knowledge of what is specifically implied by the broad headings that must be used — 'visual disturbance', 'facial weakness' or 'brainstem symptoms', for example. With individual case reports a difficulty may occasionally arise in accepting the clinical diagnosis, but the autopsy rate in multiple sclerosis is low and it is not possible to confine consideration to proven cases.

INITIAL SYMPTOMS

The initial symptoms and signs of multiple sclerosis have been analysed in many series, comprising several thousand cases. All such studies are inevitably subject to varying degrees to numerous sources of error. Of these the most important is the retrospective nature of the enquiry. Many patients are, of course, seen and fully documented in what proves to have been the first episode of multiple sclerosis, but however typical the clinical features and laboratory data, the diagnosis of clinically definite multiple sclerosis is scarcely permissible at this stage. In other patients the diagnosis is not even suspected after apparently trivial or evanescent symptoms recalled uncertainly following some more obviously significant event. It is beyond dispute that important and clearly recorded symptoms may not be remembered at all but how often the initial symptoms are expunged from the memory cannot be known. Even if remembered, the significance of poorly described sensory symptoms or dizziness cannot easily be determined. It is reasonable to assume that the longer the time that has elapsed between onset and questioning the more inaccurate will be the replies. The duration of the illness at the time of inclusion in the series may therefore be expected to influence the result. This defect may, of course, be partially or wholly repaired by consulting medical records, but other people's clinical notes, even if not prematurely destroyed, are seldom quite as precise as one would wish.

The effect of the combination of failure of recall and lack of records is almost certainly illustrated by the considerable difference between the clinical features of the initial attacks of multiple sclerosis occurring in soldiers before enlistment and those actually observed during their term of service. The former were much more likely to be recorded as monosymptomatic and minor symptoms were far less frequent.[1]

Comparison between different series is not straightforward. Patients are selected differently: hospital inpatients only,[2] or men in the US Armed

Forces[1] and therefore passed fit for service on recruitment, or autopsied cases only.[3] Series approximating to population studies[4,5] are inevitably heavily based on hospital records. Diagnostic criteria have varied, 'possible' cases being included[4-6] or excluded[2] or only included if 'strong possible'.[1] In the widely cited figures of Poser et al[5,7,8], for example, the proportion of definite cases is only 41%. The headings under which symptoms and signs are listed are tantalisingly different. Visual failure may be combined with double vision[3] or symptoms vaguely linked as affections of the cranial nerves 'V and/or VII'.[5] Lhermitte's sign may not be distinguished from other sensory symptoms,[5] or may not be mentioned at all.[1] Cerebellar disturbance may be implied by abnormalities of balance[1] or gait[2], by tremor and ataxia[3] and often no distinction is made from vertigo.

Despite these problems of comparison a considerable degree of agreement can be discerned. Wilson[9] reviewed some early reports and his own material and concluded that motor symptoms were a presenting symptom in 46.2%, paraesthesiae in 22.8%, ataxia, tremor or dysarthria in 10.2%, ocular and visual trouble in 14.3%, giddiness in 9%, sphincter impairment in 9.3% and fits in 1.1%. Only the principle symptoms were listed, the percentages totalling some 112%, allowing for only a small proportion of patients with more than one major symptom at the onset. The calculation to the nearest decimal point adds an air of unreality to these necessarily approximate figures. The small size of the series analysed, the extremely eminent and therefore highly experienced Kinnier Wilson himself contributing only 100 personal cases, strongly suggests that the material was heavily biased towards the more severe and thus more easily recognised forms of the disease. McAlpine,[10] in a more realistic review of published reports, found that the incidence of initial symptoms was roughly as follows:

1. weakness in one or more limbs 40%
2. optic neuritis 22%
3. paraesthesiae 21%
4. diplopia 12%
5. vertigo 5%
6. disturbance of micturition 5%.

Other symptoms at the onset were reported in less than 5%. He was unable to interpret the significance of 'unsteadiness in walking' or 'lack of balance' in some reported series as the cause was not defined.

McAlpine's own series[10] was large, personally observed and seen within three years of the presumed clinical onset. The proportion in whom weakness formed part of the presentation was not very different from reported figures, being 39%. There was, however, much greater recognition of paraesthesiae as an initial symptom, being present in 40%. Optic neuritis occurred in 29%. McAlpine distinguished polysymptomatic (55%) and monosymptomatic (45%) onset. In the former, weakness was present in 50% but in only 26% of those with a single initial symptom. Optic neuritis was more common in isolation but cerebellar ataxia did not occur without more widespread symptoms.

Series published subsequently have shown little deviation from these figures. Leibowitz and Alter[11] from Israel reported pure motor symptoms in 38% and combined motor and sensory symptoms in a further 8%. Their figure for sensory symptoms in isolation was much lower than in European series, being only 13% and optic neuritis at the onset was also much less common at 14%. Kurtzke et al[1] found very different proportions in their two groups of patients, men in whom the first attack occurred before joining the army and those in whom it occurred during service. In the former, motor symptoms were present in some 40% as in other series, but in those in whom the onset was recorded the figure was much higher at 67.5%. There was, in fact, a greater incidence of all recorded symptoms in men in whom the onset was observed during their service, indicating a great increase in evidence of multiple lesions.

Nearly all authors have acknowledged that the onset may be polysymptomatic although the percentages for different symptoms given by Adams et al[12] and more recently by Thompson et al[13] add up neatly to 100% indicating a single symptom per patient. The combinations most commonly encountered were analysed by Kurtzke et al.[1] They recognised symptoms as affecting 'major' systems: motor, co-ordination, sensory or brainstem, all others, including vision and sphincter control, being 'minor'. In their more closely observed

Table 2.1 Symptoms at the onset in two series of patients with clinically definite multiple sclerosis. Percentage figures (to the nearest whole number), referring either to those patients with monosymptomatic onset, or to the whole series, as relevant, are given in brackets. Visual loss indicates impaired acuity, sometimes progressive, not attributable to a recognised episode of optic neuritis. Pain includes headache not associated with optic neuritis. Ataxia was not necessarily of cerebellar origin.

	Series A		Series B	
Total	169		377	
Male	57(34)		127(34)	
Female	112(66)		250(66)	
Mean age at onset	31.5 years		30.6 years	
Monosymptomatic	135(79)		252(67)	
	Individual symptoms			
	Isolated	Combined	Isolated	Combined
Weakness	47(28)	64(38)	46(12)	129(34)
Sensory loss	19(11)	31(18)	51(14)	176(39)
Paraesthesiae	10(6)	15(9)	23(6)	115(31)
Optic neuritis	24(14)	38(22)	67(18)	156(41)
Diplopia	14(8)	17(10)	23(6)	66(18)
Vertigo	4(2)	7(4)	7(2)	26(7)
Ataxia	9(5)	16(9)	7(2)	43(11)
Paroxysmal	2	2	9(2)	20(5)
Myokymia	1	1	0	0
Dementia	1	1	2	7(2)
Epilepsy	1	1	0	0
Visual loss	1	1	4	9(2)
Falling	1	1	0	0
Bladder	0	6(4)	3	13(3)
Lhermitte	0	2	5	15(4)
Pain	0	1	3	15(4)
Facial palsy	0	0	1	1
Impotence	0	2	1	3

group, onset with involvement of a single major system, as defined, occurred in only 13.7%, motor involvement being most common. The most frequent combinations were involvement of all four systems in 13.7% motor and sensory in 11.5%; motor, co-ordination and sensory in 11.5%; and co-ordination and brainstem in 10.3%. The incidence of visual disturbance at the onset was remarkably low. Information was incomplete but loss of visual acuity was found at the onset in only 25.6% and visual loss without disturbance of a major system in only 1.3% in this group. This contrasts with McAlpine's finding that in 36% of patients with monosymptomatic onset the initial symptom was blurred vision, although more widespread physical signs might be present.

In a recent account[14] of 193 patients onset was monosymptomatic in 110 (57%). All symptoms were attributed to disturbance of the visual system, the posterior columns of the spinal cord, the pyramidal tracts, brainstem or cerebellum; certainly an oversimplification. The analysis of the frequency with which these systems were involved in different combinations appears to be distorted by arithmetical errors.

Two personal clinic series of clinically definite cases (Table 2:1), by the criteria of McAlpine,[15] may be compared and contrasted, one (Series A) being derived from experience in the early 1960s and the second (Series B) in the decade before

1987. Although the demographic characteristics of the two series are almost identical it is evident that the passage of some two decades had led the observer to pay much greater attention to sensory and paroxysmal symptoms as early evidence of the disease.

Information on the onset of the disease derived from autopsy-proven cases is biased by small numbers and selected material. The series of 111 cases collected by Poser et al[16] was derived from three countries and its unrepresentative nature is suggested by the reversal of the usual female preponderance in the cases from Norway and the USA. In histologically proven cases neither early[17] nor late[18] onset of disease was found to be related to significant differences in initial symptoms.

As multiple sclerosis has been recognised with increasing frequency in different geographical areas it has become apparent that symptomatology, including that of the onset, may vary between regions. The most remarkable difference is in the greater frequency of optic neuritis in oriental cases. Kuroiwa et al[19] compared the onset symptoms in 488 cases of multiple sclerosis from 6 Asian countries with those of 177 cases in Hungary. In the former, visual loss was present at the onset in 41.7% of cases, being bilateral in 15.6%, the comparable figures for Hungary being 19.9% and 4%.

Any large series includes a small proportion of patients in whom the onset has taken a more unusual form: vertigo, facial palsy, sphincter disturbance, epilepsy or paroxysmal phenomena, for example. When such symptoms occur in isolation their import can often only be recognised retrospectively.

Prodromal symptoms

Abb & Schaltenbrand[20] emphasised the common occurrence of prodromal symptoms, described as pseudo-rheumatic and pseudo-neurasthenic. These non-specific symptoms of limb pains, fatigue, irritability, poor memory and weight loss might be dismissed as insignificant were it not for the claim that abnormalities may be found in the CSF at this stage before the appearance of overt neurological disease. The opportunity to confirm these observations seldom arises as such symptoms are not regarded as an indication for lumbar puncture. Inevitably some patients will have experienced such symptoms before the clinical onset of multiple sclerosis. Identical symptoms are common in those who do not immediately develop this, or indeed any other disease. In personal experience the initial episode of multiple sclerosis is not preceded by recognisable prodromata.

SYMPTOMS AND SIGNS IN THE COURSE OF MULTIPLE SCLEROSIS

The incidence of individual symptoms and signs in the course of the disease can be expressed in several ways. In any series large enough to be worth analysing there will naturally be a very wide variation in duration of disease at the time of reporting. The proportion of patients displaying a certain feature can be related to the mean duration in the series or can be calculated, most approximately, for a given duration, from the observed increasing rate of positive findings with the passage of time from the onset. In multiple sclerosis, a remitting disease, it may also be possible to state the proportion of those who have, at any time up to the point of recording, suffered from a particular symptom, whether or not it is still present. Analyses confined to patients who have died of multiple sclerosis or its consequences, in whom the whole duration of the disease can be studied, should in theory provide more precise figures. In practice such series are small and clinical details may be poorly recorded or observed, particularly in the later years of the disease. It is therefore unrealistic to expect precise figures and in any case great precision, if attainable, would scarcely add to understanding of the disease process.

In the well known series of 46 autopsied cases reported by Carter et al[3] some of the findings are difficult to understand. Although all the patients had ocular manifestations only 93% are said to have been weak. It is not easy to understand how multiple sclerosis could prove fatal without some form of weakness being observed. To some degree, therefore, the accuracy of these figures must be suspect, but in general they confirm the importance of weakness, ataxia, ocular and visual signs, sphincter disturbance and increased spinal reflex activity in the established disease.

In three reports, results where comparable, are very similar. In Shepherd's[4] series the mean duration was 14.4 years. Signs of pyramidal disease, presumably including weakness and appropriate reflex changes, were present in 83.7%, sensory changes in 80.6%, cerebellar signs in 67%, brainstem involvement in 65%, sphincter disturbance in 56.4% and mental changes in 30.5%.

Poser et al[5] used slightly different categories. In their very large series, signs of upper motor neurone involvement were present in 80%, weakness in 78%, sensory change in 73%, optic nerve signs in 48%, ocular signs in 14%, brainstem and cerebellar involvement in 77%, cerebral (mainly mental) abnormalities in 36% and autonomic disturbance, presumably mainly of the sphincters, in 56%. In their smaller series, less hospital orientated, all percentages for these categories were somewhat lower, with the exception of optic nerve involvement, which was higher at 53%. While these two series were most carefully documented it is not easy to determine the nature of the surveys. The figures for observation at 11 years from onset are identical with those given for the whole course of the disease and it becomes apparent that the results published are those for a cross section at a *mean* duration of 11 years. The difficulty with the diagnostic criteria has already been mentioned.

The clinical features of the series of British and Japanese patients described by Shibasaki et al[2] are much more minutely subdivided but in both national groups the same preponderance of weakness (80% and 80% respectively) with increased tendon reflexes (87% and 92%), extensor plantars (84% and 67%), absent abdominal reflexes (77% and 62%) is evident. Other prominent features common to both groups were paraesthesiae (84% and 77%), sphincter disturbance (74% and 58%), ataxia (84% and 58%), optic atrophy (71% and 70%) and diplopia (39% and 35%). Notable differences were as follows:

	Percentage of patients affected	
	British	Japanese
Tonic seizures	4	28
Girdle sensation	9	27
Transverse cord lesion	5	28
Dysphagia	3	23
Lhermitte's sign	15	42

indicating more severe involvement of the spinal cord and a greater tendency to at least one form of paroxysmal symptom. This latter difference has often been reported from Japan[21,22] and is also apparent in patients in Taiwan, where 28% were reported as having tonic seizures.[23] The comparison of symptoms in the course of the disease in Asian and Hungarian patients[19] is invalidated by the much greater age and duration of disease in the latter.

INDIVIDUAL SYMPTOMS AND SIGNS

Certain symptoms and signs — weakness, spasticity, ataxia, sensory loss, loss of bladder control — are present in virtually every advanced case of multiple sclerosis. At the other extreme are symptoms so unusual that it is difficult to accept them as due to multiple sclerosis without the histological proof so often lacking. In other circumstances it may be impossible to distinguish symptoms due to multiple sclerosis from those resulting from separate conditions occurring in random or in significant association: narcolepsy, spasmodic torticollis or the restless legs syndrome, for example. It is often only by the relative frequency of reported observations that symptoms can be attributed to multiple sclerosis and this may be done without even a single example verified at autopsy. Once this attribution is accepted, sufficiently characteristic symptoms, such as facial myokymia or unilateral painful tonic spasms, may strongly suggest the diagnosis of multiple sclerosis even when occurring in isolation. When reading accounts of unusual symptoms it must be remembered that even a diagnosis of clinically definite multiple sclerosis may be wrong.

Weakness

Weakness of the limbs is a constant feature of advanced multiple sclerosis. It is, of course, possible to establish a diagnosis of clinically definite multiple sclerosis at a stage when no weakness is present, thus accounting for the figures of rather more than one third of cases in whom no weakness was present at the time of reporting.[24, 25] There is little to be gained by attempting to apportion with any precision the number of limbs affected[25] as this is also obviously greatly influenced by the duration and severity of the disease at the time of examination. The commonest distribution is certainly weakness of both lower limbs, usually asymmetrical, followed in decreasing order of frequency by weakness of one lower limb, and one lower limb and one upper limb, nearly always on the same side. Weakness of one arm without weakness of the legs is uncommon and isolated weakness of both arms is distinctly rare.

The mode of onset varies greatly. Often the initial complaint is of fatigue or of weakness only on exertion, gradually increasing until evident weakness is constantly present. Two well documented examples are described by Ferrari et al.[26] In these patients, who had experienced what the authors call 'intermittent pyramidal claudication' for a number of years, there were no abnormal signs on examination at rest, except absence of the abdominal reflexes. On exercise, weakness, spasticity and extensor plantar reflexes rapidly appeared, reversible with rest. At the other extreme is the 'apoplectic' onset of hemiparesis or an acute or subacute myelitis.

One of the most taxing diagnostic problems is presentation with slowly progressive hemiparesis. This begins with weakness of the lower limb, obviously of upper motor neurone type, but conceivably attributable to a lesion at any level from the lower spinal cord to the opposite motor cortex. With the passage of time the upper limb on the same side is involved but in progressive hemiplegia in multiple sclerosis the face is seldom or perhaps never affected and it is highly probable that the responsible lesion is in the lateral column of the cervical spinal cord. Many years may elapse before more widespread signs develop.

Kurtzke[25] has drawn particular attention to acute respiratory weakness as a cause of death in relapse of multiple sclerosis and believes that this should be considered in any sudden deterioration in clinical state, particularly if the arms are weak. The warning signs are rapid shallow breathing and obvious restriction of respiratory movement. Cooper et al[27] described severe weakness of the diaphragm, recovering after assisted ventilation. Acute ventilatory failure in multiple sclerosis appears to be more common in the acute severe form of the disease encountered in Japan. A midline medullary lesion was a constant finding in 4 such cases,[28] but the spinal cord was also involved. In the patient described by Rivzi et al[29] there appeared to be a defect of automatic respiration: as she fell asleep breathing would stop. The diagnosis of multiple sclerosis, however, appeared doubtful.

Chronic respiratory weakness is common in established disease and its effects may be aggravated by the greatly increased energy cost of walking with spastic legs.[30] Smeltzer et al,[31] however, found normal pulmonary function in ambulant patients but marked respiratory weakness in bedridden or chairbound patients with upper limb involvement.

Pyramidal signs

In an early case of multiple sclerosis presenting with tiredness or slight dragging of one leg after walking some distance, it may be difficult or impossible to detect any weakness of the limb on ordinary clinical examination. Nevertheless, some abnormalities of the reflexes can usually be found. Kinnier Wilson,[19] writing on multiple sclerosis, stated 'loss of the abdominals is without question proof that pyramidal function is no longer intact: it distinguishes a high proportion of all cases . . at an opening phase'.

The importance of the abdominal reflexes was first noted by von Strümpell[33] who found them absent in 67% in a small series. The majority of reports concerned with abdominal reflexes do not take into account the stage of the disease at which the observations were made. Accordingly there is little accurate information about their behaviour in the early phase of the disease or even in normal subjects. De Morsier[34] observed that in multiple sclerosis the reflexes might be lost and then return. Nevertheless, absence of the abdominal reflexes has assumed undue prominence as a useful diagnostic sign in multiple sclerosis. On reflection, however, there are only two circumstances in which examination of these reflexes could be of real value. If it could be shown that the reflexes were frequently lost in multiple sclerosis in the absence of other traditional signs of pyramidal tract disease, early diagnosis would be facilitated. It would also be helpful if retention of abdominal reflexes in the presence of other pyramidal signs did not occur in multiple sclerosis. There appears to have been no serious study of either of these possibilities and the importance attached to these reflexes in multiple sclerosis may be regarded as exaggerated.

In the form of the disease which begins with slowly progressive spastic weakness of one lower limb, an extensor plantar reflex may also often be found on the other side, despite strenuous denial of relevant symptoms.[35]

In established disease exaggerated tendon reflexes and extensor plantar reflexes are usually present. In the upper limbs the biceps and supinator jerks may be associated with finger flexion and Hoffman's sign is often present. These phenomena are not necessarily pathological but asymmetry is frequent and the phenomenon of 'inversion' may be seen whereby a tendon jerk, usually the supinator, is absent but the fingers flex.

The jaw jerk is a sign of limited value largely because of a lack of any objective method at the bedside of estimating whether it is increased or not. It is, of course, often exaggerated in multiple sclerosis, but also in other conditions and in agitated subjects. In the lower limbs tendon reflexes may become clonic, not only during conventional examination but spontaneously. Ankle clonus on putting the ball of the foot to the ground is the most usual form and is distressing to some patients but is usually intermittent. In extreme examples spontaneous patellar clonus may be continuous for prolonged periods, even when the posture is not exerting stretch on the quadriceps muscles, as when lying flat in bed.

Spasticity

The concept of spasticity has expanded far beyond the resistance to passive movement by which it is usually estimated and includes a complex disorder of voluntary movement.[36,37] This rather than weakness no doubt accounts for much of the disability resulting from an upper motor neurone

lesion in multiple sclerosis, particularly affecting the lower rather than the upper limbs. Nevertheless the increase in tone is an important factor. A weak leg held rigidly extended at the knee is a more useful prop in standing or walking than if tone or stretch reflex activity was reduced or abolished. In contrast, a further aspect of increased extensor tone whereby the foot is held plantar flexed, impedes walking. Persistent reduction of tone to the precise degree that facilitates movement has proved impossible to achieve (Ch. 9), but can sometimes be attained briefly, showing that this therapeutic aim is at least worth pursuing.

In multiple sclerosis, particularly in the progressive stage, increased extensor tone may be exaggerated as extensor spasms. These are particularly prone to occur in bed at night or when trying to rise in the morning. The legs are held rigidly extended usually for several minutes. These spasms are inconvenient rather than disabling and are seldom painful. As the disease progresses flexor tone begins to take over. When walking this may result in falling without warning. With increasing disability the distressing condition of paraplegia in flexion is threatened. In contrast to extensor spasm, flexor spasms are frequently painful. They occur in bed or when sitting and may make it impossible for the patient to use a wheelchair. Adoption of the flexed posture increases in frequency and becomes permanent, reinforced by contractures in the ilio-psoas and hamstring muscles. Painful spasms may continue. Adductor spasm usually develops during the phase of increased extensor tone but persists into flexion and is an important cause of distress. Care of sphincter function is rendered particularly difficult. Flexor and adductor spasm is increased by the persistent stimulation afforded by bedsores or urinary infection, both unfortunately prone to occur in these patients.

This description naturally only applies to the helpless bedridden case of multiple sclerosis and no follow-up studies have shown what proportion of patients with clinically definite multiple sclerosis enter this state. Such patients are usually either cared for at home by devoted relatives or are in units for the disabled where they are seldom examined by a neurologist.

Depression or absence of deep reflexes

Deep reflexes may be diminished or even lost in multiple sclerosis; nor is this surprising in view of the pathological evidence of occasional invasion of the posterior root entry zone, the posterior horn, and more rarely the anterior horn or anterior root, through all of which the spinal reflex pathway passes. Depression of reflexes in the upper limbs is more common than in the lower limbs. The triceps jerk is more frequently affected in this way than any other deep reflex of the upper extremity. In the lower limb the ankle jerk is lost more frequently than the knee jerk. Bonduelle et al[38] noted an absence, sometimes temporary, of one or more deep reflexes in 13% of multiple sclerosis patients in whom amyotrophy was absent. Garcin et al[39] attributed permanent loss of tendon reflexes to a lesion in the posterior horn of the spinal cord. The possible involvement of the peripheral nervous system is discussed on p. 118.

Muscle wasting — lower motor neurone lesions

In advanced multiple sclerosis the hand muscles often appear to be symmetrically wasted to a degree greater than expected even in the debilitated state of the patient. There is little evidence on whether this common finding is due to central lesions, decubitus pressure on peripheral nerves or to disuse. Davison et al[40] found such wasting in 11 of 20 cases examined post mortem. In only one case was there wasting affecting the lower limbs. They attributed their findings to loss of anterior horn cells involved in plaques and cited earlier similar observations. In 110 patients observed clinically muscle atrophy was seen in 17, again usually of hand muscles, but they also reported wasting of pectoral muscles, glutei, deltoid, sternomastoid and masseter muscles. In three cases there was wasting of the tongue, a remarkable finding not confirmed by personal observation. Fasciculation was not mentioned but was commented on by McAlpine.[10] Fisher et al[41] found atrophy of hand muscles in 9 of 150 patients. Wasting was unilateral in 6 and was judged to be severe in 2 patients. Electrophysiological investigation showed no

evidence of the denervation that would have occurred with loss of anterior horn cells. Paty & Poser[42] described, unfortunately not in detail, remarkable instances of widespread neurogenic atrophy and fasciculation, followed by partial remission and attributed to multiple sclerosis.

Garcin et al[39] also described loss of anterior horn cells, not always associated with clinically observed wasting. Barnard & Jellinek[43], in a most complex case, described unilateral wasting of the right hand muscles with loss of tendon reflexes in that arm associated with focal loss of myelinated fibres and of anterior horn cells at the 7th cervical segment. Whether focal weakness of lower motor neurone type can occur as an acute relapse with subsequent remission is uncertain. Noseworthy & Heffernan[44] described a patient who presented with acute weakness of the muscles controlling the right ankle. Denervation was demonstrated and the myelogram was normal. Subsequent developments were certainly suggestive of multiple sclerosis, including Lhermitte's sign, sensory symptoms in one arm and an extensor left plantar reflex. The weakness of the right leg recovered.

Lower motor neurone involvement in central lesions of the spinal cord is therefore well attested in multiple sclerosis but the wasted hand muscles not uncommonly observed are probably not due to this cause. Pronounced focal signs of radicular distribution should only be accepted as due to multiple sclerosis on strong clinical evidence of multiple lesions and exclusion of other causes. Motor neurone disease may occasionally develop in a patient already suffering from multiple sclerosis.[45]

Fatigue

Excessive fatigue is a common complaint of patients with multiple sclerosis. Although physical disability can undoubtedly contribute, it is not the whole cause as it can afflict those with mild disease. Fatigue is, of course, common enough even in the apparently healthy and the frequency and severity of pathological fatigue in multiple sclerosis patients is naturally difficult to estimate. Some feel constantly tired but the more frequent complaint is of fatigue following ordinary exertion, not always easy to distinguish from weakness. Freal et al[46] recorded this symptom in 78% of patients. In a controlled study Krupp et al[47] found that fatigue was present in 28 of 33 patients with multiple sclerosis but also in 17 of 32 controls. Fatigue was not related to depression or to degree of disability and in 10 patients it had been the first symptom, although retrospective assessment must present difficulties. The adverse effect of heat was the only factor that differentiated pathological fatigue from that in normal subjects. A minor degree of relief of this symptom was demonstrated in a carefully conducted trial of amantadine,[48] and was attributed to increased release of noradrenaline. In individual cases the response is not impressive.

Sensory symptoms and signs

The scattered lesions of multiple sclerosis naturally result in a great variety of sensory symptoms and signs but certain common patterns can be recognised.

Prodromal symptoms

McAlpine[10] believed that the onset of multiple sclerosis might rarely be preceded by paraesthesiae in the extremities, occurring at rest and relieved by movement. This may indeed be true, but 'pins and needles' are a banal experience in normal people or may result from many comparatively trivial conditions of the peripheral nervous system.

The sensory relapse

Purely sensory symptoms are common at the onset or in early relapse. Sanders et al[49] noted paraesthesiae as an isolated initial symptom in 28 of 127 patients. The sensations were often described as occurring in brief frequent episodes, not easy to distinguish from those regarded as prodromal by McAlpine. The most usual pattern of a clearly recognisable attack is for abnormal sensations to begin in one foot and in the course of a few days spread to involve the whole of both lower limbs, the buttocks and perineum and a variable area on the trunk. The sensations described are tingling, often said to be less pronounced than the familiar 'pins and needles', and numbness. The latter is a word used by patients in many contexts often unrelated to loss of sensation and must be interpreted with caution. In the typical sensory attack of multiple sclerosis, loss of perineal sensation is the most obtrusive as the normal sensation of micturition or defaecation may be lost, although control remains normal. Vaginal sensation is also diminished.

In a purely sensory attack of this kind there is no interference with walking or any other function. Examination by conventional methods will not reveal any loss of cutaneous sensation as light touch is felt and a pinprick is experienced as sharp. On enquiry, however, both these stimuli may be felt to be in some way different from normal. The pinprick may feel 'distant' or 'as if there was something between the pin and my skin'. The tickle sensation normally elicited by cotton wool may be absent. These apparently bizarre responses will cause no surprise to the neurologist but are naturally often misinterpreted by those no longer accustomed to examining the nervous system. A young woman with unusual symptoms, not supported by recognised physical signs, with normal strength and reflexes, is liable to be diagnosed as suffering from a psychogenic disorder.

These symptoms clearly arise from plaques in the sensory pathways of the spinal cord. McAlpine[10] believed that the posterior columns were usually involved, less commonly the spinothalamic tracts, but opportunities for verification are obviously rare. In a relapse of the kind described above, somatosensory evoked potentials (SEP) that are believed to use the posterior columns are normal (personal observation). The pathogenesis of the positive symptoms, the paraesthesiae, is considered in Chapter 8.

The usual course of a sensory episode of multiple sclerosis is towards complete remission within six to eight weeks, although in patients in whom the pattern of the disease is that of frequent attacks for many years without disability, these sensory episodes may clear within ten days. Indeed, intelligent and observant patients with established multiple sclerosis may recognise sensory symptoms of a similar nature, although more sharply localised, lasting for no more than one or two days, apparently unrelated to exercise, infection or environmental temperature. Naturally the symptoms and their spread and distribution are not stereotyped. The onset may be symmetrical; further areas, particularly in the upper limbs, may be involved as the early symptoms are resolving. Paraesthesiae may spread to the face. Motor signs may develop. Despite all these variants the typical episode can often be recognised immediately from the patient's description.

Another entirely distinct form of sensory relapse involves loss of position sense in one or both hands. This develops rapidly, the complaint being that of loss of use, the useless hand. Cutaneous sensation is intact and there is no weakness or reflex change but position sense is lost, often not only in the fingers but in the large joints of the limb. It is not unknown for this too to be dismissed as 'hysterical'. Clinical localisation to a lesion in the posterior columns of the spinal cord is confirmed by absent spinal somatosensory evoked potentials and by magnetic resonance imaging.[50] Remission, not always complete, is usual.

Established disease

Both types of sensory attack described above more commonly but not exclusively occur early in the disease. Persistent paraesthesiae are extremely common, occurring in 84% of patients in one series.[49] The distribution may be diffuse or closely localised, a common site being the ulnar two digits of one or both hands. This segmental distribution may cause diagnostic confusion.

Other sensory symptoms are also common. A constricting feeling around some part of a lower limb is interpreted as being due to a plaque in the posterior column of the spinal cord although seldom accompanied by loss of position sense. The complaint is of 'a string round my toe'; 'like a bandage'; 'as if my leg was in plaster'. The hand in particular may feel swollen or 'twice its normal size'. A symptom that I have encountered rarely in multiple sclerosis and in no other condition is a sensation of vibration throughout the body present on resting after mild exertion. Strange sensations referred to the skin include heat or even burning or, in contrast, the limb feels cold or wet.

Loss of thermal sensation in particular may be observed by the patient as in the bath or as in my patient whose first symptom was that the lavatory seat only felt cold on one side.

Persistent dense loss of cutaneous sensation is a rare finding in multiple sclerosis except in the severely disabled patient or where, exceptionally, there has been a transverse spinal cord lesion. A persistent bilateral sensory level should therefore prompt an anxious review of the diagnosis to ensure that no cause of spinal cord compression has been overlooked. In the patient with moderate disability but still ambulant and not in relapse, cutaneous sensory changes are usually limited to blunting of all forms of sensation and impaired two-point discrimination asymmetrically in the extremities, particularly the fingers. This pattern is relatively common and it is not easy to explain how sensory changes, not of segmental distribution but with a transverse upper border, could result from central lesions. Vibration sense is nearly always absent at the ankles in the presence of any degree of spastic weakness of the legs. Halonen et al[51] noted an increased perception threshold for vibration in at least one limb in 38% of patients rather vaguely described as having 'mild' multiple sclerosis. This loss of vibration sense is often remarkably localised so that, for example, the fifth finger is affected but no change can be detected in the other digits. In the patient presenting with progressive spastic weakness of the lower limbs, vibration sense is often impaired but this is of little diagnostic help.

Sensory symptoms can naturally also arise from lesions of the brain stem, facial paraesthesiae being particularly common. More complex abnormalities, including sensory neglect,[52] can result from cerebral lesions.

A woman of 51 developed right sided optic neuritis with partial recovery. In the course of the next two years she sustained a rapid series of severe relapses of multiple sclerosis, including bilateral optic neuritis, paraplegia and cerebellar ataxia, with some remission on ACTH. She then had a further relapse with left hemiparesis, hemianopia and tactile inattention. CT scan showed massive demyelination in the right parietal white matter. The signs of cerebral disease resolved but, following further relapses she died 2½ years from the onset following a generalised fit. The diagnosis was confirmed at autopsy.

Restless legs

Patients with multiple sclerosis, being predominantly women and often relatively immobile, are prone to the restless legs syndrome. A complaint of unpleasant paraesthesiae at rest should suggest this diagnosis. Correction of any iron deficiency present will often effect a cure. Clonazepam, 0.5 mg at bedtime and again during the day if necessary is often remarkably successful treatment.

Pain

Pain is frequently listed among the initial symptoms of multiple sclerosis or as occurring in the course of the disease, but the nature of the pain is seldom particularised. Thus Carter et al[3] in their study of cases coming to autopsy reported pain in 11%. Shibasaki et al[2] reported pain in 37% of British and 35% of Japanese cases of multiple sclerosis, while Poser[53] simply included pain under sensory disturbance. Nevertheless persistent pain in multiple sclerosis is one of the most difficult problems encountered in pain relief clinics.

Clifford & Trotter[54], from a review of the notes of 317 patients, found that pain persisting for more than 2 weeks had been recorded in some 29% of cases. Pain had been the initial symptom in 7 of 69 patients seen within 3 years of the onset. Many of the forms of pain they distinguish are well recognised: pain in optic neuritis, in trigeminal neuralgia and painful reflex spasms, for example. Low back pain, sometimes with sciatica, is frequent and can be related to abnormal posture, spasm of the spinal musculature or osteoporosis linked to immobility. Fractures of the femur from this cause are, however, usually painless.[55] Clifford & Trotter's[54] figure of 12 of 317 patients with backache is probably lower than that in the 'normal' population. They did not recognise any instance of paroxysmal pain, except that of trigeminal neuralgia. Root pain is rare in multiple sclerosis and, particularly when accompanied by appropriate focal signs, should prompt a search for other causes.

In a similar retrospective review[56] of 159 patients, 55%, were recorded as experiencing pain due to the disease at some time. Fifteen had acute pain; 7 trigeminal neuralgia, 2 painful tonic seizures and 2 paroxysmal burning extremity pain. Four patients reported Lhermitte's sign as painful. Chronic pain was much more frequent. In addition to the expected frequency of back pain and painful reflex spasms in the legs, dysaesthetic limb pain, worse at night and aggravated by heat, was also common. In personal experience, this is the most characteristic and intractable form of pain apparently due to multiple sclerosis. Sometimes as the presenting symptom, the pain begins in both feet and extends gradually up the legs. The pain is persistent and aggravated by walking. It is accompanied by loss of vibration sense and, somewhat later, by signs of mild paraparesis. The diagnosis of multiple sclerosis in such cases is, of course, at first far from obvious, and only revealed by the passage of time. Similar pain may affect both lower and upper limbs in established disease. The response to antidepressant drugs is frequently disappointing.

Even more distressing but fortunately rare is diffuse pain involving the entire trunk and lower limbs and described as 'electric', but constant and not elicited by neck flexion or any other movement. Such pain, that it would be difficult not to accept as 'genuine', may persist for over a decade despite the most energetic treatment. These forms of persistent pain have not been well studied and indeed may be said to have been neglected.[57] Well-read patients complain that pain receives little attention in popular or learned accounts of multiple sclerosis.

Lhermitte's sign

This sensation is undoubtedly a symptom but was described as Lhermitte's sign, apparently for the first time by Read[58] and the title has been universally accepted. According to Kanchandani & Howe[59] it was first described by Marie & Chatelin[60] in 1917 in a patient with a head wound and was related to neck injury by Babinski & Dubois.[61] It was not until 1924 that Lhermitte et al[62] reported the symptom during the first attack of multiple sclerosis.

The common form of Lhermitte's sign consists of an electric feeling passing down the back to the legs on flexing the neck. Although most patients compare the sensation to an electric shock, other descriptions may be given, especially tingling, pins and needles and occasionally pain. All are agreed that it is unpleasant. The spread of the sensation is usually downwards, terminating either at the lower end of the spine or passing down both legs, but there are variations. All four limbs may be affected or, rarely, the arms alone. Even more unusual is unilateral involvement either of the leg or of both limbs on one side. I have encountered one patient who insisted that the sensation passed down the front of the trunk and some patients state that the shock may be felt as passing up the spine. The sensation is always brief, estimated as lasting about two seconds.[59]

Neck flexion, sometimes only of slight degree, is by far the most common precipitating cause, although other brusque movements may have the same effect, in particular coughing, laughing or expansive movements of the limbs. It can usually be fatigued and does not recur after from one to six repetitions of the movement.

Lhermitte's sign is common in multiple sclerosis. Müller[24] reported it in only 1% of patients either at the onset or in the course of the disease, but this is far below common clinical experience and later reports. Kanchandani & Howe[59] found that 38% of patients with clinically definite multiple sclerosis had experienced this symptom at some stage and 33% of patients in all diagnostic categories. It had been present in the first attack in more than half, and in two patients had been the initial symptom. Shibasaki et al[2] found a remarkable racial difference, Lhermitte's sign having occurred in 15% of British and in 42% of Japanese cases at the time of reporting.

Multiple sclerosis is undoubtedly the commonest cause of Lhermitte's sign but it can occur in other conditions. Radiation myelopathy[63] should not cause diagnostic confusion and subacute combined degeneration of the spinal cord,[64] where the sign is present in perhaps a quarter of the patients, is usually in an older age group. As originally observed, it may be a sequel to trauma to the head and neck. It is sometimes claimed that Lhermitte's sign occurs in cervical spondylotic myelopathy but this must be a great rarity and its occurrence in this context should suggest the coexistence of multiple sclerosis.

The pathogenesis of Lhermitte's sign is briefly discussed on page 237 and more thoroughly reviewed by Kanchandani & Howe,[59] who conclude that a combination of a lesion of the cervical spinal cord and a mechanical factor is required to produce the electric sensation. Whether demyelination is an essential feature of the responsible lesion is not certain. Demyelination with preservation of axons occurs in radiation myelopathy and myelin is lost in subacute combined degeneration, but it is not known whether myelin damage with axonal preservation is found in the early stages. Clinical opinion that the responsible lesion is in the posterior columns of the spinal cord has been confirmed by MRI[50] but Lhermitte's sign may occur without sensory loss and with normal SEP (personal observation).

The mechanical factor appears to be stretch of the spinal cord. Cord compression can scarcely be responsible as, if this could occur at all in young adults, it would be on extension of the neck, causing folding of the ligamentum flavum.

Few patients find Lhermitte's sign sufficiently unpleasant to warrant treatment. Ekbom[65] found that it could be abolished by carbamazepine, an interesting finding, as Shibasaki & Kuroiwa[66] found that 64% of patients with painful tonic spasms, responsive to this drug, also had Lhermitte's sign. It has proved difficult to substantiate Ekbom's results as the condition often persists for no more than two months, or less, and is in any case not sufficiently unpleasant as to incline the patients to take tablets regularly. In a few patients Lhermitte's sign recurs for a few weeks at a time over many years, in personal experience not associated with other evidence of disease activity.

In a young adult with no history of trauma to the neck, Lhermitte's sign, even in the absence of any other symptoms or signs, is a strong indication of multiple sclerosis.

Cerebellar symptoms and signs

Symptoms of cerebellar dysfunction are undoubtedly common in multiple sclerosis but in many series the difficulty in distinguishing the signs of such disease from those of weakness, spasticity, sensory loss and vertigo, is acknowledged. These difficulties are reflected in clinical practice. A patient may have a 'spastic-ataxic' gait, walking unsteadily with stiff legs and feet placed too far apart, but to what extent cerebellar ataxia contributes is necessarily uncertain. Conventional tests of co-ordination such as the heel-knee-shin test are poorly performed by weak or spastic legs. The different components of cerebellar inco-ordination are more easily demonstrated in the upper limbs. Kurtzke[25] thought that the frequency of cerebellar deficit was second only to that of cortico-spinal involvement, being present in 84% of personally examined male cases attending one hospital. Thygesen[67] found ataxia in 37% of closely observed attacks.

Cerebellar signs at the onset of the disease are distinctly uncommon although at the time of first examination, a different matter, McAlpine[10] found such signs in 37% of his patients. Nystagmus may certainly be seen in an initial attack but is usually associated with internuclear ophthalmoplegia and therefore not a direct result of cerebellar involvement. A patient presenting with a pure cerebellar syndrome is unlikely to have multiple sclerosis. The early appearance of cerebellar ataxia is an indication of a bad prognosis and cerebellar signs are frequently persistent, without important remission.

In the lower limbs cerebellar ataxia naturally affects the gait, but spasticity and weakness are usually more important causes of disability. Truncal ataxia is seldom sufficiently severe as to be obvious when sitting but certainly contributes to the frequent complaint of poor balance. Cerebellar inco-ordination in the upper limbs may be extremely disabling, particularly when combined with any significant degree of intention tremor. This famous sign, a member of Charcot's original triad, may be of diagnostic importance when slight, the wavering of the finger as it approaches the target being highly characteristic. Severe degrees of intention tremor may render the hands useless and voluntary movement may be so disturbed by violent deviations of the arms that the patient is virtually unapproachable.

Dysarthria is uncommon at the onset of the disease, speech being affected in 3–5% in the series of Shibasaki et al.[2] Later in the disease dysarthria is common, but is not always of cerebellar type. The classical scanning speech is a comparative rarity and usually only heard in advanced disease. Lesser degrees of slurring dysarthria are common but less distinctive. In contrast, Miller[68] attributed cessation of lifelong stuttering in two multiple sclerosis patients to progressive involvement of the cerebellum. Nystagmus, as already indicated, need not necessarily be the result of cerebellar disease. A common form of nystagmus in multiple sclerosis, probably the result of damage to the cerebellum or its immediate connections, is symmetrical horizontal gaze nystagmus. This appears well within the field of binocular vision and the jerking movement is towards the periphery.

MENTAL CHANGES

A common question from patients trying to come to terms with the idea of a disease of the nervous system is: 'Will it affect my mind?' Whatever it may seem right to reply, the true answer is complex. It was already evident to Charcot[69] that the memory was often severely impaired and affect and intellect blunted. In the absence of standardised tests the presence and degree of dementia in multiple sclerosis remained controversial, although attempts were made to identify a specific 'dementia polysclerotica'.[70] However, the Association for Research into Nervous and Mental Disease decided in 1921[71] that there was no particular psychic disorder characteristic of multiple sclerosis, a declaration sometimes misinterpreted as meaning that mental changes are not characteristic of the disease.[72] In 1926, Cottrell & Wilson[73] wrote a highly influential paper, the effects of which can still be detected. They examined 100 unselected patients and by simple questioning found that 63 were euphoric, with a positive sense of mental wellbeing. No less than 84 had an unjustified feeling of physical health — eutonia. Lability of emotional expression was almost universal. Ten of the patients were, however, severely depressed. These changes were attributed to periventricular lesions and were thought to be quite independent of intellectual impairment that was judged to be present in only 2 patients. The association of euphoria with multiple sclerosis has proved ineradicably memorable among those who see and know little of the disease, and has been regarded even by experts as a valuable early diagnostic sign. In most instances, however, any inappropriate sense of wellbeing is a manifestation of admirable stoicism in the face of adversity.

In contrast to the virtual absence of dementia detected in the patients in this famous paper, Ombredane[74], a few years later, found intellectual deterioration in 36 of 50 patients with multiple sclerosis and commented that the changes were often not apparent in ordinary converse or on routine examination. The first controlled investigation of the psychiatric aspects of multiple sclerosis was that of Pratt[75] in 1951. It is now accepted that intellectual impairment is common in multiple sclerosis and the phenomenon has been intensively investigated with ever increasing sophistication of methods of testing and analysis of results.

Dementia

Surridge[72] using formal testing, found that 40.7% of 108 patients had mild intellectual loss; 13.9% were moderately and 6.5% severely impaired. All but 2 euphoric patients were demented and there was a strong correlation between the degree of euphoria and that of dementia. The patients examined were relatively severely disabled. This is of some importance, as Matthews et al[76] found that intellectual function in multiple sclerosis patients with mild disability was no different from control, a conclusion challenged by later reports. Marsh[77] found that physical disability on the Kurtzke scale was not correlated with the Wechsler IQ, while Poser[53] found that all forms of mental disorder in multiple sclerosis were correlated with severe disability and long duration of disease. In a more thorough investigation, Peyser et al[78] found evidence of intellectual deterioration in 29 of 53 patients. They emphasised that failure in the tests was not due to depression or fatigue and confirmed that dementia was often difficult to detect on routine neurological examination. Beatty & Grange[79] found that their patients had particular difficulty in the storing of new material, without impairment of verbal IQ.

These early findings have been greatly elaborated with not wholly consistent results. Rao et al[80] in a controlled study of 44 multiple sclerosis patients found that 9 had moderate to severe impairment of memory, particularly retrieval of linguistic and spatial material. Nineteen patients had mild defects and 16 were normal. Mental changes were *not* correlated with duration of disease or severity of disability, but there was a possible relationship to impaired upper limb function. Truelle et al[81] found that 55% of patients with multiple sclerosis for less than 5 years and 54% of those graded 0–2 on the Kurtzke scale had marked memory impairment.

Ivnik[82] could find no differences from control that could with confidence be attributed to duration of symptoms of the disease. Grant et al,[83] however, concluded that intellectual defect, notably memory failure, was related to what they defined as years of 'active disease'; that is to say years in which symptoms had been present for a week or longer. This measure certainly appears to be open to a number of sources of error and indeed the authors had to revert to time-since-onset to make comparisons with other series. Results are expressed as mean score values in the individual tests which are compared to controls, but the numbers of patients found to be abnormal are not stated. They agree that learning and short-term memory may be impaired early in the disease and that these functions are likely to be more disturbed during relapse.

Early cognitive impairment in patients with mild physical disability was confirmed by Van den Burg et al.[84] In their study of 40 patients with Kurtzke DSS 1–4, including relapsing/remitting and progressive disease, they found 7 patients definitely impaired, 5 of whom were in the progressive stage. They made the point, however, that much depends on the standards of normality in the tests used. If 'dubious' abnormalities were included, 15 patients would be regarded as impaired. The suggestion that patients in the progressive stage are more prone to dementia was also made by Heaton et al,[85] although their progressive patients were older and more disabled than those with remitting disease. Lyon-Caen et al[86] examined intellect and memory function within 2 years of the onset in 21 patients with multiple sclerosis and 9 with isolated optic neuritis. Some evidence of cognitive impairment was found in 18 subjects, including 6 with optic neuritis. The changes were generally slight and unrelated to degree of disability.

In contrast to these generally depressing findings, a group of socially integrated out-patients with stable multiple sclerosis were found to function no differently from controls in tests of visuospatial problem solving, conceptual reasoning and sorting behaviour.[87] Comparison with other groups presents difficulties because of different criteria of selection but the result dispels the gathering opinion that early loss of cognitive function is inevitable.

There is general agreement as to the nature of the cognitive defect. Speech functions are scarcely disturbed, even in severely disabled patients,[88] with the result that quite severe dementia may pass unnoticed in casual contact. Heaton et al[85] found that clinical assessment of mental state, as opposed to formal testing, was wrong in 41% of their patients. Litvan et al[89] found that impaired long-term verbal memory was associated with slowing of information processing, as judged by a timed calculation test. This appeared not to be closely related to the level of general intelligence. The difficulties are in learning and in recall, admirably summed up by Van den Burg et al[84] as: 'Slowness in acquiring new information from the outside world and in responding to its demands'. Charcot himself could scarcely have expressed it better.

Recent contributions[89,90] appear to be primarily directed to exploring the neural basis of memory and intellect, particularly the concept of subcortical and cortical dementia. Defects attributed to both these states occur in multiple sclerosis.[91,92] As a possible practical result of their investigation into 'working memory', Litvan et al[89] suggest that memory might be improved in patients with multiple sclerosis by 'forced encoding' but do not describe the proposed method or any results.

While it may certainly be necessary and advantageous to the patient to indicate to relatives the probability or presence of these failings there is no indication for routine formal examination of cognitive function. Patients so tested are apt to want to know the results and will not be encouraged by any suggestion that they are losing their reason or by the evident deterioration in test results in serial studies.[93]

Severe dementia may occasionally be an early or even the presenting symptom. Young et al[94] described five cases, in four of whom behavioural or intellectual changes had been the initial symptom. In two of these, mental symptoms had been present for several years before overt evidence of multiple sclerosis appeared. In both, the initial psychiatric diagnosis had been that of depression, but intellect was found to be gravely impaired as soon as it was tested. In these five cases the predominant physical signs indicated disease involving the brainstem, but apart from noting the association, no conclusions could be drawn. Franklin et al[95] also emphasise that cognitive impairment, out of proportion to physical disability may be overlooked for long periods. Dementia was often associated with gait disturbance similar to that seen in normal pressure hydrocephalus.

The lesion responsible for the cognitive defects has proved elusive. Where anatomical verification has been possible, in both chronic and relatively acute cases, dementia has been related to widespread cerebral lesions.[96,97] Barnard & Triggs[98] were impressed by the relatively severe atrophy of the corpus callosum in such cases. Rao et al,[99] using CT scanning, found that ventricular dilatation was not strongly correlated with cognitive defect; seven patients with dilated ventricles performed normally in a battery of tests, while five with normal ventricles performed badly. The only radiological correlation with impairment was with the width of the IIIrd ventricle, probably incriminating periventricular lesions. However, using MRI, defects in recent memory, reasoning and language function were strongly related to total lesion area, but again enlargement of the lateral ventricles was not found to be relevant.[100] Using MRI, Huber et al[101] could find no correlation of mental impairment with the number of visible lesions, the degree of cerebral atrophy or the position of the lesions. Medaer et al,[102] from the extent of lesions seen on MRI, could distinguish patients with normal cognitive function from those impaired, but could not separate those with mild changes from the severely demented. It is possible that when no correlation is found between extent of lesions and degree of cognitive deficit, the tests have been inappropriate. Franklin et al[103] devised a test battery, including figure copying, trail making, verbal learning and numerical attention, with results strongly correlated with lesion number and size. The suspected importance of temporal lobe damage in the causation of defective memory has been confirmed by Brainin et al[104] who found that all patients with severe memory defects had bilateral medial temporal lobe lesions, while in those with normal or slightly impaired memory, such lesions were absent or unilateral.

Affective disorder

Controlled studies of the affective state in multiple sclerosis have not unexpectedly shown that depression is more common than euphoria. Surridge[72] compared 108 multiple sclerosis patients under the age of 40 years with 39 patients with muscular dystrophy. He found mild depression in 16.5% in multiple sclerosis, moderately severe in 6.5% and severe depression in 3.7%. A further 3.7% were euphoric and in 7.4% there were marked swings of mood. Depression was no more common in multiple sclerosis than in the controls and Surridge concluded that in the majority, the depressed mood was a reaction to the knowledge of the disease and disability rather than a specific symptom.

Whitlock & Siskind[105] compared 40 patients with multiple sclerosis with much more closely matched control subjects with neuromuscular disease of comparable severity. The multiple sclerosis patients were highly significantly more depressed than the controls. This was not correlated with duration of illness, degree of disability or drug intake. The authors were particularly impressed by the relative frequency of depression in the multiple sclerosis patients before the onset of the disease. They concluded that in some patients, severe affective disorder may be a presenting or complicating feature of the disease. The implications of these two alternatives are different: the former suggesting that depression is caused by the disease process, while the latter leaves the question of causation open.

The presentation of multiple sclerosis as a depressive illness was described by Goodstein & Ferrell,[106] but their case reports do not indicate that the diagnosis was in a higher category than clinically possible. In an extensive review of published reports, they found few indications that depression might precede physical symptoms or that such depression might be the initial symptom of the disease.

Baretz & Stephenson[107] examined 40 patients with multiple sclerosis of whom 13 were overtly depressed, 19 had concealed depression and 4 had elevation of mood. They firmly attributed the presence and degree of depression to disability and circumstance, many of the patients being in hospital or chronic care. In contrast, Joffe et al[108] found that 14 of 100 consecutive patients already attending a multiple sclerosis clinic were suffering from major depression and that no less than 47 had so suffered in the past. In addition, 9 patients had had minor depression, 4 were intermittently depressed, 2 had hypomania and 13 bipolar affective disorder. This astonishing excess of depressive illness was not related to degree of disability and the findings have been challenged by Rao & Leo.[109] Apart from the lack of a control series, the most serious criticism is that the methods employed to establish the presence of depression or mania took no account of the physical symptoms of the disease. Fatigue, loss of interest, sleep disturbance and weight gain due to lack of activity, that were scored as depressive symptoms, are common in multiple sclerosis for other reasons. Certain apparently manic symptoms could well arise from cognitive impairment and emotional lability.

The question of whether depression in multiple sclerosis is reactive or a direct result of cerebral plaques may be of practical importance with regard to treatment. The problem has, however, proved difficult to resolve. Dalos et al,[110] not surprisingly, found that emotional disturbance was much more marked in acute relapse than in static disease. They were unable to determine whether this preceded, accompanied or followed relapse. In a controlled epidemiological study,[111] however, emotional problems were found to be independent of the severity or stage of progression of the disease, but patients were not specifically examined before and after relapse. Of the psychosocial disability observed, 80% was not accounted for by any of the factors explored.

Attempts at excluding the role of cerebral plaques in the causation of depression by examining 'spinal' cases of multiple sclerosis are not entirely realistic, as the presence of cerebral lesions can never be wholly excluded. Schiffer et al[112] compared the incidence of depressive episodes in 15 patients with 'cerebral' multiple sclerosis with those in 15 'spinal' cases, the groups being equally disabled. Depression was far more common in the cerebral group. McIvor et al[113] studied a large group of patients with spinal multiple sclerosis. Those with chronic depression were not included and the WAIS was used to exclude dementia. Depression was more frequent in older patients with greater disability and no remissions and, in particular, with a poor perceived level of social support. The authors drew the conclusion that depressing circumstances cause depression in multiple sclerosis.

Rabins et al[114] examined the structural brain correlates of emotional disorder in multiple sclerosis. Patients judged, on clinical grounds, to have isolated spinal cord involvement were less often depressed than those with cerebral or cerebellar symptoms. Depression was unrelated to functional disability but was correlated with the degree of neurological involvement, assessed largely by walking speed, a measure not clearly demarcated from that of disability. The association of euphoria and dementia was confirmed. The authors concluded by supporting both hypotheses of the cause of depression: unspecified brain lesions and emotional reaction to disease. Honer et al[115] compared the cerebral lesions seen by MRI in 8 patients with multiple sclerosis and psychiatric disorder, 6 being depressed, with those in control patients matched for duration and severity of disease, but without mental symptoms. Dementia was said to have been excluded. There was no difference in the total area of lesions seen in the two groups, but the temporal lobe was more often involved in the psychiatric cases. On this evidence it would be difficult to establish a strong case for the temporal lobe origin of depression in these patients. It had previously been shown[116] that depression and anxiety were much more frequent in patients with multiple sclerosis than in those with temporal lobe epilepsy.

Occasional reports of mania[117,118] or rapidly cycling bipolar affective disorder[119] do not demonstrate a convincing causal relationship with the accompanying multiple sclerosis. Schiffer et al[120] concluded that bipolar disorder occurred in multiple sclerosis at approximately twice the expected rate, but the calculation was not based on observed prevalence of the disorder in the control population.

There is little evidence on the effects of treatment of depression in multiple sclerosis. Schiffer[121] in a small study, found that treatment in some variety was more likely to be effective in the presence of clinically active disease, even when this was progressive.

The evidence is inconclusive, but it is probable that depression in multiple sclerosis is not caused by the disease process but is a reaction to the prospect or actuality of chronic progressive disability and isolation.

Schizophrenia

Schizophrenia is a common disease and not surprisingly sometimes occurs in those also suffering from multiple sclerosis. In 1969 Davison & Bagley,[122] in a comprehensive review, accepted 39 reported cases of this association. They concluded that the incidence of schizophrenia was not increased in multiple sclerosis, but that the clustering of the onset of the mental disease around the time of onset of the multiple sclerosis suggested that they were not unconnected. In 61.5% of their acceptable cases, the onset of schizophrenia was between 2 years before to 2 years after the onset of multiple sclerosis. The paranoid-hallucinatory form of schizophrenia was much more common than hebephrenia. Conclusions on the frequency of the association of the two diseases based almost entirely on single case reports cannot be relied on. Consulting some of the more accessible early references[123-125] suggests that the distinction from dementia often presented unresolved difficulties.

That acute mental symptoms leading to admission to hospital with a diagnosis of schizophrenia can be the initial manifestation of multiple sclerosis is strongly suggested by the two cases described by Matthews.[126] In both, the onset was acute. In the first case, speech suddenly became repetitive and rapid, she refused all food and simply lay in bed. She then developed bizarre movements, rocking of the body, head banging and cycling with the legs. That there might be an organic cause was suggested by recurrent spontaneous fits following electroconvulsant therapy. When transferred to a neurological unit there were no abnormal signs on formal examination. She was alert and mobile but did not speak at all. The CSF repeatedly contained an excess of lymphocytes. She recovered completely within 2 months, but 3 years later developed optic neuritis followed by a succession of typical relapses of multiple sclerosis.

In the second case, the onset was with extreme apathy. Within a few days she became completely withdrawn and refused to eat. Both plantar reflexes were extensor and there was an increased lymphocyte count in the CSF. Over the course of 3 months she recovered completely, but 2 years later developed bilateral optic atrophy and delayed visual evoked potentials. Both patients were incontinent of urine which would be unusual in acute schizophrenia.

Psychiatric disorder is uncommon at the onset of multiple sclerosis. Logsdail et al[127] examined this aspect in 76 patients presenting with symptoms of a single lesion of the type commonly seen in multiple sclerosis, comparing the results with those in control subjects with chronic rheumatic or neurological disease, not affecting the brain. Some 50% of the multiple sclerosis patients had disseminated lesions on MRI scanning. Psychiatric abnormalities were rather more common in the multiple sclerosis patients, but the difference did not reach statistical significance. The authors thought that much of the disturbance found was the result of environmental factors such as perceived lack of support. They did not mention the stress of being submitted to MRI scanning, following often apparently trivial symptoms, as being possibly contributory.

Two cases of multiple sclerosis presenting as chronic psychosis, without abnormal neurological signs, have recently been reported.[128] Histological confirmation was obtained in one case and in the other the appearances on MRI and the presence of oligoclonal IgG in the CSF strongly supported the diagnosis. The psychiatric state was not typical of schizophrenia and included insomnia, aggressive behaviour and intermittent confusion. These cases are, perhaps, most remarkable for the long dur-ation of disabling disease without the appearance of the usual signs of multiple sclerosis, although details of physical examination were not given.

Langworthy[129] reported that 16 of 199 patients with multiple sclerosis that he had carefully followed had been admitted to mental hospitals. This is a high figure considering that Brown & Davis,[130] writing before the days of psychotropic drugs, found only 3 cases of multiple sclerosis in 6700 insane patients in the Manhattan State Hospital. They believed, however, that patients with multiple sclerosis would be incapable of carrying out actions that might lead to commitment. The examples Langworthy gave are mostly of paranoid ideas, belligerence, sexual inhibition and unreasonable behaviour. If focal or diffuse lesions of multiple sclerosis can indeed cause schizophrenia, this would be of great importance to the study of the latter disease, but any causal connection with chronic schizophrenia is at present tenuous. Behavioural disturbance, not satisfying diagnostic criteria for schizophrenia, certainly occurs in multiple sclerosis, and may reasonably be attributed to the disease.

Hysteria

It is a source of some astonishment that patients already labouring under some disability from undoubted multiple sclerosis not infrequently develop additional burdens from hysterical symptoms. This strange phenomenon has long been recognised and has in the past led to controversy, largely based on differing opinions held on the pathogenesis of hysteria.[131,132] It might be thought difficult to recognise hysterical signs in the presence of so much that is organic but the experienced neurologist will have no difficulty in picking up the bizarre gait, the fluctuating weakness, the sensory loss that changes sides when the patient turns over, the finger unerringly placed on the point of the chin in the finger-nose test. In the undoubted presence of numerous lesions to which no symptoms can be ascribed, it is tempting, but I feel sure incorrect, to attribute such findings to unrecognised organic disease. It is best not to become excited by such findings or to pay too much attention to them. Certainly no attempt at treatment should be made. The symptoms have developed no doubt in response to some need which may be detected in the course of enquiry but which can seldom be fulfilled. Caplan & Nadelson[133] present two very instructive case histories of patients with undoubted mild multiple sclerosis who became incapacitated by non-organic symptoms. They mention a common feature of such cases, very active involvement in the affairs of the Multiple Sclerosis Society. There is nothing to be gained and perhaps much to be lost in disturbing this way of life.

APHASIA

Aphasia is uncommon in multiple sclerosis and, indeed, Kurtzke[25] wrote that he had never seen a well-documented example. He regarded the presence of aphasia as evidence against the diagnosis. The frequency of aphasia in representative reported series has been 1% by Poser,[53] 1% by Kahana et al[133] and one of 145 cases.[135]

The advent of CT scanning has led to the increasing recognition of multiple sclerosis presenting in a manner clinically and radiologically indistinguishable from a malignant brain tumour (p. 63) and in such cases aphasia is commonly present if the dominant hemisphere is involved. As early as 1902, Gussenbauer[136, 137] reported such a case, where the history and findings, that included aphasia, strongly indicated a left hemisphere tumour, but at post mortem only multiple sclerosis plaques were found. Remitting aphasia has been described in a number of such cases.[138–140] Aphasia may be accompanied by alexia and agraphia.[141] Apraxia for speech — aphemia — without aphasia has been described as the presenting symptom of multiple sclerosis,[142] but the clinical diagnosis has been disputed.[143]

EPILEPSY

Fits or seizures appear in virtually every list of symptoms of multiple sclerosis either at the onset or in the course of the disease. The proportion of patients affected is never large but epilepsy is perhaps a surprising effect of a disease process predominantly affecting white matter. Tables of symptoms are naturally not accompanied by clinical descriptions either of the evidence of multiple

sclerosis or the nature of the seizures. There are a number of possible sources of error.

Epilepsy is common in young adults, certainly much more common than multiple sclerosis, and coincidental association must occur. Two such cases were described by Matthews.[144] In one patient, epilepsy had begun at the age of 12 and symptoms of multiple sclerosis at 41, while in the other patient epilepsy at 14 had been followed by multiple sclerosis at the age of 20. The possibility that the chronic recurrent major fits had been the initial symptom of multiple sclerosis must be discarded, as in both patients the EEG contained symmetrical 3 per second spike and wave discharges.

In another patient in this series in whom psychomotor fits developed in the course of clinically definite multiple sclerosis a temporal lobe astrocytoma found at autopsy was thought to be the cause, although numerous multiple sclerosis plaques were also present.

In the past there has certainly been confusion with unilateral tonic seizures[145] now thought unlikely to be epileptic as this word is normally understood. In earlier reports these paroxysmal symptoms have sometimes been regarded as Jacksonian motor fits.

Nevertheless there remains a small proportion of patients in whom the diagnosis both of epilepsy and of multiple sclerosis can be established and a causal connection accepted.

Early reports were reviewed by Matthews.[144] Writing in 1962, 65 case reports were found in which both the grounds for the diagnosis of multiple sclerosis and some description of the fits were given. It was evident that the sources of error described above had not been entirely avoided. The paucity of post mortem confirmation so often found in clinical studies of multiple sclerosis was particularly pronounced, only seven reports being found. In one, the diagnosis did not appear to be multiple sclerosis and one patient could not be said with certainty to have had epilepsy. Two patients certainly had both conditions but the relation between the two was obscure: for example, one patient had sustained a serious closed head injury some years before the onset of the fits. In the remaining three cases a causal connection could be accepted but both the clinical features and pathological findings were unusual, severe dementia and extremely extensive demyelination of the hemispheres being prominent. It is not easy to reconcile these findings with the estimate of Drake & Macrae,[146] reviewing the same series, that fits occurred in 4.1% of cases of multiple sclerosis.

In tabulated lists of symptoms the incidence of fits has ranged from the 1% found by Müller,[24] 1.8% of Abb & Schaltenbrand,[20] to 2 and 5% in British and Japanese cases respectively.[2] In an elaborate study of 2400 case notes, Elian and Dean[147] found 27 patients with multiple sclerosis and epilepsy, 1.1% that they regarded as higher than the expected figure of 0.5%. In other reports devoted specifically to the relation of multiple sclerosis and epilepsy higher figures are generally found: 2.4%,[148] 3%,[149] 3.5%,[150] 4.5%,[151] 6%,[146] and even 8% of 125 cases,[152] although this last figure is attributed to the series being derived from a special hospital. Against such results must be placed that of Ritter & Poser[153] of only five cases of epilepsy in 812 patients, a proportion of 0.6%, little different from the conventionally accepted figure of 0.5% for the general population.

Where epilepsy can reasonably be attributed to multiple sclerosis virtually any type of fit can occur, although naturally classical petit mal should be excluded.[148] Tonic-clonic major fits, with or without a focal onset, are the most common, but fits of presumed temporal lobe origin or focal motor fits are also reported.[149] Wilson & MacBride[154] described epilepsia partialis continuans and Boudouresques et al[155] reported an extraordinary case of focal status epilepticus involving clonic lateral movement of the eyes. The diagnosis was confirmed at autopsy. Generalised status epilepticus may also occur.[149]

The immediate cause of fits in multiple sclerosis is naturally not easy to determine. In the comparatively rare neuropathological studies the significant findings have appeared to be either plaques immediately beneath the cerebral cortex[146,148] or massive demyelination of cerebral white matter. It has been assumed that the oedema and inflammation of an acute plaque or the gliosis of a chronic lesion may in some way initiate the excessive neuronal discharge leading to an epileptic fit but the details are of course obscure.[155]

The circumstances under which fits occur in multiple sclerosis are of some importance. In most reported series epilepsy had preceded the onset of other symptoms of multiple sclerosis in a small number of patients. This occurred in 1 of 17 of the patients described by Cendrowski & Majkowski.[149] In 2 of Drake & Macrae's[146] 13 cases, focal epilepsy preceded other symptoms and Trouillas & Courjon[152] state that in 4 of their 10 cases, epilepsy was the sole initial manifestation. With generalised fits the possibility of chance association in such cases must be considerable. In 10 of the 21 cases of epilepsy and multiple sclerosis reported by Kinnunen & Wikström[150], the epilepsy preceded the onset of multiple sclerosis. In 3 of these, epilepsy dated from established causes of epilepsy in childhood. In 2 further patients presenting with epilepsy the CSF had been examined and increased production of IgG noted several years before the onset of multiple sclerosis. In 3 patients epilepsy and multiple sclerosis developed at about the same time and in 8 the onset of epilepsy was later. Two thirds of the patients had partial seizures.

A number of authors[146, 149, 152] have found that their cases fall into two groups. In one fits are chronic but infrequent, unrelated to any detectable activity of the disease and easily controlled by anticonvulsants. In these patients the epilepsy is never a serious problem and may not even need treatment. In nearly half of Kinnunen & Wikstrom's patients the epilepsy had resolved.[150] In the other group the fits are associated with rapidly increasing disability, particularly mental disorder, and are difficult or impossible to control. Status epilepticus is a constant threat and often fatal. Another category can be identified in whom one or several fits occur during an acute relapse, not being followed by recurrent epilepsy.[145, 148] Status epilepticus maybe a terminal event in severely disabled patients.[156]

There are certain practical implications. Should multiple sclerosis be considered in the differential diagnosis of the cause of epilepsy in the young adult without other evidence of neurological disease? From the reports cited above it seems that this must be so, particularly with focal motor fits. In a comparatively early investigation of 1000 cases of epilepsy beginning at or after the age of 20, multiple sclerosis was thought to be present in

2.4%.[157] In personal experience this has been an extremely rare event.

In acute relapse, particularly with prominent focal cerebral symptoms, epilepsy is an acceptable symptom and should not be taken as evidence in favour of tumour or abscess. Chronic epilepsy in multiple sclerosis is usually easily controlled and failure of treatment should lead to consideration of the correctness of the diagnosis. Intractable epilepsy in multiple sclerosis carries an extremely poor prognosis for survival.

MULTIPLE SCLEROSIS MIMICKING BRAIN TUMOUR

The clinical features of multiple sclerosis may closely mimick those of a brain tumour. Even when such symptoms develop in the course of long established disease, a tumour may be mistakenly diagnosed,[158] the distinction being far more difficult at the onset of the disease. The presentation is that of a rapidly progressive focal cerebral lesion, usually with hemiplegia, focal or generalised fits and aphasia if the dominant hemisphere is involved. Headache and confusion are common. Papilloedema has not been described, but bilateral optic neuritis may add to the diagnostic difficulties.[139]

CT scan, far from providing the solution, shows solidly or ring enhancing space occupying lesions, indistinguishable from glioma or metastases.[138, 139] Bilateral frontal lesions closely resemble the appearances of a glioma of the corpus callosum.[159] Biopsy is less informative than might be supposed, the main feature of the histology being sheets of astrocytes, seldom with any evidence of inflammation.[139, 140] Unless white matter is included in the specimen and stained to show demyelination with preserved axons, the diagnosis of multiple sclerosis may not be made. Diagnosis is eventually confirmed by the partial or complete resolution of the clinical and radiological abnormalities, or, with progressive disease, at autopsy. Two of the cases described by Hunter et al[139] were children 10 and 11 years old respectively, but the subsequent relapsing course of the disease is in favour of multiple sclerosis rather than acute disseminated encephalomyelitis. One child was given radiotherapy for the presumed glioma, the biopsy later being thought to show cerebral Whipple's disease, before multiple sclerosis was eventually diagnosed.

ALTERED CONSCIOUS LEVEL

It is unusual for the level of consciousness to be disturbed in multiple sclerosis, except for the coma that is often a terminal event. Kurtzke[25] believes that this is sometimes the result of unrecognised acute respiratory failure but usually no immediate cause is evident. In a personal case, a women of 26 who died in coma after a total duration of disease of 4 months, there was massive demyelination of the brainstem, a reasonable explanation for the effect on conscious level. Castaigne et al[160, 161] described recurrent episodes of coma accompanied by fever, apparently in the absence of infection, in patients with advanced multiple sclerosis. Recurrent stupor for periods of one or two days, with an increase in signs of brainstem involvement, is occasionally seen in severely disabled patients, but the immediate cause has not been determined. Ringel et al[162] describe a single episode of coma with absent pupillary and brainstem reflexes following a respiratory arrest, with recovery to the previous state.

Persistent hypothermia causing intermittent confusion and stupor has recently been described[163] and attributed to a hypothalamic lesion.

A woman of 32 had an acute illness with headache, vertigo and ataxia, that she was told was 'viral encephalitis'. Her gait remained ataxic and bilateral extensor plantar reflexes were noted the following year. When 37, she developed sensory ataxia of the left arm and thereafter had slowly increasing difficulty in walking. She was excellently cared for at home. However, during a cold spell, she became slow and confused and when admitted a week later was stuporose. Rectal temperature was 31.8°C and pulse rate 60. Gradual warming over two days restored her temperature which remained stable. She became fully alert but it was evident that her disabilities had greatly increased during this episode and she showed little recovery.

Partial recovery from catastrophic relapse may lead to a persistent vegetative state, in the case described below following status epilepticus.

A man of 23 developed vertigo and paroxysmal itching of both upper arms. He recovered, but two years later had right-sided optic neuritis, deafness and facial numbness. Vision in both eyes progressively deteriorated and when 28 he developed increasing cerebellar ataxia, becoming helpless the following year. When 31, he was admitted in coma with frequent generalised fits. These were controlled with intravenous diazepam but he remained in a vegetative state with frequent focal motor fits until his death three years later. Permission for autopsy was not obtained.

PAROXYSMAL SYMPTOMS

An increasing variety of paroxysmal symptoms has been recognised in multiple sclerosis. These are brief episodes, almost stereotyped for the individual patients, occurring frequently and often triggered by movement or sensory stimuli. This description would, of course, include flexor spasm but the clinical context is entirely different.

Trigeminal neuralgia

The first paroxysmal symptom to be identified in multiple sclerosis was trigeminal neuralgia. This, of course, occurs far more frequently in patients who do not have multiple sclerosis or indeed any other identifiable disease. The first recognition that it occurs more frequently in multiple sclerosis and could be a symptom of the disease was by Oppenheim[164] who published the post mortem findings showing pontine plaques. Guillain[165] among others endorsed this finding and Harris[166] reported 23 patients with trigeminal neuralgia and spastic paraparesis, most of whom probably had multiple sclerosis. The first detailed description was that of Parker[167] who justly stated that in earlier reports 'symptoms were not subjected to the minute scrutiny that modern clinical experience has demanded'. He described four undoubted cases of multiple sclerosis in whom trigeminal neuralgia had developed later, in three many years after the onset of the disease. He obtained a post mortem examination in one patient, confirming the diagnosis. Estimates of the frequency of the association have shown little variation. Harris[168] found that 3% of his patients with trigeminal neuralgia had multiple sclerosis; Ruge et al[169] 2.2%; Rushton & Olafson[170] 2%; and Jensen et al[171] 2.7%, this last figure being adjudged to be 20–50 times higher than that in the general population. Approximately 1% of patients with multiple sclerosis have trigeminal neuralgia,[169,170] but this is only at the time of reporting and the true frequency is probably higher as neuralgia is prone to develop late in the disease course.

The age of onset is significantly lower than in idiopathic trigeminal neuralgia, being on average five years earlier.[170] Jensen et al[171] found that trigeminal neuralgia associated with multiple sclerosis occurred before the age of 50 in 59% of cases while in idiopathic trigeminal neuralgia the proportion was 32%. Onset of neuralgia even at an advanced age can be the result of multiple sclerosis as the highly dramatic case reported by Daum et al.[172] A woman of 64 developed neuralgia, a little atypical in extent and duration of attacks. She had no obvious clinical evidence of multiple sclerosis but while the plantar reflex was being elicited she died of a pulmonary embolus. Multiple sclerosis was found at post mortem.

In the majority of patients other evidence of multiple sclerosis precedes the onset of trigeminal neuralgia. In one series the neuralgia came first in 2 of 24 cases while in 1 patient the two developed simultaneously.[171] The time interval between neuralgia and other symptoms was up to five years. When the conditions developed in the more usual order, that is to say, with established multiple sclerosis first, the interval can be much longer, up to 30 years.[173]

Most authors believe that the character of the pain has not differed from that in the idiopathic form of neuralgia in any way except that it is much more often bilateral: in 14% of Harris's 50 cases[174], 4 of 35 in the series from the Mayo Clinic[170] and 5 of 16 cases reported by Brisman.[175] Friedlander & Zeff[176] suggested that trigeminal neuralgia in multiple sclerosis was less often triggered but this is not general experience. Jensen et al[171] reported that in about one quarter of their patients the pain was atypical with paroxysms lasting for several minutes and persistent pain between attacks.

Signs of trigeminal nerve involvement in these patients are quite exceptional. Harris[168]described some interesting cases where dense loss of sensation on one side of the face accompanied by unilateral loss of taste and followed by complete remission had preceded trigeminal neuralgia and evidence of multiple sclerosis by many years. Paraesthesia on the face, not related in time or situation to the neuralgia, had occurred in 7 of the 35 cases reported by Rushton & Olafson.[170] Some signs of brainstem disease were present in 17 of 24 cases examined by Jensen et al.[171]

A number of autopsies have been reported[164, 167,172,173,177] and in all plaques have been present in the pons. The entry zone of the trigeminal nerve appears to be the most consistent site of demyelination and has been demonstrated at biopsy[178] but lesions in the descending root and nucleus of the nerve may also be important. Possible pathogenetic mechanisms are discussed on page 235.

The course of trigeminal neuralgia in multiple sclerosis is very seldom described. Temporary remission can certainly occur,[177] but I have found no description of permanent spontaneous recovery, nor has this occurred in personal cases. The response to carbamazepine is initially excellent as in idiopathic neuralgia, but this drug aggravates many symptoms of multiple sclerosis, particularly weakness of the legs, and is therefore not tolerated in high doses. Alcohol injection was successful in the hands of experts.[174] Brett et al[179] had excellent results with percutaneous radiofrequency rhizotomy. Brisman[175] found response to treatment similar to that in idiopathic neuralgia.

No case of glossopharyngeal neuralgia appears to have been described in multiple sclerosis.

Dysarthria and ataxia

Paroxysmal dysarthria and ataxia in multiple sclerosis was first described in 1946 by Parker[180] but attracted little attention until the much fuller account by Andermann et al[181] in 1959. In contrast to trigeminal neuralgia that is only rarely related to multiple sclerosis, this form of paroxysmal symptom is highly characteristic of this disease. There have been many later descriptions.[182–189]

The attacks are sudden in onset. If the patient is talking at the time or attempting to do so, speech is slurred. There is no doubt of the dysarthric nature of the change but there is little time to analyse its nature. It is accompanied by other symptoms of which the most common is ataxia. Again precise examination is difficult but the signs are usually clearly localised to the limbs on one side. The arm becomes clumsy and walking is affected so that the patient staggers and may fall. In a personal case the initial symptom of multiple sclerosis was that of repeated falls when bicycling to work, the result of paroxysmal ataxia. Sometimes, particularly as it affects the legs, the ataxia appears to be bilateral. As far as can be judged in the brief time available for examination, the ataxia is of cerebellar type. Accompanying sensory symptoms are also common with paraesthesiae following a stereotyped pattern in each patient, for example, affecting one side of the face and the digits of the opposite hand. The symptoms can all be attributed to disordered function of the brainstem and cerebellum.

The attacks are brief, seldom lasting for as long as 20 seconds. They are usually frequent, occurring every half hour or more often. Harrison & McGill[183] recorded six attacks each lasting 15–20 seconds while the patient was writing a page. In a personal case the patient correctly stated that throughout the day an attack would occur 'every alternate minute'. It is difficult to determine the degree to which they are triggered by external stimuli. Many attacks appear to be spontaneous but others are precipitated by movement, particularly walking, and perhaps by talking. One of my patients believed that changing his train of thought would trigger an attack. In another patient who initially had paroxysmal dysarthria and ataxia as described above, the attacks became simplified to a momentary unsteadiness of one leg while walking. This would occur on average every six paces, causing her to limp as the left foot came to the ground. Like some other forms of paroxysmal symptoms, dysarthria and ataxia can easily be induced by overbreathing, often after only a few forced respirations.

There are few estimates of the incidence of paroxysmal dysarthria. Espir & Millac[190] found 8 examples in approximately 600 cases of multiple sclerosis, definite or suspected, compared with 9 patients with trigeminal neuralgia. In a personal series of 377 patients, paroxysmal ataxia with or without dysarthria had occurred in 14 (3.7%). Almost certainly many instances are overlooked. The symptoms, although remarkable enough, are very much less unpleasant than trigeminal neuralgia and remit completely after a few weeks or months. They may be referred to by the patient simply as 'dizziness' only revealed more exactly on close questioning. The paroxysms may occur as the initial symptom of multiple sclerosis,[188] in the absence of physical signs[191] or more usually during the relapsing and remitting stage of the disease. They are so characteristic that the diagnosis of multiple sclerosis must be strongly suspected even if further evidence of the disease is not apparent. Indeed Wolf & Assmus[189] regarded them as pathognomonic. The differential diagnosis is with transient ischaemic attacks involving the brain-stem, but the extreme brevity and frequency of the paroxysms are distinctive. The response to treatment is described below.

Tonic seizures

Tonic seizures were first recognised as a characteristic feature of multiple sclerosis in 1958.[145]. Earlier descriptions can be found but the remarkable attacks were not recognised for what they were. Determan[192] described identifiable tonic seizures in a patient he believed to be suffering from the neurological effects of influenza, but the partial Brown-Séquard syndrome was more probably the result of multiple sclerosis. Redlich[193] described two cases of what he regarded as hemitetany in multiple sclerosis and Störring[194] included two cases of unilateral tonic seizures in his series of epilepsy due to multiple sclerosis. He referred to these as Jacksonian epilepsy but specifically mentioned the 'Pfötchenstellung', the tetanic posture of the hand. Guillain et al[195] also described painful unilateral tonic spasm in a patient with a form of neuromyelitis optica. At autopsy three necrotic lesions were found, and a diagnosis of multiple sclerosis cannot be regarded as certain. Possible examples were briefly described by Williams et al[196] and by Fugelsang-Frederiksen & Thygesen.[197]

The original description was confirmed in a further four cases by Joynt & Green[198] and it has since become apparent that these strange attacks are relatively common. The original description was of 4 cases seen within two years, 2 of them being patients of the same general practitioner. As these were the only cases of multiple sclerosis under his care, he came to regard tonic seizures as a usual feature of the disease. Exactly how commonly they occur is not easy to establish as they are probably sometimes described by patients and their medical attendants as cramps. In British cases, tonic seizures had occurred in 4% of 204 cases at the time of reporting.[190] Espir et al[190] found 8 cases in 600 patients with definite or suspected multiple sclerosis. In a personal series of 377 patients, tonic seizures had occured in 14 (3.7%), a frequency identical to that of paroxysmal dysarthria and ataxia. In Japan, however, tonic seizures are much more common, occurring in 17%[66] or even 28% of cases.[226]

Tonic seizures usually conform to the general pattern of paroxysmal symptoms in appearing suddenly, occurring frequently and eventually remitting completely. Different patterns have been described, with seizures occurring in repeated clusters[199] or infrequently over several years.[186] The individual seizures are often triggered, apparently by movement, but it is naturally difficult to determine whether it is the motor activity or the consequent sensory stimulation, such as that resulting from putting the foot to the floor, a common trigger, that is effective.

Attacks may also occur spontaneously and can be induced by overbreathing.

Seizures are usually stereotyped for individual patients, although there may be degrees of severity and extent of the spasm. The spasm may be preceded by sensory symptoms, characteristically affecting the limbs or trunk on the side opposite the muscular spasm. These may be described as burning or tingling but are always unpleasant. The tonic contraction may affect one or both limbs on one side and often the face. Nearly always, spasm begins in one limb but spread is rapid. The posture adopted is often that of tetany but there are variations: the fingers may be flexed at distal joints rather than extended, the upper limb is flexed at the elbow and usually abducted at the shoulder. The lower limb is extended at all joints. The face is contracted, probably involuntarily, but it may also be contorted by pain. Pain in the affected limbs may indeed be extremely severe but is not invariable, some patients merely complaining of discomfort.

In all cases personally observed tonic seizures have been unilateral and this appears to be the case in Europe and North America. However, in Japan tonic seizures are not only more frequent but are often more severe, being bilateral and intensely painful.[66] In the only reported case from Africa, the spasm was also bilateral. Tonic seizures may occur concurrently with other paroxysmal symptoms, particularly with dysarthria and ataxia.[186]

The duration of tonic seizures may be as long as two minutes and the frequency does not attain that sometimes seen in paroxysmal dysarthria. Their pathophysiology is discussed on p. 235. It is unlikely that tonic seizures of this kind occur only in multiple sclerosis, but journals now seldom allow space for descriptions of purely clinical phenomena. Earlier reports of forms of 'subcortical epilepsy' were reviewed by Matthews.[145] Durston & Milnes[201] described similar attacks in patients thought to have relapsing encephalomyelitis but the dividing line from multiple sclerosis is imprecise. In context, tonic seizures are unmistakable evidence of multiple sclerosis and on one occasion led to my telling a patient that this was the diagnosis, in the complete absence of physical signs.

A woman of 26 had experienced two episodes of optic neuritis six and five years earlier, with complete recovery of vision and normal optic discs. One year before being seen she had Lhermitte's sign for some three months. She was referred because of right sided tonic seizures affecting mainly the upper limb but frequently triggered by putting the right foot to the ground. The attacks were unpleasant but not painful. There were no abnormal physical signs. However, after 20 deep breaths a typical tonic seizure was induced exactly as in her spontaneous attacks. The history was thought to be pathognomonic and at her urgent request the diagnosis was discussed.

Paraesthesiae

Sensory symptoms ranging from tingling to severe pain may accompany tonic seizures and the former commonly form part of the brainstem syndrome of paroxysmal dysarthria. It is not therefore surprising that paroxysmal paraesthesiae or dysaesthesia can occur in isolation but being entirely subjective, these are much more difficult to recognise. In a personal example[186] the initial symptom of clinically definite multiple sclerosis was an extremely severe quivering sensation beginning on the right side of the face and spreading to the right arm, index finger and thumb. These attacks lasted a few seconds but built up to such extreme frequency that his doctor had to be summoned twice in one night. The sensations, which he insisted were not painful, responded immediately to treatment with carbamazepine. Evidence of multiple sclerosis was not long delayed but to anyone unfamiliar with the paroxysmal symptoms of the disease, diagnosis was scarcely possible at the onset. Osterman & Westerberg[185] mentioned a patient with episodes of numbness as the initial symptom of multiple sclerosis but did not elaborate on how this sometimes misleading word should be interpreted. Espir & Millac[190] described a paroxysmal burning sensation in one lower limb and mentioned two less convincing cases of isolated sensory paroxysms. It is probable that the paroxysmal nature of sensory symptoms is only detected when obtrusive. Segmental paroxysmal dysaesthesiae appear to be relatively common in Japan, as Yabuki & Hayabara[202] were able to report 7 examples.

Pain

Paroxysmal pain has been reported rather more frequently[190,185,203] as an isolated or virtually isolated symptom. The pain characteristically involves a stereotyped segment of one limb, more usually the arm, but has been described in the perineum.[204] It is sometimes less easy to characterise as paroxysmal in that the duration of attacks may be longer and the response to carbamazepine is less assured. There is also room for diagnostic confusion with other forms of episodic limb pain unrelated to multiple sclerosis but sometimes responding to appropriate treatment.

Here is an example of paroxysmal pain following a different form of paroxysm at the onset of multiple sclerosis.

A woman of 28 presented with a 3-month history of attacks occurring about six times a day in which she experienced a strange sensation in the left upper lip and side of the nose accompanied by inability to use the right hand for about 30 seconds. If she was walking, the right leg would drag for a few steps.

Speech was not affected. Examination showed only minimal clumsiness of the right hand but multiple sclerosis was suspected and carbamazepine prescribed. These attacks stopped almost immediately but she then began to experience daily attacks of pain, beginning in the left side of the neck and spreading to the left upper arm. The pain would build up slowly, eventually becoming very severe and lasting for about one hour. There were no additional abnormal signs. Some improvement followed increased doses of carbamazepine but severe attacks continued about once a week for 6 months. Three years later she developed internuclear ophthalmoplegia and an ataxic gait. Oligoclonal IgG was present in the CSF.

Itching

Paroxysmal itching in multiple sclerosis was first described by Osterman & Westerberg[185] in 1976 although itching was mentioned as an initial sensory symptom by McAlpine.[10] Subsequent reports[202,205,206] have confirmed the paroxysmal nature of the symptom although, as with pain, the natural history may differ in some respects from the accepted pattern in that in some patients the attacks are more prolonged, 20 minutes or longer, and the response to carbamazepine is sometimes disappointing. Itching has been described in the upper and lower limbs and on the face and trunk.

In a personal series of 377 patients, 17 experienced paroxysmal itching, in one as an isolated initial symptom. Itching affected the upper limbs alone in 8, usually one shoulder region or a localised area of the forearm. In 5, the lower limbs were affected, most commonly one or both thighs. One patient had itching of one side of the scalp. In the remaining 3 patients, more than one area was involved: right face and shoulder, left forearm and abdominal wall and right side of the neck, and bilaterally on the trunk and arms. In 9 patients, changes in cutaneous sensation were present in the affected area.

Paroxysms may be spontaneous or induced by sensory stimulation or movement. The itching is intense, leading to vigorous but ineffective scratching to the extent of excoriating the skin. One patient used a wire brush in an attempt to control the itch. Between the paroxysms there may be persistent dysaesthesia or even some blunting of cutaneous sensation in the same area. In one case reported by Yamamoto et al[206] either or both shoulders would be affected, unlike the usual constant form of paroxysmal symptoms.

Itching may be associated, either simultaneously or in sequence, with other paroxysmal symptoms including tonic seizures or trigeminal neuralgia.[206]

Diplopia

Diplopia may occur with other symptoms of brainstem disturbance in paroxysmal dysarthria. It has also been described as occurring as an isolated symptom.[185] Both as an initial symptom or during the course of the disease, diplopia is peculiarly difficult to recognise as paroxysmal. Momentary double vision is a common complaint in those who believe, incorrectly, that they are developing multiple sclerosis and may also occur with fatigue in patients with latent squint. In established multiple sclerosis, fatigue and changes in environmental temperature will also cause transient recurring diplopia. In convincing cases double vision has occurred many times a day and has lasted for up to a minute. Dysjunctive movement was illustrated by Matthews[186] as forming part of a complex paroxysm of brainstem signs. Paroxysmal ocular flutter may cause blurred vision.[207]

Akinesia

Paroxysmal loss of use of one or more limbs is also encountered. There is naturally some difficulty in distinguishing such symptoms from those of ataxia or even from some of the less severe forms of tonic seizure. This remarkable symptom is usually, however, instantly recognisable even in the total absence of evidence of multiple sclerosis. This is exemplified by the man of 25 who complained of frequent sudden episodes of complete inability to take a further step. This usually occurred almost immediately he had risen to his feet. In observed attacks he would stand quite still for a few seconds before stepping out again. The attacks were immediately abolished by carbamazepine. There was no other evidence suggestive of multiple sclerosis. Zeldowicz[208] described 12 patients with 'paroxysmal motor episodes' in all as the first symptom of multiple sclerosis, in fact with a mean interval of nine years before the appearance of further signs of the disease. There are other causes for transient weakness or unexplained falls but many of these case descriptions closely resemble those of Castaigne et al[209] and Matthews[186] where the relation to multiple sclerosis was more obvious.

The legs are most commonly affected, usually both simultaneously, but the attacks are so brief that even when witnessed it is not possible to determine the exact nature or extent of the disordered function. Castaigne et al[209] described one patient with paroxysmal akinesia of one arm produced by playing the piano.

It is surprising that the paroxysmal symptoms of multiple sclerosis have proved so long in discovery and no doubt other forms remain to be described: paroxysmal unproductive coughing is a possible example.[210]

Natural history

The time scale of paroxysmal symptoms is usually that of a relapse of multiple sclerosis. Symptoms appear suddenly and continue with great intensity for from two days to some three months and then remit completely. Other patterns can, however, be recognised by the alert physician. Infrequent 'cramps' occurring on walking may be recognisable as tonic seizures on detailed enquiry. Paroxysms, when occurring frequently, can usually be provoked by overbreathing. Toyokura et al[211] made the interesting observation that rebreathing from a bag was ineffective.

A curious feature seldom remarked on is the tendency for individual patients to have more than one form of paroxysm in the course of their disease: ataxia and tonic seizures, akinesia and tonic seizures, and trigeminal neuralgia and dysarthria or itching have all been observed. It is possible that very slight metabolic differences, perhaps a lowered ionic calcium, might be responsible for this tendency and perhaps for the racial predilection to paroxysmal symptoms shown by natives of Japan and China.

Treatment

Some relief of paroxysmal symptoms can be obtained from anticonvulsant agents including phenytoin and even phenobarbitone.[145] This does not, of course, imply that the symptoms are epileptic as these drugs have complex actions. Phenytoin, for example, is of some benefit in idiopathic trigeminal neuralgia where an epileptic origin can scarcely be considered. Far more effective, however, is carbamazepine[190] that had previously been used as an anticonvulsant and as incomparably the best medical treatment of trigeminal neuralgia. The response in many forms of paroxysmal symptom would be remarkable in any context and particularly so in the intractable condition multiple sclerosis. Within an hour of the first dose of 100 mg, paroxysmal ataxia or tonic seizures that have been occurring 50 or 100 times a day may stop completely.[212] The response, particularly with pain or itching, is sometimes less impressive but even there some alleviation occurs. Carbamazepine has side effects and is poorly tolerated by patients with multiple sclerosis with motor disabilities. If necessary, acetozolamide[203] is an effective alternative. As paroxysmal symptoms remit, spontaneously successful treatment may be reduced after a suitable interval and stopped if there is no return of symptoms.

NARCOLEPSY

That narcolepsy should be a symptom of multiple sclerosis is so improbable that Kurtzke thought that the occurrence of the two conditions in the same patient must be coincidence. However the number of such cases reported can now leave little doubt of a significant connection.[213–215] Ekbom[215] described an extraordinary series of cases of the association of familial multiple sclerosis with narcolepsy. In two families, the pattern was of multiple sclerosis in one or more siblings and a further sibling with both multiple sclerosis and narcolepsy. In another family, three siblings had multiple sclerosis and a fourth had narcolepsy without evidence of multiple sclerosis. Such an association does not, of course, necessarily indicate that the narcolepsy was caused by multiple sclerosis. Familial occurrence is more readily explicable since the discovery that virtually all patients with classical narcolepsy are HLA DR2 positive,[216,217] this HLA antigen also being unduly common in multiple sclerosis (p. 309).

The case described by Schrader et al[218] does indeed suggest a causal connection. The patient, a monozygotic twin, whose sister was normal, had a very long history of clinically definite but comparatively mild multiple sclerosis. At the age of 56 she developed narcolepsy and cataplexy. These episodes were witnessed and investigated and the only unusual feature was the great frequency of cataplectic attacks, up to 40 a day. Idiopathic narcolepsy would not develop at this age and the authors suggest that the symptoms might arise from a plaque in the reticular activating system. The possibility of the syndrome being a form of paroxysmal symptom was raised but the response to carbamazepine was not examined. Poirier et al[219] found that symptoms suggestive of narcolepsy were remarkably common in multiple sclerosis patients but in not a single case investigated could this diagnosis be confirmed.

ADVENTITIOUS MOVEMENTS

Intention tremor is well recognised as a characteristic feature of multiple sclerosis. It is almost universally attributed to disordered function of the cerebellum or its connections, although Gordon Holmes,[220] whose knowledge of the clinical signs of cerebellar lesions was unrivalled, did not consider that such exclusive localisation was possible. As described on page 55, it may become totally disabling in a few patients with multiple sclerosis. At other end of the scale it is common to find 'slight intention tremor' recorded as evidence of multiple sclerosis in patients not suffering from any form of organic nervous disease. Properly interpreted it is, however, an important physical sign but too much attention should not be paid to slight tremor in the non-dominant hand in an anxious patient.

Tremor at rest or on sustained posture is very much less common. Titubation when the head is held erect may occur in patients with severe ataxia and may be regarded as part of the cerebellar syndrome. Tremor at rest was recorded in 4.6% of cases by Abb & Schaltenbrand[20] but was not otherwise described, and McAlpine[10] did not mention this form of tremor at all. Fog & Linnemann[221] reported that 2 of 73 patients carefully studied had Parkinsonian tremor, remitting in one

case. Chi-Chen Mao et al[222] described two patients in whom the features of Parkinson's disease appeared some years after the onset of multiple sclerosis. There was a reasonable therapeutic response to levodopa but apparently the parkinsonism did not remit.

A variety of other forms of involuntary movement have been described in multiple sclerosis, usually as single case reports, unavoidably not always supported by anatomical demonstration of the diagnosis.

Athetosis was said to have occurred in 2 of the 46 autopsy-proven cases of Carter et al.[3] Bachman et al[223] described two remarkable cases. Their first patient, with clinically definite multiple sclerosis, developed oro-facial dyskinesia and dystonic movements of the limbs of such severity as to induce muscle hypertrophy. Their second patient, whom the diagnosis was eventually confirmed at autopsy, had choreo-athetosis and intention tremor. Grigoresco's[213] patient had narcolepsy and unilateral chorea, the diagnosis of multiple sclerosis being confirmed. Generalised chorea in multiple sclerosis has recently been described by Chi-Chen Mao et al.[222] In the remitting choreoathetosis reported in three cases by Sarkari,[224] the diagnosis of multiple sclerosis was much less assured and systemic lupus appears more probable.

Thiery & de Reuck[225] described monoballism affecting the arm in a confirmed case of multiple sclerosis. The movements as described were more stereotyped than those usually seen in ballism. The subthalamic nucleus was not found to be involved by plaques. Mouren et al[226] described the late onset of hemiballismus in classical multiple sclerosis confirmed at autopsy. Riley & Lang[227] have described hemiballismus in a patient with clinically definite multiple sclerosis, responsive to tetrabenazine and to steroids, but returning when treatment was stopped. A lesion in the region of the opposite subthalamic nucleus was shown by MRI.

Myoclonus of different types has been described in isolated cases. The patient reported by Hassler et al[228] had 'intention myoclonus'. Severe jerking of both arms, head and trunk were induced by movement, but it is not clear whether they were present at rest. The movements were reduced by stereotactic surgery but this was followed by inability to swallow. The diagnosis was confirmed at autopsy, the myoclonus being attributed to lesions involving the red nucleus. Mouren et al[229] and Herrmann & Brown[230] have described palatal myoclonus in multiple sclerosis and there is a brief reference to episodic segmental myoclonus.[231]

Spasmodic torticollis associated with multiple sclerosis was described by Guillain & Bize[232] and has occasionally been reported since,[233,234] although a causal connection has not been established. Focal dystonia and writer's cramp have also been described.[234]

HEADACHE

Headache appears in most lists of symptoms of multiple sclerosis but with remarkable variations in frequency and usually without any attempt to define the type of headache or how it is thought to be related to multiple sclerosis. Abb & Schaltenbrand[20] reported headache in 32.5% of patients but their information was obtained largely by correspondence. In the comparative study of autopsy proven cases of multiple sclerosis from different countries,[16] headache did not appear at all as a symptom in British cases, in 19% of those from Norway and 12% of patients in the USA. Poser[53] does not include headache in the list of symptoms analysed. Kurtzke[25] found headache common in the onset bout, but remarked that it was usually associated with visual or brainstem signs.

Clifford & Trotter[54] reported that 17 of 317 patients with multiple sclerosis suffered from severe headache but this was not thought to be due to the disease. Migraine has been thought to be unduly common in multiple sclerosis[235] and Freedman & Gray[236] found that in 44 of 1113 cases, onset or relapse had been heralded by headache that they regarded as of vascular type. Seventeen of these patients had a previous history of migraine. Headache was most commonly associated with signs of a progressive posterior fossa lesion, sometimes causing diagnostic difficulty.

Bonduelle & Albaranès[135] defined the type of headache that they attribute to multiple sclerosis, in 5.5% of their cases. They excluded vague discomfort around the orbit in optic neuritis but it is not clear whether they included the by no means vague frontal pain sometimes experienced in this condition. They accepted headache of recent onset preceding or accompanying definite signs of relapse. In three patients headache was the initial symptom.

In the absence of definitions nothing can be learnt from the comparison of different series, as differences will depend on methods of enquiry and interpretation and perhaps on relative national fortitude.

Headache is certainly a feature of acute 'pseudotumorous' multiple sclerosis[237] and in such cases does not differ from that of other causes of raised intracranial pressure. Kahana et al[134] do not mention headache as a symptom of 'cerebral' multiple sclerosis.

REFERENCES

1. Kurtzke J F, Beebe G W, Nagler B, Auth T L, Kurland L T, Nefzger M D 1968 Studies on natural history of multiple sclerosis. 4: Clinical features of the onset bout. Acta Neurologica Scandinavica 44: 467–499
2. Shibasaki H, McDonald W I, Kuroiwa Y 1981 Racial modification of clinical picture of multiple sclerosis; comparison between British and Japanese patients. Journal of the Neurological Sciences 49: 253–271
3. Carter S, Sciarra D, Merritt H H 1950 The course of multiple sclerosis as determined by autopsy proven cases. Research Publications of the Association for Research into Nervous and Mental Disease 28: 471–511
4. Shepherd D I 1979 Clinical features of multiple sclerosis in north-east Scotland. Acta Neurologica Scandinavica 60: 218–230
5. Poser S, Wikström J, Bauer H J 1979 Clinical data and identification of special forms of multiple sclerosis with a standardised documentation system. Journal of the Neurological Sciences 40: 159–168
6. McAlpine D, Compston N D, Lumsden C E 1955 Multiple sclerosis. Livingstone, Edinburgh
7. Bauer H J 1978 Problems of symptomatic therapy in MS. Neurology 28(2): 8–20
8. Kelly R 1985 In: Vinken P J, Bruyn G W, Klawans H L (eds) Handbook of clinical neurology, Vol 47 Elsevier, Amsterdam, p 53
9. Wilson S A K 1940 Neurology. Edward Arnold, London, p 156
10. McAlpine D (ed) 1972 In: Multiple sclerosis: a reappraisal. Churchill Livingstone; Edinburgh
11. Leibowitz U, Alter M 1973 Multiple sclerosis: clues to its cause. North-Holland, Amsterdam

12. Adams D K, Sutherland J M, Fletcher W B 1950 Early clinical manifestations of disseminated sclerosis. British Medical Journal 2: 431–436

13. Thompson A J Hutchinson M, Brazil J, Feighery C, Martin E A 1986 A clinical and laboratory study of benign multiple sclerosis. Quarterly Journal of Medicine 58: 69–80

14. Sanders E A C M, Bollen E L E M, van der Velde E A 1986 Presenting signs and symptoms in multiple sclerosis. Acta Neurologica Scandinavica 73: 269–272

15. McAlpine D (ed) 1972 In: Multiple sclerosis, a reappraisal. Churchill Livingstone, Edinburgh, p 202

16. Poser C M, Presthus J, Hörsdal O 1966 Clinical characteristics of autopsy-proven multiple sclerosis. Neurology 16: 791–798

17. Izquierdo G, Lyon-Caen O, Marteau R, Martinez-Parra, Lhermitte F, Hauw P P 1986 Early onset multiple sclerosis: a clinical study of 12 pathologically proven cases. Acta Neurologica Scandinavica 73: 493–497

18. Lyon-Caen O, Izquierdo G, Marteau R, Lhermitte F, Caostaigne P, Hauw J J 1985 Late onset multiple sclerosis: a clinical study of 16 pathologically proven cases. Acta Neurologica Scandinavica 72: 56–60

19. Kuroiwa Y, Shibasaki H, Tabira T, Itoyama Y 1982 Clinical picture of multiple sclerosis in Asia. In: Kuroiwa Y, Kurland L T (eds) Multiple Sclerosis East and West. Kyushu University Press

20. Abb L, Schaltenbrand G 1956 Statistische Untersuchung zum Problem der multiplen Sklerose. II: Mitteilung. Das Krankheitsbild der multiplen Sklerose. Deutsche Zeitschrift für Nervenheilkunde 174: 199–218

21. Kuroiwa Y, Shibasaki H 1973 Clinical studies of multiple sclerosis in Japan. Part I: A current appraisal of 83 cases. Neurology 23: 609–617

22. Satayoshi E, Saku N, Sunohara N, Kinoshita M 1976 Clinical manifestations and the diagnostic problem of multiple sclerosis in Japan. Neurology 26/6 (2): 23–25

23. Hung T-P, Landsborough D, Hsi M-S, 1976 Multiple sclerosis among Chinese in Taiwan. Journal of the Neurological Sciences 27: 459–484

24. Müller R 1949 Studies on disseminated sclerosis with special reference to symptomatology, course and prognosis. Acta Medica Scandinavica 133 (suppl. 222): 1–214

25. Kurtzke J F 1970 Clinical features of multiple sclerosis. In: Vinken P J, Bruyn G W (eds) Handbook of clinical neurology, Vol 9. North-Holland, Amsterdam, pp 161–216

26. Ferrari M D, Hilkens P H E, Kremer B, Polder T W 1988 Intermittent pyramidal claudication as presenting and sole symptom in multiple sclerosis. Journal of Neurology, Neurosurgery and Psychiatry 51: 147–148

27. Cooper C B Trend P St J, Wiles C M 1985 Severe diaphragm weakness in multiple sclerosis. Thorax 40: 633–634

28. Yamamoto T, Imai T, Yamasaki M 1989 Acute ventilatory failure in multiple sclerosis. Journal of the Neurological Sciences 89: 313–324

29. Rivzi S S, Ishikawa S, Faling L J, Schlessinger L, Satia J, Seckel B 1974 Defect in automatic respiration in a case of multiple sclerosis. American Journal of Medicine 56: 433–436

30. Olgiati R, Jacquet J, Di Prampero P E 1986 Energy cost of walking and exertional dyspnea in multiple sclerosis. American Review of Respiratory Diseases 134: 1005–1010

31. Smeltzer S C, Utell M J, Rudick R A, Herndon 1988 Pulmonary function and dysfunction in multiple sclerosis. Archives of Neurology 45: 1245–1249

32. Wilson S A K 1940 Neurology. Edward Arnold, London, p 165

33. Strümpell A von 1896 Zur Pathologie der multiplen Sklerose. Neurologishes Zentralblatt 15: 961–964

34. Morsier G de 1971 Sur 1351 cas de névraxite (sclérose en plaques). Revue Neurologique 125: 103–118

35. Ferguson F R, Liversedge L A 1959 A clinical aphorism in the diagnosis of multiple sclerosis. Lancet 1: 1159–1160

36. Dimitrijevic M R, Nathan P W 1967 Studies of spasticity in man. 1: some features of spasticity. Brain 90: 1–30

37. Dimitrijevic M R, Nathan P W 1967 Studies of spasticity in man. 2: analysis of stretch reflexes in spasticity. Brain 90: 333–358

38. Bonduelle M, Bouygues P, Chaumont P 1964 Amyotrophies et abolition des réflexes dans la sclérose en plaques. Semaine des Hôpitaux de Paris 40: 814–821

39. Garcin R, Lapresle J, Fardeau M 1962 Documents pour servir a l'étude des amyotrophies et des abolitions durable des réflexes tendineux observeés dans la sclérose en plaques. Revue Neurologique 107: 417–431

40. Davison C, Goodhart S P, Lander J 1934 Multiple sclerosis and amyotrophies. Archives of Neurology and Psychiatry (Chicago) 31: 270–289

41. Fisher M, Long R R, Drachman D A 1985 Hand muscle atrophy in multiple sclerosis. Archives of Neurology 40: 811–815

42. Paty D W, Poser C 1984 Clinical symptoms and signs of multiple sclerosis. In: Poser C M (ed) The diagnosis of multiple sclerosis. Thieme–Stratton, New York, p 39

43. Barnard R O, Jellinek E H 1967 Multiple sclerosis with amyotrophy complicated by oligodendroglioma. History of recurrent herpes zoster. Journal of the Neurological Sciences 5: 441–445

44. Noseworthy J H, Heffernan I P M 1980 Motor radiculopathy — an unusual presentation of multiple sclerosis. Canadian Journal of Neurological Sciences 7: 207–209

45. Hader W J, Rozdilsky B, Nair C P 1986 The concurrence of multiple sclerosis and amyotrophic lateral sclerosis. Canadian Journal of Neurological Sciences 13: 66–69

46. Freal J E, Kraft G H, Coryell J K 1984 Symptomatic fatigue in multiple sclerosis. Archives of Physical Medicine and Rehabilitation 65: 135–138

47. Krupp L B, Alvarez L A, LaRocca N G, Scheinberg L C 1988 Fatigue in multiple sclerosis. Archives of Neurology 45: 435–437

48. Canadian MS Research Group 1987 A randomised controlled trial of amantadine in fatigue associated with multiple sclerosis. Canadian Journal of Neurological Sciences 14: 273–278

49. Sanders E A C M, Arts R J H M 1986 Paraesthesiae in multiple sclerosis. Journal of the Neurological Sciences 74: 297–305

50. Miller D H, McDonald W I, Blumhardt L D et al

1987 Magnetic resonance imaging in isolated noncompressive spinal cord syndromes. Annals of Neurology 22: 714–723

51. Halonen P, Panelius M, Halonen J-P, Lang H 1986 Vibration perception threshold in patients with mild multiple sclerosis. Acta Neurologica Scandinavica 74: 63–65

52. Graff-Radford N R, Rizzo M 1987 Neglect in a patient with multiple sclerosis. European Neurology 26: 100–103

53. Poser S 1978 Multiple sclerosis: an analysis of 812 cases by means of electronic data processing. Springer, Berlin

54. Clifford D B, Trotter J L 1984 Pain in multiple sclerosis. Archives of Neurology 41: 1270–1272

55. Cocksedge S, Freestone S, Maryin J F 1984 Unrecognised femoral fractures in patients with paraplegia due to multiple sclerosis. British Medical Journal 289–309

56. Moulin D E, Foley K M, Ebers G C 1988 Pain syndromes in multiple sclerosis. Neurology 38: 1830–1834

57. Aring C D 1973 Pain in multiple sclerosis. Journal of the American Medical Association 223: 547

58. Read C F 1932 Multiple sclerosis and Lhermitte's sign. Archives of Neurology and Psychiatry 27: 227–228

59. Kanchandani R, Howe J G 1982 Lhermitte's sign in multiple sclerosis: a clinical survey and review of the literature. Journal of Neurology, Neurosurgery and Psychiatry 45: 308–312

60. Marie P, Chatelin C 1917 Sur certains symptomes d'origine vraisemblement radiculaires chez les blessés du crâne. Revue Neurologique 32: 336

61. Babinski J, Dubois R 1918 Douleurs à forme de décharge électrique, consécutives aux traumatismes de la nuque. Presse Médicale 26: 64

62. Lhermitte J, Bollak, Nicholas M 1924 Les douleurs à type de décharge électrique consécutives à la flexion céphalique dans la sclérose en plaques. Revue Neurologique 42: 56–62

63. Boden G 1948 Radiation myelitis of the cervical spinal cord. British Journal of Radiology 21: 464–469

64. Gautier-Smith P C 1973 Lhermitte's sign in subacute combined degeneration of the cord. Journal of Neurology, Neurosurgery and Psychiatry 36: 861–863

65. Ekbom K 1971 Carbamazepine: a new symptomatic treatment for the paraesthesiae associated with Lhermitte's sign. Zeitschrift für Neurologie 200: 341–344

66. Shibasaki H, Kuroiwa Y 1974 Painful tonic seizure in multiple sclerosis. Archives of Neurology 30: 47–51

67. Thygesen P 1953 The course of disseminated sclerosis: a close-up of 105 attacks. Rosenkilde and Bagger, Copenhagen

68. Miller A E 1985 Cessation of stuttering with progressive multiple sclerosis. Neurology 35: 1341–1343

69. Charcot J M 1898 In: Bourneville (ed) Lecons sur les maladies du systèm nerveux, Vol 1. Louis Bataille, Paris, pp 237–238

70. Seiffer W 1905 Ueber psychische, inbesondere intelligenzstörungen bei multipler Sklerose. Archiv für Psychiatrie und Nervenkrankheiten 40: 252–303

71. Research Publications of the Association for Research in Nervous and Mental Disease 1922, Vol 2, p 129

72. Surridge D 1969 An investigation into some psychiatric aspects of multiple sclerosis. British Journal of Psychiatry 115: 749–762

73. Cottrell S S, Wilson S A K 1926 The affective symptomatology of disseminated sclerosis. Journal of Neurology and Psychopathology 7: 1–50

74. Ombredane A 1929 Sur les troubles mentaux de la sclérose en plaques. Thèse de Paris

75. Pratt R T C 1951 An investigation of the psychiatric aspects of disseminated sclerosis. Journal of Neurology, Neurosurgery and Psychiatry 14: 326–336

76. Matthews C G, Cleeland C S, Hopper C L 1970 Neuropsychological patterns in multiple sclerosis. Diseases of the Nervous System 31: 161–170

77. Marsh G G 1980 Disability and intellectual function in multiple sclerosis patients. Journal of Nervous and Mental Disease 168: 758–762

78. Peyser J M, Edwards J R, Poser C M, Filskov S B 1980 Cognitive function in patients with multiple sclerosis. Archives of Neurology 37: 577–579

79. Beatty P A, Grange J J 1977 Neuropsychological aspects of multiple sclerosis. Journal of Nervous and Mental Disease 164: 42–50

80. Rao S M, Hammeke T A, McQuillen M P, Khatri B O, Lloyd D 1984 Memory disturbance in chronic progressive multiple sclerosis. Archives of Neurology 41: 625–631

81. Truelle J L, Palisson E, LeGall D, Stip E, Derouesne C 1987 Troubles intellectuels et thymiques dans la sclérose en plaques. Revue Neurologique 143: 595–601

82. Ivnik R J 1978 Neuropsychological test performance as a function of the duration of MS-related symptomatology. Journal of Clinical Psychiatry 39: 304–307

83. Grant I, McDonald W I, Trimble M R, Smith E, Reed E 1984 Deficient learning and memory in early and middle phases of multiple sclerosis. Journal of Neurology, Neurosurgery and Psychiatry 47: 250–255

84. Van den Burg W, van Zomeren E A, Minderhoud J M, Prange A J A, Meijer N S A 1987 Cognitive impairment in patients with multiple sclerosis and mild physical disability. Archives of Neurology 44: 494–501

85. Heaton R K, Nelson L M, Thompson D S, Burks J S, Franklin G M 1985 Neuropsychological findings in relapsing-remitting and chronic-progressive multiple sclerosis. Journal of Consulting and Clinical Psychology

86. Lyon-Caen O, Jouvert R, Hauser S, Chauno M-P, Benoit N, Widlöcher D, Lhermitte F 1986 Cognitive function in recent-onset demyelinating disease. Archives of Neurology 43: 1138–1141

87. Jennekens-Schinkel A, van der Velde E A, Sanders E A C M, Lanser J B K 1989 Visuospatial problem solving, conceptual reasoning and sorting behaviour in multiple sclerosis out-patients. Journal of the Neurological Sciences 90: 187–202

88. Staples D, Lincoln N B 1979 Intellectual impairment in multiple sclerosis and its relation to functional abilities. Rheumatology and Rehabilitation 18: 153–160

89. Litvan I, Grafman J, Vendrell P, Martinez J M, Juqué C, Vendrell J M, Barraquer-Bordas J L 1988 Multiple memory defects in patients with multiple sclerosis. Archives of Neurology 45: 607–610

90. Litvan I, Grafman J, Vendeil P, Martinez J M 1988 Slowed information processing in multiple sclerosis.

Archives of Neurology 45: 281–285

91. Beatty W W, Goodkin D E, Monson N, Beatty P A, Hertsgaard D 1988 Anterograde and retrograde amnesia in patients with chronic progressive multiple sclerosis. Archives of Neurology 45: 611–619

92. Jennekens–Schinkel A, Sanders E A C M 1986 Decline in cognition in multiple sclerosis: dissociated deficits. Journal of Neurology, Neurosurgery and Psychiatry 49: 1354–1360

93. Vowels L M 1988 A longitudinal study of neuropsychological function in multiple sclerosis. An update on multiple sclerosis. IFMSS Conference, Rome, VII/2

94. Young A C, Saunders J, Ponsford J R 1976 Mental change as an early feature of multiple sclerosis. Journal of Neurology, Neurosurgery and Psychiatry 39: 1008–1013

95. Franklin G M, Nelson L M, Filley C M, Heaton R K 1989 Cognitive loss in multiple sclerosis. Case reports and review of literature. Archives of Neurology 46: 162–167

96. Bergin J D 1957 Rapidly progressive dementia in disseminated sclerosis. Journal of Neurology, Neurosurgery and Psychiatry 20: 285–292

97. O'Malley P P 1966 Severe mental symptoms in disseminated sclerosis: a neuropathological study. Journal of the Irish Medical Association 55: 115–127

98. Barnard R O, Triggs M 1974 Corpus callosum in multiple sclerosis. Journal of Neurology, Neurosurgery and Psychiatry 37: 1259–1264

99. Rao S M, Glatt S, Hammeke T A, McQuillen M P, Khatri B O, Rhodes A M, Pollard S 1985 Chronic progressive multiple sclerosis. Relationship between cerebral ventricular size and neuropsychological impairment. Archives of Neurology 41: 678–682

100. Rao S M, Leo G-J, Haighton V M, St Aubin–Faubert P, Bernadin L 1989 Correlation of MRI with neuropsychological testing in multiple sclerosis. Neurology 39: 161–166

101. Huber S J, Paulson G W, Shuttleworth E C et al 1987 Magnetic resonance imaging correlates of dementia in multiple sclerosis. Archives of Neurology 44: 732–736

102. Medaer R, Nelissen E, Appel B, Swerts M, Geutjens J, Callaert H 1986 Magnetic resonance imaging and cognitive functions in multiple sclerosis. Journal of Neurology 235: 86–89

103. Franklin G M, Heaton R K, Nelson L M, Filley C M, Seibert C 1988 Correlation of neuropsychological and MRI findings in chronic progressive multiple sclerosis. Neurology 38: 1826–1829

104. Brainin M, Goldenburg G, Ahlers C, Reisner T, Neuhold A, Decke L 1988 Structural brain correlates of anterograde memory defects in multiple sclerosis. Journal of Neurology 235: 362–365

105. Whitlock F A, Siskind M M 1980 Depression as a major symptom of multiple sclerosis. Journal of Neurology, Neurosurgery and Psychiatry 43: 861–865

106. Goodstein R K, Ferrell R B 1977 Multiple sclerosis presenting as depressive illness. Diseases of the Nervous System 38: 127–131

107. Baretz R M, Stephenson G R 1981 Emotional responses to multiple sclerosis. Psychosomatics 22: 117–127

108. Joffe R T, Lippert G P, Gray T A, Sawa G, Horvath Z 1987 Mood disorder and multiple sclerosis. Archives of Neurology 44: 376–377

109. Rao S M, Leo G J 1988 Mood disorder and multiple sclerosis. Archives of Neurology 45: 247–248

110. Dalos N P, Rabins P V, Brooks B R, O'Donnell P 1983 Disease activity and emotional state in multiple sclerosis. Annals of Neurology 13: 573–577

111. Harper A C, Harper D A, Chambers L W, Cino P M, Singer J 1986 An epidemiological description of physical, social and psychological problems in multiple sclerosis. Journal of Chronic Diseases 39: 305–310

112. Schiffer R B, Caine E D, Bamford K A, Levy 1983 Depressive episodes in patients with multiple sclerosis. American Journal of Psychiatry 140: 1498–1500

113. McIvor G P, Riklan M, Reznikoff M 1984 Depression in multiple sclerosis as a function of length and severity of illness, age, remissions and perceived social support. Journal of Neuropsychology 40: 1028–1033

114. Rabins P V, Brooks B R, O'Donnell P et al 1986 Structural brain correlates of emotional disorder in multiple sclerosis. Brain 109: 585–597

115. Honer W G, Hurwiyz T, Li D K B, Palmer M, Paty D W 1987 Temporal lobe involvement in multiple sclerosis patients with psychiatric disorders. Archives of Neurology 44: 187–193

116. Schiffer R B, Babigian H M 1984 Behavioral disorders in multiple sclerosis, temporal lobe epilepsy and amyotrophic lateral sclerosis. An epidemiological study. Archives of Neurology 41: 1067–1069

117. Peselow E D, Fieve R R, Deutsch S I, Kaufman M 1981 Coexistent manic symptoms and multiple sclerosis. Psychosomatics 22: 824–825

118. Kemp K, Lion J R, Magram G 1977 Lithium in the case of a manic patient with multiple sclerosis — a case report. Diseases of the Nervous System 38: 210–211

119. Kellner C H, Davenport Y, Post R M, Ross R J 1984 Rapidly cycling bipolar disorder and multiple sclerosis. American Journal of Psychiatry 141: 112–113

120. Schiffer R B, Wineman M, Weitkamp L R 1986 Association between bipolar affective disorder and multiple sclerosis. American Journal of Psychiatry 143: 94–95

121. Schiffer R B 1987 The spectrum of depression in multiple sclerosis. An approach for clinical management. Archives of Neurology 44: 596–599

122. Davison K, Bagley C R 1969 Schizophrenia-like psychoses associated with organic disorders of the central nervous system; a review of the literature. In: Herrington R M (ed) British Journal of Psychiatry Special Publication 4, pp 113–184

123. Dercum F X 1912 A case of cerebrospinal sclerosis, presenting unusual symptoms suggesting paresis. Journal of the American Medical Association 59: 1612–1614

124. Knoblauch A 1908 Ein Fall von multipler Sklerose, kompliziert durch eine chronische Geistesstörung. Monatschrift für Psychiatrie und Neurologie 24: 238–250

125. Lannois M 1903 Troubles psychiques dans un cas de sclérose en plaques. Revue Neurologique 11: 876–884

126. Matthews W B 1979 Multiple sclerosis presenting with acute remitting psychiatric symptoms. Journal of Neurology, Neurosurgery and Psychiatry 42: 859–862

127. Logsdail D S J, Callanan M M, Ron M A 1988 Psychiatric morbidity in patients with clinically isolated lesions of the type seen in multiple sclerosis: a clinical and MRI study. Psychological Medicine 18: 355–364

128. Kohler J, Heilmeyer H, Volk B 1988 Multiple sclerosis presenting as chronic atypical psychosis. Journal of Neurology, Neurosurgery and Psychiatry 51: 281–284

129. Langworthy O R, Kolb L C, Androp S 1941 Disturbance of behaviour in patients with multiple sclerosis. American Journal of Psychiatry 98: 242–248

130. Brown S, Davis T K 1922 The mental symptoms of multiple sclerosis. Archives of Neurology and Psychiatry 7: 629–634

131. Langworthy O R 1950 A survey of the maladjustment problems in multiple sclerosis and the possibilities of psychotherapy. Research Publications of the Association for Research in Nervous and Mental Disease 28: 598–611

132. Aring C D 1965 Observations on multiple sclerosis and conversion hysteria. Brain 88: 663–674

133. Caplan L R, Nadelson T 1980 Multiple sclerosis and hysteria. Lessons learnt from their association. Journal of the American Medical Association 243: 2418–2420

134. Kahana E, Leibowitz U, Alter M 1971 Cerebral multiple sclerosis. Neurology 21: 1179–1185

135. Bonduelle M, Albaranès R 1962 Etude statistique de 145 cas de sclérose en plaques. Semaine des Hôpitaux 38: 3762–3773

136. Gussenbauer C 1902 Erfahrungen über die osteoplastische Schädestrepanation wegen Hirngeschwülsten. Wiener Klinische Wochenschrift 15: 175–182

137. Gussenbauer C 1902 Hirnsklerose and Herderscheinung. Wiener Klinische Wochenschrift 15: 964–965

138. Sagar H J, Warlow C P, Sheldon P W E, Esiri M M 1982 Multiple sclerosis with clinical and radiological features of cerebral tumour. Journal of Neurology, Neurosurgery and Psychiatry 45: 802–808

139. Hunter S B, Ballinger W E, Rubin J J 1987 Multiple sclerosis mimicking primary brain tumour. Archives of Pathology and Laboratory Medicine 111: 464–468

140. Mastrostefano R, Occhipinti E, Bigotti G, Pompili A 1987 Multiple sclerosis plaque simulating cerebral tumour: case report and review of the literature. Neurosurgery 21: 244–246

141. Day T J, Mastaglia F L 1987 Alexia with agraphia in multiple sclerosis. Journal of the Neurological Sciences 78: 343–348.

142. Herderscheê D, Stam J, Derix M M A 1987 Aphemia as a first symptom of multiple sclerosis. Journal of Neurology, Neurosurgery and Psychiatry 50: 499–500

143. Poser C M 1987 Aphemia as a first symptom of multiple sclerosis. Journal of Neurology, Neurosurgery and Psychiatry 50: 1388

144. Matthews W B 1962 Epilepsy and disseminated sclerosis. Quarterly Journal of Medicine 31: 141–155

145. Matthews W B 1958 Tonic seizures in disseminated sclerosis. Brain 81: 193–206

146. Drake W E, Macrae D 1961 Epilepsy in multiple sclerosis. Neurology 11: 810–816

147. Elian M, Dean G 1977 Multiple sclerosis and epilepsy. In: Perry J K (ed) Epilepsy, the 8th International Symposium. Raven Press, New York, p 341–344

148. Boudouresques J, Khalil R, Cherif A A et al 1975 Epilepsie et sclérose en plaques. Revue Neurologique 131: 729–735

149. Cendrowski W, Makowski J 1972 Epilepsy in multiple sclerosis. Journal of the Neurological Sciences 17: 389–398

150. Kinnunen E, Wikström J 1986 Prevalence and prognosis of epilepsy in patients with multiple sclerosis. Epilepsia 27: 729–733

151. Hopf H C, Stamatovic A M, Wahren W 1970 Die cerebralen Anfällen bei der multiplen Sklerose. Journal of Neurology 198: 256–279

152. Trouillas P, Courjon L 1972 Epilepsy with multiple sclerosis. Epilepsia 13: 325–333

153. Ritter G, Poser S 1974 Epilepsie und multiple Sklerose. Münchener Medizinischer Wochenschrift 116: 1984–1986

154. Wilson S A K, McBride H J 1925 Epilepsy as a symptom of disseminated sclerosis. Journal of Neurology and Psychopathology 6: 91–103.

155. Boudouresques J, Khalil R, Roger J et al 1980 Etat du mal epileptique en sclérose en plaques. Revue Neurologique 136: 777–782

156. Allison R S 1950 Survival in disseminated sclerosis: a clinical study of a series of cases first seen twenty years ago. Brain 73: 103–120

157. Sheehan S 1956 One thousand cases of late onset epilepsy. Irish Journal of Medical Science No 390: 261–272

158. Abbott R J, Howe J G, Currie S, Holland J 1982 Multiple sclerosis plaque mimicking tumour on computed tomography. British Medical Journal 285: 1616–1617

159. Reith K G, DiChiro G, Cromwell L D et al 1981 Primary demyelinating disease simulating glioma of the corpus callosum. Journal of Neurosurgery 55: 620–624

160. Castaigne P, Escourolle R, Laplane D, Augustin P 1966 Comas transitoires avec hyperthermie au cours de la sclérose en plaques. Revue Neurologique 114: 147–150

161. Castaigne P, Escourolle R, Laplane D, Augustin P 1966 Comas transitoires avec hyperthermie au cours de la sclérose en plaques. Encéphale 55: 191–211

162. Ringel R A, Riggs J E, Brick J F 1988 Reversible coma with prolonged absence of pupillary and brainstem reflexes: an unusual response to a hypoxic-ischemic event in MS. Neurology 38: 1275–1278

163. Sullivan F, Hutchinson M, Bahandeka S, Moore R E 1987 Chronic hypothermia in multiple sclerosis. Journal of Neurology, Neurosurgery and Psychiatry 50: 813–815

164. Oppenheim H 1911 Textbook of nervous diseases, 5th edn, Vol 1, trans. Bruce R Foulis, London, p 337

165. Guillain G 1924 Rapport sur la sclérose en plaques. Revue Neurologique 41: 648–683

166. Harris W 1927 Sensory changes in spinal cord and medullary lesions. Brain 50: 399–412

167. Parker H L 1928 Trigeminal neuralgic pain associated with multiple sclerosis. Brain 51: 46–62

168. Harris W 1950 Rare forms of paroxysmal trigeminal neuralgia and their relation to disseminated sclerosis. British Medical Journal 2: 1015–1019

169. Ruge D, Brochner R, Daris L 1958 A study of the treatment of 637 patients with trigeminal neuralgia. Journal of Neurosurgery 15: 528–536

170. Rushton J G, Olafson R A 1965 Trigeminal neuralgia associated with multiple sclerosis. Archives of Neurology 13: 383–386

171. Jensen P S, Rasmussen P, Reske-Nielsen E 1982

Association of trigeminal neuralgia with multiple sclerosis: clinical and pathological features. Acta Neurologica Scandinavica 65: 182–185

172. Daum S, Vogein-Rappoport, Gruner J, Foncin J F 1960 Sclérose en plaques revélée à l'age de 64 ans par une néuralgie trigeminale. Etude anatomo-clinique. Revue Neurologique 102: 500–503

173. Garcin R, Godlewski S, Lapresle J 1960 Névralgie du trijumau et sclérose en plaques (à propos d'une observation anatomo-clinique) Revue Neurologique 102: 441–451

174. Harris W 1940 An analysis of 1433 cases of paroxysmal trigeminal neuralgia (trigeminal tic) and the end results of Gasserian alcohol injection. Brain 63: 209–224

175. Brisman R 1987 Trigeminal neuralgia and multiple sclerosis. Archives of Neurology 44: 379–381

176. Friedlander A H, Zeff S 1974 Atypical trigeminal neuralgia in patients with multiple sclerosis. Journal of Oral Surgery 32: 301–303

177. Olafson R A, Rushton J G, Sayre G P 1966 Trigeminal neuralgia in a patient with multiple sclerosis. An autopsy report. Journal of Neurosurgery 24: 755–759

178. Lazar M L, Kirkpatrick J B 1979 Trigeminal neuralgia and multiple sclerosis: demonstration of the plaque in an operative case. Neurosurgery 5: 711–716

179. Brett D C, Ferguson G G, Ebers G C, Paty D W 1982 Percutaneous trigeminal rhizotomy. Treatment of trigeminal neuralgia secondary to multiple sclerosis. Archives of Neurology 39: 219–221

180. Parker H L 1946 Periodic ataxia. Collected papers of the Mayo Clinic 38: 642–645

181. Andermann F, Cosgrove J B R, Lloyd-Smith D, Walters A M 1959 Paroxysmal dysarthria and ataxia in multiple sclerosis. A report of two unusual cases. Neurology 9: 211–216

182. Espir M L E, Watkins S M, Smith H V 1966 Paroxysmal dysarthria and other transient neurological disturbances in disseminated sclerosis. Journal of Neurology, Neurosurgery and Psychiatry 29: 323–330

183. Harrison M, McGill J I 1969 Transient neurological disturbances in disseminated sclerosis: a case report. Journal of Neurology, Neurosurgery and Psychiatry 32: 230–232

184. Miley C E, Forster F M 1974 Paroxysmal signs and symptoms in multiple sclerosis. Neurology 24: 458–461

185. Osterman P O, Westerberg C-E 1975 Paroxysmal attacks in multiple sclerosis. Brain 98: 189–202

186. Matthews W B 1975 Paroxysmal symptoms in multiple sclerosis. Journal of Neurology, Neurosurgery and Psychiatry 38: 617–623

187. Netsell R, Kent R R 1076 Paroxysmal ataxic dysarthria. Journal of Speech and Hearing Disorders 41: 93–109

188. Perks W H, Lascelles R G 1976 Paroxysmal brain stem dysfunction as presenting symptoms of multiple sclerosis. British Medical Journal 2: 1175–1176

189. Wolf P, Assmus H 1974 Paroxysmale Dysarthrie und Ataxie: ein pathognomisches Anfallssyndrom bei Multipler Sklerose. Journal of Neurology 208: 27–38

190. Espir M L E, Millac P 1970 Treatment of paroxysmal disorders in multiple sclerosis with carbamazepine (Tegretol). Journal of Neurology, Neurosurgery and Psychiatry 33: 528–531

191. Twomey J A, Espir M L E 1980 Paroxysmal symptoms

as the first manifestation of multiple sclerosis. Journal of Neurology, Neurosurgery and Psychiatry 43: 269–304

192. Determan H 1892 Zwei Fälle von Rückensmarkerkrankung nach Influenza. Deutsche Zeitschrift für Nervenheilkunde 2: 106–120

193. Redlich E 1929 Zur Klinik der Hemitetanie mit Erörterungen über den Auslösungsort der tetanische Krämfe. Zeitschrift für die gesamte Neurologie und Psychiatrie 120: 236–264

194. Störring G 1940 Epilepsie und multiple Sklerose. Archiv für Psychiatrie und Nervenkrankheiten 112: 45–75

195. Guillain G, Alajouanine T, Bertrand I, Garcin R 1928 Sur une forme anatomo-clinique de neuromyelite optique avec crises toniques tetanoides. Annales de Médecine 24: 24–57

196. Williams G H, Nosik W A, Hunter J A 1952 Convulsions as manifestations of multiple sclerosis. Journal of the American Medical Association 150: 990–992

197. Fugelsang-Frederiksen V, Thygesen P 1952 Seizures and psychopathology in multiple sclerosis. Acta Psychiatrica et Neurologica Scandinavica 27: 17–41

198. Joynt R J, Green D 1962 Tonic seizures as a manifestation of multiple sclerosis. Archives of Neurology 6: 293–299

199. Heath P D, Nightingale S 1982 Clusters of tonic seizures as an initial manifestation of multiple sclerosis. Annals of Neurology 12: 494–495

200. Dumas M, Girard P L, Ndiaye I P, Gueye M 1977 Manifestations motrices paroxystiques au cours d'une sclérose en plaques chez une Noire africaine. Bulletin de la Société de Médecine Afrique de Langue Francaise 22: 30–34

201. Durston J H J, Milnes J N 1970 Relapsing encephalomyelitis. Brain 93: 715–730

202. Yabuki S, Hayabara T 1979 Paroxysmal dysesthesia in multiple sclerosis. Folia Psychiatrica et Neurologica Japonica 33: 97–104

203. Voiculescu V, Pruskauer-Apostol B, Alecu C 1975 Treatment with acetozolamide of brain-stem and spinal paroxysmal disturbances in multiple sclerosis. Journal of Neurology, Neurosurgery and Psychiatry 38: 191–193

204. Miró J, Garcia-Moncó, Leno C, Berciano L 1988 Pelvic pain: an undescribed manifestation of multiple sclerosis. Pain 32: 73–75

205. Osterman P O 1976 Paroxysmal itching in multiple sclerosis. British Journal of Dermatology 95: 555–558

206. Yamamoto M, Yabuki S, Hayabara T, Otsuki S 1981 Paroxysmal itching in multiple sclerosis: a report of three cases. Journal of Neurology, Neurosurgery and Psychiatry 44: 19–22

207. Francis D A, Heron J R 1985 Ocular flutter in suspected multiple sclerosis: a presenting paroxysmal manifestation. Postgraduate Medical Journal 61: 333–334

208. Zeldowicz L 1961 Paroxysmal motor episodes as early manifestations of multiple sclerosis. Canadian Medical Association Journal 84: 937–941

209. Castaigne P, Cambier J, Masson M et al 1970 Les manifestations motrices paroxystiques de la sclérose en plaques. Presse Médicale 78: 1921–1924

210. Jacôme D E 1985 La toux diabolique: neurogenic tussive crises. Postgraduate Medical Journal 61: 515–516

211. Toyokura Y, Sakuta M, Nakanishi T 1976 Painful tonic seizures in multiple sclerosis. Neurology 26 (6 pt 2): 18–19
212. Castaigne P, Cambier J, Barbizet J, Brunet P, Poirier J 1974 Crises sensitivo-motrices d'origine spinale au cours d'une sclérose en plaques à poussée aigue terminale. Revue Neurologique 130: 261–271
213. Grigoresco D 1932 Contribution à l'étude des troubles dus à des lésions des noyaux gris dans la sclérose en plaques. Revue Neurologique 58: 27–45
214. Berg O, Hanley J 1963 Narcolepsy in two cases of multiple sclerosis. Acta Neurologica Scandinavica 39: 252–257
215. Ekbom K 1966 Familial multiple sclerosis associated with narcolepsy. Archives of Neurology 15: 337–344
216. Juji T, Satake M, Honda Y, Doi Y 1984 HLA antigens in Japanese patients with narcolepsy. All the patients were DR2 positive. Tissue Antigens 24: 316–319
217. Langdon N, Walsh K I, van Dam M, Vaughan R W, Parkes D 1984 Genetic markers in narcolepsy. Lancet 2: 1178–1180
218. Schrader H, Gotlibsen O B, Skomedal G N 1980 Multiple sclerosis and narcolepsy/cataplexy in a monozygotic twin. Neurology 30: 105–108
219. Poirier G, Montplaisir J, Dumont M, Duquette P, Décary F, Pleines J, Lamoureux G 1987 Clinical and sleep laboratory study of narcoleptic symptoms in multiple sclerosis. Neurology 37: 693–695
220. Holmes G 1946 Introduction to clinical neurology. Livingstone, Edinburgh
221. Fog T, Linnemann F 1970 The course of multiple sclerosis in 73 cases with computer designed curves. Acta Neurologica Scandinavica 46 (suppl 47): 1–175
222. Chi-Chen Mao, Gancher S T, Herndon R M 1988 Movement disorders in multiple sclerosis. Movement Disorders 3: 109–116
223. Bachman D S, Laó-Velez C, Estanol B 1976 Dystonia and choreoathetosis in multiple sclerosis. Archives of Neurology 33: 590
224. Sarkari N B S 1968 Involuntary movements in multiple sclerosis. British Medical Journal 2: 738–740
225. Thiery E, de Reuck J 1974 Monoballism in multiple sclerosis. Acta Neurologica Belgica 74: 241–249
226. Mouren P, Tatossian A, Toga M, Poinso Y, Blumen G 1966 Etude critique du syndrome hémiballique. Encéphale 55: 212–274
227. Riley D, Lang A E 1988 Hemiballismus in multiple sclerosis. Movement Disorders 3: 88–94
228. Hassler R, Bronisch F, Mandringer F, Riechert T 1975 Intention myoclonus of multiple sclerosis, its patho-anatomical basis and stereotaxic relief. Neurochirurgica 18: 90–106
229. Mouren P, Tatossian A, Giraud F, Stiglioni L, Verne P, Poinso Y 1962 Le 'nystagmus du voile du palais' (le syndrome myorhythmique du carrefour aéro-digestif). Revue d'Oto-Neuro-Opthalmologie 34: 273–304
230. Herrmann C, Brown J W 1967 Palatal myoclonus: a reappraisal. Journal of the Neurological Sciences 5: 473–492
231. Mouren P, Tassinari C A, Roger J, Poinso Y 1965 Episodes de myoclonies de type squelettique dans un cas de sclérose en plaques. Revue Neurologique 113: 270
232. Guillain G, Bize R 1933 Sur un cas de sclérose en plaques avec torticollis spasmodique. Revue Neurologique 40: 133–138
233. Matthews W B 1985 In: McAlpine's multiple sclerosis. Churchill Livingstone, Edinburgh, p 118
234. Coleman R J, Quinn N P, Marsden C G 1988 Multiple sclerosis presenting as adult onset dystonia. Movement Disorders 3: 329–332
235. Watkins S M, Espir M 1966 Migraine and multiple sclerosis. Journal of Neurology, Neurosurgery and Psychiatry 32: 35–37
236. Freedman M S, Gray T A 1989 Vascular headache: a presenting symptom of multiple sclerosis. Canadian Journal of Neurological Sciences 16: 63–66
237. Nelson M J, Miller S L, McLain W, Gold L H A 1981 Multiple sclerosis: large plaque causing mass effect and ring sign. Journal of Computer Assisted Tomography 5: 892–894

3. Symptoms and signs (contd)

ANOSMIA

Loss of sense of smell is seldom complained of in multiple sclerosis and perhaps seldom looked for. I have encountered it twice, on each occasion accompanying widespread symptoms in an initial attack of multiple sclerosis. The complaint was of loss of sense of taste and bilateral anosmia was found. Remission of this symptom occurred in both cases.

Ansari[1] looked for concealed impairment of the sense of smell in multiple sclerosis but on detailed examination of 40 patients no difference from control was observed. Pinching,[2] in the course of developing a more sophisticated method of testing sense of smell, detected symptomless abnormalities in 15 of 22 multiple sclerosis patients.

OPTIC NEURITIS

Optic neuritis is of great significance to many aspects of multiple sclerosis. The clinical features are briefly described in the consideration of the differential diagnosis from other conditions of the optic nerve and retina (Ch. 6). The possible prognostic significance of optic neuritis at the onset of multiple sclerosis with respect to the eventual severity of the disease is discussed on page 157. The clinical details and their implications merit a more extensive account.

The optic nerves and chiasma are particularly vulnerable in multiple sclerosis. This was recognised towards the end of the last century by Parinaud[3] but the most notable early contribution was the classical paper of Uhthoff[4] on the ophthalmic and visual findings in 100 cases of multiple sclerosis. He found a high incidence of optic atrophy in chronic disease and optic neuritis in five patients. He observed the central scotoma and the severity of the loss of visual acuity. He also recorded that the optic disc might be normal in appearance in spite of a past history of visual disturbance, and also that histological changes could be found in the optic nerve in the absence of any ophthalmoscopic abnormality in life.

The term 'optic neuritis' is used throughout this discussion. 'Retrobulbar neuritis' is certainly useful in the description of individual cases with characteristic visual symptoms but a normal optic nerve head but, especially in some earlier accounts, has led to the unjustified exclusion of cases with papillitis.

Frequency of optic neuritis in multiple sclerosis

The frequency with which distinct episodes of optic neuritis are recorded either at the onset or in the course of multiple sclerosis naturally depends on the diagnostic criteria adopted. A classical attack of optic neuritis is easily recognisable but the significance of brief transient episodes of slight blurring of vision is much less easy to determine. The use of VEP has, however, demonstrated that such symptoms, lasting for no more than two or three days, may be accompanied by evidence of persistent damage to the optic nerve.[5] The frequency of overt symptoms of visual disturbance, however slight, will always be much lower than those of concealed visual loss or clinically entirely inapparent optic nerve lesions revealed by VEP, psychophysical tests or histology. Studies of epidemiological and even aetiological significance of optic neuritis are not unnaturally based on recorded unmistakable attacks but the implications of these are unlikely to differ in any important respect from those of plaques in the optic nerve producing slight symptoms or even none at all. Figures for frequency must therefore be regarded as approximate and reflecting the clinical criteria accepted by individual investigators.

The frequency of visual failure at the onset of multiple sclerosis, either alone or with other signs, as recorded in general surveys of initial symptoms, is described on page 43. In a study specifically directed to this question, Wikström et al[6] found that the optic nerve was involved in the first attack in 34.7% of 1271 patients and that optic neuritis was an isolated initial feature in 16.6%. These figures are somewhat higher than those from smaller series from Europe. As an isolated initial event it occurred in 18.4% of males and 15.5% of females. The mean age of onset in patients with optic neuritis alone or in combination was 2 years younger than that of the whole series. Wikström et al[6] expressed the opinion that optic neuritis in the initial attack reflects more precisely than other symptoms the beginning of the disease. This is unlikely to be so. When VEP were recorded in patients with recent isolated optic neuritis and no other history of visual disturbance prolonged latency was found in the unaffected eye in 6 out of 28 patients,[7] presumably indicating earlier symptomless attacks. Further evidence of preexisting silent lesions in patients presenting with optic neuritis is provided by multi-modal evoked potential recording,[8] MRI[9–11] and even by neuropsychological testing.[12]

The frequency of visual failure in the course of multiple sclerosis in a number of large series from Europe, the USA and Japan is discussed on page p. 46. Overt attacks become distinctly less frequent as the disease enters the progressive stage, but as involvement of the optic nerve is known to be virtually constant in severe multiple sclerosis, the significance of individual episodes becomes less important.

Clinical features

The clinical features of optic neuritis have been reviewed in detail by Perkin & Rose.[13] The mean

age at which optic neuritis without apparent cause occurs was not thought to differ from that of the onset of multiple sclerosis, with a peak early in the fourth decade. The age range is rather more extensive and the special problem of optic neuritis in childhood is discussed later (p. 121). Isolated optic neuritis over the age of 50 becomes increasingly difficult to distinguish from ischaemic papillitis, both in published series and personal cases. The sex distribution of unexplained optic neuritis in all recent reports has shown female preponderance[14–16] of the same order as that of multiple sclerosis.

Optic neuritis occurs with approximately equal frequency in the two eyes. Of large series, Kurland et al[17] reported 73 left eyes affected and 70 right; Rischbieth[18] 51 left and 48 right; Perkin & Rose[13] 87 left and 83 right. Bilateral optic neuritis must be considered separately as it has different connotations.

Pain is usually present at some stage, most commonly preceding the onset of visual symptoms but sometimes simultaneously or developing subsequently. The pain is felt in the eye or is supraorbital and sometimes accompanied by unilateral or generalised headache. It varies in intensity, sometimes only being mentioned after direct enquiry but sometimes distressingly severe. It is often aggravated by movement of the eye or is only present on movement. The absence of pain does not exclude the diagnosis as this has been reported in 20–87% of cases.[13] Pain may persist for several weeks but subsides before maximum recovery of vision is attained. The severity or duration of the pain does not appear to influence the prognosis for recovery of vision, nor is it related to the presence of papillitis. Perkin & Rose[13] believe that the pain is due to stretching of the meninges surrounding the swollen optic nerve. Relief of pain often follows treatment with steroids or ACTH.[19] Tenderness of the eyeball nearly always accompanies pain. That pain in the eye without visual loss can be due to optic neuritis may be suspected. Patients who have experienced optic neuritis may describe similar pain in the same eye or on the opposite side with no deterioration in acuity, visual field or VEP. In such cases anxiety and apprehension cannot be excluded as a cause.

Patients can nearly always date the onset of the

awareness of visual loss with precision. To what extent this accurately reflects the true onset may be doubted as uniocular impairment of vision may only be noted when the other eye is fortuitously closed, an action that is seldom performed except when rubbing the eye. This observation is, however, more relevant to chronic progressive visual failure but it is nonetheless not infrequent even in apparently acute optic neuritis. Other patients, more observant or more severely affected, are immediately aware of any abnormality of vision with both eyes open. The onset is often described as being sudden during waking hours or may be first noticed on waking from sleep.

Progressive deterioration of vision is, however, common, even when the onset is reported as sudden. If patients with optic neuritis can be seen by an interested and instructed observer within a few days of the onset, and this is unexpectedly difficult to achieve, the duration of progression can be accurately timed. Personal experience of such cases agrees with that of Perkin & Rose, whose patients were seen comparatively late.[13] The period from onset of visual symptoms to maximum loss of acuity is most commonly 3–7 days, longer progression for more than 2 weeks being quite exceptional. Deterioration by no means always proceeds at a steady rate.

The initial visual symptom is nearly always that of simple blurring of vision. This is sometimes qualified by descriptions suggesting more positive phenomena such as a haze or mist over the eye, but probably these are used as illustrative of the difficulty in seeing clearly. The shimmering 'heat haze' effect so common in migraine is encountered very exceptionally. Movement phosphenes,[20] a bright flash on eye movement in the dark, have not occurred at or before the onset of optic neuritis in cases seen personally but may develop later, particularly during the stage of improvement.

The patient may be aware of the nature of the field defect and this is particularly so in the 5% of cases where the initial defect is not central. An altitudinal defect, spreading within a few days to generalised blurring of vision, may be clearly described. In the initial stages it is uncommon for the patient to observe that vision is clear in the periphery in the presence of a central scotoma.

The degree of loss of visual acuity as recorded by the means generally available, the Snellen chart and Jaeger test or their equivalent, varies from none at all to loss of perception of light. A complaint of complete blindness in the affected eye at the time of presentation is rarely substantiated, the patient naturally making no clear distinction between loss of all useful vision and blindness. The figure of five out of 165 cases[13] in whom there was no perception of light when the patient presented, is higher than in personal experience. The degree of visual impairment naturally depends on the time from onset when the patient was seen, given the natural tendency to improvement.[21] An acuity of between 6/36 and detection of hand movements is the most usual finding in patients seen about a week from the onset. An acuity of 6/6 or better may either indicate that recovery has occurred or simply reflect the inadequacy of the Snellen chart as a test of visual function.[22]

The optic disc is normal in appearance in approximately 50% of affected eyes examined soon after the onset, the criterion of retrobulbar neuritis. Slight blurring of the disc edge, particularly on the nasal side and often subject to disagreement between observers, is present in some 20–30%. Complete loss of the disc margins is seen in a further 15–20% and haemorrhages have been reported in very varied proportions, from 2%[21] to 16.7%[23] of the total, always associated with obscuration of the disc margins. The haemorrhages are linear, radiating from the disc. The fundal appearances are naturally not static, slight swelling being observed to progress to severe papillitis or, much more commonly, swelling is seen to subside over the course of several weeks. Perivenous sheathing has been reported in 6 of 50 patients specifically examined for vascular abnormalities.[24] If there have been previous attacks of optic neuritis, pallor of the disc may be evident.

In the great majority of affected eyes the visual field defect is either a central scotoma or generalised impairment of the whole field. The size of the scotoma of course varies with the stimulus used but is usually large, sometimes breaking through to the periphery in some section. Perkin & Rose[13] present examples of less usual defects, altitudinal, arcuate or even one example of peripheral constriction of the field, in addition to central defects extending to horizontal or altitudinal hemianopia. They also show an example of generalised diminution of vision in one eye with a small temporal scotoma in the other; a junctional defect indicating a plaque where the optic nerve joins the chiasma, involving the crossing fibres that form a loop in the ipsilateral nerve.

These results are in general conformity with those of other large reported series.[14,21,23,25,26] That only a small proportion of field defects differ greatly from the accepted central scotoma is not unexpected. Involvement of the central field by a plaque in the optic nerve is almost inevitable because of the large proportion of the fibres in the nerve that are concerned with central vision and their location in the centre of the nerve. Strategically placed small lesions could, at least in theory, avoid encroachment on these fibres, but peripheral constriction of the field is difficult to explain as an effect of multiple sclerosis and may occasionally be the result of other forms of disease of the optic nerve. Hutchinson[14] excluded from consideration cases without involvement of the central field, perhaps rather an extreme view, but avoiding possible confusion with conditions irrelevant to the investigation of the relation of optic neuritis to multiple sclerosis. Optic neuritis in childhood is discussed in Chapter 4.

The pupils

A lesion of the optic nerve may be expected to interrupt to some degree the afferent arc of the pupillary light reflex. In optic neuritis with gross loss of acuity the pupil is relatively dilated in approximately two thirds of cases and even with lesser degrees of visual loss the pupil may be larger. Simply observing the response of the pupil to a bright torch is an imprecise clinical gesture often leading to the conclusion that the reaction is 'sluggish'. The intriguing sign known as the Marcus Gunn pupil is more convincing. The torch shone into the normal eye causes bilateral pupillary constriction. When the light is rapidly switched to the abnormal eye the pupil is seen to be dilating after the consensual reaction from the other eye. The direct light reflex is impeded by the optic nerve lesion and the illusory effect is that of seemingly inducing pupillary dilatation. This sign is sometimes present when acuity has

returned to normal. It is now customary to talk of 'an afferent pupillary defect' but considerable caution is required in the interpretation of supposed minor degrees of abnormality of the direct light reflex.

Lhermitte et al[27] have described monocular blindness in a patient with multiple sclerosis with preservation of the direct and consensual light reflex of the pupil. No satisfactory explanation of this remarkable phenomenon was advanced.

Visual evoked potentials

In acute optic neuritis with severe reduction of acuity, no response to pattern reversal stimulation can usually be recorded although flash responses may be obtainable. Fixation is often difficult or impossible because of the central scotoma and the methods in general use do not stimulate the peripheral field from which some response might be obtained. With less severe loss of optic nerve function a greatly delayed low amplitude potential can sometimes be obtained. An absent or abnormal response is not, however, always found. Even in the acute stage while vision is still considerably impaired, although improving, a normal response is occasionally obtained.[7]

Recovery

It is the rule for good visual acuity to be regained after an initial attack of optic neuritis although there are unfortunate exceptions. The onset of improvement is difficult to time precisely as the patient may not be aware of a shrinking scotoma or a change from perception of hand movements to being able to read 6/60. Patients seen again two weeks after their first examination will almost invariably have made measurable recovery. The mean time to reach 6/6 vision, in those who achieved this, was 8 weeks in one series.[13] In another[21] 50% of patients had recovered to 6/6 or 6/9 by one month. Earl & Martin,[28] using a different criterion, found that optimal acuity was achieved after a mean of two months from onset. As these are mean figures, improvement can continue for considerably longer but at a decelerating rate. No further recovery can be expected after six months and in most cases improvement does not continue for more than three months from the onset.

Where neuritis of known or presumed other causes such as Leber's atrophy or ischaemic papillitis has been excluded, approximately 70–75% of eyes will recover 6/6 or 6/9 vision.[14,21] The prognosis for this degree of recovery has been found to be somewhat less good in patients over 45 in some series[28,29] while others have found no difference in the final result[13,21] although recovery may be slower.[21] The degree of initial visual loss does not appear to influence the prognosis, at least in a first attack. The proportion of patients left with vision worse than 6/12 is approximately 14% with less than 5% worse than 6/60.[13]

Recovery of normal visual acuity does not mean full recovery of function of the optic nerve, nor complete freedom from symptoms. Abnormal VEP may demonstrate persistent abnormalities of conduction and psychophysical tests may demonstrate disturbance of function fully sufficient to account for the common symptom of slight dulling of the visual image, apparently a lack of the normal contrast.[22] There may be a spontaneous complaint of lack of appreciation of the brightness of colours but colour blindness, even if demonstrable on testing, is seldom noticed by the patient.

Persistent intolerance of bright light, an occasional complaint, may be related to an inadequate pupillary reaction. Better vision at dusk[30] despite normal acuity indicates some persistent disturbance of function in fibres serving central vision (see Chapter 9).

Movement phosphenes[20] may occur in the acute stage of optic neuritis but in personal experience are much more common as fleeting symptoms during the later stages of recovery.

Uhthoff's phenomenon

Uhthoff in 1890[4] described temporary blurring of vision induced by exercise in patients with multiple sclerosis. The pathophysiology of this symptom and of the similar effects of heat on vision and other functions is discussed in Chapter 9. This may be the first and only indication of an optic nerve lesion in the absence of other evidence of optic neuritis, although the VEP may be abnormal. As usually encountered, violent exertion such

as playing squash induces monocular blurred vision, preventing continuation of the game and persisting for many minutes. In acute optic neuritis this effect is seldom noticed but it is common during the recovery stage. In one series[13] 11% of patients observed blurring on exertion but 20% claimed a similar effect of emotional disturbance. Menstruation, increased environmental temperature, eating a hot meal and smoking were other features observed. When severe and bilateral, Uhthoff's syndrome can be disabling.

Blurred vision after a hot bath may be a persistent symptom but Uhthoff's syndrome, exercise induced, usually slowly improves or patients learn to avoid it.

Residual signs

Temporal pallor of the optic disc, either as a sequel to recognised optic neuritis or as a sign of clinically silent optic nerve damage, is universally recognised. Unfortunately the detection of such pallor and its acceptance as a sign of disease is subject to a number of sources of error. The temporal half of the disc is normally paler than the nasal half. There is often a deep pale cup particularly in the temporal half of the disc. The disc in myopic eyes is pale. Even when all these factors have been discounted there is considerable observer disagreement. It is a common experience to be astonished at one's previous note of pathological temporal pallor when observing what appears to be a normal optic disc. With practice and stern resolve not to accept doubtful degrees of relative pallor the sign is undoubtedly useful but on no account should it be used in isolation as evidence of multiple lesions of the CNS.

Pallor of the whole optic disc is also commonly seen. The figures given for the proportion of patients with 'optic atrophy' are almost impossible to assess as much depends on definition and the standards adopted for the normal appearance of the disc. A common definition of optic atrophy in other conditions is that of visual impairment with pallor of the disc. Following optic neuritis, a pale disc may often accompany normal visual acuity. If atrophy is taken to mean simply disc pallor then this can be detected following a single episode of optic neuritis in approximately 50–60% of eyes.[13,26,31,32] There is no close relationship be-tween the presence or degree of optic nerve pallor and acuity. A pale disc is, however, present when there is severe permanent visual loss.

Sanders et al[33] examined various aspects of visual function in 53 patients examined at least 6 months after an attack of optic neuritis, bilateral in 8. Of the total of 106 eyes, 45 were not known to have been affected, 33 had recovered normal acuity and 28 had some degree of persistent visual loss and were recorded as 'not recovered'. Sub-clinical abnormalities were found in 43% of 'unaffected' eyes; in particular, 27% had impaired contrast sensitivity. The optic disc was judged to be pale in 76% of eyes that had recovered normal acuity. Vision in 30% of these eyes was subjective-ly fogged and colours appeared pale in 15%. All abnormalities were much more frequent in the presence of persistent loss of acuity, impaired con-trast sensitivity reaching 100%.

Persistent change in visual fields, colour vision and VEP are discussed in Chapters 8 and 9.

Persistent abnormality of the direct light reflex on ordinary clinical testing is relatively uncommon in most reported series. Perkin & Rose,[13] in con-trast, found an abnormal reaction in over 50% but their definition of abnormality was imprecise. Figures of between 10% and 20% are more usual.[32,34] Kirkham & Coupland,[35] using an in-genious method of examination, found that an abnormal pupillary reaction was the most constant sign of optic neuritis in the past in eyes with acuity of 6/12 or better, being found in 74%. A slit lamp beam was raised until it overlapped the lower margin of the pupil. The light reaching the retina caused pupillary constriction, thus cutting off the light and allowing pupillary dilatation. This self-perpetuating cycle was timed and was characteristically slowed in the majority of affected eyes.

The risk of developing multiple sclerosis

This is obviously a matter of the greatest practical importance. Anyone who rapidly and painfully loses the sight of one eye is entitled to ask what has happened and what is going to happen next. A young woman is seen with unmistakable unilateral optic neuritis with no other symptoms or signs. She wishes to marry, to insure her life to cover payments on a mortgage and to have children. Vision rapidly recovers and she is quite well. She surely cannot marry unless her future husband realises at least something of the future prospects. Life insurance companies will make en-quiries and to the girl's astonishment, refuse to accept her. A married childless woman may apply to adopt a baby but find her application rejected on the grounds of some half-forgotten episode of blurred vision. What can or should be said in such circumstances is highly individual to the patient and to the physician, but the factual basis for ad-vice must be available.

This has been remarkably difficult to establish. Ebers[36] has rehearsed the pertinent evidence for regarding isolated demyelinating optic neuritis as a *forme fruste* of multiple sclerosis. Optic neuritis is unduly common in the families of patients with multiple sclerosis.[37] The incidence[38] and sex dis-tribution of the two conditions are very similar. The changes in the CSF are often identical to those in multiple sclerosis, although oligoclonal bands of IgG are found in a smaller proportion.[39] MRI scanning at the time of presentation with optic neuritis has shown additional lesions in 61% of 35 patients.[9] It could not be claimed that every instance of isolated optic neuritis is a form of mul-tiple sclerosis as many other causes are known, including post-infective demyelination,[40] systemic lupus,[41] sarcoidosis[42] and syphilis,[43] for example. The pathology may well be different but it may not be possible to determine that this is so on clinical grounds. Ebers[36] and also Kahana et al[44] have accepted that recurrent optic neuritis is suf-ficient evidence of disseminated disease to warrant a clinical diagnosis of multiple sclerosis, provided of course, that no other cause is evident. These views are entirely rational and may well be correct, but they do not answer the patients' questions about the future: what are the risks of developing overt clinical multiple sclerosis and can the out-come be foretold?

The evidence up to 1985 has been critically, perhaps overcritically, reviewed by Kurtzke.[45] At first sight it would seem simple, although tedious, to follow a population of patients with optic neuritis to see how many of them develop multiple sclerosis. There are, however, many obstacles.

Diagnostic criteria for optic neuritis must be strictly defined as there are a number of sources of error (Ch. 6). The criteria for the diagnosis of multiple sclerosis have not been standardised, some surveys including possible or even latent cases in varying proportions.[46-49] The majority of surveys have been retrospective, based on discovering the subsequent course of patients who have been recorded as attending hospital with optic neuritis. Dependence on other peoples' notes of patients' recollections is apt to be unreliable. There have been very few attempts at population surveys. The length of follow-up necessary to obtain useful information almost invariably leads to failure to trace an important proportion of patients.

Kurtzke, in his penetrating review,[45] detected flaws in many of the published series and his tables, derived from these series, make a clear distinction between the proportion of those patients traced who developed multiple sclerosis and the proportion of *the whole-series* who did so. He was inclined to reject as almost certainly erroneous all studies that claimed over 40% of patients progressing to multiple sclerosis, without regard to the length of follow-up. Some of these reports must certainly be suspected of errors of selection or reporting. McAlpine's[50] statement that in Lynn's[51] series 85% of those followed for more than 5 years had progressed was never subsequently repeated or published in detail. Hutchinson[14] and also probably Rischbeith[18] included established cases of multiple sclerosis with a history of initial optic neuritis. Haller et al,[52] who claimed 80% progression within 2 years, have not published detailed results. Nikoskelainen & Riekkenen[47] (56% progression), Nikoskelainen et al[53] (75%) and Perkin & Rose[13] (58%) included some patients who already had signs of disseminated disease. Bradley & Whitty,[48] who reported progression in 52% of traced patients and 41% of all cases, conducted a retrospective study. Kurtzke[45] objected to this series as derived from a single hospital and therefore not of wide application. Landy[54] found in a prospective study 54% progression in all cases and in 62% of those traced but admitted cases with simultaneous optic neuritis and disseminated symptoms.

Kurtzke was rather less unhappy with studies reporting progression rates between 30% and 40%[15,26,49,55,56] but placed most reliance on those with even lower figures.[57-59] He makes a strong point when contrasting the results of population studies with those from hospital or clinic. For instance, Kinnunen[38] in an area of Finland found progression in 19% of traced patients and in 17% of the whole series over a mean of 9 years. The district he studied was contiguous with that from which extremely high figures had been obtained in hospital series.[53,60] Percy et al[60] found 17% progression over a mean of 18 years in the population of Rochester, but a higher figure of 32% had earlier been reported for patients attending the Mayo Clinic.[61] Alter et al[62] in Hawaii and Kahana et el[44] in Israel found somewhat higher figures of 29% and 26% respectively, but they both included recurrent optic neuritis as multiple sclerosis. The lowest reported proportion of progression to multiple sclerosis was that of Kurland et al[17] who found only 13% of 138 cases after a prolonged follow-up of from 12–18 years. Kurtzke[45] suggested that this might be considered as equivalent to a population survey but this claim is difficult to sustain for a study confined to males.

Since Kurtzke's critique there have been further significant contributions, the most important being an extension of the admirable prospective study of Cohen et al.[15] In the original report, 60 of 67 patients diagnosed as having optic neuritis of unknown cause were followed for at least 5 years, a mean of 7.1 years. Optic neuritis was fully defined and was bilaterally simultaneous in two patients. Two patients originally accepted were later diagnosed as having neuroretinitis, which is not thought to be related to multiple sclerosis.[63,64] The authors were clearly alert for symptoms or signs of pre-existing multiple sclerosis, as 42 such patients were rejected. During the follow-up period 28% developed definite and 7% probable or possible multiple sclerosis. The combined figure of 35% would, of course, be reduced to 31% if all those who refused follow-up had proved not to have multiple sclerosis.

Six patients who had not developed multiple sclerosis by 1977 died before the further follow-up survey in 1985,[65] evidence suggesting that these patients had not developed disseminated disease. All but one of the surviving 54 subjects were either examined or contacted. A further 14 were found to have progressed to multiple sclerosis, the proportion of traced cases to have progressed being 58%, and of the total series 52%. A much higher risk of multiple sclerosis in females noted in the original study was confirmed: 69% of women and 33% of men had progressed. A higher risk of progression in women had previously only been reported by Kinnunen.[38] These findings may well be relevant to the very low progression rate in the all-male series of Kurland et al.[17]

Francis et al[66] have reported an extended follow-up of the series originally described by Compston et al.[49] This was not a prospective study, the subjects being derived from a survey of clinical records. In the first report, 58 of 146 patients had developed multiple sclerosis, in various categories of diagnostic certainty from definite to latent, after a follow-up period ranging from 1 month to 23 years, with a mean of 47 months. The date of the original attack of optic neuritis was apparently sometimes derived from the patient's recollection. On further follow-up after a mean period of 11.6 years, of the 88 patients who had uncomplicated optic neuritis in the original report 21 were lost, 24 had progressed to multiple sclerosis and 43 were still classified as isolated optic neuritis. The total known to have progressed was 82 of the original 146 patients but, certainly in the first report, latent multiple sclerosis was diagnosed on the strength of abnormal sensory or auditory evoked potentials, in the absence of clinical evidence of disseminated disease. No doubt a number of the untraced patients had also developed multiple sclerosis, but the observed progression rate was 56%. The authors believed that their figures approximated to the 85% progression of Lynn's series[50,51] but this calculation was based on the proportion of traced cases rather than that of the total series. A number of risk factors were assessed but the sex distribution of the patients was not mentioned.

In a prospective study of 82 patients followed for a mean of 57 months, Hely et al[67] found that 32% had progressed to multiple sclerosis, again with a higher risk in females. It is not stated whether these comprised all patients with isolated optic neuritis seen between 1975 and 1983 or only those that could be traced. The range of follow-up

extended to 22 years and must, in some cases, have been dated from an earlier unobserved episode of optic neuritis.

A prospective study from Japan[16] contained a high proportion (45%) of bilateral and presumably simultaneous optic neuritis and the age ranged from 5 to 69 years, both factors that might reduce the risk of progression (see below). Only 7 of 84 (8.3%) cases had progressed to multiple sclerosis after a mean follow-up period of 5.2 years. The proportion of those progressing after unilateral optic neuritis can be calculated as 13%.

The results of a number of studies have been subjected to actuarial analysis, permitting prediction beyond the mean follow-up period. Hutchinson[14] calculated a 77.8% risk of multiple sclerosis within 15 years of optic neuritis, but this series was affected by entry bias and, according to Kurtzke[45] contained an arithmetical error, the correct figure being 67%. Hely et al[67] predicted 47% progression within 7 years. Rizzo & Lessell[65] calculated that in their series 74% of the women and 33% of the men would have developed multiple sclerosis within 15 years and Francis et al[66] predicted 75% progression in the same period. In a population based study Kinnunen[38] calculated 38% progression in 9 years in an area of Finland with a high risk of multiple sclerosis, and 24% in a medium risk area.

Kurtzke[45] has pointed out that as the numbers become smaller, particularly as a result of untraced cases, the precision of actuarial analysis is much reduced. Nevertheless, the observed proportion of cases of optic neuritis progressing to multiple sclerosis on prospective follow-up in those of European stock is consistently much higher than that found in population surveys. Problems of case selection and ascertainment are no doubt responsible, but the conflicting figures do not provide a very sound basis for advice to individual patients. Those who seek advice are naturally patients attending a clinic with isolated optic neuritis and it is from such patients that nearly all the data have been derived. It seems realistic, therefore, to conclude that the higher predictive figures are more likely to be applicable in this context than Kurtzke's[45] more hopeful prognostication that only approximately one third will ever develop multiple sclerosis. Which answer enshrines the 'true'[68] picture remains uncertain.

Time relationships

If isolated optic neuritis in the absence of other detectable cause is accepted as the initial episode of multiple sclerosis it must be expected that the interval before the first relapse will show great variation. This interval certainly ranges from a few weeks to recorded instances of over 20 years[69,70] or even 37 years[71] but it would be useful if some pattern could be detected. To be able to say that after so many years of freedom from evidence of widespread disease the risk was reduced to some small percentage would be of practical value. As might be expected from the differing criteria and standards of the largely retrospective studies already discussed, no very clear guidance can be given.

The preponderance of admittedly somewhat flawed evidence originally suggested that if definite multiple sclerosis is to follow optic neuritis, it will do so more commonly, or even much more commonly, within the first four or five years. In some series, indeed, no further cases have developed after this period[60,55] even with prolonged follow-up. Hyllested[72] found that all 'serious' cases became apparent within this period and in Bradley & Whitty's[48] much more detailed report, virtually all definite cases had also occurred within the first four years, but probable cases continued to be diagnosed for two decades.

In a prospective study, Landy[54] found that the risk of progression was much higher in the first 2 years, while 92% of those who progressed in the prospective study of Hely et al[67] did so within 4 years, but the follow-up period was relatively brief. Cohen et al[15] found that no patient developed multiple sclerosis more than 6 years from the onset of optic neuritis, but in the later review of this series,[65] multiple sclerosis continued to develop at an approximately steady rate. This was also found by Hutchinson[14] and in the serial follow-up reports of Compston et al[49] and Francis et al.[66] An increase in the proportion of patients who have developed multiple sclerosis over the years, as earlier indicated by McAlpine[50] and by

Taub & Rucker[61] certainly occurs, but on balance, probably at a declining rate.

Other prognostic factors

In most reports the sex of the patient with isolated optic neuritis does not influence the prognosis for the development of multiple sclerosis[48,67] but, as already noted, Rizzo & Lessell[65] and Kinnunen[38] found a much higher risk in women.

There is also disagreement over the effect of age. In all series the numbers of patients over 45 or 50 with optic neuritis are small and the figures are not amenable to statistical treatment. There is also an increasing risk of diagnostic confusion with ischaemic papillitis. Optic neuritis over the age of 50 can certainly herald the onset of multiple sclerosis[48] but in personal experience very rarely does so. Optic neuritis between the ages of 21 and 40 was found by Cohen et al[15] and by Hely et al[67] to be significantly more likely to be followed by multiple sclerosis, confirmed by further follow-up.[65]

There is no indication that any other clinical feature of an attack of optic neuritis can be related to subsequent multiple sclerosis. Laterality,[67] pain,[48] acuity and degree of recovery,[15,17,48] character of visual field change and the appearance of the optic disc[15] all appear to be without relevance. A possible effect of race resulting in a lesser risk in Japanese[16] has already been referred to.

The month of onset of optic neuritis has also been considered significant, but evidence is conflicting. Taub & Rucker[61] found that optic neuritis in the summer months was more than twice as dangerous as onset between November and March and a similar difference in the seasons was found by Hutchinson[14] (see also Ch. 4). No increased risk of developing multiple sclerosis from optic neuritis in any specific season was noted by Kurland et al,[17] Perkin & Rose[13] or Bradley & Whitty.[48] In Japan the winter months carried a worse outlook[16] but numbers were small. Compston et al[49] found that the combination of optic neuritis in the winter with the determinant BT101 predisposed to subsequent multiple sclerosis.

The time scale of multiple sclerosis has so far prevented full evaluation of the predictive value of laboratory investigations. Using evoked potentials, blink reflex, high dose contrast CT scanning and CSF examination, Feasby & Ebers[8] found evidence of at least one unsuspected lesion in 27 of 36 patients with optic neuritis, but whether these findings foretold multiple sclerosis is not known. Sanders et al[73] similarly investigated 30 patients. Abnormalities were found in 16, including 6 with abnormal scans. No follow-up was reported. Sandberg-Wollheim[59] examined the CSF in 61 patients with optic neuritis, of whom 51% showed pleocytosis, 41% oligoclonal IgG and 18% increased IgG. After a mean follow-up period of 2.6 years, 11 patients had progressed to multiple sclerosis, of whom 5 had originally shown pleocytosis and oligoclonal bands. Nikoskelainen et al[53] carried out a similar investigation but apparently only 28 of their cases had isolated idiopathic optic neuritis and the results in these cases are not reported separately. They concluded, however, that increase in IgG and oligoclonal bands were strong risk factors for progression to multiple sclerosis.

The results reported by Stendahl-Brodin & Link[56] are much more clear-cut. They found that 11 of 30 patients with optic neuritis had CSF oligoclonal IgG. Six years later, 9 of these patients had developed multiple sclerosis, while only 1 of the 19 who had not shown oligoclonal bands had done so. Moulin et al,[39] when considering the predictive value of CSF electrophoresis, included 33 cases of optic neuritis, 10 with oligoclonal bands and 23 without. They did not present separate figures for optic neuritis but indicated that the rate of progression to multiple sclerosis was similar to that in the whole series and was much more frequent if oligoclonal bands had been found.

Magnetic resonance imaging has shown silent lesions in a high proportion of patients with isolated optic neuritis, but follow-up has been necessarily brief. None of those with MRI abnormalities had progressed to multiple sclerosis in the series reported by Jacobs et al[10] and only one in that of Johns et al.[11] In a more extensive study[74] serial scans were performed on 53 patients with isolated optic neuritis, 34 of whom showed abnormalities on the first scan. Over a mean of 12 months, 12 of these developed disseminated clinical disease and a further 7 showed new lesions on MRI without clinical relapse. In contrast, none of the 19 patients in whom MRI was initially normal relapsed, although in 3 patients, new lesions were seen on MRI. The other end of the scale is illustrated by the report[75] of 10 patients who had presented with unilateral optic neuritis 9–14 years earlier, and who had developed no further signs of disease. MRI showed changes of multiple sclerosis in 4, and 3 patients had bilateral abnormalities of visual evoked potentials.

It is unfortunately plain that while positive findings on examination of the CSF and CT or MRI scanning increase the probability of progression to clinical multiple sclerosis, the possibility of progression cannot be ruled out by normal results in these investigations.

Bilateral optic neuritis

Involvement of both optic nerves in rapid succession has been regarded by some authorities as being too atypical for inclusion in series of optic neuritis.[17] There is little reason for such exclusion and difficulties of definition arise. Cohen et al[15] include two cases of 'simultaneous' bilateral optic neuritis. If this means that the effects of acute optic neuritis in each eye overlapped in time, this is certainly not at all unusual at the onset or during the course of multiple sclerosis. The precisely simultaneous *onset* of optic neuritis is, however, quite rare and, particularly if symmetrical, would justify some diagnostic circumspection. It is, however, obviously important to know whether bilateral concurrent visual failure from optic neuritis or any other combination of bilateral defect carries a worse or indeed a better prognosis for the eventual development of multiple sclerosis. Arbitrary periods between episodes must be chosen and have varied from two weeks[14] to three months.[21] The category of bilateral and sequential used by Compston et al[49] is difficult to distinguish from recurrent optic neuritis if no time interval is specified, and the term 'simultaneous' is not further detailed. As it is known that the apparently unaffected optic nerve is sometimes already abnormal in the complete absence of symptoms,[7] the definition of bilateral optic neuritis becomes increasingly obscured.

The frequency of isolated bilateral optic neuritis as variably defined naturally bears no relationship to the frequency of overt episodes later in the course of the disease. Early reports suggested that bilateral examples were very rare[76,77] and recently Perkin & Rose[13] only observed one example in their 148 cases. This has not, however, been general experience. Bradley & Whitty reported 19.2% of cases becoming bilateral within 3 months.[21] Hely et al[67] found bilateral optic neuritis, defined as both eyes being affected within 4 weeks, in 9 of 82 patients. Hutchinson[14] reported that 19% of 144 patients had bilateral optic neuritis within 2 weeks. From Japan, bilateral involvement, apparently concurrent, was present in no less than 45.2%.[16]

It is difficult to detect any possible influence of bilateral optic neuritis on subsequent development of multiple sclerosis. Kurland et al[17] and Bradley & Whitty[21] found no such effect, while Hutchinson[14] found a somewhat increased risk. In the small number of Japanese cases observed to develop multiple sclerosis after isolated optic neuritis, this was bilateral in only one patient, despite the relatively greatly increased incidence of bilateral involvement.[16] There is, therefore, certainly no strong evidence that bilateral concurrent optic neuritis is particularly liable to herald multiple sclerosis. It is indeed possible that the reverse is true. Bilateral truly simultaneous optic neuritis occurs in acute disseminated encephalomyelitis, which cannot with certainty be regarded as identical with multiple sclerosis in view of the rarity of relapse.

Heirons & Lyle[78] reviewed a series of bilateral optic neuritis in adults and children and a further report on the great majority of these patients was published 25 years later.[79] Of the 6 adults with acute simultaneous bilateral optic neuritis, one had died of 'neuromyelitis optica' and one had been thought to have early probable or latent multiple sclerosis but died from cerebrovascular disease at the age of 76. The remainder had not developed multiple sclerosis. Of the 7 with progressive simultaneous bilateral neuritis, one developed multiple sclerosis. Only 2 of these patients regained normal vision. Of 20 adults with sequen-

tial bilateral neuritis within 3 months, 2 were lost to follow-up and one was excluded on mistaken diagnosis. Seven had been diagnosed as having multiple sclerosis. In contrast, Hutchinson[14] found that bilateral simultaneous optic neuritis increased the risk of multiple sclerosis, while recurrent attacks did not.

Recurrent optic neuritis

Overt optic neuritis can occur or recur at any stage of multiple sclerosis although more commonly before a progressive stage is reached. The significance of recurrent optic neuritis in the absence of other signs of disease is of interest with respect to the risk of developing multiple sclerosis, the other important question being that of the risk to vision. In published accounts the distinction between bilateral consecutive and recurrent optic neuritis is not always sharply drawn. Bradley & Whitty[21] deliberately excluded further episodes affecting the same eye from the category of recurrent neuritis, but even with this proviso found on follow-up a recurrence rate of 19%. It is not, however, clear how many of these occurred after the appearance of other evidence of multiple sclerosis. Hutchinson's[14] recurrence rate was 24%. Perkin & Rose[13] obtained a past history of earlier attacks of optic neuritis in 30 of their cases seen in a second or subsequent attack but it is not clear how many of these patients already had overt multiple sclerosis. By far the most common combination was that of a single episode in each eye, this being so in 14 cases. A further 8 patients had experienced two separate episodes in the same eye. In the remaining 8, multiple attacks had occurred, in 1 patient no less than eight. From this material it was obvious that more than one attack affecting the same optic nerve reduced the chance of obtaining 6/9 vision to approximately 60%. Almost identical figures were found by Hutchinson.[14] Full recovery of visual acuity is possible after multiple attacks of neuritis affecting the same eye[80] but pallor of the optic nerve head is usually present.

Recurrent optic neuritis is regarded by Ebers[36] as justifying a diagnosis of multiple sclerosis and was originally reported in two series[15,49] as increasing the risk of progression to disseminated disease.

In extended study of these two series[65,66] the increased risk was not, however, confirmed, in conformity with other series.[14,67]

Progressive visual failure

Progressive visual failure in multiple sclerosis is poorly documented. It was recorded in 7 of 52 patients with visual symptoms and in 25 of 185 patients with evidence of optic nerve involvement in two series.[31,81] Ashworth[82] reported 9 cases of chronic optic neuritis and in 2 of the 3 cases described in detail, the diagnosis of multiple sclerosis seems assured. In 2 patients an earlier episode of acute optic neuritis had been followed by recovery, with subsequent progressive loss of vision. Matthews & Small[5] recorded decline in visual acuity in 19 eyes in 51 patients over a period of 2–42 months (mean 18 months). In only 7 eyes could this be related to a recognisable episode of optic neuritis. No detailed longitudinal study appears to have been published, although a great deal of relevant data must be available.

Progressive visual failure as the presenting feature of multiple sclerosis has been carefully documented by Ormerod & McDonald.[83] In the five cases described the onset was unilateral, but after a variable interval the other eye was also affected, usually before the appearance of disseminated symptoms. The possibilities of diagnostic error were emphasised and are discussed in Chapter 6.

Severity of multiple sclerosis following optic neuritis

The possible and disputed relation of early or initial symptoms of the disease to ultimate prognosis is discussed in Chapter 5. Onset with optic neuritis has been variously reported as affecting prognosis adversely,[84] as linked to a benign course[77,85,86] or being without effect.[87,88] Wikström et al[6] and Sanders et al[89] considered that the initial course following optic neuritis was benign but that no long term difference could be detected. The latter attributed this effect to the relatively long symptom-free remission after optic neuritis, which occurred on average 5 years earlier than other presenting symptoms. The most impressive comparison is that

between McAlpine's[50,90] patients with unrestricted and restricted mobility on prolonged follow-up. Of the former, 37% had presented with optic neuritis, not always isolated. Of those presenting with optic neuritis alone, 57% were unrestricted, as opposed to 27% presenting in some other form, assessed after a similar period. Comparisons have been drawn with the much higher rates of disability reported in other series[91] but these are unrealistic. If optic neuritis is to be shown to be associated with any particular course of multiple sclerosis, comparison should be with patients with other forms of *monosymptomatic* onset, not affecting mobility: diplopia, facial myokymia, trigeminal neuralgia or purely sensory symptoms, for example.

Conclusion

Only partial answers can be given to the questions posed by optic neuritis. In the absence of other discoverable cause, optic neuritis is almost certainly due to a plaque of multiple sclerosis. The chances of multiple lesions developing are less if optic neuritis occurs in childhood, especially if bilateral. Multiple sclerosis is also less likely to become overt with optic neuritis after the age of 50, perhaps because of faulty diagnosis. The risk of multiple sclerosis is probably greatest during the first five years after optic neuritis but some risk persists, perhaps indefinitely. The risk to vision is much greater with recurrent attacks. There are objections to all these statements but I suspect that optic neuritis differs from other attacks of multiple sclerosis only in being more obtrusive and more easily recognised.

OTHER LESIONS OF THE VISUAL PATHWAYS

The retina

Atrophy of retinal nerve fibres in multiple sclerosis has been detected by Frisén & Hoyt[92] in patients without visual symptoms. This may be attributed to subclinical axonal degeneration in the optic nerve. Sharpe & Sanders[93] observed demyelination of myelinated retinal nerve fibres in one case, which they also attributed to retrograde axonal degeneration from the optic nerve lesion. Whether the neural apparatus of the retina is more directly involved in multiple sclerosis is uncertain. McDonald[94] considered the possibility that the prolonged latency of the VEP might be due in part to synaptic delay in the retina.

The electroretinogram (ERG) in multiple sclerosis has been investigated by a number of observers with conflicting results. Feinsod et al[95] found abnormalities of amplitude, either increased or reduced, in some patients and Paty et al[96] also found occasional enhanced potentials. This finding is traditionally attributed to loss of central inhibitory impulses and does not imply intrinsic retinal disease. Ikeda et al[97] found no increase in latency of the ERG. This was confirmed by Coupland & Kirkham[98] but only in patients with no history of optic neuritis. In those with a history of visual involvement, the mean ERG latency was prolonged but there was much overlap with normal values. These authors suggested the possibility of transynaptic retinal degeneration.

Plant et al[99] discussed these varied results, which are greatly influenced by the technique employed. Using pattern stimulation, they found no evidence of a lesion more peripheral than the site of origin of the ERG, presumed to be the ganglion cell layer of the retina.

The chiasma

The optic chiasma is a common site of multiple sclerosis plaques and it is not surprising that characteristic visual field changes are occasionally found. That these are not more frequent is probably explained by the multiplicity of lesions of the anterior visual pathway.

Sacks & Melen[100] described bitemporal hemianopia in three patients with presumed multiple sclerosis. In their first case the clinical evidence for the diagnosis was acceptable and the field defect cleared in two patients. The patients were naturally investigated to exclude any cause of chiasmal compression. Spector et al[101] described six patients with evidence of a chiasmal lesion and presumed multiple sclerosis. Field defects varied from bitemporal hemianopia to bitemporal scotomata or evidence of a junctional lesion. They recom-

mended visual field testing of the apparently unaffected eye in optic neuritis and evaluation of central fields with a red objective. Their patients were women with relatively minor evidence of multiple sclerosis. The prognosis for recovery of vision was good. Ashworth[82] described one patient with progressive visual loss as the first symptom in whom the bitemporal scotomata indicated a chiasmal lesion. Such changes should only be accepted as due to multiple sclerosis after exhaustive investigation.

Hemianopia

Homonymous hemianopia is surprisingly rare in multiple sclerosis considering how commonly plaques occur in the optic radiation. The paper by Savitsky & Rangell[102] is an excellent example of the difficulties encountered in attempting to confirm that an unusual symptom is in fact caused by multiple sclerosis. They found no example of homonymous hemianopia in 50 observed and verified personal cases nor in 415 clinical cases. Hemianopia did not occur in 217 reported verified cases of multiple sclerosis. In a detailed review, alternative or additional diagnoses were indicated for the few published examples. The case of Hawkins & Behrens[103] is clinically acceptable and convincing CT scanning evidence for a plaque in an appropriate site, associated with hemianopia, was presented by Beck et al[104] in three patients.

In personal experience homonymous hemianopia has only been seen in acute relapse, associated with other evidence of involvement of the cerebral hemisphere (see Ch. 2).

Ocular movements

Subclinical abnormalities of ocular movement may be detected by specific tests in a high proportion of patients with multiple sclerosis, as described in Chapter 8. Clinical symptoms and signs of involvement of the oculo-motor system are also very common. Representative figures for diplopia reported at the onset are 13% by Müller[91] and Poser[105] and 11% in British and 8% in Japanese patients[106] but 22% in the US Army series.[107] As an isolated symptom it is also common at the onset.

In the course of the disease, diplopia has been recorded in 35%,[108] 38%[91] and in 39% in British and 35% in Japanese cases.[106] Poser[105] and Kurtzke[107] found rather lower figures of 20% and 19% respectively. In many series diplopia is included in such terms as 'ocular disturbance' or 'brainstem symptoms' and not recorded separately.

Diplopia, in what proves to be the onset of the disease, may not be accompanied by any ocular palsy detectable on ordinary clinical examination. Usually, however, there is either a VIth nerve palsy or some elements of an internuclear palsy. An isolated IIIrd nerve palsy should not immediately suggest a diagnosis of multiple sclerosis[109] but has been observed at the onset.[110] Isolated IVth nerve palsy has not been described. In acute relapse VIth nerve palsy is again common. Persistent diplopia is usually a symptom of internuclear ophthalmoplegia, but patients often refer to oscillopsia as 'seeing double'. Ptosis is rare in multiple sclerosis, being reported in 5% in one series[111] and complete ptosis I have never seen. Partial bilateral ptosis may occur in relapse, affecting the brainstem and Horner's syndrome may also occur (p. 100).

Uhthoff[4] first observed an essential feature of internuclear ophthalmoplegia, that the internal rectus muscle may not act on lateral movement of the eye but does so on convergence. Wilson[112] gave a clear description of the full syndrome, with weakness of each internal rectus and nystagmus on lateral gaze limited to the abducting eye. This disturbance of ocular movement has been attributed to a lesion in the medial longitudinal fasciculus interrupting fibres running from the VIth to the IIIrd nerve nucleus and thus disrupting conjugate gaze.

Internuclear ophthalmoplegia is a common phenomenon in multiple sclerosis. Cogan[113] claimed that when unilateral it was nearly always due to infarction of the brainstem and that in multiple sclerosis it was characteristically bilateral. This is not borne out in clinical practice as the unilateral type is also commonly found in multiple sclerosis.[107] Incomplete forms also occur frequently. Adduction may appear to be full but there is nystagmus of the abducting eye — the so-called ataxic nystagmus. The defect of adduction may be confined to relative slowness of movement.[114] Muri & Weinberg[115] describe detailed clinical methods of detecting the various elements of internuclear palsy. Of 100 consecutive patients with definite multiple sclerosis attending a rehabilitation centre examined in this way, 34 were found to have internuclear ophthalmoplegia, 14 bilateral and 20 unilateral. Sixteen patients had full adduction but with delayed saccades. Persistent dissociated nystagmus was found in only one patient.

The presence of this form of ocular palsy is strong presumptive evidence of multiple sclerosis but it is not pathognomonic. Bilateral internuclear ophthalmoplegia may occur in conditions that could well be mistaken for multiple sclerosis including the Chiari malformation and brainstem and IVth ventricular tumours.[114,116,117] Cogan et al[118] found that in multiple sclerosis the symptoms most commonly associated with internuclear palsy were trigeminal neuralgia, optic neuritis, homonymous field defects, depression and facial palsy. These observations suggest a highly specialised practice.

Other forms of defective conjugate gaze are less common and less distinctive. They include paresis of lateral and upward gaze.[91,119] Bilateral paralysis of voluntary lateral gaze with normal eye movement on caloric vestibular stimulation has been ascribed to multiple sclerosis lesions in the pons.[120] Midbrain lesions may cause complex abnormalities of ocular movement including paralysis of upgaze, vertical nystagmus, convergence spasm and convergence-retraction nystagmus.[121] Multiple sclerosis is the commonest cause of the one-and-a-half syndrome in which there is gaze palsy to one side and internuclear palsy to the other,[122] due to a lesion in the tegmentum of the pons ipsilateral to the gaze palsy.[123]

Internuclear ophthalmoplegia may remit completely in the early stages of the disease. It is present to some degree, without causing symptoms, in many chronic cases of multiple sclerosis.

Nystagmus is a classical sign of multiple sclerosis but in reported series is seldom separated from other brainstem signs. Shibasaki et al[106] found nystagmus present at the time of reporting in 56% of British and 50% of Japanese cases. The commonest form is that of symmetrical horizontal gaze nystagmus with the fast movement directed towards the periphery. This can sometimes be difficult to distinguish from the effects of fatigue, lack of co-operation or the normal tendency of the eyes to drift towards the centre when held in extreme lateral gaze. Nystagmus of this type should not be held to be abnormal, particularly in the sense of indicating multiple lesions of the CNS, unless it is consistently present in the field of binocular gaze.

Many other forms of nystagmus are encountered in multiple sclerosis of which some merit more detailed description. Jelly nystagmus[124] is normally only detectable on inspection of the fundus with an ophthalmoscope when the optic disc can be seen to be jerking rapidly from side to side over a small range. This should not be confused with the other form of nystagmus sometimes first seen when looking at the fundus — latent nystagmus.[125] This condition, where nystagmus only occurs when one eye is covered, as by the ophthalmoscope, has no known relation to CNS disease.

Sharpe et al[126] described convergence-induced nystagmus in multiple sclerosis and showed that it could be distinguished from the congenital form by being dysjunctive with the eyes moving in opposite directions. Most forms of nystagmus in multiple sclerosis are jerking in type but pendular nystagmus also occurs,[127] being found in 25 of 644 cases. It was strongly correlated with head tremor, and was thought to be due to impaired cerebellar function.

Keane[128] described the rare condition of periodic alternating nystagmus with downward beating nystagmus in a case of rapidly fatal multiple sclerosis. Plaques in the floor of the IVth ventricle were thought to be responsible. Nystagmus does, of course, accompany prolonged episodes of vertigo in multiple sclerosis. Oscillopsia may not be complained of even in the presence of severe nystagmus. It may accompany vertical nystagmus when it can be a severe disability if exacerbated by downward gaze. It is present in pendular nystagmus[127] and in convergence-induced nystagmus.[126]

THE TRIGEMINAL NERVE

Trigeminal neuralgia is described on page 64.

Paralysis of the motor division of the Vth nerve in multiple sclerosis is described by Oppenheim[129] but I have never seen this.

Numbness of the face frequently accompanies the more widespread symptoms of a predominantly sensory relapse. Sensory loss may be difficult to detect and the corneal reflex is usually normal. Isolated persistent facial numbness is unlikely to be due to multiple sclerosis and should be remembered as a symptom of systemic lupus erythematosus. Marked loss of facial sensation may occur in severe brainstem attacks.

THE FACIAL NERVE

Facial palsy

Facial weakness is listed in virtually every general account of the clinical features of the onset or course of multiple sclerosis. There is reasonable agreement on the frequency of facial weakness at the onset. In the US Army series[130] this was present in 2.1%. Leibowitz & Alter[131] recorded 4% with facial weakness at the onset, Müller[91] 5%, Shibasaki et al[106] 2% in British and 3% in Japanese cases, Hung et al[132] 4% (1 case) in Taiwan, Bonduelle & Albaranès[133] 4.8% and Kelly[134] 1.4%. The reported frequency of facial weakness in the course of the disease has been far more varied: 2.6% in the US Army series,[130] 11%,[7] 14.4%,[135] 10%.[105,133] In the series confirmed at autopsy,[108] facial weakness had been observed at some point in no less than 52%.

Despite these figures indicating that facial weakness is a relatively common finding in multiple sclerosis, there is a remarkable lack of clear clinical description. It is almost certain that different authors have adopted different criteria. For example, the 52% of patients with facial weakness reported by Carter et al[108] do not appear to have had acute facial palsy. It is seldom possible to determine whether the facial palsies listed have actually been observed or merely reported by the patients. Upper motor and lower motor neurone forms of palsy are usually not distinguished. Facial palsy has been claimed to be an early isolated symptom.[133,136,137] The incidence of idiopathic Bell's palsy is not exactly known but is certainly much more than ten times that of multiple sclerosis. A minute description of how, if at all, facial palsy as the initial symptom of multiple sclerosis, differs from the idiopathic condition is obviously needed.

Ivers & Goldstein[137] personally observed lower motor neurone facial palsy in 3 patients, in 2 of whom it was the initial event. In a further 4 patients, 'Bell's palsy' had occurred in the past. Bonduelle & Albaranès[133] provided more details: 15 of the 145 patients had sustained facial palsy, sometimes recurrent. The palsy was always 'périphérique' and sudden or rapid in onset. The descriptive term presumably does not imply a lesion of the peripheral portion of the nerve, as in all but two instances facial palsy was accompanied by other cranial nerve palsies, usually ocular. Sense of taste was not mentioned. Recovery was good with only slight sequelae, again not described in detail. Thygesen[138] remarked that facial weakness in multiple sclerosis was usually slight and that, unless accompanied by ocular palsies, it was often difficult to determine whether it was upper or lower motor neurone in type. McAlpine[139] stated that absence of pain, preservation of taste and usually rapid recovery distinguish the facial palsy from the idiopathic form but none of these features is in any way distinctive.

In extensive experience I have not seen an example of facial palsy convincingly attributable to multiple sclerosis that might be mistaken for idiopathic Bell's palsy. Evidence of facial palsy in the past with faulty reinnervation shown by synkinesis is certainly encountered, as indeed in the population without multiple sclerosis. Facial palsy can now be investigated in some detail: EMG, neuronography, gustatometry, stapedius reflex, enquiry into subjective loss of taste or hyperacusis, impaired salivation and lacrymation and the detection of sequelae. As occasion arises these techniques should be applied to facial weakness in multiple sclerosis.

Taste

Decrease or loss of sense of taste on one or both sides of the tongue is an occasional complaint.

Kahana et al,[140] in a study of cranial nerve lesions, found one example of loss of taste in 295 patients. McAlpine[139] observed that this complaint was common in patients with paraesthesiae or loss of sensation on the face, and isolated examples of this have been described as an incidental finding.[141–143] The apparent association with trigeminal rather than facial nerve involvement may be partially explained by the frequent use by patients of the word 'numbness' to describe weakness, stiffness or other abnormalities, particularly of the face. Detailed testing of taste in these patients is not reported. As noted above, it is difficult to find full descriptions of facial palsy resulting from multiple sclerosis. In one such report, for example,[144] where taste was lost on the side of the palsy, the diagnosis of multiple sclerosis was far from certain and the facial palsy was probably due to herpes zoster.

Cohen[145] described a patient whose probable multiple sclerosis was preceded by two episodes of loss of taste, but at the time of examination taste was normal.

Catalanotto et al,[146] using an extremely sophisticated test, found that patients with multiple sclerosis were significantly less sensitive to the tastes of salt and quinine, but not to those of sucrose or citric acid. They did not consider that these strange findings were reflected in recognisable symptoms.

Facial hemispasm

This phrase is used imprecisely. Bonduelle & Albaranès,[133] however, leave no doubt that of their 6 cases of facial hemispasm, 3 were post-paralytic and presumably synkinesis. In their other 3 cases there was no preceding palsy and the spasm was of short duration, of eight days to one month. It was observed in only one case and the description given is specifically that of facial myokymia and not of facial hemispasm or clonic facial spasm, as usually implied. The facial hemispasm reported in three cases by Thiébaut et al[147] also did not follow facial palsy but is difficult to interpret. The EMG as illustrated was not that of facial myokymia.

Myokymia

The term 'myokymia' has been used to describe a

number of different forms of rapidly flickering muscular contraction, being first applied to benign fasciculation of the calf muscles.[148] Facial myokymia is, in most instances, a highly distinctive condition, although minor degrees may be difficult to recognise. The association with multiple sclerosis was observed by Oppenheim[149] and by Kino[150] but attracted little attention until the later reports of Andermann et al[141] and Matthews.[151] The condition is briefly described in Chapter 8 where its possible pathogenesis is considered.

When occurring as a symptom of multiple sclerosis or as an isolated event, the onset is sudden and can usually be dated precisely by the patient although a few fail to notice any abnormality. The complaint is of 'stiffness' of the face so that certain movements may be difficult to perform, although there is no weakness. Patients in the habit of observing their own reflections in the glass can detect that the face is 'drawn up' on the affected side; the palpebral fissure is slightly narrowed and the naso-labial fold deepened. Flickering in the muscles is not always remarked. There is no pain.

Slight contraction, apparently of all the muscles of one side of the face, is accompanied by extraordinarily rapid flickering that passes over the face in undulating waves too fast and complex for visual analysis. Only when an episode is subsiding can there be any possibility of confusion with the benign myokymia of the eyelids that commonly occurs in fatigue.

The EMG findings are described on p. 238.

Facial myokymia is not pathognomonic of multiple sclerosis and was first reported as a sign of an intrinsic brainstem tumour by Lambert et al.[152] In 1979 Waybright et al[153] reviewed published reports of 50 cases of which 31 were thought to have multiple sclerosis and 15 pontine glioma, in the remaining cases myokymia occurring as an isolated event. They added a further 14 cases: 8 having multiple sclerosis and 2 tumours in the posterior fossa. They also described myokymia in the Guillain-Barré syndrome with facial palsy, an unexpected finding with a presumed peripheral lesion. They also reported the first autopsy on a patient with myokymia and a pontine glioma. The nucleus of the facial nerve was not involved in the tumour but loss of corticobulbar fibres was considered as a possible causative factor, as already postulated by Sethi et al.[154] No autopsy on a patient with multiple sclerosis and myokymia has been reported.

It is obviously important to be able to distinguish facial myokymia due to multiple sclerosis from that due to brainstem tumour. In multiple sclerosis or presumed multiple sclerosis, where myokymia is an isolated symptom, remission nearly always occurs within a week to six months, but this distinction is not absolute as prolonged myokymia has been described in multiple sclerosis.[109] Recurrent attacks of myokymia sometimes occur after a long interval. If facial weakness is present with myokymia the cause is unlikely to be multiple sclerosis. I have not seen simultaneous involvement of both sides of the face in multiple sclerosis but each side may be affected in rapid succession.[151]

Facial myokymia is a relatively minor symptom but nobody likes having an even mildly distorted face. I have not found that it responds to carbamazepine but some improvement can be obtained with clonazepam.

THE AUDITORY NERVE

Deafness as a symptom of multiple sclerosis has been regarded as unusual but unless bilateral or obtrusive, may be overlooked or discounted. That remitting or persistent deafness can occur was recognised by Hess[155] and by Oppenheim[129] and Beck[156] compared transitory deafness to the visual symptoms of multiple sclerosis. There have been many isolated case reports but the topic of overt deafness in multiple sclerosis was reviewed by Daugherty et al.[157] They described hearing loss in 9 patients but did not indicate what proportion of their patients this represented. Deafness formed part of the initial episode in 4 patients but in 1 occurred 11 years after the onset. Hearing loss was bilateral in 2 patients. It was accompanied by tinnitus in four patients and by vertigo in three. Brainstem or cerebellar signs were present in all patients and were often severe.

Despite the complaint of deafness, this was not always easy to demonstrate. Pure tone audiograms were abnormal in 7 patients without any specific pattern. Other tests were performed in the majority of the patients, including the acoustic reflex decay, word discrimination, binaural fusion and dichotic sentence testing. It seems that no test was abnormal in all 9 patients and it is difficult to determine from the description which test was abnormal in any particular patient. Brainstem auditory potentials were abnormal in 6 of the 7 patients examined. Improvement in hearing was noted in 7 patients but the period of observation was evidently brief.

Fischer et al[158] described the acute onset of deafness in 10 patients, unilateral in 8 and bilaterally simultaneous or consecutive in 2. Seven patients had tinnitus and 5 had vertigo. Most had extensive signs of more widespread disease, especially of the cerebellum, but in 2 patients the auditory symptoms occurred in isolation. Hearing was restored within 3 months. The authors[159] were surprised that in 2 cases, Wave 1 of the auditory evoked potential was absent, suggesting a peripheral lesion, if the presumed origin of this wave is correct.

In personal experience, unilateral or bilateral deafness, evidently due to a brainstem lesion, is rapid or even sudden in onset and is followed by remission.

The detection of concealed hearing loss as a sign of MS has been hampered by the frequency with which this is also found in control subjects. Von Leden & Horton[160] compared 100 cases of multiple sclerosis with 100 controls and found some degree of hearing loss in 46 of the former and 18 of the latter. There was marked dissociation between any complaint of deafness and the abnormalities found. Dayal & Swisher[161] found abnormalities of pure tone threshold in 59% of patients with multiple sclerosis but also in 27% of matched controls. Apart from patients with overt deafness, multiple sclerosis has little effect on pure tone thresholds,[162] but hearing loss, specifically for shifts of tone frequency,[163] may be detected. This may account for the occasional complaint of difficulty in hearing speech with normal conventional audiometry.[164]

Hearing loss due to bilateral temporal lobe lesions has been described in multiple sclerosis by Tabira et al.[165] Apparently total deafness was accompanied by normal brainstem auditory potentials but virtually absent cortical potentials. With recovery of hearing, the evoked potentials reverted to normal.

THE VESTIBULAR SYSTEM

Acute vertigo is not uncommon in the initial episode of multiple sclerosis, sometimes as an isolated symptom, and it may occur during relapse. In the absence of any agreed definition of vertigo its frequency cannot be more precisely stated, as dizziness, giddiness and unsteadiness are not clearly distinguishable from tables of symptoms.

In its most unpleasant form, vertigo in multiple sclerosis is of acute onset and is prostrating. On lying perfectly still it may subside but is immediately aggravated by any movement of the head. Vomiting is frequent and walking, when attempted at all, is extremely unsteady. Nystagmus is seen and is also increased by head movement. There is no mistaking this condition for some form of nonspecific dizziness. An acute attack of this kind is indistinguishable from 'vestibular neuronitis' unless there are other signs of CNS involvement. The duration of the attack is variable, from a few days to several weeks.

A curious feature is the frequency with which vertigo is a symptom in the rare cases of multiple sclerosis with onset of symptoms in childhood.[166]

Other forms of evident vertigo, as opposed to less definitely recognisable sensations affecting equilibrium, occur in multiple sclerosis. Postural vertigo, induced by getting out of bed,[167] may be coincidental when it exactly resembles the common benign form.

In patients with multiple sclerosis not specifically selected because of a history of vertigo, caloric vestibular reactions are often abnormal, the frequency depending to a large extent on the interpretation. Thus Noffsinger et al[168] found 7% of unilateral canal paresis and 11% directional preponderance using the Hallpike and Fitzgerald method in which nystagmus is observed visually. Using electronystagmography interpreted by Jongkee's formula, a very much higher proportion of abnormal results was obtained including hyperexcitability in 48%. In patients who proved to have multiple sclerosis specifically referred for neuro-otological investigation, presumably highly selected for symptoms and signs of brainstem disorder, Aantaa et al[169] found abnormal caloric reactions in 32 out of 50 but did not remark on hyperexcitability.

Grénman[170] exhaustively investigated vestibular and auditory function and eye movement control in 70 mildly disabled multiple sclerosis patients and found abnormalities, especially of smooth pursuit, in nearly all. Caloric vestibular reactions were abnormal in 40%. It was concluded that completely normal results in the extensive battery of tests employed would be against the diagnosis of multiple sclerosis. Any relation of these abnormalities to actual symptoms or overt signs was not clearly stated.

BRAINSTEM LESIONS

Plaques involving the brainstem may occasionally produce acute life-threatening symptoms[171] of which the following case of the locked-in syndrome is an example.

A woman of 41 was admitted with a five-day history of illness beginning with hiccough and vomiting, followed by diplopia, numbness of the face and arm, vertigo, tinnitus and headache. She then became dysarthric, deaf in both ears and developed right-sided weakness. She continued to deteriorate and within a further four days had become quadriplegic, mute, totally deaf, as far as could be judged, and unable to swallow. Vertical eye movement was preserved. Pupils became constricted and she developed periodic respiration but she was conscious as she could imitate eye movements. She did not require assisted ventilation, however, and in the course of the next six weeks made a spontaneous partial recovery. She was emotionally labile and had slight restriction of lateral gaze. She was ambulant with some persistent weakness and ataxia of all limbs. The plantars remained extensor. The CSF contained between 15 and 30 lymphocytes/mm³ and a total protein of 0.25 g/l, of which 22% was IgG. CSF electrophoresis was not available at that time. Extensive investigation excluded as far as possible vascular causes for this illness. There was a past history of weakness of both legs for a period of three weeks three years before her severe illness. Some six months after leaving hospital she had a further episode of weakness of both legs so that she was unable to walk. The tendon reflexes were increased and plantars extensor.

The diagnosis of multiple sclerosis is highly probable in this case and the locked-in syndrome with partial recovery has been described in multiple sclerosis with eventual confirmation of the diagnosis.[172] That even with such a severe lesion of the lower brainstem she did not require assisted ventilation lends support to Kurtzke's view[107] that respiratory paralysis, fatal or otherwise, in multiple sclerosis is seldom or never due to involvement of the respiratory centre but to paralysis of respiration resulting from a cervical cord lesion. Even in fatal cases it may be difficult to attribute respiratory failure to specific lesions. For example, in the rapidly fatal case of bulbar paralysis reported by Guillain & Alajouanine,[173] a plaque was also found in the cervical spinal cord. Convincing temporary paralysis of automatic respiration has, however, been reported in proven multiple sclerosis.[174]

Bonduelle & Albaranès[133] mention that a lateral medullary syndrome may occur in multiple sclerosis and I have seen an example of this.

Dysphagia is relatively uncommon in ambulant patients with multiple sclerosis. In patients affected to the point of helplessness, the ability to swallow may be lost and survival is an indication of the level of nursing care.

Persistent hiccough as a symptom of multiple sclerosis has been described in three patients[175] all of whom had symptoms and signs of lesions involving the brainstem but also more widespread disease. Lack of descending inhibitory impulses was the suggested mechanism. Carbamazepine proved extremely successful treatment in one case. Hiccough accompanied by vomiting as the first symptom of multiple sclerosis and attributed to a brainstem lesion has also been described.[176]

THE AUTONOMIC NERVOUS SYSTEM

The bladder

By far the most important disturbance of autonomic function in multiple sclerosis is loss of bladder control. Of 297 cases examined by Miller et al,[177] 78% had experienced such symptoms at some time and in 52% they had persisted for more than 6 months at the time of examination. Of these cases, 60% had urgency of micturition and 50%

frequency; 10% had been incontinent and 2% had suffered from recurrent retention. In a personal series of 377 patients, at the time of last examination, 96 had urgency and 22 hesitancy of micturition; 75 were troubled by incontinence. During the earlier course of the disease, 138 had experienced urgency and 91 had been incontinent. Hesitancy was common, but retention requiring catheterisation was only occasional. Such figures are naturally dependent on the stage at which the patients are examined. Bladder symptoms at the onset were present in only 13 patients.

These impersonal figures give but a pale indication of the impact of disordered bladder function on the patients' lives. Isolated episodes of retention or incontinence may occasionally be recognised in retrospect as the first evidence of the disease. The common story, however, is for urgency of micturition to occur in even mild relapses involving the spinal cord. If there is remission, bladder function is restored, but with persistent mild motor disability, urgency also persists. Leaving the home involves constant awareness and anxiety about the distance from the nearest lavatory. Only small quantities of urine are passed and urgency may be very uncomfortably accompanied by hesitancy. Frequency is usual. Typically, persistent urgency leads to incontinence, fear of an 'accident', often restricting the activity of ambulant patients. Nocturia may cause serious sleep deprivation and, in the disabled, exhaustion from struggling out of bed several times each night. Nocturnal enuresis eventually ensues.

With increasing disability, the nature of the incontinence changes, large quantities of urine being passed without warning and, in those confined to bed or chair, sometimes without sensation, leading to a final state of continuous dribbling. Acute retention can occur at any stage of the disease but usually resolves, although recurrence is common.

In general terms, the degree of bladder disorder is related to the severity of signs of motor and sensory impairment[178] and total disability, but there are many exceptions. Parity has been identified as a significant risk factor for incontinence in women.[179] At the onset it is possible that acute bladder symptoms may present without other signs of disease but persistent incontinence as an isolated feature is very unlikely to be due to multiple sclerosis.

The relation of these symptoms to disordered function and what can be attempted in mitigation are discussed in Chapter 9.

The bowel

Faecal incontinence or urgency is relatively uncommon, although extremely distressing. Constipation is common in advanced disease. This is probably not simply some presumed non-specific effect of inactivity. Glick et al[180] have demonstrated absence of the normal post-prandial increase in colonic motility in advanced multiple sclerosis. They demonstrated by means of somatosensory evoked potential recordings that the peripheral sensory pathways were intact, but not those of the CNS, a not unexpected finding.[181] Distension of the lower bowel is uncomfortable and may occasionally lead to grotesque abdominal bloating. A loaded rectum may also appear to interfere with bladder function.

Paralysis of gastric function[182] and functional pyloric obstruction[183] have been described in multiple sclerosis, both presenting with vomiting, and in one case as the initial symptom. Vomiting in multiple sclerosis is usually an accompaniment of vertigo or headache in acute relapse.

Sexual function

Erectile impotence was a symptom in 44% of patients examined by Miller et al.[177] When judged to be due to multiple sclerosis, erectile impotence was always associated with impaired bladder function. In most general accounts of the symptoms of multiple sclerosis, sexual function, of great significance to the patients, is barely mentioned or concealed under 'autonomic' disorder. It is naturally often difficult to determine whether impotence is psychogenic or physical in origin and sexual function in women is notably difficult to evaluate. It may be suspected, however, that full enquiry is often neglected and that patients are in any case reluctant to discuss such matters with a doctor who may show little interest. This is unfortunate, as effective treatment for both neurogenic and psychogenic impotence is now available (Ch. 9).

The question arises as to whether impotence in the absence of any other clinical evidence of multiple sclerosis can be the initial symptom of the disease. Although impotence is usually associated with prolonged disease it can certainly occur in the first episode, even when this is not severe. I am doubtful whether it occurs in complete isolation.

Vas[184] investigated impotence in some detail. He assessed 37 men with multiple sclerosis on two occasions a year apart. All patients were mobile. On the first examination 21 were normally potent, 13 partially and three totally impotent. A year later there had been slight changes in these figures, but sufficient to show that total impotence can remit although only in one case. There was a clear relationship of impotence with sphincter disturbance and also with duration of the disease. The bulbocavernosus reflex was usually absent. Vas also related sexual function to sweating. In men totally impotent, thermoregulatory sweating was absent below the waist. In partial impotence sweating was usually absent below the groin. These findings were confirmed almost exactly by Cartlidge.[185]

Sexual dysfunction in women with multiple sclerosis is less well documented. Lundberg[186] conducted a detailed investigation of 25 women with multiple sclerosis producing little disability and compared the results with those in matched controls suffering from migraine. Of the multiple sclerosis patients, 13 had major sexual problems; loss of libido was usually associated with alteration of genital sensation, often transitory. Difficulties probably related to disordered autonomic function were less evident but lack of vaginal secretion occurred in 3.

In a study of 74 ambulant patients and matched controls,[187] sexual function in those over 50 years of age was not very different in the two groups. Of the patients under 50, 48% of the men and 44% of the women had serious sexual problems and in 20% sexual activity had stopped altogether. In men, erectile impotence was the main problem, but difficulties of ejaculation and orgasm were also common. In women, lack of lubrication and failure of orgasm predominated, and in both sexes fatigue and sensory defects were important. These difficulties were not related to age, duration of disease or degree of motor disability but were strongly correlated with disordered function of bladder and bowel and with a frequent and unexplained complaint of coldness of the legs.

Sweating

Partial loss of thermoregulatory sweating was found in 20 of 50 patients examined by Cartlidge[185] and 23 of 60 by Noronha et al.[188] In the latter series there were two patients who could not be induced to sweat at all by the methods used, including intravenous pilocarpine. In two patients sweating occurred only on the face. Despite these severe abnormalities, spinal reflex sweating that can be induced in paraplegic patients by bladder disturbance did not occur in the seven patients investigated, presumably indicating surviving spinal cord function.

Cardiovascular reflexes

There have been a number of detailed controlled studies of cardiovascular reflexes in multiple sclerosis.[189-191] Abnormalities can be found in a number of tests: response to deep breathing, exercise, the Valsalva manoeuvre, hand grip and assuming the upright posture. No consistent pattern can be discerned, however, and there is no correlation with disturbance of bladder function. The abnormalities found appear to be entirely symptomless. The only patient in these series who suffered from syncope was found not to have postural hypotension[191] and, in contrast to the effects of spinal cord trauma, this is rarely a problem in multiple sclerosis, but may occur in acute relapse affecting the brainstem.[192]

More alarming cardio-respiratory problems are occasionally reported with brainstem lesions from probable or clinically definite multiple sclerosis. Paroxysmal atrial fibrillation has accompanied a pontine lesion demonstrated by MRI.[193] Other abnormalities in patients with lesions of the pons or medulla have included acute pulmonary oedema and transient hypertension with bradycardia of 40 per minute.[192]

Horner's syndrome

Bamford et al[194] described Horner's syndrome, localised by pharmacological means to a lesion of central or intermediate sympathetic fibres, in three clinically definite cases of multiple sclerosis. They did not comment on the possibility of recovery. Although in the title of their paper they refer to Horner's syndrome as being 'unusual' in multiple sclerosis they stated that it occurs in from 2–3% of their patients.

The hypothalamus

The possible involvement of the hypothalamus in multiple sclerosis has been relatively neglected, particularly in view of the frequent localisation of plaques around the third ventricle. Kamalian et al[195] described a patient who presented with rapid unexplained weight loss accompanied by numbness of one arm and leg. Her condition rapidly deteriorated until her death less than two years from the onset. She was found to have multiple sclerosis including plaques in the lateral hypothalamus, considered likely to be the cause of her emaciation. Bignami et al[196] described a different syndrome of acute depression, organic mental changes and hyperthermia related to acute multiple sclerosis plaques found to be involving the whole of the hypothalamus.

Apple et al[197] described a patient with presumed but atypical multiple sclerosis in whom inappropriate secretion of antidiuretic hormone occurred during an acute attack involving headache, vomiting, weakness and total blindness. The serum sodium fell to 109 mEq/l although she was not dehydrated. On salt supplementation and steroids, vision began to improve in 48 hours, but few subsequent details are given.

Fever

Fever now seldom receives any mention as a feature of multiple sclerosis, but in descriptions of the disease from the last century, episodes of hyperpyrexia were regarded as characteristic. For example, Loomis[198] mentioned high fever associated with loss of consciousness and Bristowe[199] claimed that the temperature might rise to 109°F (43.8°C). By the time Kinnier Wilson[200] wrote his textbook, however, such extravagant ideas were no longer mentioned but a mild degree of fever during relapse was regarded as common. It is doubtful how much attention is now paid to this aspect in what are, in areas of high prevalence, regarded as routine relapses. In China, however, where multiple sclerosis is probably rare and individual episodes are evidently more closely observed on this account, fever in excess of 41°C was recorded for up to three months during acute episodes in 3 of 57 cases and minor rises in temperature were common.[201]

It is, of course, probable that some episodes of hyperpyrexia, particularly those recorded from the last century, have been due to septicaemia from urinary infection. However, Castaigne et al[202] have reported repeated episodes of coma and hyperpyrexia, sometimes with nuchal rigidity, in the absence of detectable infection. These attacks lasted for one or two days. The diagnosis was confirmed at autopsy in one case. The authors were more concerned with the disturbance of consciousness than with the fever and believed that plaques involving thalamo-tegmental connections might be responsible.

CONCLUSION

No account of the symptoms and signs of multiple sclerosis can be more than selective and incomplete. The extraordinary variety of clinical features is well illustrated by the most recent report of multiple sclerosis discovered accidentally at autopsy.[203] Twelve cases were evenly divided between those in whom no neurological symptoms had ever been recorded, those with gross signs in whom a diagnosis of multiple sclerosis had never even been considered and those in whom multiple sclerosis had been considered but rejected. The clinical indications must be recognised before sophisticated diagnostic techniques can be applied or understood.

A complaint is often expressed that descriptions of the clinical features of multiple sclerosis are 'anecdotal'. This is certainly true but is scarcely avoidable, the anecdotes being case histories and the presumably preferred statistical approach no more than a collection of such histories. Clinical medicine is inevitably and rightly anecdotal.

REFERENCES

1. Ansari K A 1976 Olfaction in multiple sclerosis. European Neurology 14: 138–145
2. Pinching A 1977 Clinical testing of olfaction reassessed. Brain 100: 377–388
3. Parinaud H 1884 Troubles oculaires de la sclérose en plaques. Journal de la Santé Publique 3: 3–5
4. Uhthoff W 1890 Untersuchungen über die bei der multiplen Herdsklerose vorkommenden Augenstörungen. Archiv für Psychiatrie und Nervenkrankheiten 21: 55–116 and 303–410
5. Matthews W B, Small D G 1979 Serial recordings of visual and somatosensory evoked potentials in multiple sclerosis. Journal of the Neurological Sciences 40: 11–21
6. Wikström J, Poser S, Ritter G 1980 Optic neuritis as initial symptom in multiple sclerosis. Acta Neurologica Scandinavica 61: 178–185
7. Matthews W B, Small D G, Small M, Pountney E 1977 Pattern reversal evoked visual potential in the diagnosis of multiple sclerosis. Journal of Neurology, Neurosurgery and Psychiatry 40: 1009–1010
8. Feasby T E, Ebers G C 1982 Risk of multiple sclerosis in isolated optic neuritis. Canadian Journal of Neurological Science 9: 269
9. Ormerod I E C, McDonald W I, Du Boulay G H et al 1986 Disseminated lesions at presentation in patients with optic neuritis. Journal of Neurology, Neurosurgery and Psychiatry 49: 124–127
10. Jacobs L, Kinkel P R, Kinkel W R 1986 Silent brain lesions in patients with isolated idiopathic optic neuritis. Archives of Neurology 43: 452–455
11. Johns K, Lavin P, Elliot J H, Partain C L 1986 Magnetic imaging of the brain in isolated optic neuritis. Archives of Ophthalmology 104: 1486–1488
12. Lyon-Caen O, Jouvert R, Hauser S et al 1986 Cognitive function in recent-onset demyelinating disease. Archives of Neurology 43: 1138–1141
13. Perkin G D, Rose F C 1979 Optic neuritis and its differential diagnosis. Oxford University Press, Oxford
14. Hutchinson W M 1976 Acute optic neuritis and the prognosis for multiple sclerosis. Journal of Neurology, Neurosurgery and Psychiatry 39: 283–289
15. Cohen M M, Lessell S, Wolf P A 1979 A prospective study of the risk of developing multiple sclerosis in uncomplicated optic neuritis. Neurology 29: 208–213
16. Isayama Y, Takahashi T, Shimoyoma T, Yamadori A 1982 Acute optic neuritis and multiple sclerosis. Neurology 32: 73–76
17. Kurland L T, Beebe G W, Kurtzke J F et al 1966 Studies on the natural history of multiple sclerosis. 2. The pogression of optic neuritis to multiple sclerosis. Acta Scandinavica 42 (suppl 19): 157–176
18. Rischbieth R H C 1968 Retrobulbar neuritis in the state of South Australia. Proceedings of the Australian Association of Neurologists 5: 573–575
19. Rawson M D, Liversedge L A 1966 Treatment of acute retrobulbar neuritis with corticotrophin. Lancet 2: 1044–1046
20. Davis F A, Bergen D, Schauf C, McDonald W I, Deutsch W 1976 Movement phosphenes in optic neuritis: a new clinical sign. Neurology 26: 1100–1104
21. Bradley W G, Whitty C W M 1967 Acute optic neuritis: its clinical features and their relation to prognosis for recovery of vision. Journal of Neurology, Neurosurgery and Psychiatry 30: 531–538
22. Reagan D, Silver R, Murray T J 1977 Visual acuity and contrast sensitivity in multiple sclerosis — hidden visual loss. Brain 100: 563–579
23. Nikoskelainen E 1975 Symptoms, signs and early course of optic neuritis. Acta Ophthalmologica 53: 254–272
24. Lightman S, McDonald W I, Bird A C, Francis D A, Hoskins A, Batchelor J R, Halliday A M 1987 Retinal venous sheathing in optic neuritis. Its significance for the pathogenesis of multiple sclerosis. Brain 110: 405–414
25. Marshall D 1950 Ocular manifestations of multiple sclerosis and relationship to retrobulbar neuritis. Transactions of the American Ophthalmological Society 48: 487–525
26. Hyllested K, Møller P M 1961 Follow-up of patients with a history of optic neuritis. Acta Ophthalmologica 39: 665–662
27. Lhermitte F, Guillaumat L, Lyon-Caen O 1984 Monocular blindness with preserved direct and consensual pupillary reflex in multiple sclerosis. Archives of Neurology 41: 993–994
28. Earl C J, Martin B 1967 Prognosis in optic neuritis related to age. Lancet 1: 74–76
29. Sandberg H O 1972 Acute retrobulbar neuritis — a retrospective study. Acta Ophthalmologica 50: 3–8
30. Carroll F D 1940 Retrobulbar neuritis. Observations on one hundred cases. Archives of Ophthalmology 24: 44–54
31. Kahana E, Leibowitz V, Fishback N, Alter M 1973 Slowly progressive and acute visual impairment in multiple sclerosis. Neurology 23: 729–733
32. Nikoskelainen E 1975 Later course, prognosis of optic neuritis. Acta Ophthalmologica 53: 273–291
33. Sanders E A C M, Volkers A C W, van der Poel J C, van Lith 1986 Estimation of visual function after optic neuritis: a comparison of clinical tests. British Journal of Ophthalmology 70: 918–924
34. Rosen J A 1965 Pseudoisochromatic visual testing in the diagnosis of disseminated sclerosis. Transactions of the American Neurological Association 90: 283–284
35. Kirkham T H, Coupland S G 1981 Multiple regression analysis of diagnostic predictions in optic nerve damage. Canadian Journal of Neurological Sciences 8: 67–72
36. Ebers G C 1985 Optic neuritis and multiple sclerosis. Archives of Neurology 42: 702–704
37. Ebers G C, Cousin H K, Feasby T E, Paty D W 1981 Optic neuritis in familial multiple sclerosis. Neurology 31: 1138–1142
38. Kinnunen E 1983 The incidence of optic neuritis and its prognosis for multiple sclerosis. Acta Neurologica Scandinavica 68: 371–377
39. Moulin D, Paty D W, Ebers G C 1983 The predictive value of cerebrospinal fluid electrophoresis in 'possible' multiple sclerosis. Brain 106: 809–816
40. Miller D H, Kay R, Schon F, McDonald W I, Haus L F, Hughes R A 1986 Optic neuritis following chickenpox in adults. Journal of Neurology 233: 182–184
41. Dutton J J, Burde R M, Klingele T G 1982 Autoimmune retrobulbar optic neuritis. American Journal of Ophthalmology 94: 11–17
42. Piéron R, Coulaud J M, Debure A, Mafart Y,

Lesorbre B 1979 Névrite optique et sarcoïdose. Semaine des Hopitaux 55: 137–139

43. Graveson G S 1950 Syphilitic optic neuritis. Journal of Neurology, Neurosurgery and Psychiatry 13: 216–224

44. Kahana E, Alter M, Feldman S 1976 Optic neuritis in relation to multiple sclerosis.

45. Kurtzke J F 1985 Optic neuritis or multiple sclerosis. Archives of Neurology 42: 704–710

46. Rose F C 1970 The aetiology of optic neuritis. Clinical Science 39: 17P

47. Nikoskelainen E, Riekkenen P 1974 Optic neuritis — a sign of multiple sclerosis or other diseases of the central nervous system. A retrospective study of 116 patients. Acta Neurologica Scandinavica 50: 690–718

48. Bradley W G, Whitty C W M 1966 Acute optic neuritis: prognosis for development of multiple sclerosis. Journal of Neurology, Neurosurgery and Psychiatry 31: 10–18

49. Compston D A S, Batchelor J R, Earl C J, McDonald W I 1978 Factors influencing the risk of multiple sclerosis developing in patients with optic neuritis. Brain 101: 495–512

50. McAlpine D 1964 The benign form of multiple sclerosis: results of a long-term study. British Medical Journal 2: 1029–1032

51. Lynn B 1959 Retrobulbar neuritis. A survey of the present condition of cases occurring over the last fifty six years. Transactions of the Ophthalmological Societies of the United Kingdom 50: 262–267

52. Haller P, Patzold U, Eckert G 1980 Optic neuritis in Hannover: an epidemiologic and serogenetic study. In: Bauer H J, Poser S, Ritter G (eds) Progress in multiple sclerosis research. Springer, Berlin, pp 546–548

53. Nikoskelainen E, Frey H, Salmi A 1980 Prognosis of optic neuritis with special reference to cerebrospinal fluid immunoglobulins and measles virus. Annals of Neurology 9: 545–550

54. Landy P J 1983 A prospective study of the risk of developing multiple sclerosis in optic neuritis in a tropical and subtropical area. Journal of Neurology, Neurosurgery and Psychiatry 46: 659–661

55. Collis W J 1965 Acute unilateral retrobulbar neuritis. Archives of Neurology 13: 409–412

56. Stendahl-Brodin L, Link H 1983 Optic neuritis: oligoclonal bands increase the risk of multiple sclerosis. Acta Neurologica Scandinavica 67: 301–304

57. Appen R E, Allen J C 1974 Optic neuritis under 60 years of age. Annals of Ophthalmology 6: 143–146

58. Tatlow W F T 1948 The prognosis of retrobulbar neuritis. British Journal of Ophthalmology 32: 488–497

59. Sandberg-Wollheim M 1975 Optic neuritis: studies on the cerebrospinal fluid in relation to clinical course in 61 patients. Acta Neurologica Scandinavica 52: 167–178

60. Percy A K, Nobrega F T, Kurland L T 1972 Optic neuritis and multiple sclerosis. Archives of Ophthalmology 87: 135–139

61. Taub R G, Rucker C W 1954 The relationship of retrobulbar neuritis to multiple sclerosis. American Journal of Ophthalmology 32: 488–497

62. Alter M, Good J, Okihiro M 1973 Optic neuritis in Orientals and Caucasians. Neurology 23: 631–639

63. Maitland C G, Miller N R 1984 Neuroretinitis. Archives of Ophthalmology 102: 1146–1150

64. Parmley V C, Schiffman J S, Miller N R, Dreyer R F, Hoyt W F 1987 Does neuroretinitis rule out multiple sclerosis? Archives of Neurology 44: 1045–1048

65. Rizzo J F, Lessell S 1988 Risk of developing multiple sclerosis after uncomplicated optic neuritis: a long-term prospective study. Neurology 38: 185–189

66. Francis D A, Compston D A S, Batchelor J R, McDonald W I 1987 A reassessment of the risk of multiple sclerosis developing in patients with optic neuritis after extended follow up. Journal of Neurology, Neurosurgery and Psychiatry 50: 758–765

67. Hely M A, McManis P G, Doran T J, Walsh J C, McLeod J G 1986 Acute optic neuritis: a prospective study of risk factors for multiple sclerosis. Journal of Neurology, Neurosurgery and Psychiatry 49: 1125–1130

68. Mcdonald W I 1983 The significance of optic neuritis. Transactions of the Ophthalmological Societies of the United Kingdom 103: 230–246

69. Adie W J 1930 Acute retrobulbar neuritis in disseminated sclerosis. Transactions of the Ophthalmological Societies of the United Kingdom 50: 262–267

70. Mackay R P 1953 Multiple sclerosis: its onset and duration. Medical Clinics of North America 37: 511–521

71. McAlpine D, Compston N 1952 Some aspects of the natural history of disseminated sclerosis. Quarterly Journal of Medicine 21: 135–167

72. Hyllested K 1966 On the prognosis of retrobulbar neuritis. Acta Ophthalmologica 44: 246–252

73. Sanders E A C M, Reulen J P H, Hogenhuis L A H 1984 Central nervous system involvement in optic neuritis. Journal of Neurology, Neurosurgery and Psychiatry 47: 241–249

74. Milier D H, Ormerod I E C, McDonald W I et al 1988 The early risk of multiple sclerosis after optic neuritis. Journal of Neurology, Neurosurgery and Psychiatry 51: 1569–1571

75. Kinnunen E, Larsen A, Ketonen L, Koskimies S, Sandström A 1987 Evaluation of central nervous system involvement in uncomplicated optic neuritis after prolonged follow-up. Acta Neurologica Scandinavica 76: 147–151

76. Adie W J 1932 The aetiology and symptomatology of disseminated sclerosis. British Medical Journal 2: 997–1000

77. McIntyre H D, McIntyre A P 1943 Prognosis of multiple sclerosis. Archives of Neurology and Psychiatry 50: 431–438

78. Heirons R, Lyle T K 1959 Bilateral retrobulbar neuritis. Brain 82: 56–67

79. Parkin P J, Hierons R, McDonald W I 1984 Bilateral optic neuritis: a long-term follow up. Brain 107: 951–964

80. Scott G I 1961 Ophthalmic aspects of demyelinating diseases. Proceedings of the Royal Society of Medicine 54: 38–42

81. Schlossman A, Phillips C C 1954 Optic neuritis in relation to demyelinating disease. American Journal of Ophthalmology 37: 487–494

82. Ashworth B 1957 Chronic retrobulbar and chiasmal neuritis. British Journal of Ophthalmology 51: 698–702

83. Ormerod I E C, McDonald W I 1984 Multiple sclerosis presenting with progressive visual failure. Journal of Neurology, Neurosurgery and Psychiatry 47: 943–946

84. Poeck K, Markus P 1964 Gibt es eine gutartige Verlaufsform der multiplen Sklerose? Münchener Meizinischer Wochenschrift 106: 2190–2197

85. Kraft G H, Freal J E, Coryell J K, Hanan C L, Chitnis N 1981 Multiple sclerosis: early prognostic guidelines. Archives of Physical Medicine and Rehabilitation 62: 54–58

86. Poser S, Raun N E, Poser W 1982 Age at onset, initial symptomatology and the course of multiple sclerosis. Acta Neurologica Scandinavica 66: 355–362

87. Shepherd D J 1979 Clinical features of multiple sclerosis in north-east Scotland. Acta Neurologica Scandinavica 60: 218–230

88. Leibowitz U, Alter M 1968 Optic nerve involvement as initial manifestation of multiple sclerosis. Acta Neurologica Scandinavica 44: 70–80

89. Sanders E A C M, Bollen E L E M, van der Velde E A 1986 Presenting symptoms and signs in multiple sclerosis. Acta Neurologica Scandinavica 73: 269–272

90. McAlpine D 1972 In: Multiple sclerosis: a reappraisal. Churchill Livingstone, Edinburgh, p 215

91. Müller R 1949 Studies on disseminated sclerosis with special reference to symptomatology, course and prognosis. Acta Medica Scandinavica 133 (suppl 222): 1–214

92. Frisén, Hoyt W F 1974 Insidious atrophy of retinal nerve fibres in multiple sclerosis: funduscopic identification in patients with and without visual complaints. Archives of Ophthalmology 92: 91–97

93. Sharpe J A, Sanders M A 1975 Atrophy of myelinated nerve fibres in the retina in optic neuritis. British Journal of Ophthalmology 59: 229–232

94. McDonald W I 1977 In: Desmedt J E (ed) Visual evoked potentials in man: new developments. Oxford University Press, London, pp 427–437

95. Feinsod M, Abramsky O, Auerbach E 1973 Electrophysiological examination of the visual system in multiple sclerosis. Journal of the Neurological Sciences 20: 161–175

96. Paty J, Brenot Ph, Henry P, Faure J M A 1976 Potentials évoqués visuels et sclérose en plaques. Revue Neurologique 132: 605–621

97. Ikeda H, Tremain K E, Sanders M D 1978 Neurophysiological investigation in optic nerve disease: combined assessment of the visual evoked response and electroretinogram. British Journal of Ophthalmology 62: 227–239

98. Coupland S G, Kirkland T H 1982 Flash electroretinogram abnormalities in patients with multiple sclerosis. Canadian Journal of Neurological Sciences 9:325–330

99. Plant G T, Hess R F, Thomas S J 1986 The pattern evoked electroretinogram in optic neuritis: a combined psycho-physical and electrophysiological study. Brain 109: 469–490

100. Sacks J G, Melen O 1975 Bitemporal visual field defects in presumed multiple sclerosis. Journal of the American Medical Association 234: 69–72

101. Spector R H, Glaser J S, Schatz N J 1980 Demyelinative chiasmal lesions. Archives of Neurology 37: 757–762

102. Savitsky N, Rangel L 1950 On homonymous hemianopia in multiple sclerosis. Journal of Nervous and Mental Disease 111: 225–231

103. Hawkins K, Behrens M M 1975 Homonymous hemianopia in multiple sclerosis with report of bilateral case. British Journal of Ophthalmology 59: 334–337

104. Beck RW, Savino P J, Schatz N J, Smith C H, Sergott R C 1982 Plaque causing hemianopsia in multiple sclerosis identified by computed tomography. American Journal of Ophthalmology 94: 229–234

105. Poser S 1978 Multiple sclerosis: an analysis of 812 cases by means of electronic data processing. Springer, Berlin

106. Shibasaki H, McDonald W I, Kuroiwa Y 1981 Racial modification of clinical picture of multiple sclerosis: comparison between British and Japanese patients. Journal of the Neurological Sciences 49: 253–271

107. Kurtzke J F 1970 Clinical manifestations of multiple sclerosis. In: Vinken P J, Bruyn G W (eds) Handbook of clinical neurology, Vol 9. North-Holland, Amsterdam, pp 161–216

108. Carter S, Sciarra D, Merritt H H 1950 The course of multiple sclerosis as determined by autopsy proven cases. Research Publications of the Association for Research into Nervous and Mental Disease 28: 471–511

109. Green W R, Hackett E R, Schlezinger N S 1964 Neuro-ophthalmologic evaluation of oculomotor nerve palsies. Archives of Ophthalmology 72: 154–167

110. Uitti R J, Rajput A H 1986 Multiple sclerosis presenting as isolated oculomotor palsy. Canadian Journal of Neurological Sciences 13: 270–272

111. Poser C M, Presthus J, Hörsdal O 1966 Clinical characteristics of autopsy-proven multiple sclerosis. Neurology 16: 791–798

112. Wilson S A K 1906 Case of disseminated sclerosis with weakness of each internal rectus and nystagmus on lateral deviation limited to the outer eye. Brain 29: 298

113. Cogan D G 1956 Neurology of the ocular muscles, 2nd edn. Thormas, Springfield

114. Cogan D G 1970 Internuclear ophthalmoplegia, typical and atypical. Archives of Ophthalmology 84: 583–589

115. Muri R M, Weinberg O 1985 The clinical spectrum of internuclear ophthalmoplegia in multiple sclerosis. Archives of Neurology 42: 851–855

116. Cogan D G, Wray S H 1970 Internuclear ophthalmoplegia as an early sign of brainstem tumors. Neurology 20: 629–633

117. Schraeder P L, Cohen M H, Goldman W 1981 Bilateral internuclear ophthalmoplegia associated with fourth ventricular tumor. Journal of Neurosurgery 54: 403–405

118. Cogen M S, Kline L B, Duvall E R 1987 Bilateral internuclear ophthalmoplegia in systemic lupus erythematosus. Journal of Clinical Neuro-Ophthalmology 7: 69–73

119. Savitsky N, Rangell L 1950 The ocular findings in multiple sclerosis. Research Publications of the Association for Research into Nervous and Mental Disease 26: 403–413

120. Joseph R, Pullicino P, Goldberg C D S, Rose F C 1985 Bilateral pontine gaze palsy. Nuclear magnetic resonance findings in presumed multiple sclerosis. Archives of Neurology 421: 93–94

121. Costantino A, Black S E, Carr T, Nicholson R L, Noseworthy J H 1986 Dorsal midbrain syndrome in multiple sclerosis with magnetic imaging correlation. Canadian Journal of Neurological Sciences 13: 62–65

122. Wall M, Wray S H 1983 The one-and-a-half syndrome — a unilateral disorder of the pontine tegmentum: a study of 20 cases and review of the literature. Neurology 33: 971–980

123. Martyn C N, Kean D 1988 The one-and-a-half

syndrome. Clinical correlation with a pontine lesion demonstrated by nuclear magnetic resonance imaging in a case of multiple sclerosis. British Journal of Ophthalmology 72: 515–517

124. Wilson S A K 1940 Neurology. Edward Arnold, London, p 161

125. Sorsby A 1931 Latent nystagmus. British Journal of Ophthalmology 15: 1–18

126. Sharpe J A, Hoyt W F, Rosenberg M A 1975 Convergence evoked nystagmus. Congenital and acquired. Archives of Neurology 32: 191–194

127. Aschoff J V C, Conrad B, Kornhuber H H 1974 Acquired pendular nystagmus with oscillopsia in multiple sclerosis. Journal of Neurology, Neurosurgery and Psychiatry 37: 570–577

128. Keane J R 1974 Periodic alternating nystagmus with downward beating nystagmus. Archives of Neurology 30: 399–402

129. Oppenheim H 1914 Der Formenreichtum der multiplen Sklerose. Deutsche Zeitschrift für Nervenheilkunde 52: 169–239

130. Kurtzke J F, Beebe G W, Nagler B, Auth T L, Kurland L T, Nefzger M D 1968 Studies on natural history of multiple sclerosis. 4: Clinical features of the onset bout. Acta Neurologica Scandinavica 44: 467–499

131. Leibowitz U, Alter M 1973 Multiple sclerosis — clues to its cause. North-Holland, Amsterdam

132. Hung T-P, Landsborough D, Hsi M-S 1976 Multiple sclerosis amongst Chinese in Taiwan. Journal of the Neurological Sciences 27: 459–484

133. Bonduelle M, Albaranès R 1962 Etude statistique de 145 cas de la sclérose en plaques. Semaine des Hôpitaux 38: 3762–3773

134. Kelly R 1985 Clinical aspects of multiple sclerosis. In: Vinken P J, Bruyn G W, Klawans H L, Koetsier J C (eds), Handbook of clinical neurology, Vol 47. Elsevier, Amsterdam, p 53

135. Abb L, Schaltenbrandt G 1956 Statistische Untersuchungen zu, Problem der multiplen Sklerose. Deutsche Zeitschrift für Nevenheilkunde 174: 199–218

136. Oppenheim H 1911 Textbook of nervous diseases, Vol 1. Trans Bruce R Foulis, Edinburgh

137. Ivers R R, Goldstein N P 1963 Multiple sclerosis: a current appraisal of symptoms and signs. Mayo Clinic Proceedings 38: 457–466

138. Thygesen P 1953 The course of disseminated sclerosis: a close-up of 105 attacks. Rosenkilde and Bagger, Copenhagen

139. McAlpine D (ed) 1972 Multiple sclerosis: a reappraisal. Churchill Livingstone, Edinburgh

140. Kahana E, Leibowitz U, Alter M 1973 Brainstem and cranial nerve involvement in multiple sclerosis. Acta Neurologica Scandinavica 49: 269–279

141. Andermann F, Cosgrove J B R, Lloyd-Smith D L, Gloor P, McNaughten F L 1961 Facial myokymia in multiple sclerosis. Brain 84: 31–44

142. Harris W 1935 Paroxysmal neuralgic tic as sequel of trigeminal neuritis. British Medical Journal 1: 1112–1114

143. Gutmann L, Hartwel G T, Martin J D 1969 Transient facial myokymia. Journal of the American Medical Association 209: 389–391

144. Schaeffer H 1933 Paralysie faciale périphérique. Sclérose en plaques. Revue Neurologique 60: 619–622

145. Cohen L 1965 Disturbance of taste as a symptom of multiple sclerosis. British Journal of Oral Surgery 2: 184–185

146. Catalanotto F A, Dore-Duffy P, Donaldson J O, Testa M, Peterson M, Ostrom K M 1984 Quality-specific taste changes in multiple sclerosis. Annals of Neurology 16: 611–615

147. Thiébaut F, Isch F, Isch-Treussard C, Ebtinger-Jouffroy J 1960 Hémispasme facial dans la sclérose en plaques: étude clinique et électromyographique. Revue Oto-Neuro-Ophtalmologique 32: 162–166

148. Schultze F 1895 Beitrage zur Muskelpathologie. 1. Myokymie (Muskelwogen) besonders an den Unterextremitäten. Deutsche Zeitschrift für Nervenheilkunde 6: 65–70

149. Oppenheim H 1917 Uber den facialen Typus der multiplen Sklerose. Neurologisches Zentralblatt 36: 142–143

150. Kino F 1928 Muskelwogen (Myokymie) als Fruhsymptom der multiplen Sklerose. Deutsche Zeitschrift frr Nervenheilkunde 104: 31–41

151. Matthews W B 1966 Facial myokymia. Journal of Neurology, Neurosurgery and Psychiatry 29: 35–39

152. Lambert E H, Love J G, Mulder D W 1961 Facial myokymia and brain tumor. Electromyographic studies. Newsletter of the American Association for Electromyography and Electrodiagnosis 8: 8

153. Waybright E A, Gutmann L, Chou S M 1979 Facial myokymia. Pathological features. Archives of Neurology 36: 244–245

154. Sethi P K, Smith B H, Kalyanaraman K 1974 Facial myokymia: a clinicopathological study. Journal of Neurology, Neurosurgery and Psychiatry 37: 745–749

155. Hess K 1887 Uber ein Fall von multipler Sklerose des Cenralnervensystems. Archiv für Psychiatrie und Nervenkrankheiten 19: 64–87

156. Beck O 1910 Gehörorgan und multiple Sklerose. Monatsschrift für Ohrenheilkunde und Laryngo-Rhinologie 44: 1161–1172

157. Daugherty W T, Lederman R J, Nodar R H, Conomy J P 1983 Hearing loss in multiple sclerosis. Archives of Neurology 40: 33–35

158. Fischer C, Joyeux O, Haguenauer J P, Maugière F, Schott B 1984 Surdité et acouphènes lors de poussées dans 10 cas de sclérose en plaques. Revue Neurologique 140: 117–125

159. Fischer C, Mauguière F, Ibanez V, Confavreux C, Chazot 1985 The acute deafness of definite multiple sclerosis: B A E P patterns. Electroencephalography and Clinical Neurophysiology 61: 7–15

160. Von Leden H, Horton B T 1948 The auditory nerve in multiple sclerosis. Archives of Otolaryngology 48: 51–57

161. Dayal V S, Swisher L P 1967 Pure tone audiometry thresholds in multiple sclerosis. Laryngoscope 77: 2169–2177

162. Cohen M, Rudge P 1984 The effect of multiple sclerosis on pure tone thresholds. Acta Oto-Laryngology 97: 291–295

163. Quine D B, Regan D, Berverley K I, Murray T J 1984 Patients with multiple sclerosis experience hearing loss specifically for shifts of tone frequency. Archives of Neurology 41: 506–508

164. Quine D B, Regan D, Murray T J 1984 Degraded discrimination between speech-like sounds by patients

with multiple sclerosis and Friedreich's ataxia. Brain 107: 1113–1122

165. Tabira T, Tsuji S, Nagashima T, Nakajima T, Kuroiwa Y 1981 Cortical deafness in multiple sclerosis. Journal of Neurology, Neurosurgery and Psychiatry 44: 433–436

166. Molteni R A 1977 Vertigo as a presenting symptom of multiple sclerosis in childhood. American Journal of Disease in Childhood 131: 553–554

167. Berkowitz B W 1985 Matutinal vertigo. Clinical characteristics and possible management. Archives of Neurology 41: 874–877

168. Noffsinger D, Olsen W O, Carhart R, Hart C W, Sahgal V 1972 Auditory and vestibular aberrations in multiple sclerosis. Acta Oto-Laryngologica 303 (suppl 303): 1–63

169. Aantaa E, Reikkenen P J, Frey H J 1973 Electronystagmographic findings in multiple sclerosis. Acta Oto-Laryngologica 75: 1–5

170. Grénman R 1985 Involvement of the audiovestibular system in multiple sclerosis. Acta Oto-Laryngologica (suppl 420): 1–95

171. Forti A, Ambrosetto G, Amore M et al 1982 Locked-in syndrome in multiple sclerosis with sparing of the ventral portion of the pons. Annals of Neurology 12: 393–394

172. Seeldrayers P A, Borenstein S, Gerard J-M, Flament-Durant J 1987 Reversible capsulo-tegmental locked-in state as first manifestation of multiple sclerosis. Journal of the Neurological Sciences 80: 153–160

173. Guillain G, Alajouanine T 1928 La forme aigue de la sclérose en plaques. Bullein de l'Académie de Médecine (Paris) 99: 366–376

174. Bloor J W, Johnson R J, Canales L, Dunn D P 1974 Reversible paralysis of automatic respiration. Archives of Neurology 34: 686–689

175. McFarling D A, Susac J O 1979 Hoquet diabolique: intractable hiccups as a manifestation of multiple sclerosis. Neurology 29: 797–801

176. Birkhead R, Friedman J H 1987 Hiccups and vomiting as initial manifestations of multiple sclerosis. Journal of Neurology, Neurosurgery and Psychiatry 50: 232–233

177. Miller H, Simpson C A, Yeates W K 1965 Bladder dysfunction in multiple sclerosis. British Medical Journal 1: 1265–1269

178. Awad D S A, Gajewski J B, Sogbein S K, Murray T J, Field C A 1984 Relationship between neurological and urological status in patients with multiple sclerosis. Journal of Urology 132: 499–502

179. Swash M, Snooks S J, Chalmers D H K 1987 Parity as a factor in incontinence in multiple sclerosis. Archives of Neurology 44: 504–508

180. Glick M E, Meshkinpour H, Haldeman S, Bhatia N N, Bradley W E 1982 Colonic dysfunction in multiple sclerosis. Gastroenterology 83: 1002–1007

181. Haldeman E, Glick M, Bhatia N N, Bradley W E, Johnson B 1982 Colonometry, cystometry and evoked potentials in multiple sclerosis. Archives of Neurology 39: 698–701

182. Gupta Y K 1984 Gastroparesis with multiple sclerosis. Journal of the American Medical Association 252: 42

183. Graves M C 1981 Gastric outlet obstruction in a patient with multiple sclerosis. Annals of Neurology 10: 397–398

184. Vas C J 1969 Sexual impotence and some autonomic disturbances in men with multiple sclerosis. Acta Neurologica Scandinavica 45: 166–183

185. Cartlidge N F E 1972 Autonomic function in multiple sclerosis. Brain 95: 661–664

186. Lundberg P O 1981 Sexual dysfunction in female patients with multiple sclerosis. International Rehabilitation Medicine 3: 32–34

187. Minderhoud J M, Leemhuis J G, Kremer J, Laban E, Smits P M L 1984 Sexual disturbances arising from multiple sclerosis. Acta Neurologica Scandinavica 70: 299–306

188. Noronha M J, Vas C J, Aziz H 1968 Autonomic dysfunction (sweating responses) in multiple sclerosis. Journal of Neurology, Neurosurgery and Psychiatry 31: 19–22

189. Senaratne M P J, Carroll D, Warren K G, Kappagoda T 1984 Evidence for cardiovascular autonomic nerve dysfunction in multiple sclerosis. Journal of Neurology, Neurosurgery and Psychiatry 47: 947–952

190. Sterman A B, Coyle P K, Panesci D J, Grimson R 1985 Disseminated abnormalities of cardiovascular autonomic functions in multiple sclerosis. Neurology 35: 1665–1668

191. Pentland B, Ewing D J 1987 Cardiovascular reflexes in multiple sclerosis. European Neurology 26: 46–50

192. Giroud M, Guard O, Dumas R 1988 Anomalies cardio-respiratoires dans la sclérose en plaques. Revue Neurologique 144: 284–288

193. Chagnac Y, Martinovits G, Tadmor R, Goldhammer Y 1986 Paroxysmal atrial fibrillation associated with an attack of multiple sclerosis. Postgraduate Medical Journal 62: 385–387

194. Bamford C R, Smith M S, Sibley W A 1980 Horner's syndrome, an unusual manifestation of multiple sclerosis. Canadian Journal of Neurological Sciences 7: 65–66

195. Kamalian N, Keesey R E, ZuRhein G M 1975 Lateral hypothalamic demyelination and cachexia in a case of 'malignant' multiple sclerosis. Neurology 25: 25–30

196. Bignami A, Gherardi D, Gallo D 1961 Sclerosi a placche acuta a localizzazone ipotalamica con sintomatologia psichica di tip malinconico. Rivista di Neurolgia 31: 240–268

197. Apple D, Keinees K, Biehl J P 1978 The syndrome of inappropriate antidiuretic hormone secretion in multiple sclerosis. Archives of Internal Medicine 138: 1713–1714

198. Loomis A L 1885 A textbook of practical medicine, 3rd edn. Wm Wood, New York, p 1015

199. Bristow J S 1876 A treatise on the theory and practice of medicine, 1st edn. Smith Elder, London, p 1005

200. Wilson S A K 1940 Neurology. Edward Arnold, London, p 168

201. Baoxun Z, Xuiqin I, Yupu G, Yinchang Y, Huifen H 1981 Multiple sclerosis: a clinical study from Beijing, China. European Neurology 20: 394–400

202. Castaigne P, Escourolle R, Laplane D, Augustin P 1966 Comas transitoires avec hyperthermie au cours de la sclérose en plaques. Revue Neurologique 114: 147–150

203. Phadke J G, Best P V 1983 Atypical and clinically silent multiple sclerosis: a report of 12 cases discovered unexpectedly at autopsy. Journal of Neurology, Neurosurgery and Psychiatry 46: 414–420

4. Some aspects of the natural history

FACTORS ASSOCIATED WITH ONSET OR RELAPSE

As with any important disease, there is a natural tendency on the part of both patient and physician to search for precipitating causes. If energetically pursued this search is seldom in vain as, in retrospect, events that would normally be accepted as commonplace assume unnatural proportions when related in time to the onset of disease. Minor trauma, transient infections, fatigue and emotional disturbance are scarcely rare in everyday life. Nearly all studies of such possible precipitating or aggravating factors in multiple sclerosis have been retrospective with all the inherent disadvantages of this method.

In considering the role of such factors as have from time to time been incrimated the question naturally arises as to whether the disease may be *caused* by these agents. This assumes great medico-legal significance in relation to trauma and will be considered in more detail under that heading. In general there has been a tacit, but sometimes explicit agreement that it is not reasonable to believe that, for example, a bereavement can *cause* multiple sclerosis, but that symptoms that may develop immediately after such an event, if causally related at all, are merely precipitated and that the disease process was already established. This assumption has received considerable support from the results of MRI in patients presenting with a single initial symptom, but in whom multiple lesions are already visible.

When considering the effects of a putative triggering factor, a number of reputed questions may be asked. Can the agent precipitate the onset of the disease? Can it trigger a relapse? Is there any long-term or continuing effect on prognosis? Advances in techniques of investigation have narrowed the distinction between onset of clinical symptoms and clinical relapse, but we do not yet know enough to state that from the point of view of pathogenesis they are identical.

Infection

In the present context the question is not whether infection by some specific agent is the 'cause' of multiple sclerosis, but whether transient systemic infection can precipitate the onset or relapse of the disease. As with other such possible factors, most of the evidence is derived from retrospective studies. McAlpine[1] summarised the early reports as suggesting that the onset was preceded by some infective disease, usually imprecisely diagnosed, in about 10% of cases. McAlpine & Compston[2] found no instance of an exanthem in the three months before the onset in their 250 cases. Seasonal variations in rates of onset and relapse provide conflicting evidence of doubtful relevance. In Switzerland[3] disease activity was shown to be at a peak in the winter, when respiratory infections are common, but this was not so in Ohio[4] or Arizona[5] where risk was greatest in spring and summer. This was clearly shown in a prospective study of exacerbations. In Newcastle-upon-Tyne there was no significant seasonal trend.[6] Taub & Rucker[7] found that optic neuritis was less frequent in the winter, while Compston et al[8] showed that optic neuritis in patients who subsequently developed multiple sclerosis was more frequent in winter, but only in HLA DR2 positive subjects. Optic neuritis in children was found to be much more common in the month of April in a British series.[9] All these findings may be quite unrelated to the incidence of infection.

The relationship of upper respiratory infection to onset and exacerbation in 92 patients was examined by Gay et al.[10] They were particularly concerned with infection of the paranasal sinuses as an element in their hypothesis of an oral spirochaete as the cause of multiple sclerosis.[11] The retrospective data were obtained from general practice records, an excellent source for determining the frequency of infections, but necessarily often imprecise as to the diagnosis of sinusitis. Their results indicate that nasopharyngeal infection, whether sinusitis or not, was recorded highly significantly more often in patients with multiple sclerosis than in several control groups. Sinusitis was recorded in 69.5% of patients and in 17.4% of matched controls. Infection was predictably common in winter and peaks of both onset and relapse of multiple sclerosis followed after a lag of one month. First recorded attacks of sinusitis and of multiple sclerosis tended to occur in January and February respectively, while in subsequent attacks, the equivalent peaks were in March and May. Similar results were obtained in the same way by Callaghan[12] in a smaller group of patients, but in a population study in France[13] the incidence of sinusitis in multiple sclerosis patients did not differ from that in controls (see also p. 31). Sibley et al[14] reported that in a prospective study upper respiratory infection, not specifically sinusitis, was significantly less frequent in multiple sclerosis patients than in controls.

Excluding the specific implications of sinusitis, an association of common infections of the type generally assumed to be viral with exacerbation of multiple sclerosis receives support from prospective observations. Miller et al[15] found that one third of relapses were preceded by banal infections. Sibley et al[16] followed 170 patients at monthly intervals. The risk period from infection was defined rather widely as from 2 weeks before symptoms to 5 weeks afterwards. The relapse rate in this period was increased threefold. Of infections, 9% were related to relapse and 27% of relapses were related to infection. The relative infrequency of infections in multiple sclerosis patients, particularly in the more disabled, observed by Alter & Speer,[17] was confirmed and attributed either to enhanced immunity or to a sheltered life.

The role of infection appears to be established but not its mode of action. Sibley favours a post-infective reaction as in acute disseminated encephalomyelitis. A different possible explanation lies in the action of infection in stimulating production of gamma interferon, that has been shown, in attempted therapeutic use, to induce relapse,[18] presumably through its action of increasing immune responses. A specific viral effect is not essential as most viral infections are rapidly followed by bacterial invasion and Morris[19] has suggested that a cross reaction between bacterial antigens and human brain proteins might precipitate relapse.

Vaccination

The occurrence of acute disseminated encephalomyelitis after different forms of vaccination is well recognised. Largely on this account there has been some apprehension about the wisdom of patients with multiple sclerosis receiving prophylactic injections of any kind.

Early case reports of multiple sclerosis developing or relapsing immediately after vaccination against a great variety of infections were reviewed by Miller et al[20] who added nine personal observations, mostly of the onset of the disease. Certainly the cases described are remarkable, with symptoms developing within a few hours of the injection. There was no attempt at a controlled study and it was recognised that most patients with multiple sclerosis can be vaccinated with impunity. In whatever manner the investigation had been conducted it would have been impossible to deny that in these particular patients vaccination might have been responsible for precipitating the onset or relapse of the disease. The advice given was that patients with multiple sclerosis should avoid vaccination unless there was thought to be grave risk of infection.

Sibley & Foley[21] reported on small numbers of patients with established multiple sclerosis vaccinated against influenza, measles and poliomyelitis, using the Sabin vaccine. One of 24 patients given influenza vaccine developed optic neuritis 24 hours later, an event thought to be fortuitous. No other ill effects were noted. In a much larger series,[22] 93 patients received 209 doses of influenza vaccine with one subsequent relapse. Nevertheless, doubts remained and Rabin[23] reported a single case of a patient with a history of optic neuritis 7 years previously who became blind and paraplegic following influenza vaccination.

Apprehension was particularly keen concerning the ·use of swine-influenza vaccine that had apparently led to an increased incidence of the Guillain–Barré syndrome, sometimes accompanied by chronic or progressive disease of the central nervous system.[24] However, controlled trials in multiple sclerosis[25,26] showed that relapse was rather more common in the group receiving placebo. Kurland et al[27] concluded that the vaccine given to 45 million people had caused no known or reported increase in the incidence of multiple sclerosis.

These results certainly go far to allay anxiety and it is plain that if vaccination is harmful to patients with multiple sclerosis this is a rare event. As already indicated, there is no way of completely exonerating vaccination as an occasional precipitating or aggravating factor. What advice should therefore be given? If there has been any hint of exacerbation following previous vaccination, further inoculations should not be given. Necessary prophylactic injections before venturing into areas of high risk should normally be given. With influenza there is a complex balance between possible risks of vaccination, evidently very low, and the risks to the patient with multiple sclerosis of an attack of influenza, not necessarily avoided by vaccination. Advice may be irrationally influenced by recent personal experience and the author's inclination is to advise against influenza vaccination.

Pregnancy

The possible precipitating factor most thoroughly studied is childbirth. Early opinion was that pregnancy was a grave hazard for the woman with multiple sclerosis and early termination was regarded by some as mandatory, although the risks of induced abortion were not shown to be any less. Modern ideas are very different.

An effect of pregnancy in triggering the *onset* of multiple sclerosis has seldom been examined in isolation, although the onset bout is the only one necessarily free from bias from a decision not to have children because of the disease or from unknown differential effects of disease severity. Leibowitz et al[28] examined the possibility that pregnancy might predispose to multiple sclerosis, or at least its clinical expression. They compared women with multiple sclerosis with age-matched healthy controls, 2 for each patient. Control subjects were given an artificial 'age of onset' identical with that of the patient with whom they were matched. Sixty per cent of the patients and 56% of controls had been pregnant at least once before the age of onset. Of patients, 16% had last been pregnant in the year before onset, compared with 8% of controls. The proportions were reversed in the period 1–2 years before onset. The authors concluded that in a woman in the 'premorbid stage', the clinical onset might be advanced by up to 2 years by pregnancy. The recent acceptance that lesions may long precede symptoms is in keeping with this proposal, but the influence of pregnancy, although statistically significant, remains problematical. The study was naturally retrospective and the method of control appears somewhat contrived.

Tillman,[29] who is sometimes credited with the first demonstration that the supposed adverse effect of pregnancy had been overstressed, separated onset from relapse. His figures and percentages are difficult to unravel but in his series of 145 women who had never been pregnant, the onset was in pregnancy in 10, and in a further 11 in the 6 months following delivery.

Andersen,[30] using the detailed information from the Göteborg series, found that there was only 1 instance of onset of multiple sclerosis in the nine months of pregnancy compared with 9 in the same period following childbirth. Onset during pregnancy was significantly less frequent than expected, being higher than expected, but not significantly so, in the succeeding nine months.

Korn-Lubetzki et al[31] in their study of 199 pregnancies in 66 women with multiple sclerosis included with relapses 36 onset bouts, but their exact relationship to childbirth was not particularised.[32]

Frith & McLeod[33] reporting on 85 pregnancies in 52 women with multiple sclerosis mention pregnancy-related onset of the disease in 4:2 during pregnancy and 2 in the puerperium. These were presumably not regarded as relapses. Events were only recorded after 1980, so the true incidence of onset related to pregnancy in these women cannot be determined. Poser & Poser[34] make no distinction between onset and relapse and Millar et al,[35] Schapira et al[36] and Ghezzi & Caputo[37] do not mention onset related to pregnancy. The evidence is not extensive but it is probable that pregnancy has an effect on the onset of multiple sclerosis similar or identical to its effect on relapse.

Relapse

The relationship of pregnancy to relapse has been much more thoroughly examined. In Tillman's[29] series, 52 women with multiple sclerosis experienced 70 pregnancies. In 5 patients there was a relapse during pregnancy and no less than 22 relapsed in the 6 months after delivery. From the abbreviated case histories it is difficult to obtain a clear idea of the definition of an exacerbation. Tillman concluded that women with mild remittent symptoms or those in complete remission were not adversely affected by pregnancy and childbirth, but that exacerbation occurred in those with unstable or progressive disease.

In a highly influential retrospective study, Millar et al[35] concentrated on the relapse rate. Of the population series of 262 women, 111 were unmarried and had not been pregnant, and 151 were married, of whom 70 had experienced 170 pregnancies after the onset of multiple sclerosis. There were 45 relapses in the pregnancy year (the nine months of pregnancy and 3 months puerperium). Only 6 relapses occurred in pregnancy, the remaining 39 being in the puerperium. The relapse rate for the pregnancy year was 0.265, more than double the observed mean rate for both single and married women (0.104) and slightly

higher than that observed in young women within 5 years of the onset, when relapse is frequent. The significant excess of relapses during the pregnancy year was accompanied by a significant deficiency in non-pregnancy years. Of several possible explanations, the authors favoured the view that the puerperium may provoke relapse which would, in any case, have occurred later. It was suggested that this 'anticipation' was the result of the stresses of labour. In this series, the mean relapse rate of 0.104, equivalent to a relapse every 10 years, with which the rate in the pregnancy year was compared, is remarkably low.

In a similar study, Schapira et al[36] confirmed some of these findings. The mean relapse rate in women with no pregnancies (0.137) was significantly lower than that in women who had been pregnant (0.171). The mean relapse rate in pregnancy years rose to 0.250 and in women who had first been pregnant before the onset of multiple sclerosis it was 0.395. They did not find a reduction below the expected level in non-pregnancy years that had been the basis for the theory of anticipation of relapse. Again there was a preponderance of relapse in the puerperium. They concluded that there was a 1 in 4 risk of relapse in a pregnancy year, the risk being some 50% greater than in a non-pregnancy year. In this study also the relapse rates observed unrelated to pregnancy were unexpectedly low for a group of young women.

Ghezzi & Caputo[37] compared pregnancy-related relapse frequency with that in 100 women with multiple sclerosis who had not been pregnant. The mean relapse rate in the controls was 0.29, a rather more realistic figure than those in the two studies cited above. The rate in women who had been pregnant was not significantly different. During 206 pregnancies there were 34 relapses when 45 would have been expected. In the 3 months after childbirth, 91 relapses occurred: a great excess over the expected 15. In the post-pregnancy year, there was a significant reduction of relapse rate below that expected, affording some support for anticipation of relapse. The apparent protective effect of pregnancy was even more marked in the series reported from Israel.[31] The mean relapse rate for women between the ages of 20 and 38 was 0.29. In pregnancy, the rate of relapse plus onset fell progressively from 0.22 in the first trimester, 0.17 in the second and 0.04 in the third, with an immediate increase to 0.8 in the 3 months following delivery. It would have been helpful for purposes of comparison if relapses had been separated from onset bouts, but it was evident that there had been no overall increase during the pregnancy year and also that the relapse rate in the puerperium was much higher than in the non-pregnant state. The conclusion from these findings was the reverse of the anticipation theory: pregnancy was thought to have postponed relapse until the puerperium.

The Australian series[33] was notable for a much closer definition of pregnancy, as gestation of more than 20 weeks was required. The pregnancies examined were also limited to those occurring within a set period of some 7 years, so that the full obstetric history of a number of the women was presumably not considered. Clinical data for this restricted period were, however, evidently abundant and reliable. The 52 women acted as their own controls, the relapse rate in non-pregnancy and pregnancy periods of 15 months being compared. The annual relapse rate in non-pregnancy periods was 0.53 and in pregnancy periods 0.38, the difference not being significant. There was a significant reduction in the number of relapses compared with those expected in the first two trimesters, but, in contrast to the report from Israel, there was no reduction in third trimester. Relapses in the 6 months following delivery, unlike all other studies, were not significantly increased. The relapse rates found in this investigation much more closely resemble those to be expected in young women and increase confidence in the accuracy of the observations, but the lack of an increase in relapse in the puerperium is surprising and not supported by any other study.

Nelson et al[38] retrospectively examined the effect of childbirth in 111 women who had completed 191 pregnancies after the onset of multiple sclerosis. There had been 19 relapses during pregnancy and 65 in the nine months after childbirth, 44 of these occurring in the first three months. Women who became pregnant during the progressive stage of the disease were excluded, so it was not possible to examine Tillman's[29] view that such pregnancies carried a high risk.

Progress

More important and much more difficult to investigate is whether pregnancy increases the risk or hastens the onset of disability. Millar[39] referred to the completion of a review of patients seen previously by himself and Allison.[40] There were 377 women concerning whom information was adequate: 139 single, 109 married with children born after the onset of the disease, and 129 married women without children born after the onset. In these three categories 110 women had died during a ten-year interval. The remaining 267 women were graded according to disability (Grades 1-6). Relatively fewer single women and relatively more married women with pregnancies came into the first three, less disabled grades. This may have been because marriage and pregnancy are more likely in the less disabled women, or the prognosis may actually be better for women who have children after the onset.

Andersen[30] also found that in women with two children born after the onset of multiple sclerosis, disability was less pronounced. The explanation that women with mild disease would be likely to have more children was thought probable. Schapira et al[36] found that women who were pregnant before the onset of multiple sclerosis become more disabled in the early stages of the disease than married women without children, but that this difference did not persist. Poser & Poser[34] made a special study of the rate of progression in a large group of women. Using the progression index (Kurtzke DSS score divided by the duration of the disease in years) there was no significant difference in prognosis for disability between those never pregnant, pregnant only before the disease, pregnant during the disease, those with one pregnancy and those with no children, those with one child and those with more than one. As these authors found a marked increase in onset, relapse or deterioration in the months succeeding childbirth, the conclusion must be that the ill-effects of the puerperium do not alter the subsequent course of the disease.

Thompson et al,[41] in their retrospective study of 178 women with multiple sclerosis, concentrated on the long-term outcome. They found no significant difference in disability between women with no children, those with one child and those with more than one. For those with onset of the disease during pregnancy, disability was significantly less pronounced, but there was no difference in disability between those with onset before or after a first completed pregnancy. There appears to be no controlled follow-up study comparing women who relapsed in the puerperium and those who did not.

If, as seems highly probable, pregnancy exerts a protective effect that is rapidly lost after delivery, a metabolic, hormonal or immunological influence may be presumed. The topic, with particular respect to natural immunosuppression in pregnancy, is reviewed by Birk & Rudick.[42] There is no evidence that other obvious possible risk factors, breast feeding[38] or fatigue resulting from lack of help with the new baby,[43] have any adverse effect.

There are, of course, many other problems concerned with pregnancy and multiple sclerosis apart from the risk of exacerbation.[42] Fertility is not reduced, but deliberate decision on family limitation on account of the disease is common, being a factor in 18% of 435 women in one series.[38] There is no increased risk of spontaneous abortion or stillbirth. An association between maternal multiple sclerosis and infantile arthrogryposis multiplex has been suggested[44] but is exceedingly rare. The rate of induced abortion is high. There are no specific complications of labour and no contraindication to breast feeding. Care of the infant by a disabled mother may be an intractable problem.[43] Heredity is discussed on page 304.

The risks of pregnancy and labour are certainly much less than originally feared but it is not yet known whether Tillman[29] was right in advising against pregnancy in progressive or active disease, however this might be estimated. A large family seems inadvisable but, after explaining the increased risk of relapse in the puerperium found by most observers, a woman with multiple sclerosis desiring to have a child can be encouraged to do so.

Menstruation

Investigation of the effect of menstruation on symptoms of the disease[2] showed a tendency towards improvement during menstruation and the first half of the cycle. In some patients this effect is obvious, but in a few there is temporary deterioration of function during the menstrual period.

Oral contraceptives

No prospective study appears to have been published on the possible effect of the use of oral contraceptives on the course of the disease. In a large retrospective study[45] there was no evidence that the Pill increased disability.

Trauma

Trauma, while much more common than pregnancy, is often a somewhat less well-defined event and its relationship to multiple sclerosis remains problematical. This might not be suspected from confident opinions expressed in medico-legal reports. The evidence that multiple sclerosis may be precipitated or aggravated by trauma is almost entirely based on single case reports, but there are almost insuperable obstacles to obtaining scientifically respectable data.

In ignorance of the 'cause' of multiple sclerosis it clearly cannot be proven that trauma might not play a part in precipitating or aggravating the disease in some patients. Some highly suggestive case histories have been published. McAlpine[1] described the onset of mainly sensory symptoms shortly after trivial injury to the limbs or after tooth extraction under local anaesthesia. Miller's[46] two most convincing cases sustained painful injuries, one electrical, and developed sensory loss, initially in the same area, within six days, with later clinically definite multiple sclerosis. He also described the onset of optic neuritis within a few hours of mild head injury. That such cases occur is undeniable: their meaning remains obscure.

McAlpine was naturally much influenced by the results of his own partially controlled investigation.[2] In 250 cases of multiple sclerosis, a history of trauma, not specifically to the nervous system, within three months of the onset of symptoms was obtained in 14% and in the majority there was a correlation between the site of the injury and that of the initial symptoms. In a control series of 250 patients with other diseases a similar history of injury was obtained in 5.2%. As McAlpine acknowledged, there are obvious, and indeed fatal defects in such a retrospective comparison. Patients with a numb leg are much more likely to remember an injury to that leg than a patient with acute appendicitis. Kelly[47] reported that 65 of 980 personal cases had experienced relapse or deterioration following trauma but details such as time relationships, the nature of the trauma, selection of cases and incidence of trauma not followed by relapse are essential for the interpretation of such figures.

Bamford et al[48] carried out a controlled retrospective and prospective trial in which 130 patients with multiple sclerosis were followed for a maximum of $3\frac{1}{2}$ years. Every form of physical trauma was noted and the relapse rate and rate of deterioration recorded for the six months following each event and compared with the course of the disease in the non-risk periods. No significant differences were found. It has never been supposed that trauma commonly precipitates relapse and nor is it possible by any form of trial to exclude trauma as an occasional trigger. A larger and more prolonged prospective trial might have been more informative, but would have been extremely burdensome to carry out. It was not, of course, possible to examine prospectively the role of trauma in precipitating the onset of multiple sclerosis, but retrospective data from these patients, compared with matched healthy controls, showed no difference in the pattern or frequency of preceding trauma. Perhaps the most important finding was that following head injury, deterioration was more rapid than expected in 9 instances, but less rapid in 14, the rate being unaltered in 6.

Mechanisms by which trauma to the central nervous system might precipitate or aggravate the symptoms of multiple sclerosis have been suggested. Both Miller[46] and McAlpine[1] thought that experimental work showing that peripheral stimulation caused circulatory changes in the spinal cord might be relevant. Such changes, if indeed they occur, would be unlikely to cause the formation of a plaque and resulting symptoms within a few hours. Some effect of peripheral stimulation must be postulated, however, if it is believed that trauma to a limb, with no possibility of damage to the central nervous system, can result in onset or relapse of multiple sclerosis.

The postulated modes of action of closed trauma to the brain and spinal cord are somewhat more convincing. Poser[49] believed that trauma and other triggering factors act by altering the safety factor for conduction in partially demyelinated plaques. It is well known that many plaques, even strategically sited, do not cause symptoms and conduction sufficient for function is evidently maintained. This can be altered by changes in ambient temperature and no doubt by many other factors of the internal environment. Trauma might act by disturbing a delicately held balance, with immediate failure of conduction and appearance of symptoms. A difficulty in accepting this theory, so attractive in accounting for the rapidity of onset sometimes observed, is ignorance of the relevant factors that might be affected by a blow on the head.

An alternative theory, also propounded by Poser,[50] concentrates on the blood/brain barrier. It has long been known that the barrier may be broken in multiple sclerosis plaques but imaging techniques, particularly MRI, have provided highly significant detail (see p. 243). In the formation of new plaques, the barrier is breached at an early stage, perhaps even as an initial event. Of course, it is not known whether breaching the barrier is the cause of the plaque, by admitting some harmful agent, or is a consequence of inflammatory change within the plaque. If the former were true, traumatic breaking of the barrier might lead to the formation of new plaques, although the nature of the circulating noxious agent, if such there be, remains obscure.

In severe head injury the blood/brain barrier is obviously broken, but personal experience of a large series of veterans who have survived penetrating head wounds has not revealed any instance of multiple sclerosis. Closed head injury is very much more common in most communities and in fatal cases it is not surprising to find extensive brain damage, particularly of the white matter.[51] In such cases, microscopic haemorrhagic lesions are also present and these have been described in five cases following comparatively minor concussive head injury, where death has resulted from respiratory or other causes not directly related to the trauma.[52] Similar lesions in the spinal cord are not known to result from minor injuries. Ommaya et al[53] showed that in cats, fluorescein leaked into the brain at the site of a blow to the head, but also in the brainstem and cervical spinal cord if the neck was not immobilised. The blows were, however, sufficiently severe to cause subarachnoid bleeding, skull fracture and even death from respiratory arrest. Leakage of horseradish peroxidase through the barrier has also been produced in experimental animals by relatively minor trauma, admittedly applied directly to the brain.[54,55] In none of these studies was the state of the blood/brain barrier followed for more than a few hours. Electrolytic cerebral lesions in animals with experimental allergic encephalomyelitis can induce focal plaques at the site of injury and precipitate relapse,[56,57] although the relevance of these findings to the human disease is perhaps a little remote. Fresh plaques sometimes form around the needle tracks in patients with multiple sclerosis treated by stereotactic surgery[58] but this is not invariable.[59] Such procedures damage a great deal more than the blood/brain barrier. There is, however, sufficient tangential evidence to permit the elaboration of a theory that cerebral concussion could initiate or aggravate multiple sclerosis plaques through an action on the blood/brain barrier. There is no evidence that trauma not involving the nervous central nervous system could exert such an effect.

That multiple sclerosis can be discovered at autopsy in people who have never had symptoms of neurological disease has long been known[60] and has recently been confirmed.[61,62] Extrapolation from the small number of such cases found to calculate a figure for an entire population can only be approximate but perhaps one fifth of cases of multiple sclerosis remain clinically silent.[62] It is inescapable that a small proportion of the vast numbers of people who sustain closed head injuries will already be carrying lesions of multiple sclerosis that have caused no symptoms. If the theory outlined above is correct, the clinical onset of the disease might be precipitated, but there is now no suggestion that trauma can cause the disease.

If scientific interest were the only spur, we might rest content with this hypothetical explanation of what is, after all, an unproven phenomenon, but the demands of adversarial litigation are more insistent. For how long after injury is the risk of onset or relapse increased? If there had been no injury would the symptoms have occurred anyway and, if so, when? Is the course and ultimate prognosis of the disease altered? Anyone with knowledge of the disease knows that answers to these questions can be based only on conjecture, aided by fragile theoretical considerations and common sense.

There is no means of discovering the duration of the breakdown in the blood/brain barrier resulting from the microscopic vascular lesions occurring in concussion, but an analogy may be drawn from larger, radiologically visible lesions. Weisberg[63] found that in 40 cases of cerebral infarction, enhancement on the CT scan, indicative of breach of the blood/brain barrier, did not persist for longer than 42 days from the time of the stroke. There is no obvious reason why repair should take longer in minute traumatic vascular lesions. It is difficult to believe that symptoms of multiple sclerosis beginning more than 6 weeks after head injury are related to the trauma but, of course, it could be argued that breach of the blood/brain barrier might not be detectable by CT scanning. On entirely different grounds, Poser[50] also concluded that the time limit of a triggering effect of trauma was 6 weeks.

The question of whether the symptoms of multiple sclerosis would have developed if there had been no injury is often answered boldly in court but there are no data on which to base an opinion. Claims that the majority of people with multiple sclerosis never develop symptoms and that external triggers are therefore very important have been based on the statistically frail evidence of 5 unsuspected cases in 2400 autopsies.[61] There is, however, even less evidence that a given patient would necessarily have developed symptoms after some stated period. One reads with amazement of judgements that, because of injury, the onset of multiple sclerosis has been advanced by a precise number of years.

If an analogy can be drawn with childbirth, the only triggering factor to have been thoroughly studied, it is unlikely that onset or relapse following trauma will adversely affect the long-term prognosis or that trauma could be held responsible for progressive deterioration. I have heard it stated in court that myelin basic protein released from plaques induced by trauma will further exacerbate the disease by inducing an autoimmune reaction, ignoring the fact that no auto-antigen has been identified in multiple sclerosis.

In summary, a hypothesis can be constructed linking concussive head injury with onset or relapse of multiple sclerosis up to six weeks from the time of injury, but thereafter with rapidly diminishing probability. Minor injury to the spinal cord is much more difficult to define but could be held similarly responsible. The hypothesis is based on the unproven primary role of breach of the blood/brain barrier in the pathogenesis of the plaque. It is impossible to give a scientific answer to the question as to what would have happened if there had been no injury; it is not inevitable that symptoms of multiple sclerosis would have developed. It is the uncertainty on this point that frequently leads to compromised decisions. Neurologists will form their own opinions but would hope to avoid making pronouncements unsupported by evidence. The course of multiple sclerosis following trauma has not been examined systematically but does not appear to follow any distinctive pattern.

Surgical operations and anaesthesia

The natural tendency to attribute the onset or aggravation of disease to stress is particularly relevant to the possible risks of elective surgery. The neurologist will often be asked whether a patient known to have multiple sclerosis should be submitted to necessary but not vital surgery, such as hernia repair, and if so what form of anaesthesia should be used.

Uncontrolled observations are of little help except that a frequent and obvious temporal correlation between operations and onset of relapse could be detected. Keschner[64] reported on 31 patients undergoing major surgery with closely related relapse in only one in whom laminectomy had been performed. This at least shows that the great majority of such operations are not followed by relapse. A further 31 patients had minor surgery and symptoms increased in 4. Ridley & Schapira[65] studied retrospectively the immediate and long term course of 40 patients who had 57 operations under general anaesthesia. Operation was followed by improvement on 2 occasions and by deterioration on 8, the remaining 47 not being followed by any change. In the long term, deterioration in static disability was noted a year later on 8 occasions. In a restrospective controlled study, McAlpine & Compston[2] reported an increase in relapse rate within three months following operations compared with controls. The difference was not remarkable but it was concluded that surgery was detrimental. In a retrospective investigation covering the whole period before the onset of multiple sclerosis, no increase in surgical procedure was found compared with control subjects attending hospital with other diseases.[17]

Bamford et al[48] included surgical operations in their controlled investigation of trauma as an aggravating factor. There appeared to be no influence of surgery on the course of the disease as equal numbers of patients submitted to surgery subsequently progressed more slowly and more rapidly than expected.

The effects of surgery can scarcely be separated from those of anaesthesia. Keschner[64] advised against spinal anaesthesia as one patient relapsed following a minor pelvic operation in which this procedure was used. Baskett & Armstrong[66] suggested that barbiturate anaesthetics might be harmful and Siemkowicz[67] described marked deterioration immediately following general anaesthesia in 5 of 15 patients, but could not relate this to any particular drug. In the case reports it is noteworthy that deterioration was brief in 4 instances and usually accompanied post-operative infection and fever. Bamford et al[68] questioned 44 patients with multiple sclerosis about their past experience following general or spinal anaesthesia and hospital records were obtained where possible. One of 42 patients having 88 general anaesthetics had a post-operative relapse. In a small number of patients there was a 10% aggravation of symptoms of multiple sclerosis in the month following spinal anaesthesia. One patient had caudal anaesthesia on three occasions without ill effect. Local anaesthesia was used so frequently that the small number of occasions on which deterioration appeared to follow was not thought significant.

There is therefore some suspicion that spinal

anaesthesia may be harmful in multiple sclerosis. This was approached from another aspect by Sténuit & Marchand[69] who reviewed a large series of patients receiving spinal anaesthesia. Of the 29 who had complications there were 19 cases of multiple sclerosis of whom two had a definite relapse.

Lumbar puncture

There is a long-standing tradition that lumbar puncture and a fortiori myelography and pneumo-encephalography may aggravate the symptoms of multiple sclerosis and precipitate a relapse. It is difficult to establish how this arose. Henner in 1957[70] simply stated that it was 'une notion admise'. He further stated that lumbar puncture aggravated the disease in 70% of cases, that pneumo-encephalography often had an unfavourable effect and that spinal anaesthesia was always deleterious. He believed that cisternal puncture carried a much lower risk. He did not mention myelography. In contrast, Schapira,[71] in a retrospective study of 250 patients, found that in 231 the procedure was not followed by any immediate change in clinical state, 14 patients improved and 5 became worse. In 100 patients the clinical course of the disease in the month following LP was compared with that in the corresponding month one year earlier and one year later. The only patient who had greatly deteriorated following LP had disease which had progressed although less rapidly during both the periods used for comparison. Eight patients improved following LP and had not been improving a year earlier. It was concluded that lumbar puncture had no detectable effect on the course of multiple sclerosis.

Tourtellotte et al[72] stated that the removal of 20 ml of CSF at lumbar puncture had no ill effect on the course of multiple sclerosis in the following three months. Later Tourtellotte[73] reported that 144 lumbar punctures were performed on seven patients for experimental purposes with no adverse effect on the disease. Similarly Weisner[74] found no immediate effect of LP on the clinical state.

The possible effects of myelography have been less well documented. Schapira[71] found no ill effects in five patients. Weisner,[74] although reporting no adverse effect of pneumo-encephalography in 50 patients, did not mention myelography.

The evidence therefore suggests that there are no contra-indications to diagnostic lumbar puncture or myelography in patients suspected of having multiple sclerosis.

Emotional stress

If the effects on the course of multiple sclerosis of finite physical events such as lumbar puncture, surgical operations and pregnancy have proved so difficult to estimate in retrospect, it is not to be expected that any conclusive answers can be given on the influence of emotional stress. It is true that presumed causes of stress can be graded and in an approximate sense measured, but it is a matter of common observation that disasters are borne very differently by different individuals. There are also many methods of sorting people according to psychological type but the introduction of an increasing number of variables renders precise conclusions increasingly difficult.

Many remarkable examples of the apparent onset of symptoms following emotional shock or grief have been recorded. Perhaps the most famous is that contained in a small diary bearing the title 'The Case of Augustus d'Este', now in the library of the Royal College of Physicians of London, from which extracts were published by Firth in 1948.[75] At the age of 22, the first entry occurs:

In the month of December 1822 I travelled from Ramsgate to the Highlands of Scotland for the purpose of passing some days with a Relation for whom I had the affection of a son. On arrival I found him dead. I attended his funeral; there were many persons present and I struggled *violently not to weep*: I was however unable to prevent myself from doing so. Shortly after the funeral I was obliged to have my letters read to me, and their answers written for me, as my eyes were so attacked that when fixed upon minute objects indistinctness of vision was the consequence. Until I attempted to read, or to cut my pen, I was not aware of my eyes being in the least attacked. Soon after I went to Ireland, and without anything having been done to my eyes, they completely recovered their strength and distinctness of vision.

Subsequent entries in the diary leave no doubt about the diagnosis.

The multiplication of similar accounts in retrospective uncontrolled studies can do no more than in the case of physical trauma, that is to say to indicate that in some patients, emotional stress precedes the onset of multiple sclerosis or subsequent relapse and that possibly such patients are predisposed to react in this way.[76,77] Charcot[78] recognised that long-continued grief or vexation might play a part in precipitating multiple sclerosis but also considered that these factors might influence the occurrence of other neurological diseases. In Moxon's[79] excellent description of the disease in a small series of cases, he described one patient who ascribed the commencement of her ailment to a shock received on the occasion of her sister's confinement, when she saw the doctor come into the room with hands covered with blood and was told that her sister was dead. At the time of the shock she had at once an hysterical fit, soon followed by weakness of the legs; this disability disappeared but returned in six months. The occasional relationship between emotional shock and the onset of disease was also recognised by McAlpine[80] and by Adams et al.[81] Braceland & Giffin[82] abandoned an attempt at a controlled study, as it was found that in both multiple sclerosis and controls: 'Any and all types of situations, recent and remote, were alleged to be the cause of the symptoms, either by the patient or, more often, by his immediate family'.

The first successful attempt at a controlled investigation was that of Pratt[83] who studied 100 patients with multiple sclerosis and 100 control cases, nearly all of whom had organic nervous disease. By the methods used he found no difference in premorbid personality between patients and controls. Emotional stress in the month preceding onset was rather more common in the multiple sclerosis patients, but the difference was not significant. The incidence of emotional stress preceding relapse was similar to that preceding onset of the other neurological diseases studied. Pratt was impressed by the occasional striking instance of onset or relapse related to stress but his figures plainly showed that this was an occasional sequence of events. Alter et al[84] used healthy controls and could find no conclusive difference in the incidence of emotional stress preceding the onset of multiple sclerosis. In a case-control study Warren et al[85] found that 79% of patients with multiple sclerosis had been exposed to unusual stress in the two year period before onset of the disease, compared with 54% of hospital controls.

Sibley[86] has reported the results of a prospective study of the effects of stress on relapse or deterioration of multiple sclerosis. Causes of stress were categorised, but individual events were not included unless regarded as stressful by the patient. The period of risk was defined as the duration of the stress plus a further three months, with conditions laid down on the handling of repeated stressful episodes. The mean relapse rates in the risk and non-risk periods were compared. No significant increase was found following family bereavements, illness other than multiple sclerosis causing stress, marital and other conflicts or stress concerned with work. Taking all forms of stress together there was, however, a significant increase during risk periods. Sibley thought that this probably resulted from concurrent reporting of job- and home-related stress and relapse, permitting patient bias. In patients exposed to frequent stress, the disease did not progress more rapidly then in those with less stressful lives, when patients with similar degrees of disability were compared. It was concluded that stress probably did not influence the course of multiple sclerosis. In a study of patients with relapsing/remitting disease, Franklin et al[87] found that the risk of relapse was significantly increased in patients experiencing negative and uncontrollable events during the period of observation.

In a meticulously performed investigation[88] of 39 patients with multiple sclerosis of recent onset compared with 40 matched normal control subjects, it was found that 77% of patients had experienced defined threatening events or marked difficulties compared with 35% of controls. As the authors recognise, there is an important difference between the two groups, the controls being questioned about events in the year before interview and the patients about the year before the onset of their disease, in fact two or three years earlier. The increase in distressing events was largely in the six months before the onset of symptoms of multiple sclerosis. Concern is expressed about such events being forgotten by patients, but the common tendency to remember unpleasant or striking events as much closer in time than in fact they were is not mentioned and there was no opportunity for independent verification. The adverse influence of stress must be regarded as probable but by no means proven.

Exertion, fatigue and heat

The temporary aggravation or induction of symptoms of multiple sclerosis by exertion or heat has long been known and the pathophysiology of these effects is discussed on page 239. It is certainly alarming to step into a hot bath and to become too weak to get out again until the water has chilled and it is not unnatural for patients to fear that such events mean that the disease has advanced. There is, however, little to suggest that unaccustomed exertion or high ambient temperature induce relapse. Detels et al[89] considered that the unduly rapid course of the disease in California might be due to the hot climate: a difficult hypothesis to test. Permanent deterioration following the hot bath diagnostic test for multiple sclerosis, sunbathing and use of a hair dryer was described by Berger & Sheremata,[90] but Davis[91] believed that any prolonged effect was due to heating someone already entering a relapse. Sibley et al[14] reported preliminary negative results of the effects of unaccustomed exercise on relapse. The avoidance of excessive fatigue commonly advised will contribute to comfort, but is unlikely to mitigate the course of the disease.

THE PERIPHERAL NERVOUS SYSTEM

It is commonly stated or assumed that multiple sclerosis exclusively affects the central nervous system but there is growing evidence that this is not so. Early clinical evidence of an association between peripheral neuritis and multiple sclerosis was reviewed by Wartenberg[92] who inclined strongly to the view that episodes of mononeuritis, including sciatica and meralgia paraesthetica, could herald multiple sclerosis. He also suspected that the distinctive migrant sensory neuritis that he described was related and, indeed, the symptoms in one of his cases of 'neuritis' were unmistakably those of a sensory attack of multiple sclerosis. Hasson et al[93] reported that in 4 of 6 autopsies of multiple sclerosis cases in whom the peripheral nervous system had been examined, distal demyelination was present. This distribution in no way resembled the plaques of central lesions. From this account it is not easy to determine whether clinical evidence of peripheral neuropathy had been detected. Lumsden[94] found evidence of Wallerian degeneration in peripheral nerves in 'not unexpected places' but in 13 cases nothing that satisfied the criterion of 'discontinuous demyelination extending laterally across fasciculi'. However, Argyrakis[95] found ultrastructural changes of peripheral paranodal demyelination in two cases at autopsy. No clinical or electrophysiological data were presented. Motor[96] and sensory[97] nerve conduction velocities have been found to be normal in multiple sclerosis but Hopf & Eysholdt[98] reported an increase in the mean relative refractory period in a group of 36 patients. This was not related to age or drugs and suggested mild persistent demyelination. This finding was confirmed on sural nerve biopsies by Pollock et al[99] who found a generalised reduction of myelin lamellae and many internodes with 50% reduction of myelin thickness in 8 of 10 patients. The sural nerve is notoriously subject to external trauma but only one of their patients was severely disabled. There was no clinical evidence of peripheral neuropathy. The occasional absence of wave 1 of the BAEP in multiple sclerosis has been interpreted as indicating involvement of the auditory nerve.[100]

Weir et al[101] produced further evidence of peripheral involvement. Using single fibre EMG, increased jitter was found in 6 of 15 cases of multiple sclerosis, 2 of whom were said also to be suffering from previously undiagnosed peripheral neuropathy, although the clinical features were not described. In a further communication,[102] 3 patients had overt peripheral neuropathy accompanied by a reduction in motor unit numbers and in motor conduction velocity. Some abnormality in motor unit potentials was found in 12 of 19 patients with clinical neuropathy. The authors believed that these findings indicated patchy denervation and re-innervation in the intramuscular nerve network.

In 1977 Schoene et al[103] described 4 patients shown at autopsy to have both multiple sclerosis and hypertrophic peripheral neuropathy with characteristic 'onion bulb' formations, indicative of repeated demyelination. The clinical history and physical signs in 3 patients had been of central nervous system disease with only occasional hints of peripheral involvement such as loss of tendon reflexes, as commonly seen in advanced multiple sclerosis. In the remaining patient, the initial sensory symptoms had been diagnosed, perhaps correctly, as those of peripheral neuropathy, but the subsequent course was typical of multiple sclerosis. Isolated cases had been reported in the past,[104–107] usually regarded as an interesting coincidence, and, as in the more recent case of Rosenberg & Bourdette,[108] peripheral neuropathy had not been suspected in life. The association has, however, been demonstrated by sural nerve biopsy, most remarkably in a child[109] whose illness began with optic neuritis and paraplegia at the age of 9. In a subsequent relapse, slight wasting of the upper limbs was noted and motor nerve conduction velocity, previously normal, was found to be slow. Onion bulb formation was found in a sural nerve biopsy. A very high level of CSF total protein in a patient with otherwise typical multiple sclerosis may provide an early indication of co-existing hypertrophic neuropathy.[110] Less convincing clinical descriptions of the 'polyneuritic' onset of multiple sclerosis have been published.[111,112]

Two series of cases of chronic demyelinating neuropathy associated with MRI evidence of cerebral demyelination have recently been reported. In the 6 patients described by Thomas et al,[113] the original presentation was with symptoms of multiple sclerosis, with the later appearance of peripheral wasting, occasional loss of tendon reflexes and peripheral nerve hypertrophy. Peripheral and central motor and sensory conduction were slow and sural nerve biopsy showed loss of large myelinated fibres and onion bulbs. The CSF total protein was higher than acceptable for multiple sclerosis in 5 cases. Central lesions were shown by CT in 3 and by MRI in all 5 patients examined. Visual evoked potentials were also delayed in most patients. These latter findings were not unexpected, as the clinical diagnosis of multiple sclerosis was not in doubt. In contrast, in only one of the patients described by Mendell et al[114] did symptoms of central nervous disease precede those of peripheral neuropathy. Two patients presented with the Guillain-Barré syndrome, with recovery, and subsequent chronic neuropathy, accompanied by clear clinical evidence of central lesions. Three patients developed chronic demyelinating peripheral neuropathy late in life with no clinical indication of multiple sclerosis but with central lesions on MRI thought to indicate demyelination. The patients were over 70 years of age at the time of the examination and interpretation might be questioned, but strict criteria were used.

Acute demyelinating neuropathy associated with multiple sclerosis has been described less frequently. In the first patient reported by Forrester & Lascelles,[115] the Guillain-Barré syndrome preceded symptoms of multiple sclerosis by 5 years, while in their second case, acute polyneuritis occurred in a man with established disease. Best[116] described acute fatal polyneuritis where unsuspected demyelinated plaques were found in the spinal cord, optic chiasm and brainstem.

The most remarkable example of the acute and apparently simultaneous onset of multiple sclerosis and demyelinating polyradiculitis is that reported by Lassmann et al.[117] This young woman developed swelling of the legs and eyelids and numbness of the face. This was followed by further brainstem signs and by spastic paraparesis and distal wasting of the extremities. She died 12 weeks from the onset. Active plaques were present in the CNS and segmental demyelination in the peripheral nervous system. The CSF had perhaps reflected both processes with a total protein of 430 mg/100 ml and 42 cells/mm^3. The authors, not unnaturally, were unwilling to accept the association as coincidental.

As a number of authors have observed[113,114,118] the combination of central and peripheral relapsing and remitting demyelination is closely paralleled by the animal model, experimental allergic encephalomyelitis (EAE), where the degree of peripheral involvement varies with the species and mode of induction of the disease.[119] All that is lacking in multiple sclerosis is an identifiable antigen. De la Monte et al[120] reported a case in whom two episodes of peripheral and central demyelination followed two different vaccines, influenza and pneumococcal, but the clinical and pathological features were very unusual, the patient also suffering from leukaemia, and the relevance to multiple sclerosis is doubtful.

Increasing recognition of peripheral nerve disease in multiple sclerosis should not obscure the fact that in the great majority of cases examined, the pathological process appears to extend no further than the proximal nerve roots where myelin is controlled by oligodendroglia. The usual clinical features are clearly attributable to central nervous lesions and even the common wasting of the hand muscles is apparently not due to denervation.[121] Remyelination occurs readily in the peripheral nervous system but the ingenious suggestion[122] that relapse and remission in multiple sclerosis are due to fluctuations in the integrity of peripheral myelin cannot be supported.

MULTIPLE SCLEROSIS IN CHILDHOOD

Childhood multiple sclerosis is rare and only recently has it been possible to discern with any clarity the pattern of the disease with onset below the age of 10 or 15. In 1922, Wechsler[123] reviewed earlier reports in which incidence in the first decade sometimes reached 10% and considered that they were highly unreliable. In 1940, Kinnier Wilson[124] found that in reported large series, symptoms had begun below the age of 10 in 2.2%. In three clinic-based series[125–127] published between 1951 and 1963, onset in the first decade occurred in 0.3%. Poser[128] in 1978 recorded only a single case in 812 patients and Shepherd[129] found no instance of onset below 10 years of age in 464 patients in north-east Scotland. In the Canadian population study, symptoms occurred before the age of 16 in 125 of 4632 patients[130] but only 8 were affected in the first decade. Onset below the age of 10 indeed excludes the diagnosis on the Schumacher[131] criteria that have sometimes been used in population studies.[132]

These series, apparently indicating a declining rate of acceptance of childhood multiple sclerosis, inevitably have all the failings of retrospective studies and it is undeniable that even impressive

events in adult life are often forgotten and recollection of illness in childhood is obviously fallible. It also cannot be known how often, if at all, unexplained acute illness in children, with overt or suspected neurological involvement — the familiar 'virus infection' — is a manifestation of multiple sclerosis.

Relevant symptoms recalled from before the age of 15 by adults with established multiple sclerosis do not obviously differ from those commonly encountered at the onset of the remittent form at any age, sensory symptoms and vertigo being often described.[130] When the diagnosis is made in childhood, the clinical picture is far more variable. A considerable number of convincing single cases or small series, diagnosed on clinical[133–140] or pathological[141,142] grounds have been reported, with some rivalry in describing the earliest onset. Shaw & Alvord[143] reported the onset of relapsing and remitting disease at the age of 10 months. A more coherent picture of multiple sclerosis in childhood can be obtained from larger series in which modern diagnostic methods have been used, although discrepancies remain.

Bye et al[144] reported five children with age of onset ranging from 34 months to 14 years. In the three youngest children, up to the age of 9, the onset had been with an acute febrile illness in which optic neuritis with swollen discs, pyramidal and cerebellar signs, convulsions and disturbance of conscious level were prominent features. Investigations, not all performed in the initial illness, were generally compatible with demyelinating disease. Partial or complete spontaneous remission occurred but there was evidence of continued disease activity. At the time of reporting, these children were either free from neurological abnormalities or had static signs, but in all mental acuity was poor and had been shown to have deteriorated. In the two older children, aged 9 years and 9 months and 14 years respectively, the onset more closely resembled that of the usual adult form, although the younger child became steroid dependent. In both there was severe intellectual impairment.

Sheremata et al[145] reported, but apparently only in abstract, 12 cases of childhood multiple sclerosis. The mean age at onset was 9.5 years and the range 6–14 years. Nine had very severe disease and four had died after a mean disease duration of 5.8 years. The largest published series is that of Boutin et al[146] who observed multiple sclerosis in nineteen children under the age of 15 in the course of 20 years, fifteen of the children being between 10 and 15 years old. In the majority, the symptoms and course did not differ from adult disease. In three, the pattern was of spinal cord disease progressive from the onset. In all those with the remittent form, the first relapse occurred within 5 years. Isolated optic neuritis was the first symptom in three children. An acute encephalopathic onset occurred in four children, often accompanied by fever and even neck rigidity. Remission was often followed by relapse within 3 months, followed by further remissions and relapses. Intellectual impairment was frequent but not universal.

In the encephalopathic form a diagnosis of multiple sclerosis, as distinct from acute disseminated encephalomyelitis, can only be made following subsequent relapse. Alvord[147] has reviewed the difficult problem of relapsing disseminated encephalomyelitis and concluded that this diagnosis can only be made by the histopathological demonstration of exclusively perivenous demyelination, scarcely applicable for purposes of prognosis.

In conclusion, the course of multiple sclerosis with onset in childhood does not, in the majority of cases, greatly differ from that in adults, although there has been no systematic long-term assessment. In a minority the onset is with encephalomyelitis with remission and often early relapse. It is not yet clear whether younger children are particularly prone to this form of the disease. The risk of severe intellectual impairment has been emphasised in some reports, but Riikonen et al,[148] in their study of children who developed multiple sclerosis following optic neuritis, found no evidence of this. As in adults, the clinical features are sometimes extremely aberrant: chronic psychosis[142] and hypertrophic neuropathy[109] may be cited as examples.

Optic neuritis in childhood

Optic neuritis in childhood has been the subject of a number of studies.[148-153] Girls are affected more frequently than boys. The mean age of onset is around 9 years but optic neuritis has been observed at the age of three.[153] The clinical features include a high proportion of bilateral simultaneous or closely consecutive attacks, representative figures being 10 of 14 cases,[151] 13 of 21,[148] 29 of 39[153] and 11 of 21.[152] Swollen discs, usually bilaterally, occur in similar or even higher proportions. Headache or pain in the eye and loss of central vision occur in the majority although peripheral field defects may also be found.[152] Infection, specific or unidentified, or inoculation precedes optic neuritis in from 20%[154] to 46%[153] and a further possible indication of the role of infection is that onset in the month of April was more than twice as common than in any other month in a British series.[153]

The prognosis for vision is generally good. Kriss et al[153] found on follow-up that in 7% of affected eyes, acuity had returned to 6/6 or better. The worst residual acuity was, however, perception of hand movements only.[9] De Leersnyder et al[151] reported bilateral blindness in two children, although most of their patients regained normal vision. Riikonen et al[148] reported two children who were left 'practically blind'. In patients whose vision is virtually restored, pattern reversal visual evoked potentials often rapidly return to normal.[153]

Obviously of great importance is the risk of progression to multiple sclerosis. Kennedy & Carroll[149] and Kennedy & Carter[150] found 30 cases of optic neuritis under the age of 15 where no cause could be found and 8 of these (27%) were subsequently known to have developed multiple sclerosis after a mean period of 8 years. In retrospect, no feature of the original episode could have predicted the outcome. Figures for progression from other series are 10 of 21,[152] 2 of 14 (14%),[151] 9 of 21 (43%)[148] and 6 of 39 (15%).[153] All of these figures are lower than the rate of progression to multiple sclerosis in adults with optic neuritis. The discrepancies between series must in part reflect case selection and length of follow-up. In all series, some children with accompanying disseminated neurological signs have been included and these are not figures for isolated optic neuritis such as are usually presented for adults. It seems, however, that the presence of such signs does not predict whether or not multiple sclerosis will develop later. In one series,[153] 5 of 30 children with no additional signs developed multiple sclerosis compared with 1 of 9 with signs of disseminated disease at the time of the optic neuritis.

Most observers have found that, in children, progression to multiple sclerosis is much less common after bilateral than after unilateral optic neuritis. The majority of the 19 cases of bilateral optic neuritis under the age of 15 reported by Heirons & Lyle[155] and Meadows[154] were subsequently traced,[156] after an immensely long follow-up period. Multiple sclerosis was very doubtfully diagnosed in a single case. Riikonen et al[148] found that 7 of 8 children with unilateral optic neuritis progressed to multiple sclerosis, in contrast to 2 of 13 with bilateral neuritis. De Leersnyder et al[151] regarded bilateral simultaneous affection as a strong indication that multiple sclerosis would not develop. In contrast, Kriss et al[153] found no significant difference in numbers progressing following bilateral or unilateral optic neuritis, although they attribute the high rate of progression in Haller & Patzold's[152] series to the large proportion of unilateral cases. Recurrent optic neuritis is not uncommon, occurring in 6 of 30 cases,[149,150] four of whom developed multiple sclerosis. Kriss et al,[153] however, did not find that recurrent attacks, either bilateral or unilateral, increased the risk of multiple sclerosis.

The interval between optic neuritis and the first relapse in those who progress is extremely variable. In the majority of reported cases, relapse occurs within a year or two but McKay[157] recorded a patient who lost the sight of the left eye at the age of 4, with full recovery. Twenty nine years later the left eye was again affected and after a further two years, disseminated symptoms developed, leading to typical multiple sclerosis.

ASSOCIATED DISEASES

To establish a definite link between multiple sclerosis and a disease of which the cause is better known or more accessible to investigation might well prove a great advance in understanding or, at least, afford an opening to be explored. Unfortunately, associations so far detected are tenuous or with diseases no better understood than multiple sclerosis. One obvious method is to screen large series of cases of multiple sclerosis for other diseases of which the incidence and prevalence are well known. Difficulty arises from the length of follow-up and high autopsy rate needed to establish an association with a condition with a later age of onset, such as cerebral glioma. Another method is to examine series of cases of other diseases for the number who also have multiple sclerosis. Unfortunately, the prevalence of multiple sclerosis in the population from which the series is drawn is seldom precisely known. The starting point for such investigations is often simple clinical observation of a few instances of patients with both multiple sclerosis and the other disease in question.

Uveitis

A probable association between inflammation of the uveal tract — iridocyclitis and choroiditis — and multiple sclerosis was first described in 1933[158] and later supported by Garcin[159] who recorded uveitis in 15 patients with multiple sclerosis. Haarr[160] reviewed 255 cases of uveitis and found an association with multiple sclerosis in 6. Approaching the problem from the neurological aspect, Tschabitscher[161] found that 5.5% of 200 cases of multiple sclerosis had iridocyclitis and 4% had choroiditis. Bammer et al[162] found evidence of choroidal involvement in 5.5% of 602 multiple sclerosis patients and in 1.6% of patients with other neurological diseases, excluding syphilis. Archambeau et al[163] reported peripheral uveitis in 1% of 675 patients and in a much smaller study Breger & Leopold[164] found evidence of past or active peripheral uveitis in 27%.

Reports on large series are seldom accompanied by any detailed descriptions and in single case reports the diagnosis of multiple sclerosis is not always secure. In the young boy reported by Curless & Bray[165], the initial ocular symptoms were severe, with posterior uveitis and bilateral vitreous haemorrhage. Some four years later, relapsing and remitting neurological symptoms developed, strongly suggestive of multiple sclerosis and with compatible CSF findings. The cases described by Giles[166] illustrate difficulty in apportioning visual loss between the effects of optic neuritis and uveitis. A pathological examination was obtained by Arné et al.[167] Their patient developed uveitis at the age of 48. This was extremely severe and led to bilateral virtual blindness. No sheathing of veins was present. The following year she developed progressive difficulty in walking and sphincter disturbance. She had spastic weakness and inco-ordination of the limbs and sensory loss. She died aged 60. At post mortem the eyes were not examined. Plaques of demyelination were present throughout the white matter of the cerebral hemispheres.

As pointed out by Bamford et al,[168] at the time of publication of many of these studies, several specific causes of uveitis combined with disease of the central nervous system had not been clearly delineated, including sarcoidosis, Behçet's disease and primary Sjögren's syndrome, all of which may be mistaken for multiple sclerosis. In their own study they found 3 cases of peripheral uveitis, or pars planitis, in 127 patients with multiple sclerosis. The pars plana is that part of the ciliary body in contact with the vitreous anterior to the termination of the retina, the inferior segment being that affected by disease. Thorough examination of this site requires indirect ophthalmoscopy and scleral depression of the peripheral retina. Pars planitis in the absence of neurological or systemic disease is not uncommon. Its cause is unknown but naturally an autoimmune pathogenesis has been suggested. The association with multiple sclerosis remains unexplained. It seems unlikely that the disease process of multiple sclerosis should itself involve the uveal tract, but the finding of oligoclonal bands of IgG in the cerebrospinal fluid of a patient with isolated pars planitis[169] is not without interest.

Venous sheathing

Rucker[170–172] in a series of papers gave a detailed description of sheathing of the retinal veins and emphasised the particular association of this abnormality with multiple sclerosis, being present in some 10% of cases at the time of examination. The characteristic appearance is that of a white line on either side of a considerable stretch of vein, not closely approaching the optic nerve head. Haarr[173] thought that this chronic state was preceded by a more active form in which rounded exudates can be seen around dilated veins. Single exudates might resolve within a few weeks and the active stage could be observed to persist for up to two years, to be followed by the chronic condition or by complete resolution. Engell[174] also stated that periphlebitis retinae might persist for a few weeks only, but provided no evidence that this was so. The chronic changes much more frequently observed are known to persist for up to two years[175] and in one instance for 14 years.[176]

Histological examination has usually shown perivenous cuffing with lymphocytes and plasma cells,[177–179] but this appearance is not confined to the active clinical stage as described by Haarr.[173] In a case where sheathing had persisted for many years unchanged, cellular response was slight and the main finding was dense collagenous thickening of the venous walls, the arteries being unaffected.[176] It is certainly tempting to equate these vascular changes with those in recent and chronic multiple sclerosis plaques.[175,176] If this is so, it is perhaps surprising that there is so little evidence of remission of periphlebitis retinae. The fact that there is no myelin in the area of retina affected strongly suggests that the primary lesion is in the vascular endothelium. There is no explanation of why retinal veins should be selectively affected, but there is little evidence that blood vessels in other tissues beyond the central nervous system have been systematically examined.

There have been many positive reports indicating that sheathing can be seen in 10–40% of cases of multiple sclerosis.[180–183] Some series have been controlled against sex- and age-matched normal subjects, in whom no sheathing occurred. Engell & Andersen,[184] by an ingenious calculation, based on the reported incidence and duration of venous sheathing and the duration of multiple sclerosis, concluded that it probably occurred in all cases at some time. Sheathing is difficult to see and can seldom be detected by direct ophthalmoscopy through an undilated pupil[175] as the veins in the periphery of the retina are selectively affected. Fluorescein angiography will frequently demonstrate leaking of dye from the veins.[183]

Venous sheathing was found in 6 of 50 patients with isolated optic neuritis by Lightman et al.[178] In 4 of these, fluorescein angiography showed leakage at the site of sheathing, but venous leakage also occurred in 6 eyes in which sheathing had not been detected. In 6 patients, cells were seen in the vitreous or anterior chamber and in 2 of these, this was the only abnormality. No additional ocular disease was found. The abnormalities were present bilaterally or solely in the eye contralateral to the optic neuritis in 5 patients.

Periphlebitis retinae is not, however, specific for multiple sclerosis, as it is known to occur in association with many infections, notably tuberculosis, in sarcoidosis and in idiopathic pars planitis. Some legitimate confusion may arise with Eales' disease with neurological complications. The ocular features originally described were recurrent retinal and vitreous haemorrhage but venous sheathing was later recognised. The association of ocular haemorrhage and abnormal neurological signs was present in 4 of 17 patients diagnosed as having Eales' disease by White[185] and abnormalities in the CSF, without clinical evidence of CNS disease, were found in a further 3 cases. Although multiple sclerosis had been diagnosed in some of these patients, none satisfied criteria for definite diagnosis. This is also true of the three patients described by Silfverskiöld[186] who developed spinal cord lesions during active retinal vasculitis. There was partial remission but after prolonged observation no evidence of multiple lesions. The problem of distinction from multiple sclerosis was discussed by Pépin et al.[187] Autopsy has confirmed that neurological symptoms are due to vasculitis but some perivenous demyelination has also been recorded.[188]

The significance of venous sheathing for the individual patient is uncertain. Bamford et al[168] found sheathing in 14 of 127 patients; 2 of whom also had pars planitis. Sheathing was not related to relapse or degree of disability, but was considerably more common in progressive disease. Lightman et al[178] found that in patients with optic neuritis, progression to multiple sclerosis was significantly more common when venous sheathing was present, but numbers were small. Engell[174] found that venous sheathing was much more common in active or severe disease, being found in 43% of patients with rapidly progressive disease, 5% with slow progression and only in 1% of patients with static disease or in remission.

Autoimmune disease

The clustering of autoimmune diseases has been amply exemplified by myasthenia gravis where the cumulative prevalence of such diseases has been found to be 11%.[189] Autoimmunity is often assumed to have an important role in the pathogenesis of multiple sclerosis, although no antigen has been identified. Association with diseases of similar causation might therefore be expected. Two retrospective studies based on scrutiny of hospital notes have failed to demonstrate any significant association. Baker et al[190] found 9 examples of known or presumed autoimmune disease in 329 patients with multiple sclerosis (2.7%). One patient had Hashimoto's thyroiditis, two had thyrotoxicosis and one had primary myxoedema and incipient pernicious anaemia. Two patients had rheumatoid arthritis and there were single examples of pemphigus vulgaris, atrophic gastritis and autoimmune Addison's disease. In a similar study[189] the notes of 826 patients with clinically definite multiple sclerosis were examined for evidence of autoimmune disease. Here again thyroid disease was the commonest association, with 15 cases of hyperthyroidism and 4 of primary myxoedema. Eleven further cases of thyroid disease were excluded because of lack of information or localised disease unlikely to have an autoimmune cause. There were 5 cases of rheumatoid arthritis (1 also being hyperthyroid), 4 of type I diabetes mellitus, 2 of ulcerative colitis and 2 of vitiligo. There were single examples of ankylosing spondylitis, polymyalgia rheumatica, coeliac disease, primary biliary cirrhosis, chronic atrophic gastritis, alopecia universalis and cutaneous lupus erythematosus. The 2 cases of chronic demyelinating peripheral neuropathy are discussed on page 119. The cumulative prevalence of associated autoimmune disease was 4.9%, no higher than an approximate estimate for the general population. Serum autoantibodies were significantly more often present in 105 multiple sclerosis patients without recognised autoimmune disease than in control patients with other neurological diseases, matched for age and sex, but titres in both groups were generally low.

While these retrospective surveys may have

underestimated the incidence of associated disease they provide no support for autoimmunity in multiple sclerosis. Reports of association with specific diseases are still of interest.

Myasthenia gravis

The association of myasthenia and multiple sclerosis is rare but probably significant. In the two cases personally observed, the onset of myasthenia long preceded that of multiple sclerosis, but the order in which symptoms of the two diseases develops appears to be random.[191] The interval may be extremely long, as in the second case of Aita et al[192] who developed multiple sclerosis, later confirmed at autopsy, 23 years after complete remission from myasthenia following thymectomy. Only occasionally have individual symptoms resulted in diagnostic difficulty. In a patient with multiple sclerosis reported by Margolis & Groves,[193] ocular palsies and ptosis were found to respond to prostigmine and were attributed to myasthenia gravis. In another example,[194] after a nine-year history of multiple sclerosis the unusual symptoms of fatigue on chewing, ptosis and episodic dysphagia developed and responded to anticholinesterase treatment. In this case, the two diseases relapsed together, but this is unusual.

Lo & Feasby[195] described a remarkable succession of hyperthyroidism at the age of 14, myasthenia at age 25, completely relieved by thymectomy, and multiple sclerosis at age 26. The authors justifiably thought that the 10 reported cases of the association of myasthenia gravis and multiple sclerosis exceeded the bounds of chance. Bixenman & Buschbaum[196] described a similar combination, but in reverse order, multiple sclerosis being followed by euthyroid Graves' ophthalmopathy and myasthenia. Ghezzi et al[197] have since reported bilateral asynchronous optic neuritis in a patient with myasthenia gravis. Oligoclonal IgG was present in the CSF.

In an epidemiological survey[198] in an area of Finland, 94 cases of myasthenia gravis and 991 of multiple sclerosis were found, both diseases occurring in 2 women, a number in excess of that expected.

Thyroid disease

As already noted, in large series of patients with multiple sclerosis, thyroid disease is not uncommon, but apparently does not exceed the expected frequency.[189] In a personal series of 377 patients with clinically definite multiple sclerosis, 8 (2.1%) were known to have had thyroid disease; thyrotoxicosis in 3, nodular goitre requiring surgery in 2, myxoema of unknown cause in two and one patient had a non-toxic goitre. Isolated cases of Hashimoto's thyroiditis[199] and of myxoedema secondary to hypopituitarism[200] have been reported and there have been ingenious but unconvincing attempts to link multiple sclerosis with goitre of dietary origin.[201,202] Thyroid function may be disturbed but not to a greater degree than in other chronic diseases.[203]

Diabetes mellitus.

Warren & Warren[204,205] have attempted to show an increased incidence of diabetes mellitus in patients with multiple sclerosis. However, no significant difference from controls was observed unless first degree relatives, not suffering from multiple sclerosis, were included. The type of diabetes was not specified and the diagnosis in relatives was not verified. No convincing association has been shown except that admission to hospital because of diabetes was found to be more common in patients with multiple sclerosis than in the general population in a cohort studied in Sweden.[206]

Bowel disease

In a survey of 2579 women with ileostomy for ulcerative colitis, 10 were found to have multiple sclerosis.[207] The figure is difficult to interpret as the prevalence of multiple sclerosis in women of this age is only approximately known, but suggests that the disease is unduly common in these patients. Either disease might present first, or both might be diagnosed on the same hospital admission. The association has also been observed in isolated cases in men.[208] Minuk & Lewkonia[209] reported a remarkable familial association of multiple sclerosis with bowel disease, both ulcerative colitis and Crohn's disease, particularly the latter. In a population of about one million they found 17 families in whom this association occurred in first or second degree relatives, the most frequent pattern being parent and child.

An intestinal disorder in multiple sclerosis resulting in the malabsorption of fatty acids was proposed by Thompson[210] and received some support from the finding of partial villous atrophy in jejunal biopsy specimens.[211] A controlled study, however, failed to show any significant abnormality of the mucosa.[212] The low level of serum linoleic acid reported in some series of patients is rapidly corrected by dietary supplements[213] and cannot be attributed to malabsorption.

Ankylosing spondylitis

An association between ankylosing spondylitis and multiple sclerosis was first suggested by Matthews[214] who, in a series of 59 cases of spondylitis found 1 definite and 1 possible case of multiple sclerosis, the latter subsequently developing clinically definite disease. Thomas et al[215] examined 45 cases of ankylosing spondylitis and found two cases of probable multiple sclerosis and one patient with chronic progressive spastic paraparesis for which no other cause could be found. Kahn & Kusher[216] found two examples of presumed multiple sclerosis in 196 cases of ankylosing spondylitis.

These figures from series of cases of ankylosing spondylitis, naturally mainly male, indicate a prevalence of multiple sclerosis greatly in excess of expected figures. The association has been much less obvious in large series of cases of multiple sclerosis. In a personal series of 377 cases, 2 men and 1 woman had ankylosing spondylitis. Two other patients, a man and a woman, each had a son with spondylitis. It may be important that the spondylitis can be symptomless[217,218] and only detected on routine radiology.

There is a very close link between ankylosing spondylitis and HLA B27, which is not one of the tissue types more loosely associated with multiple sclerosis. In personal experience, 2 men with both diseases were HLA B27 as expected. This aspect has been further explored by Hannahan et al.[218]

Forty three of 420 patients with multiple sclerosis were HLA B27. Spinal and pelvic radiographs were available in 20 and 5 of these were found to have ankylosing spondylitis. No spondylitis was found in 43 HLA B27 blood donors.

Other autoimmune diseases

The suggested negative correlation between rheumatoid arthritis and multiple sclerosis[219] has not been substantiated.[190] There is a single report of associated systemic sclerosis.[220] Systemic lupus erythematosus is discussed in Chapter 6. Isolated examples of multiple sclerosis associated with bullous pemphigoid[221] eosinophilic vasculitis[222] and thrombocytopenic purpura[223] have been described.

Cancer

The incidence of cancer in patients with multiple sclerosis was thought by Zimmerman & Netsky[224] to be increased but this has not been confirmed. Autopsy studied series, the only reliable source of information, are unfortunately too small for any but the closest association to be detected, but none has been found.[225] Sibley et al[226] reported an unexpected finding related to the family history. There was no difference in the incidence of cancer in the near relatives of patients with multiple sclerosis and in those of control subjects. However, incidence of cancer in relatives of patients with a family history of multiple sclerosis was significantly increased. The best explanation that could be offered was a genetically determined alteration in immune response, increasing susceptibility to both diseases.

Considerable interest has been aroused by the association of primary brain tumour with multiple sclerosis. It is not known how common this is. Zimmerman & Netsky[224] were impressed by finding 2 gliomas in 50 autopsied cases of multiple sclerosis but, in contrast, Palo et al[227] found only 1 glial tumour in a survey of 2200 cases and believed the incidence to be unduly low. The number of reported cases has slowly increased. In 1963 Brihaye et al[228] could find only 4 such reports, while in 1974 the total had reached 12, with 3 additional examples described by Currie &

Urich.[229] Lynch,[230] Lahl[231] and Ho & Wolfe[232] contributed single case reports. By 1977, 20 glial tumours had been reported in varying detail, with a smaller number of tumours of non-glial tissue.

Until recently, diagnosis of the dual pathology was seldom achieved in life, undiagnosed tumours being found post mortem in patients long known to have multiple sclerosis,[233] or unsuspected plaques found in patients dying of brain tumour. Imaging techniques now permit easier recognition of tumours,[234] but difficulties of distinction from the 'pseudotumorous' presentation of multiple sclerosis persist (p. 63).

There has naturally been speculation on the possibility of glial cells in the multiple sclerosis plaque undergoing malignant change. Russell & Rubenstein[235] believed that this occurred and Anderson et al[236] described gradual transition from gliosis to glioma within plaques in two cases of multiple sclerosis and one of an atypical demyelinating disease. Gliomata in association with multiple sclerosis are said often to be multi-centric,[236,237] although intervening bands of malignant tissue may connect apparently separate lesions. The origin of gliomata in plaques has not been universally accepted and, if it occurs, does so rarely.

Other primary intracranial tumours have been described: oligodendroglioma,[238] meningioma[239] and reticulosarcoma,[240] including one patient who had received immunosuppressant treatment for multiple sclerosis.[241] I have twice seen cerebral metastases from breast cancer in women with es-tablished multiple sclerosis. The theory that plaques in some way favour the development of cerebral secondary deposits[239] does not appear to have much to recommend it.

Other associations

There are isolated instances of association with diseases that have little theoretical or even conjec-tural relationship with multiple sclerosis, including myotonic muscular dystrophy.[242] Mishra et al[243] described multiple sclerosis, proven at autopsy, in a patient with familial facioscapulohumeral dystrophy and calculated the odds against co-incidence as $1:10.^9$ Even more remarkable are the two cases where multiple sclerosis developed in patients with hypokalaemic periodic para-lysis.[244,245] The concurrence of multiple sclerosis and motor neurone disease, proven at autopsy, has also been reported[246] and two further instances have been personally observed.

Watkins & Espir[247] found that 27% of 100 patients with multiple sclerosis suffered from migraine, in contrast to 12% of control subjects.

A totally unexpected association with spon-taneous pneumothorax has been described.[248] Of 141 cases of pneumothorax, 2 patients had proven multiple sclerosis and 1 had clinically definite dis-ease. Two patients already had severe multiple sclerosis at the time of the pneumothorax but the other patient had mild disease. In a personal case, spontaneous pneumothorax accompanied the initial symptoms of multiple sclerosis.

In 1968, a man of 35 developed a left spontaneous pneumothorax, accompanied by numbness of the left arm. He was no longer able to remember whether these two events occurred precisely simultaneously. In 1977 he complained of giddiness, unsteadiness and a poor memory. When seen in 1982, he had bilateral internuclear ophthalmoplegia, an ataxic gait, bilateral extensor plantar reflexes and defective immediate recall. Visual evoked potentials were bilaterally delayed but the CSF was normal.

The results of examining a population cohort in Sweden for diseases associated with multiple sclerosis were also surprising.[208] Hospital ad-missions of 159 200 subjects born between 1911 and 1940 were scrutinised for the decade 1970–9. There were 351 cases of multiple sclerosis. Ad-mission for tuberculosis was much more common in both men and women with multiple sclerosis than in the general population. Asthma, myocar-dial infarction in younger men and diabetes in younger subjects were also significantly more common than expected. There is no obvious ex-planation for these findings. Asthma and other allergic conditions have not previously been found to occur more commonly than in control subjects.

Conclusion

With the exception of ocular and retinal abnor-malities, that may well be an integral part of the disease, review of associated pathology has failed to provide any important clue to the aetiology or pathogenesis of multiple sclerosis.

SYSTEMIC ABNORMALITIES

The difficulties inherent in investigating the pathogenesis of multiple sclerosis would be less formidable if it could be shown that the disease process was not confined to the central nervous system. Abnormalities of the immune system beyond the nervous system are described in Chapter 11. There have been many attempts to incriminate specific infection as the cause of multiple sclerosis, but no claim for the existence of an infective agent in blood, CSF, bone marrow[249] or jejunum[250] has been substantiated. The multiple sclerosis-associated agent of Carp and Henle that was thought to betray its presence by an effect on reducing the circulating polymorphonuclear leucocytes of mice,[251] could not be confirmed.[252]

Coagulation defects

Abnormalities in blood platelets and in other factors concerned in coagulation have been reported in multiple sclerosis for many years, but have excited only sporadic interest. Probably the initial impetus to the search for such changes was the vascular occlusion theory of the formation of plaques put forward by Putnam.[253]

Absolute numbers of platelets were shown to fall during relapse of multiple sclerosis and to increase again during remission, but this effect was not thought to differ from that seen in many forms of acute disease.[254] Plasma fibrinogen was found to increase during relapse, but again was not thought to be in any way characteristic or related to the cause of the disease.[255] Capillary resistance, examined by a standardised low pressure method, was reported by Shulman et al[256] to be reduced compared with normal subjects, but patients with other neurological diseases were not examined. Swank[257] described spontaneous cutaneous haemorrhages in 48 of 62 female patients observed. These would begin as small red spots and develop as subcutaneous echymoses. They were apt to appear in 'showers', particularly below a sphygmomanometer cuff or in pressure areas. No control observations were reported. The impli-

cation was that similar events, perhaps the result of vascular occlusion, could be occurring within the CNS.

Feldman et al,[258] however, could find no abnormality in a wide spectrum of tests of coagulation function and capillary resistance. The increased fibrinolytic activity of venous blood in multiple sclerosis in relapse reported by Menon et al[259] again did not appear to be related to the disease process as a similar effect had been noted in blood from hemiplegic limbs.[260] Brunetti et al[261] attributed lower levels of plasminogen and fibrinogen to a non-specific effect of a chronic immunological disease on the coagulative system.

The most consistent abnormality described has been an increase in platelet stickiness, adhesiveness or aggregation, measured in a variety of ways. First reported by Nathanson & Savitsky in 1952,[262] increased aggregation in response to various stimuli has been repeatedly confirmed.[263-265]

The majority of reports have been of increased stickiness to glass, present only in clinically active disease.[266-268] Although it was naturally tempting to believe that 'sticky' platelets might be blocking venules in the CNS, most investigators concluded, admittedly not on very secure grounds other than caution, that the phenomenon was secondary to disease activity. Wright et al[266] associated increased stickiness with low serum linoleate. The linoleate content of platelets in multiple sclerosis was found to be lower than normal, but levels were not correlated with platelet stickiness.[269] Platelet adherence to glass is a non-specific phenomenon, influenced by many factors,[270] and not necessarily related to physiological function. The possible role of any abnormality in platelet function in the pathogenesis of multiple sclerosis remains obscure. Srivastava et al[271] considered a relative increase in prostaglandin PGE_2, favouring platelet aggregation, as the immediate cause and that this might result from viral infection of the platelets, of which, however, no evidence has been found. It is probable that abnormalities of platelet behaviour are secondary to slight changes in plasma lipids, either the result of CNS damage or of chronic disease.

Haemorrhage into the substance of the CNS has rarely been reported in multiple sclerosis. Abroms et al[272] reported spontaneous intracerebral haemorrhage in two young females in whom the diagnosis of multiple sclerosis had been suspected. No source for haemorrhage was found and the usual invisible arteriovenous malformation was postulated. However, Jankovic et al[273] described cerebral and spinal haemorrhage in clinically definite multiple sclerosis, for which no structural cause could be found. There is no convincing explanation for these events.

Erythrocytes

Controversy concerning abnormalities in the red blood cells in multiple sclerosis has been of particular interest because of the implications of a widespread or universal defect of cell membranes, of obvious possible relevance to myelin. Field and colleagues[274,275] long maintained that an abnormality in the red cell membrane was responsible for the results of the diagnostic tests for multiple sclerosis that they had devised. Briefly stated, the simplified test consisted of slowing of electrophoretic mobility of red cells from multiple sclerosis patients by the addition of arachidonic or linoleic acid to the medium. The claim of 100% sensitivity and specificity for multiple sclerosis could not be confirmed by most investigators,[276–280] who failed to find any distinctive pattern of red cell mobility. Seaman et al[281] found the test positive in a blind study of 56 patients with multiple sclerosis, but negative in patients thought to have early disease, throwing doubt on the fundamental nature of the abnormality. Furthermore, they demonstrated[282] conclusively that the abnormal results were derived from the plasma. Red cells from normal control subjects, incubated with multiple sclerosis plasma gave positive results, while red cells from multiple sclerosis patients, incubated with normal plasma, did not.

Mechanical fragility of red cells was found to be increased in multiple sclerosis by Schauf et al,[283] but McCrea et al,[284] using different methods, found no difference from normal. Kurantsin-Mills et al[285] found osmotic fragility to be increased in inpatients with multiple sclerosis but not in outpatients and concluded that factors such as drugs or infection might be responsible. There have been similar disagreements on the question of red cell deformability. Brunetti et al[261] and Simpson et al[286] found the viscosity of whole blood, but not that of plasma, to be significantly increased in multiple sclerosis, and the red cell filtration rate significantly slower. These findings could be accounted for by reduced deformability of the red cells that, in turn, might lead to vascular stasis. The conclusion has been questioned[287] and red cell filtration rate has been found to be normal by other workers.[288] The remarkable excess of echinocytes observed by Simpson et al[286] was not found by Kurantsin-Mills et al,[285] apparently using identical methods.

Some suggestion of an abnormality of fatty acid composition or metabolism of the red cells in multiple sclerosis persists. Homa et al[289] found that in normal subjects there was an inverse correlation between the percentage of linoleate and arachidonate in the major fatty acid content. This was not present in red cells from multiple sclerosis patients. Van Alstine & Brooks[290] interpreted the results of partition experiments between dextran and polyethylene glycol, in the presence of fatty acids, as showing that red cells in multiple sclerosis bound saturated and unsaturated fatty acids differently from normal. There was a significant difference in the mean values between multiple sclerosis and normal, but the considerable overlap does not inspire confidence in the reality of a fundamental difference. The possible effects of chronic disease must always be taken into account and normal controls are inadequate. The same reliance on normal controls must also cast doubt on the significant reduction of linoleic and arachidonic acid in lipids of the red cell membrane found by Navarro & Segura.[291].

No systemic abnormality has been consistently linked with multiple sclerosis.

REFERENCES

1. McAlpine D, Compston N D, Lumsden C E 1955 Multiple sclerosis. Livingstone, Edinburgh
2. McAlpine D, Compston N D 1952 Some aspects of the natural history of disseminated sclerosis. Quarterly Journal of Medicine 21: 135–167
3. Wüthrich R, Rieder H P 1970 The seasonal incidence of multiple sclerosis in Switzerland. European Neurology 3: 257–264

4. Sibley W A, Foley J M 1965 Seasonal variation in multiple sclerosis and retrobulbar neuritis in northeastern Ohio. Transactions of the American Neurological Association 90: 295–297

5. Bamford C R, Sibley W A, Thies C 1983 Seasonal variation of multiple sclerosis exacerbations in Arizona. Neurology 33: 697–701

6. Schapira K 1959 The seasonal incidence of onset and exacerbations in multiple sclerosis. Journal of Neurology, Neurosurgery and Psychiatry 22: 285–286

7. Taub R B, Rucker C W 1954 The relationship of retrobulbar neuritis to multiple sclerosis. American Journal of Ophthalmology 37: 494–497

8. Compston D A S, Batchelor J R, Earl C J, McDonald W I 1978 Factors influencing the risk of multiple sclerosis developing in patients with optic neuritis. Brain 101: 495–511

9. Taylor D, Cuendet F 1986 Optic neuritis in childhood. In: Hess R F, Plant G T (eds) Optic neuritis. Cambridge University Press, Cambridge, pp 73–85

10. Gay D, Dick G, Upton G 1986 Multiple sclerosis associated with sinusitis: case-controlled study in general practice. Lancet 1: 816–819

11. Gay D, Dick G 1986 Is multiple sclerosis caused by an oral spirochaete? Lancet 2: 75–77

12. Callaghan T S 1986 Multiple sclerosis and sinusitis. Lancet 2: 160–161

13. Alperovitch A, Clanet M, Mas J L 1986 Multiple sclerosis and sinusitis. Lancet 1: 1159

14. Sibley W A, Bamford C R, Clark K 1984 Triggering factors in multiple sclerosis. In: Poser C M (ed) The diagnosis of multiple sclerosis. Thieme–Stratton, New York, pp 14–24

15. Miller H, Newell D J, Ridley A 1961 Multiple sclerosis: treatment of acute exacerbations with corticotrophin. Lancet 2: 1120–1122

16. Sibley W A, Bamford C R, Clark K 1985 Clinical viral infections and multiple sclerosis. Lancet 1: 1313–1315

17. Alter M, Speer J 1968 Clinical evaluation of possible etiologic factors in multiple sclerosis. Neurology 18: 109–116

18. Panitch H S, Hirsch R L, Schindler J, Johnson J P 1987 Treatment of multiple sclerosis with gamma interferon: exacerbations with activation of the immune system. Neurology 37: 1097–1102

19. Morris J A 1985 Clinical viral infections and multiple sclerosis. Lancet 2: 273

20. Miller H, Cendrowski W, Schapira K 1967 Multiple sclerosis and vaccination. British Medical Journal 2: 210–213

21. Sibley W A, Foley J M 1965 Infection and immunisation in multiple sclerosis. Annals of the New York Academy of Sciences 122: 457–468

22. Sibley W A, Bamford C R, Laguna J F 1976 Influenza vaccination in patients with multiple sclerosis. Journal of the American Medical Association 236: 1965–1966

23. Rabin J 1973 Hazard of influenza vaccine in neurologic patients. Journal of the American Medical Association 225: 63–64

24. Poser C M 1982 Neurological complications of swine influenza vaccination. Acta Neurologica Scandinavica 66: 413–431

25. Myers L W, Ellison G W, Lucia M, Novom S 1976 Swine-influenza vaccination in multiple sclerosis. New England Journal of Medicine 295: 1204

26. Bamford C R, Sibley W A, Laguna J F 1979 Swine influenza vaccination in patients with multiple sclerosis. Archives of Neurology 35: 242–243

27. Kurland L T, Molgaard C A, Kurland E M, Wiederholt W C, Kirkpatrick J W 1984 Swine flu vaccine and multiple sclerosis. Journal of the American Medical Association 251: 2672–2675

28. Leibowitz U, Antonovsky A, Kats R, Alter M 1967 Does pregnancy increase the risk of multiple sclerosis? Journal of Neurology, Neurosurgery and Psychiatry 30: 354–357

29. Tillman A J B 1950 The effect of pregnancy on multiple sclerosis and its management. Research Publications of the Association for Research into Nervous and Mental Disease 28: 548–582

30. Andersen O 1984 Reduced risk of MS onset during pregnancy. Acta Neurologica Scandinavica 69 (suppl 98): 370–373

31. Korn-Lubetzki I, Kahana E, Cooper G, Abramsky O 1984 Activity of multiple sclerosis during pregnancy and puerperium. Annals of Neurology 16: 228–231

32. Korn-Lubetzki I, Kahana E, Abramsky O 1985 Activity of multiple sclerosis during pregnancy and puerperium. Annals of Neurology 18: 101

33. Frith J A, McLeod J G 1988 Pregnancy and multiple sclerosis. Journal of Neurology, Neurosurgery and Psychiatry 51: 495–498

34. Poser S, Poser W 1983 Multiple sclerosis and gestation. Neurology 33: 1422–1427

35. Millar J D H, Allison R S, Cheesman E A, Merrett J D 1959 Pregnancy as a factor influencing relapse in disseminated sclerosis. Brain 82: 417–426

36. Schapira K, Poskanzer D C, Newell D J, Miller H 1966 Marriage, pregnancy and multiple sclerosis. Brain 89: 419–428

37. Ghezzi A, Caputo D 1981 Pregnancy: a factor influencing the course of multiple sclerosis? European Neurology 20: 115–117

38. Nelson L M, Franklin G M, Jones M C 1988 Risk of multiple sclerosis exacerbation during pregnancy and breast feeding. Journal of the American Medical Association 259: 3441–3443

39. Millar J H D 1961 Pregnancy as a factor influencing relapse in disseminated sclerosis. Proceedings of the Royal Society of Medicine 54: 4–7

40. Allison R S, Millar J H B 1954 Prevalence of disseminated sclerosis in Northern Ireland. Ulster Medical Journal 23 (suppl 2): 1–27

41. Thompson D S, Nelson L M, Burns A, Burks J S, Franklin J M 1986 The effects of pregnancy in multiple sclerosis: a retrospective study. Neurology 36: 1097–1099

42. Birk K, Rudick R 1986 Pregnancy and multiple sclerosis. Archives of Neurology 43: 719–726

43. Poser S, Poser M 1984 Multiple sclerosis and postpartum stress. Neurology 34: 704–705

44. Livingstone I R, Sack G H 1984 Arthrogryposis multiplex congenita occurring with maternal multiple sclerosis. Archives of Neurology 41: 1216–1217

45. Poser S, Raun N E, Wikström J, Poser W 1979 Pregnancy, oral contraceptives and multiple sclerosis. Acta Neurologica Scandinavica 55: 108–118

46. Miller H 1964 Trauma and multiple sclerosis. Lancet 1: 848–850

47. Kelly R 1985 Clinical aspects of multiple sclerosis. In:

Vinken P J, Bruyn G W, Klawans H L, Koetsier J C (eds) Handbook of clinical neurology, Vol 47. Elsevier, Amsterdam, p 64

48. Bamford C R, Sibley W A, Thies C, Laguna J F, Smith M S, Clark K 1981 Trauma as an aetiologic and aggravating factor in multiple sclerosis. Neurology 31: 1229–1234

49. Poser C M 1980 Sur le rôle des traumatismes physiques et psychologiques dans la sclérose en plaques. Revue Neurologique 136: 807–814

50. Poser C M 1987 Trauma and multiple sclerosis. An hypothesis. Journal of Neurology 234: 155–159

51. Nevin N C 1967 Neuropathological changes in the white matter following head injury. Journal of Neuropathology and Experimental Neurology 26: 77–84

52. Oppenheimer D 1978 Microscopic lesions in the brain following head injury. Journal of Neurology, Neurosurgery and Psychiatry 31: 299–306

53. Ommaya A K, Rockoff S D, Baldwin M, Friauf W S 1964 Experimental concussion. Journal of Neurosurgery 21: 249–264

54. Povlishock J T, Becker D P, Sullivan H G, Miller J D 1978 Vascular permeability alterations to horseradish peroxidase in experimental brain injury. Brain Research 153: 223–239

55. Povlishock J T, Becker D P, Miller J D, Jenkins L W, Dietrich W D 1979 The morphopathologic substrates of concussion? Acta Neuropathologica 47: 1–11

56. Clark G, Bogdanove H L 1955 The induction of the lesions of allergic meningoencephalomyelitis in a predetermined location. Journal of Neuropathology and Experimental Neurology 14: 433–437

57. Bogdanove L H, Clark G 1957 The induction of exacerbations of allergic meningoencephalomyelitis. Journal of Neuropathology and Experimental Neurology 16: 57–60

58. Gonsette R, André-Balisaux G, Delmotte 1966 La perméabilité des vaisseaux cérébaux VI: démyélinisation expérimentale provoquée par les substances agissant sur la barrière hématoencéphalique. Acta Neurologica Belgica 66: 247–262

59. Reichert T, Hassler R, Mundinger F, Bronisch F, Schmidt K 1975 Pathologic-anatomic findings and cerebral localisation in stereotactic treatment of extrapyramidal motor disturbance in multiple sclerosis. Confinia Neurologica 37: 24–40

60. Georgi W 1961 Multiple Sklerose: pathologisch-anatomische Befund multipler Sklerose bei Klinisch nicht diagnostizierten Krankheiten. Schweizerische Medizinische Wochenschrift 91: 605–607

61. Gillbert J J, Sadler M 1983 Unsuspected multiple sclerosis. Archives of Neurology 40: 533–536

62. Engell T 1989 A clinical patho-anatomical study of clinically silent multiple sclerosis. Acta Neurologica Scandinavica 79: 428–430

63. Weisberg L A 1980 Computed tomographic enhancement patterns in cerebral infarction. Archives of Neurology 37: 21–24

64. Keschner M 1950 The effects of injury and illness on the course of multiple sclerosis. Research Publications of the Association for Research into Nervous and Mental Diseases 28: 533–547

65. Ridley A, Schapira K 1961 Influence of surgical procedures on the course of multiple sclerosis. Neurology 11: 81–82

66. Baskett P J D, Armstrong R 1970 Anaesthetic problems in multiple sclerosis. Anaesthesia 25: 397–401

67. Siemkowicz E 1976 Multiple sclerosis and surgery. Anaesthesia 31: 1211–1216

68. Bamford C, Sibley W, Laguna J 1978 Anesthesia in multiple sclerosis. Canadian Journal of Neulogical Sciences 5: 41–44

69. Sténuit J, Marchand P 1968 Les sequelles de rachianesthesie. Acta Neurologica Belgica 68: 628–635

70. Henner K 1957 La ponction lumbaire semble etre contrindiquée dans la sclérose en plaques d'une façon presqu'absolue. Abstracts of Sixth International Congress of Neurology. Exerpta Medica, p 40

71. Schapira K 1959 Is lumbar puncture harmful in multiple sclerosis? Journal of Neurology, Neurosurgery and Psychiatry 22: 238

72. Tourtellotte W W, Haerer A F, Heller G Z, Somers J E 1964 Postlumbar puncture headaches. Thomas, Springfield

73. Tourtellotte W W 1970 Cerebrospinal fluid in multiple sclerosis. In: Vinken P J, Bruyn G W (eds) Handbook of clinical neurology, Vol 9. North Holland, Amsterdam, pp 324–325

74. Weisner B 1975 Do lumbar puncture and other diagnostic procedures have an unfavourable effect on the clinical course of multiple sclerosis? Acta Neurochirurgica 31: 294

75. Firth D 1941 First account of disseminated sclerosis. Proceedings of the Royal Society of Medicine 34: 381–384

76. Paulley J W 1976 Psychological management of multiple sclerosis. An overview. Psychotherapy and Psychosomatics 27: 26–40

77. Mei-Tal V, Meyerowitz S, Engel G L 1970 The role of psychosomatic process in a somatic disorder: multiple sclerosis. Psychosomatic Medicine 32: 67–86

78. Charcot J M 1877 Diseases of the nervous system. New Sydenham Society, London

79. Moxon W 1875 Eight cases of insular sclerosis of the brain and spinal cord. Guy's Hospital Reports 20: 438–481

80. McAlpine D 1946 The problem of disseminated sclerosis. Brain 69: 233–250

81. Adams D K, Sutherland J M, Fletcher W B 1950 Early clinical manifestations of disseminated sclerosis. British Medical Journal 2: 431–436

82. Braceland F J, Giffin M E 1950 The mental changes associated with multiple sclerosis: an interim report. Research Publications of the Association for Research into Nervous and Mental Diseases 28: 450–455

83. Pratt R T C 1951 An investigation of the psychiatric aspects of disseminated sclerosis. Journal of Neurology, Neurosurgery and Psychiatry 14: 326–336

84. Alter M, Antonovsky A, Leibowitz U 1968 Epidemiology of multiple sclerosis in Israel. In: Alter M, Kurtzke J (eds) The epidemiology of multiple sclerosis. Thomas, Springfield, pp 83–109

85. Warren S, Greenhill S, Warren K 1985 Emotional stress and the development of multiple sclerosis: case-control evidence of a relationship. Journal of Chronic Diseases 35: 821–831

86. Sibley W A 1987 Risk factors for multiple sclerosis — implications for pathogenesis. In: Crescenzi G S (ed) A multidisciplinary approach to myelin diseases. Plenum Press, London

87. Franklin G M, Nelson L M, Heaton R K, Burk J S,
   Thompson D S 1988 Stress and its relationship to
   acute exacerbations in multiple sclerosis. Journal of
   Neurological Rehabilitation 2: 7–11
88. Grant I, Brown G W, Harris T, McDonald W I,
   Patterson T, Trimble M R 1989 Severely threatening
   events and marked life difficulties preceding onset or
   exacerbation of multiple sclerosis. Journal of
   Neurology, Neurosurgery and Psychiatry 52: 8–13
89. Detels R, Clark V A, Valdiviezo N L, Visscher B R,
   Malmgren R M, Dudley J P 1982 Factors associated
   with a rapid course of multiple sclerosis. Archives of
   Neurology 39: 377–341
90. Berger J R, Sheremata W A 1985 Neurological deficits
   following the hot bath test in multiple sclerosis.
   Journal of the American Medical Association 253: 203
91. Davis F A 1985 Neurological deficits following the hot
   bath test in multiple sclerosis. Journal of the American
   Medical Association 253: 203
92. Wartenberg R (ed) 1958 Neuritis, sensory neuritis,
   neuralgia. Oxford University Press, New York
93. Hasson J, Terry R D, Zimmerman H M 1958
   Peripheral neuropathy in multiple sclerosis. Neurology
   8: 503–510
94. Lumsden C E 1970 The neuropathology of multiple
   sclerosis. In: Vinken P J, Bruyn G W (eds) Handbook
   of clinical neurology, Vol 9. North-Holland,
   Amsterdam, pp 217–309
95. Argyrakis A 1980 Ultrastructural changes in peripheral
   nerves in multiple sclerosis and subacute
   panencephalitis. In: Bauer H J, Poser S, Ritter G (eds)
   Progress in multiple sclerosis research. Springer,
   Berlin, pp 360–364
96. Taraschi G, Lanzi G 1962 Etude de la vitesse de
   conduction du nerf cubital dans la sclérose en plaques.
   Electroencephalography and Clinical Neurophysiology
   suppl 22: 54–55
97. Conrad B, Bechinger D 1969 Sensorische und
   motorische Nervenleitgeschwindigkeit und distale
   Latenz bei Multipler Sklerose. Archiv für Psychiatrie
   und Nervenkrankheiten 212: 140–149
98. Hopf H C, Eysholdt M 1978 Impaired refractory
   periods of peripheral nerves in multiple sclerosis.
   Annals of Neurology 4: 499–501
99. Pollock M, Calder C, Allpress S 1977 Peripheral nerve
   abnormality in multiple sclerosis. Annals of Neurology
   2: 41–48
100. Hopf H C, Maure K 1983 Wave 1 of early auditory
   evoked potentials in multiple sclerosis.
   Electroencephalography and Clinical Neurophysiology
   56: 31–37
101. Weir A, Hansen S, Ballantyne J P 1979 Single fibre
   electromyographic jitter in multiple sclerosis. Journal of
   Neurology, Neurosurgery and Psychiatry 42: 1146–1150
102. Weir S, Hansen S, Ballantyne J P 1980 Motor unit
   potential abnormalities in multiple sclerosis: further
   evidence for a peripheral nervous system defect.
   Journal of Neurology, Neurosurgery and Psychiatry
   43: 999–1004
103. Schoene W C, Carpenter S, Behan P O, Geschwind N
   1977 Onion bulb formations in the central and
   peripheral nervous system in association with multiple
   sclerosis and hypertrophic neuropathy. Brain
   100: 755–773
104. Dinkler 1904 Zur Kasuistik der multiplen Herdsklerose

105. Schob F 1923 Uber Wurzelfibromatose bei multipler
   Sklerose. Zeitschrift für die gesamte Neurologie und
   Psychiatrie 83: 481–496
106. Jellinger K 1969 Einiger morphologische Aspekte der
   multiplen Sklerose. Wiener Zeitschrift für
   Nervenheilkunde 27 (suppl 2): 12–37
107. Ketelaer C J, Leruitte A, Perier O 1966
   Histopathologie de la moelle lombo-sacreé et de la
   queue de cheval dans une série de cas vérifiés de la
   sclérose en plaques. Acta Neurologica Scandinavica 42
   (suppl 20): 33–51
108. Rosenberg N L, Bourdette D 1983 Hypertrophic
   neuropathy and multiple sclerosis. Neurology
   33: 1361–1364
109. Tachi N, Ishikawa Y, Tsuzuki A, Minami R, Sasaki
   K, Shinoda M 1985 A case of childhood multiple
   sclerosis with peripheral neuropathy. Neuropediatrics
   16: 231–234
110. Ro Y I, Alexander C B, Oh S J 1983 Multiple sclerosis
   and hypertrophic demyelinating peripheral neuropathy.
   Muscle and Nerve 6: 312–316
111. Keuter E J W 1967 Polyneuritis and multiple sclerosis.
   Psychiatrica Neurologia Neurochirurgica 70: 271–279
112. Caputo D, Ghezzi A, Zaffaroni M, Zibetti A 1982
   Polyneuritic onset in multiple sclerosis. Italian Journal
   of Neurological Sciences 4: 355–357
113. Thomas P K, Walker R W H, Rudge P et al 1987
   Chronic demyelinating peripheral neuropathy associated
   with multifocal central nervous system demyelination.
   Brain 110: 53–76
114. Mendell J R, Kolkin S, Kissel J T, Weiss K L,
   Chakeres D W, Rommohan K W 1987 Evidence for
   central nervous system demyelination in chronic
   inflammatory demyelinating polyradiculoneuropathy.
   Neurology 37: 1291–1294
115. Forrester C, Lascelles R G 1979 Association between
   polyneuritis and multiple sclerosis. Journal of
   Neurology, Neurosurgery and Psychiatry 42: 864–866
116. Best P V 1985 Acute polyradiculoneuritis associated
   with demyelinated plaques in the central nervous
   system: report of a case. Acta Neuropathologica
   67: 230–234
117. Lassman H, Budka H, Schnaberth G 1981
   Inflammatory demyelinating polyradiculitis in a patient
   with multiple sclerosis. Archives of Neurology
   38: 99–102
118. Poser C M 1987 The peripheral nervous system in
   multiple sclerosis. A review and pathogenetic
   hypothesis. Journal of the Neurological Sciences
   79: 83–90
119. Madrid R E, Wisniewski H M 1978 Peripheral nervous
   system pathology in relapsing experimental allergic
   encephalomyelitis. Journal of Neurocytology 7: 265–281
120. De la Monte S M, Ropper A H, Dickersin R, Harris
   N L, Ferry J A, Richardson E P 1986 Relapsing
   central and peripheral demyelinating disease. Unusual
   pathologic features. Archives of Neurology 43: 626–629
121. Fisher M, Log R R, Drachman D A 1985 Hand
   muscle atrophy in multiple sclerosis. Archives of
   Neurology 40: 811–815
122. Rose A 1981 Multiple sclerosis: an overview. Advances
   in Neurology 31: 3–9
123. Wechsler I S 1922 Statistics of multiple sclerosis

des Gehirns und Rückenmarks. Deutsche Zeitschrift
für Nervenheilkunde 26: 233–247

including a study of the infantile, congenital, familial, hereditary forms and the mental and psychic symptoms. Archives of Neurology and Psychiatry 8: 59–75

124. Wilson S A K (ed) 1940 Neurology. Arnold, London, p 151

125. Müller R 1951 Course and prognosis of disseminated sclerosis in relation to age of onset. Archives of Neurology and Psychiatry 66: 561–570

126. Allison R S, Millar J H D 1954 Prevalence and familial incidence of disseminated sclerosis in Northern Ireland. Ulster Medical Journal 23 (suppl 2): 1–92

127. Poskanzer D C, Schapira K, Miller H 1963 Epidemiology of multiple sclerosis in the counties of Northumberland and Durham. Journal of Neurology, Neurosurgery and Psychiatry 26: 368–376

128. Poser S 1978 Multiple sclerosis. Springer, Berlin, p 29

129. Shepherd D I 1979 Clinical features of multiple sclerosis in north-east Scotland. Acta Neurologica Scandinavica 60: 218–230

130. Duquette P, Murray T J, Pleines J et al 1987 Multiple sclerosis in childhood: clinical profile in 125 patients. Journal of Pediatrics 111: 359–363

131. Schumacher G A, Beebe G, Kibler R F et al 1965 Problems of experimental trials of therapy in multiple sclerosis. Annals of the New York Academy of Sciences 122: 552–568

132. Gudmundsson K R 1971 Clinical studies of multiple sclerosis in Iceland. Acta Neurologica Scandinavica 47 (suppl 48): 1–78

133. Gall J C Jr, Hayles A B, Siekert R G, Keith H M 1958 Multiple sclerosis in children. Pediatrics 21: 703–709

134. Bonduelle M, Bouygues P, Sallou C 1954 La sclérose en plaques chez l'enfant. Presse Médicale 62: 563–564

135. Schneider R D, Ong B H, Moran M J, Greenhouse A H 1969 Multiple sclerosis in early childhood: case report with notes on frequency. Clinical Pediatrics 8: 115–118

136. Bell M A 1977 Adult type relapsing multiple sclerosis presenting in childhood. Nursing Times 73: 294–297

137. Brandt S, Gyldensted C, Offner H, Melchior J C 1981 Multiple sclerosis with onset in a two-year-old boy. Neuropediatrics 12: 75–82

138. Andler W, Roosen K 1980 Multiple Sklerose im ersten Lebensjahrzehnt. Klinische Pädiatrie 192: 365–369

139. Low N L, Carter S 1956 Multiple sclerosis in children. Pediatrics 18: 24–30

140. Hauser S L, Bresnan M J, Reinherz E L, Weiner H L 1982 Childhood multiple sclerosis: clinical features and demonstration of changes in T cell subsets with disease activity. Annals of Neurology 11: 463–468

141. Nobel E 1912 Histologischer Befund in einem Falle von akuter multiplen Sklerose. Wiener Medizinischer Wochenschrift 62: 26–32

142. Salguero L F, Itabashi H H, Gutierrez N B 1969 Childhood multiple sclerosis with psychiatric manifestations. Journal of Neurology, Neurosurgery and Psychiatry 32: 572–579

143. Shaw C M, Alvord E C 1987 Multiple sclerosis beginning in infancy. Journal of Child Neurology 2: 252–256

144. Bye A M E, Kendall B, Wilson J 1985 Multiple sclerosis in childhood: a new look. Developmental Medicine and Child Neurology 27: 215–222

145. Sheremata W, Brown S B, Curless R R, Dunn H G 1981 Childhood multiple sclerosis: a report of 12 cases. Annals of Neurology 10: 304

146. Boutin B, Esquivel E, Mayer M, Chamet S, Ponsot G, Arthuis M 1988 Multiple sclerosis in children: report of clinical and paraclinical features of 19 cases. Neuropediatrics 19: 118–123

147. Alvord E C 1985 Disseminated encephalomyelitis: its variations in form and their relationship to other diseases of the nervous system. In: Koetsier J C (ed) Handbook of clinical neurology, Vol 47. Elsevier, Amsterdam, pp 467–502

148. Riikonen R, Donner M, Erkkilä H 1988 Optic neuritis in children and its relationship to multiple sclerosis: a clinical study of 21 children. Developmental Medicine and Child Neurology 30: 349–359

149. Kennedy C, Carroll F D 1960 Optic neuritis in children. Archives of Ophthalmology 63: 747–755

150. Kennedy C, Carter S 1961 Relation of optic neuritis to multiple sclerosis in children. Pediatrics 28: 377–387

151. De Leersnyder H, Burstin J, Ponsot G, Dulac O, Arthuis M 1981 Névrites optiques chez l'enfant. Archives Francaises de Pédiatrie 38: 563–572

152. Haller P, Patzold U 1979 Die Optikusneuritis im Kindesalter. Fortschritte der Neurologie und Psychiatrie 47: 209–216

153. Kriss A, Francis D A, Cuendet F et al 1988 Recovery after optic neuritis in childhood. Journal of Neurology, Neurosurgery and Psychiatry 51: 1253–1258

154. Meadows S P 1969 Retrobulbar and optic neuritis in childhood and adolescence. Transactions of the Ophthalmological Societies of the United Kingdom 89: 603–638

155. Heirons R, Lyle T K 1959 Bilateral retrobulbar optic neuritis. Brain 82: 56–87

156. Parkin P J, Heirons R, McDonald W I 1984 Bilateral optic neuritis. A long-term follow-up. Brain 107: 951–964

157. McKay R P 1953 Multiple sclerosis: its onset and duration. Medical Clinics of North America 511–521

158. Ter Braak J G W, van Herwaarden A 1933 Ophthalmo-encephalo-myelitis mit ungewönlichen Augenerscheinungen. Klinische Monatsblätter für Augenheilkunde 91: 316–343

159. Garcin R 1958 A propos de quelques observations d'association d'uvéite et de syndrome neurologique de type sclérose en plaques. Laval Médical 26: 422–454

160. Haarr M 1964 Changes of the retinal veins in multiple sclerosis. Acta Neurologica Scandinavica 40 (suppl 10): 17–20

161. Tschabitscher H 1958 Die klinischen und experimentallen Forschungen bei der multiplen Sklerose. Wiener Zeitschrift für Nervenheilkunde 14: 381–436

162. Bammer H G, Hofmann A, Zick R 1965 Aderhautentzündungen bei Multipler Sklerose und die sogenannte Uveoencephalomeningitis. Deutsche Zeitschrift für Nervenheilkunde 187: 300–316

163. Archambeau P, Hollenhorst R, Rucker C 1965 Posterior uveitis as a manifestation of multiple sclerosis. Mayo Clinic Proceedings 40: 544–551

164. Breger B C, Leopold I H 1966 The incidence of uveitis in multiple sclerosis. American Journal of Ophthalmology 62: 540–545

165. Curless R G, Bray P F 1972 Uveitis and multiple sclerosis in an adolescent. American Journal of Diseases of Children 123: 149–150

166. Giles C L 1970 Peripheral uveitis in patients with multiple sclerosis. American Journal of Ophthalmology 70: 17–19

167. Arné L, Vital C L, Barat M, Noble Y, Demelle B 1978 Uvéite et sclérose en plaques. Revue Neurologique 134: 395–401

168. Bamford C R, Ganley J P, Sibley W A, Laguna J F 1978 Uveitis, perivenous sheathing and multiple sclerosis. Neurology 28 (9 Pt 2): 119–124

169. Nissenblatt M J, Masciulli L, Yarian D L, Duvoisin R 1981 Pars planitis — a demyelinating disease? Archives of Ophthalmology 99: 697

170. Rucker C W 1944 Sheathing of the retinal veins in multiple sclerosis. Mayo Clinic Proceedings 19: 176–178

171. Rucker C W 1944 Sheathing of the retinal veins in multiple sclerosis. Journal of the American Medical Association 127: 970–973

172. Rucker C W 1947 Retinopathy of multiple sclerosis. Transactions of the American Ophthalmological Society 45: 564–570

173. Haarr M 1963 Retinal periphlebitis in multiple sclerosis. Acta Neurologica Scandinavica 39 (suppl 4): 270–272

174. Engell T 1986 Neurological disease activity in multiple sclerosis patients with periphlebitis retinae. Acta Neurologica Scandinavica 73: 168–172

175. Arnold A C, Pepose J S, Hepler R S, Foos R Y 1984 Retinal periphlebitis and retinitis in multiple sclerosis. I. Pathologic characteristics. Ophthalmology 91: 255–261

176. Fog T 1965 The topography of plaques in multiple sclerosis with special reference to cerebral plaques. Acta Neurologica Scandinavica 41(suppl 15): 1–161

177. Engell T, Jensen O A, Klinken L 1985 Periphlebitis retinae in multiple sclerosis. A histopathological study of 2 cases. Acta Ophthalmologica 68: 83–88

178. Lightman S, McDonald W I, Bird A C, Francis D A, Hoskins A, Batchelor J R, Halliday A M 1986 Retinal venous sheathing in optic neuritis: its significance for the pathogenesis of multiple sclerosis. Brain 110: 405–414

179. Shaw P J, Smith N M, Ince P G, Bates D 1987 Chronic periphlebitis retinae in multiple sclerosis. A histological study. Journal of the Neurological Sciences 77: 147–152

180. Wybar K C 1952 Ocular manifestations of disseminated sclerosis. Proceedings of the Royal Society of Medicine 45: 315–320

181. Orbán T 1955 Beitrag zu dem Augenhintergrundsveranderungen bei Sklerosis multiplex. Ophthalmologica 30: 387–396

182. Møller P, Hammerberg P 1963 Retinal periphlebitis in multiple sclerosis. Acta Neurologica Scandinavica 39 (suppl 4): 263–270

183. Younge R B 1976 Fluorescein angiography and retinal venous sheathing in multiple sclerosis. Canadian Journal of Ophthalmology 11: 31–36

184. Engell T, Andersen P K 1982 The frequency of periphlebitis retinae in multiple sclerosis. Acta Neurologica Scandinavica 65: 601–608

185. White R H R 1961 The aetiology and neurological complications of retinal vasculitis. Brain 84: 262–273

186. Silfverskiöld B P 1947 Retinal periphlebitis with paraplegia. Archives of Neurology and Psychiatry 57: 351–357

187. Pépin B, Goldstein B, Man H X, Hagenau M, Henault S 1978 Maladie de Eales avec manifestations neurologiques. Revue Neurologique 134: 427–436

188. Dastur O K, Singhal B S 1976 Eales' disease with neurological involvement. Part II. Pathology and pathogenesis. Journal of the Neurological Sciences 27: 323–345

189. De Keyser J 1988 Autoimmunity in multiple sclerosis. Neurology 38: 371–374

190. Baker H W G, Balla J I, Burger H G, Ebling P, MacKay I R 1972 Multiple sclerosis and autoimmune diseases. Australian and New Zealand Journal of Medicine 3: 256–260

191. Patten B, Hart A, Lovelace R 1972 Multiple sclerosis associated with defects in neuromuscular transmission. Journal of Neurology, Neurosurgery and Psychiatry 35: 385–394

192. Aita J F, Snyder D H, Reichl W 1974 Myasthenia gravis and multiple sclerosis: an unusual combination of diseases. Neurology 24: 74–75

193. Margolis L H, Groves R W 1945 The occurrence of myasthenia gravis in a patient with multiple sclerosis. North Carolina Medical Journal 6: 243–244

194. Achari A N, Trontej J V, Campoos R J 1976 Multiple sclerosis and myasthenia gravis. Neurology 25: 544–546

195. Lo R, Feasby T E 1983 Multiple sclerosis and autoimmune diseases. Neurology 33: 97–98

196. Bixenman W W, Buchsbaum H W 1988 Multiple sclerosis, euthyroid restrictive Graves ophthalmopathy and myasthenia gravis. Graefe's Archive for Clinical and Experimental Ophthalmology 226: 168–171

197. Ghezzi A, Zaffaroni M, Caputo D, Zibetti A, Mariani G 1984 A case of myasthenia gravis associated with optic neuritis. Journal of Neurology 231: 94–95

198. Somer H, Müller K, Kinnunen E 1989 Myasthenia gravis associated with multiple sclerosis. Epidemiological survey and immunological findings. Journal of the Neurological Sciences 89: 37–48

199. Roquer J, Escudero D, Herraiz J, Masó E, Cano F 1987 Multiple sclerosis and Hashimoto's thyroiditis. Journal of Neurology 234: 23–24

200. Nagashima T, Yamada K, Uono M, Nagashima K 1984 Multiple sclerosis co-existent with myxedema. An autopsy case report. Journal of the Neurological Sciences 66: 217–221

201. Campbell A M G, Crow R S, Land D W 1960 Goitre and disseminated sclerosis. British Medical Journal 1: 200–201

202. Warren T R 1984 The increased prevalence of multiple sclerosis among people who were born and bred in areas where goitre is endemic. Medical Hypotheses 14: 111–114

203. Kiessling W R, Pflughaupt K W, Haubitz I, Mertens H G 1980 Thyroid function in multiple sclerosis. Acta Neurologica Scandinavica 62: 255–258

204. Warren S A, Warren K G 1981 Multiple sclerosis and associated diseases: a relationship to diabetes mellitus. Canadian Journal of Neurological Sciences 8: 35–39

205. Warren S A, Warren K G 1982 Multiple sclerosis and diabetes mellitus: further evidence of a relationship. Canadian Journal of the Neurological Sciences 9: 415–419

206. Lindegård B 1985 Diseases associated with multiple sclerosis and epilepsy. Acta Neurologica Scandinavica 71: 267–277

207. Rang E H, Brooke B N, Hermon-Taylor J 1982 Association of ulcerative colitis with multiple sclerosis. Lancet 2: 555

208. Matthews W B 1985 In: McAlpine's multiple sclerosis Matthews W B (ed) Churchill Livingstone, Edinburgh, p 81

209. Minuk G Y, Lewkonia R M 1986 Possible familial association of multiple sclerosis and inflammatory bowel disease. New England Journal of Medicine 314: 586

210. Thompson R H S 1966 A biochemical approach to the problem of multiple sclerosis. Proceedings of the Royal Society of Medicine 59: 269–276

211. Lange M S, Shiner M 1976 Small-bowel abnormalities in multiple sclerosis. Lancet 2: 1319–1322

212. Bateson M C, Hopwood D, MacGillivray J B 1979 Jejunal morphology in multiple sclerosis. Lancet 1: 1108–1110

213. Beilin J, Pettet N, Smith A D, Thompson R H S, Zilkha K J 1971 Linoleate metabolism in multiple sclerosis. Journal of Neurology, Neurosurgery and Psychiatry 34: 25–29

214. Matthews W B 1968 The neurological complications of ankylosing spondylitis. Journal of the Neurological Sciences 6: 561–573

215. Thomas D J, Kendall M J, Whitfield A G W 1974 Nervous system involvement in ankylosing spondylitis. British Medical Journal 1: 148–150

216. Kahn M A, Kusher I 1979 Ankylosing spondylitis and multiple sclerosis. A possible association. Arthritis and Rheumatism 22: 784–786

217. Matthews W B 1985 In: McAlpine's multiple sclerosis Matthews W B (ed) Churchill Livingstone, Edinburgh, p 242

218. Hannahan P S, Russell A S, McLean D R 1988 Ankylosing spondylitis and multiple sclerosis: a possible association. Journal of Rheumatology 15: 1512–1514

219. Derini M S 1982 Multiple sclerosis and rheumatoid arthritis. Journal of Neurology, Neurosurgery and Psychiatry 45: 661

220. Trostle D C, Helfrich D, Medsger T A 1986 Systemic sclerosis (scleroderma) and multiple sclerosis. Arthritis and Rheumatism 29: 124–127

221. Simjee S, Konqui A, Ahmed A E 1985 Multiple sclerosis and bullous pemphigoid. Dermatologica 170: 86–89

222. Tanpaichitr K 1980 Multiple sclerosis associated with eosinophilic vasculitis, pericarditis and hypocomplementemia. Archives of Neurology 37: 314–315

223. Taillan B, Pedinielli F J, Blanc A P, Miletto G 1985 Association familiale sclérose en plaques-purpura thrombopénique chronique. Presse Médicale 14: 700

224. Zimmerman H M, Netsky M G 1950 The pathology of multiple sclerosis. Research Publications of the Association for Research into Nervous and Mental Disease 28: 271–312

225. Allen I V, Millar J H D, Hutchinson M J 1978 General disease in 120 necropsy-proven cases of multiple sclerosis. Neuropathology and Applied Neurobiology 4: 279–284

226. Sibley W A, Bamford C R, Lagun J F 1978 Anamnestic studies in multiple sclerosis: a relationship between familial multiple sclerosis and neoplasia.

Neurology 28 (9 Pt 2): 125–128

227. Palo J, Duchesne J, Wikström J 1977 Malignant disease among patients with multiple sclerosis. Journal of Neurology 216: 217–222

228. Brihaye J, Périer O, Sténuit J 1963 Multiple sclerosis associated with a cerebral astrocytoma. Journal of Neuropathology and Experimental Neurology 22: 128–137

229. Currie S, Urich H 1974 Concurrence of multiple sclerosis and glioma. Journal of Neurology, Neurosurgery and Psychiatry 37: 598–605

230. Lynch P G 1974 Multiple sclerosis and malignant glioma. British Medical Journal 3: 577

231. Lahl R 1980 Combination of multiple sclerosis and cerebral glioblastoma. European Neurology 19: 192–197

232. Ho K L, Wolfe D E 1981 Concurrence of multiple sclerosis and primary intracranial neoplasms. Cancer 47: 2913–2919

233. Matthews W B 1962 Epilepsy and disseminated sclerosis. Quarterly Journal of Medicine 31: 141–156

234. Nahser H-C, Vieregge P, Nau H E, Reinhardt V 1986 Coincidence of multiple sclerosis and glioma. Surgical Neurology 26: 45–51

235. Russell D S, Rubenstein L J 1971 Primary tumours of neuroectodermal origin. In: Russell D S, Rubenstein L J (eds) Pathology of tumours of the nervous system, 3rd edn. Arnold, London, p 179

236. Anderson M, Hughes B, Jefferson M, Smith W T, Waterhouse J A H 1980 Gliomatous transformation and demyelinating diseases. Brain 103: 603–622

237. Reagan T J, Freiman I S 1973 Multiple cerebral gliomas in multiple sclerosis. Journal of Neurology, Neurosurgery and Psychiatry 36: 523–528

238. Barnard R O, Jellinek E H 1967 Multiple sclerosis with amyotrophy complicated by oligodendroglioma. History of recurrent herpes zoster. Journal of the Neurological Sciences 5: 441–455

239. Spaar F W, Wikström J 1978 Multiple sclerosis and malignant neoplasms in the central nervous system. Journal of Neurology 218: 24–33

240. Castaigne P, Escourolle R, Brunet P, Gray F, Rouques C, le Bigot P 1974 Réticulosarcome cérébral primitif associé a` des lésions de sclérose en plaques. Revue Neurologique 130: 181–188

241. Ulrich J, Wütrich R 1974 Reticulum cell sarcoma of nervous system in patient treated with immunosuppressant drugs. European Neurology 12: 65–78

242. Terrence C F 1976 Myotonic dystrophy and multiple sclerosis. Journal of Neurology 213: 305–308

243. Mishra S K, Currier R D, Smith E E, Malhotra C, Bebin J, Hudson J M 1984 Facioscapulohumeral dystrophy associated with multiple sclerosis. Archives of Neurology 41: 570–571

244. Sadeh M, Ohry A, Sarova-Pinhas I, Braham J 1980 Hypokalemic periodic paralysis with multiple sclerosis. European Neurology 19: 252–253

245. Toglia, J U, Mandel S, Kosmorsky G 1982 Multiple sclerosis and hypokalemic periodic paralysis in the same patient. Archives of Neurology 39: 530–531

246. Hader W J, Rozdilsky B, Nair C P 1986 The concurrence of multiple sclerosis and amyotrophic lateral sclerosis. Canadian Journal of Neurological Sciences 13: 66–69

247. Watkins S M, Espir M 1969 Migraine and multiple

sclerosis. Journal of Neurology, Neurosurgery and Psychiatry 32: 35–37

248. Melton L J, Bartleson J D 1980 Spontaneous pneumothorax and multiple sclerosis. Annals of Neurology 7: 492

249. Mitchell D N, Porterfield J S, Micheletti R et al 1978 Isolation of an infectious agent from bone marrows of patients with multiple sclerosis. Lancet 2: 387–391

250. Woyciechowska J L, Madden D L, Sever J L 1977 Absence of measles-virus antigen in jejunum of multiple sclerosis patients. Lancet 2: 1046–1049

251. Carp R I, Licursi P C, Merz P A, Merz G S 1972 Decreased percentage of polymorphonuclear neutrophils in mouse peripheral blood after inoculation with material from multiple sclerosis patients. Journal of Experimental Medicine 136: 618–629

252. Madden D L, Krezlewicz A G, Gravell M, Sever J L, Tourtellotte W W 1977 Multiple sclerosis-associated agent. Lancet 2: 976

253. Putnam T J 1935 Studies in multiple sclerosis IV. Encephalitis and sclerotic plaques produced by venular obstruction. Archives of Neurology and Psychiatry 33: 929–940

254. Fog T, Kristensen I, Helweg-Larsen H F 1955 Blood platelets in disseminated sclerosis. Archives of Neurology and Psychiatry 73: 267–285

255. Persson I 1955 Variations in the plasma fibrinogen during the course of multiple sclerosis. Archives of Neurology and Psychiatry 74: 17–30

256. Shulman M H, Alexander I, Ehrentheil O F, Gross R 1950 Capillary resistance studies in multiple sclerosis. Journal of Neuropathology and Experimental Neurology 9: 420–429

257. Swank R L 1958 Subcutaneous haemorrhages in multiple sclerosis. Neurology 8: 497–498

258. Feldman S, Izak G, Nelken D 1957 Blood coagulation studies and serotonin determinations in serum and cerebrospinal fluid in multiple sclerosis. Acta Psychiatrica et Neurologica Scandinavica 32: 37–49

259. Menon I S, Dewar H A, Newell D J 1969 Fibrinolytic activity of venous blood of patients with multiple sclerosis. Neurology 19: 101–104

260. Menon I S, Dewar H A 1967 Increased fibrinolytic activity in venous blood of hemiplegic limbs. British Medical Journal 2: 613–615

261. Brunetti A, Ricchieri G L, Patrassi G M, Girolami A, Tavolato E 1981 Rheological and fibrinolytic findings in multiple sclerosis. Journal of Neurology, Neurosurgery and Psychiatry 44: 340–343

262. Nathanson M, Savitsky J P 1952 Platelet adhesiveness index studies in multiple sclerosis and other neurologic disorders. Bulletin of the New York Academy of Sciences 28: 462–468

263. Prosiegel M, Neu I, Pfaffenrath V, Nahme M 1982 Thrombozytenaggregation und Multiple Sklerose. Nervenarzt 53: 227–230

264. Caspary E A, Prineas J, Miller H, Field E J 1965 Platelet stickiness in multiple sclerosis. Lancet 2: 1108–1109

265. Khan S N, Belin J, Smith A D, Sidey M, Zilkha K J 1985 Response to platelet-activating factor of platelets from patients with multiple sclerosis. Acta Neurologica Scandinavica 71: 212–220

266. Wright H P, Thompson R H S, Zilkha K J 1965 Platelet adhesiveness in multiple sclerosis. Lancet 2: 1109–1110

267. Sharp A A 1965 Platelets in multiple sclerosis. Lancet 2: 1296–1297

268. Millar J H D, Merrett J D, Dalby A M 1966 Platelet stickiness in multiple sclerosis. Journal of Neurology, Neurosurgery and Psychiatry 29: 187–189

269. Gul S, Smith A D, Thompson R H S, Wright H P, Zilkha K J 1970 Fatty acid composition of phospholipids from platelets and erythrocytes in multiple sclerosis. Journal of Neurology, Neurosurgery and Psychiatry 33: 506–510

270. Bolton C H, Hampton J R, Phillipson O T 1968 Platelet behaviour and plasma phospholipids in multiple sclerosis. Lancet 1: 99–104

271. Srivastava K C, Fog T, Clausen J 1975 The synthesis of prostaglandins in platelets from patients with multiple sclerosis. Acta Neurologica Scandinavica 51: 193–199

272. Abroms I F, Yessayan L, Shillito J, Barlow C F 1971 Spontaneous intra-cerebral haemorrhage in patients suspected of multiple sclerosis. Journal of Neurology, Neurosurgery and Psychiatry 34: 157–162

273. Jankovic J, Derman H, Armstrong D 1980 Haemorrhagic complications of multiple sclerosis. Journal of Neurology, Neurosurgery and Psychiatry 43: 76–81

274. Field E J, Shenton B K, Joyce G 1974 Specific laboratory test for multiple sclerosis. British Medical Journal 1: 212–214

275. Field E J, Joyce G 1976 Simplified laboratory test for multiple sclerosis. Lancet 2: 367–368

276. Stoof J C, Vrijmoed de Vries M C, Koestler J C, Langevoort H L 1977 Evaluation of the red blood cell cytopherometric test for the diagnosis of multiple sclerosis. Acta Neurologica Scandinavica 56: 170–176

277. Forrester J A, Smith W J 1977 Screening of children at risk of multiple sclerosis. Lancet 2: 45454

278. Hawkins S A, Millar J H D 1979 Erythrocyte-electrophoretic mobility test for multiple sclerosis. Lancet 1: 165–166

279. Poser W, Poser W 1980 Multiple sclerosis: what can and cannot be done. British Medical Journal 1: 14

280. Cuypers J, Reddemann H 1980 Evaluation of the erythrocyte-UFA (E-UFA) mobility test for the diagnosis of multiple sclerosis. Journal of Neurology, Neurosurgery and Psychiatry 43: 995–998

281. Seaman G V F, Swank R L, Tamblyn C H, Zukosi C F 1979 Simplified red cell electrophoretic mobility test for multiple sclerosis. Lancet 1: 1138–1139

282. Seaman G V F, Swank R L, Zukosi C F 1979 Red cell membrane differences in multiple sclerosis are acquired from the plasma. Lancet 1: 1139

283. Schauf C L, Frischer H, Davis F A 1980 Mechanical fragility of erythrocytes in multiple sclerosis. Neurology 30: 323–325

284. McCrea S, Killen M, Thompson J, Fleming W A, McNiell T A, Millar J H D 1979 Tests on peripheral blood cells in multiple sclerosis. Ulster Medical Journal 48: 83–90

285. Kurantsin-Mills J, Samji N, Moscarello M A, Boggs J M 1982 Comparison of membrane structure, osmotic fragility, and morphology of multiple sclerosis and normal erythrocytes. Neurochemical Research 12: 1523–1540

286. Simpson L O, Brett I, Olds R J, Larking P W, Arnott M J 1987 Red cell and hemorheological changes in multiple sclerosis. Pathology 19: 51–55

287. Ernst E 1982 Letter. Journal of Neurology, Neurosurgery and Psychiatry 45: 185

288. Pollock S, Harrison M J G, O'Connell G 1982 Erythrocyte deformability in multiple sclerosis. Journal of Neurology, Neurosurgery and Psychiatry 45: 762

289. Homa S T, Belin J, Smith A D, Monro J A, Zilkha K J 1980 Levels of linoleate and arachidonate in red blood cells of healthy individuals and patients with multiple sclerosis. Journal of Neurology, Neurosurgery and Psychiatry 43: 106–110

290. Van Alstine J M, Brooks D E 1984 Cell membrane abnormality detected in erythrocytes from patients with multiple sclerosis by partition in two-polymer aqueous-phase systems. Clinical Chemistry 30: 441–443

291. Navarro X, Segura R 1989 Red blood cell fatty acids in multiple sclerosis. Acta Neurologica Scandinavica 79: 32–37

5. Course and prognosis

There are important reasons for discovering as much as possible of the natural course of multiple sclerosis. The extraordinary extent of variation must have some relation to the unknown causes of the disease. To be able to tell patients at the onset with any degree of certainty what the future holds would be a notable advance. In some parts of the world it is apparently difficult to find untreated control subjects for therapeutic trials.[1] There is little convincing evidence that any treatment they might be having influences the course of the disease, but for the comparison with the effect of a new agent, knowledge of the natural course is essential. It is to be hoped that the use of historical controls will not have to be resurrected but, if so, the information must be as accurate as possible.

Unfortunately there are serious and, in part, insuperable obstacles to the acquisition of such knowledge. The uncertainties of early diagnosis and the failure of recognition and recollection of initial symptoms render the ideal wholly prospective study from the onset impossible. One of the nearest approaches to this was McAlpine's[2] series of patients seen within three years of the known onset. In a number of large series the interval between onset and diagnosis or onset and first examination by the observer are not stated.[3] If stated, only the mean may be given without the range or any given upper limit for inclusion in the series.[4] To confine observations to patients seen soon after onset[5] immediately introduces selection, as those whose symptoms did not lead them to seek early medical advice or rapidly indicate the correct diagnosis would be excluded, with resulting complex bias. Selection, whether deliberate or imposed by circumstance, must influence any series of observations. Examples include the study of remitting cases only;[6] cases proven at autopsy;[7-9] those willing to attend for prolonged follow up;[10] men serving in the Armed Forces at the time of diagnosis;[11] or patients attending a single hospital centre.[12]

Population-based series are less subject to bias and, as expected, disclose a more optimistic picture than those drawn from hospital inpatients.[13] Even so, to state an inescapable truism, only cases diagnosed and reported can be included. Some will be wrongly diagnosed and others will not be correctly diagnosed for many years, if at all.[14-16] Some will inevitably be lost to follow-up and even the most detailed documentation is subject to considerable error.[4] After all the uncertainties of ascertainment and classification, it is easy to succumb to a welcome but spurious feeling of finality about the laboriously collected figures. Precision cannot, however, be expected and the presentation of percentage data to one or more decimal places is unrealistic. The purposes for which the figures were compiled should be remembered. For the advance of knowledge of the disease, population-based studies are clearly superior. For purposes of advising patients attending hospital or for controlling therapeutic trials conducted at a hospital, data from the often disparaged clinic series are probably more appropriate.

DIAGNOSTIC CRITERIA

Diagnostic criteria for multiple sclerosis, considered in detail in Chapter 7, have in most instances been deliberately designed for use in therapeutic trials where it is obviously necessary to go to great lengths to avoid drawing conclusions from treating patients who do not have the disease.

Accuracy of diagnosis is, of course, also highly desirable in studies of the natural course of multiple sclerosis, but there is a dilemma. If 'possible' cases are included, a number will prove not to have multiple sclerosis, while if they are excluded, many early cases will not enter the study. In the detailed Gothenburg[17] series, patients in all diagnostic categories were admitted and McAlpine[2] and Poser[4] also included patients for whom the diagnosis was 'possible'. In these series it is not easy to determine the proportions in the different categories or how these altered with the passage of time. Shepherd & Downie[18] excluded possible cases while in some series,[5,19] no diagnostic criteria were given. It would be preferable if the numbers in each category were clearly stated and, if follow-up is attempted, the numbers changing from one category to another.

It is necessary to broaden certain criteria, in particular that concerning the age of onset. The Schumacher et al[20] criteria and those of Weiner & Ellison[21] exclude patients where onset has been below the age of 10. The onset of multiple sclerosis in childhood is, however, well documented (p. 120) and to exclude such patients in the present context would be to distort the picture. The upper age limit of onset in the Schumacher criteria was 50 years, while Weiner & Ellison recommended 45 years, with extension to 55 years in some circumstances. The research protocols of Poser et al[22] require onset between 10 and 59 years. These limits would certainly include the great majority of cases of diagnosed multiple sclerosis, but would exclude the interesting groups at the two extremes of the age range.

All large series in which diagnostic criteria are stated show a sharp decline of new cases after the age of 40 but a small percentage with onset in the sixth decade and occasionally later. For example, in Shepherd's[23] 557 cases the oldest patient at onset was 61. Leibowitz et al[24] in their study of 266 cases in Israel, found that six patients reported onset after 55 and two after 60. In the series of Poskanzer et al[25] the onset was between 65 and 69 in four patients (0.3%). Noseworthy et al[26] found that of 838 patients, 79 presented after the age of 50 years and in 49 of these, the onset was probably after this age. One problem is illustrated by the word 'reported' as it is a matter of common ob-

servation that patients forget significant symptoms even sometimes when these have been sufficiently severe to warrant inpatient hospital investigation. Opportunities for misdiagnosis also increase with age, particularly in view of the common mode of presentation in older patients, progressive spastic paraparesis.

Cases of late onset in whom the diagnosis has been proven at necropsy have been described. Friedman & Davison[27] reported that of 310 cases the onset had been above the age of 40 in 41 (13%). Of 42 necropsied cases the onset was in this older group in nine, with an age range of 41–64. As Kurtzke[28] remarked, however, it is not clear how the oldest patient who presented with dementia could have given a clear account of the mode of onset. It is of interest that in only two of these nine subjects had the diagnosis been established in life, but diagnostic procedures were less advanced at the time. One patient, for example, died after laminectomy to remove a non-existent spinal cord tumour, a mistake now unlikely to occur. Jéquier[29] reported that in 15 of 515 cases the clinical onset had been after the age of 50 and described 3 patients in whom the diagnosis had been confirmed at necropsy. One was a woman of 55 who developed optic neuritis, rapidly followed by motor and sensory symptoms. She died within a few months of unrelated causes. The second case was a woman of 55 with a progressive cervical spinal cord lesion who died after two years. In the third case, relapsing and remitting multiple sclerosis developed at the age of 56, leading to death at 68.

From these examples it can be concluded that the diagnosis of multiple sclerosis can legitimately be considered in patients in whom symptoms appear to have begun in the sixth or even seventh decade. This purely practical clinical conclusion cannot, however, be taken to imply that the disease process can actually begin at such an advanced age, although naturally this possibility cannot be excluded. The impossibility of precise dating of the onset may be illustrated by reports of multiple sclerosis being found at necropsy in patients dying of other causes, often in old age, in whom the diagnosis had never been suspected and sometimes in the complete absence of relevant symptoms and signs. Georgi,[14] reported 12 such cases, most of whom died in old age, in over 15 000 autopsies. In some, possibly relevant symptoms had occurred late in life. For example, a woman who died at 81 had developed weakness of one leg at the age of 65, an event that would not immediately suggest a clinical diagnosis of multiple sclerosis. Several patients were not thought to have had any neurological symptoms at all. Georgi referred to an 'imperceptible' form of multiple sclerosis. Gilbert & Sadler[16] in 2450 autopsies in subjects over 16 years in whom the nervous system was examined found 5 unsuspected cases of multiple sclerosis. They did not state how many overt cases were included in the series, which would have provided a useful indication of relative frequency. Engell[30] reported 13 clinically silent cases found in 16 100 autopsies and calculated that in Denmark some 40 such cases would occur every year. The average number of patients with known multiple sclerosis dying annually in the same population is 150, so that in about one fifth of cases, multiple sclerosis remains clinically silent. It cannot be known, however, how often minor unrecorded symptoms may have occurred. Mackay & Hirano[31] also described two 'clinically silent' cases discovered at necropsy in patients dying of unrelated causes at the age of 68 and 71 respectively. Moriaru & Klatzow[32] also described two patients of which the more remarkable was a man of 75 who had an epileptic fit apparently due to a subarachnoid haemorrhage. On routine examination after recovery he was found to have some impairment of postural sense in the lower limbs. He died aged 79 and multiple sclerosis was found at necropsy. No cause for the subarachnoid haemorrhage was described.

Clinical assessment

Objective methods of assessing the clinical state of the patient are essential for the understanding of the natural history of multiple sclerosis. Numerous attempts have been made to fill this need with differing degrees of appreciation of the underlying purpose. The intention is to discover whether a patient is improving or deteriorating and to record the actual condition and rate of change in a manner that allows comparison with other patients. Anyone who has examined patients with multiple sclerosis in a standard manner at frequent intervals will be aware that careful measurements of function, however essential in many contexts, may show great and unpredictable variation from day to day. That walking speed has doubled can easily be recorded but may revert to the previous level in a day or two and no improvement of any importance to the patient has occurred.

Disability scales are therefore best graded in wide steps so as to record only, for example, the difference between walking with difficulty and being unable to walk at all. Any change from one grade to another may therefore be presumed to be of significance to the patient and to be a 'real' change in clinical status. Such scales are, however, far too coarse to be used to record the clinical activity of the disease. Considerable deterioration or improvement in one or in several symptoms may occur with no change in the disability grade and more detailed methods must be employed. These are, however, far more exposed to the risk of bias on the part of the patient and the observer, with difficulties and disagreements in the assessment of functional grading, and to the recording of day to day fluctuations that possibly or even probably do not reflect changes in disease activity. Some of these difficulties can be overcome by the use of methods of measuring strength, co-ordination, sensation and other functions rather than subjective grading but such methods are undoubtedly time-consuming and some important functions cannot be measured.

Disability scales are all based to a very large extent on the single function of ambulation. Inability to walk is certainly the major cause of disablement but mental disturbance and incontinence of urine are also very important. In general it is possible to trace the appearance of increasingly fine gradations as investigators have succumbed to the temptation to use this method to record slighter and inevitably less clinically important changes. Thus, Ipsen[33] had four grades: working, ambulatory, bedridden and dying, that suited a study of life expectancy and probable disability. Riser and colleagues[3] used a slightly more sensitive scale: slight disability, moderate but able to walk, confined to wheelchair, bedridden, dead. McAlpine & Compston[34] employed six grades from unrestricted to bedridden, based entirely on mobility. Hyllested[35] also used six grades rather differently defined for different purposes. Other functions besides that of ability to walk were included but immediately increase the difficulty of grading as moderate disability in mobility might well not be accompanied by the need for assistance with any other activity.

As explained in Chapter 9, the Kurtzke Disability Status Scale (DSS) in its original[36] and extended form (EDSS)[37] was designed to be used in the assessment of response to treatment. The gradation is relatively fine and assessment requires examination of the patient, being based on scoring of 7 separate functional systems. The method is a convenient and ingenious compromise between scales with wide steps and the detailed scoring systems described below. With a few reservations, including the possibility that a distinct relapse may not alter the grade, the system is well suited to the requirements of prospective follow-up and is frequently used for this purpose. It forms an essential part of the minimal disability record.[38] For large scale field studies, however, a system using coarser gradings has some advantages. The grading system of Pedersen[39] is entirely based on function and does not include physical signs such as loss of vibration sense or nystagmus. Function is graded 0–5 for the mental state, vision, sphincters, upper and lower limbs separately, and personal efficiency. A patient could have an unpleasant brainstem relapse without this being reflected anywhere but in a decline in personal efficiency.

An extended discussion on the purpose of clinical grading in multiple sclerosis[38] emphasised two conflicting needs: that for a universally accepted record of disability and the detailed information required in special circumstances. For instance, an enquiry into the social consequences of multiple sclerosis would require information very different from that relevant to a therapeutic trial. Some agreement was apparently reached on a minimal uniform record of disability but the proposals would clearly not be of universal application and the report of the symposium conveys an impression of unrealistic complexity.

Scoring systems

Various scoring systems have been devised to produce a single numerical value to express the entire clinical state. The elaborate and laborious system of Alexander[40] in which arbitrary scores were allotted to a mixture of signs, symptoms and disabilities has been abandoned.

Fog[41] also developed a numerical scoring system which does not appear to have become popular. Here again arbitrary marks are given both for specific physical signs and for degrees of disability. Dysdiadochokinesia scores one mark and dysmetria another, each scoring double if present bilaterally. Intention tremor and many other physical signs are graded according to severity with marks up to three each side.

Patzold et al[42] have also used an idiosyncratic scoring system. Poser[43] published a scoring system in which the points awarded were not arbitrary but are based on the frequency with which the symptoms and signs occurred in a series of 111 autopsy proven cases. Any occurring in less than 50% of these cases was not scored at all. Thus weakness scored the maximum of 10 marks, being present in every case, while dysarthria scored 6. The system has recently been modified[44] but still seems better adapted to the diagnosis of multiple sclerosis than to following progress as intended.

The very detailed neurologic rating scale (NRS) of Sipe et al[45] is much more sensitive but has not proved popular. Unusually, it was tested for consistency between 4 physicians who scored within 2.6% error on 5 case descriptions. The error is likely to have been considerably greater had they examined the patients.[46] The illness severity score (ISS) of Mickey et al[47] derives a single figure from the Kurtzke functional scores, DSS and figures for the course and activity of disease, with weightings obtained from observation applied to all grades of disability. The ISS has been used in therapeutic trials but is probably too fine-tuned for other uses.

Grynderup[48] conducted a comparison of a number of grading and scoring systems applied to 400 patients. The systems compared were those of McAlpine & Compston,[34] Hyllested,[35] Pedersen,[39] Kurtzke[36,37] and a most complex scheme proposed by the American Committee on medical rating of physical impairment (CMRPI). There was good agreement in ranking of patients but less conformity in indicating the course of the disease, in particular whether deterioration was accelerating or the reverse. It was possible to devise a hypothetical patient declining steadily on Hyllested's system, but with decelerating progression according to McAlpine & Compston, and Kurtzke, but accelerating according to Pedersen. There was also some disparity at the two ends of the scales allotted to different stages of disability. Thus 67% of Kurtzke's scale refers to ambulant patients and only 40% of Pedersen's. Only 5% of the CMRPI scale refers to bedridden patients, but 30% of Pedersen's.

The methods described depend almost entirely on clinical judgment. Admittedly no great acumen is required to determine whether a patient is confined to a wheelchair or not, but the exact grading, on a 6-point scale, of degrees of cerebellar dysfunction, for example, is inevitably fallible. Standard neurological examination has been compared with Kurtzke's scale and with a system of symptom scoring and in general there was good agreement between different observers and little to choose between the methods considered.[49] Tourtellotte et al[50] have led the demands for more exact methods of assessment and have described a battery of measurements of function relevant to organic nervous disease and to multiple sclerosis in particular. For details of these tests it is important to consult the original descriptions as they have been carefully devised and evaluated. Whether they are capable of providing a more reliable indication of progression or remission of disease than clinical judgment must remain uncertain in the absence of any independent criteria. Kuzma et al[51] showed that measurements of function were repeatable between different observers at different times of day in normal subjects, indicating that the actual tests were reliable. There is again the danger of paying too much attention to minutiae, but, provided the measurements are relevant and can be compared with normal values and variations they must be superior to routine neurological examination.

Progression index

Any scoring or grading system can be used to calculate a coefficient or index of progression by dividing the score by the duration of the disease.[52] Although obviously subject to error, the index has

been found to remain stable in most patients followed up.[53] Minderhoud et al[54] have introduced a 'delta progression rate' to quantify the progressive stage. This is obtained by dividing the increase in the Kurtzke EDSS from the onset of progression by the time elapsed. This index may be somewhat more accurate as 3 observers tested on 41 cases attained only 81% agreement within $\pm$ 1 year on the date of onset of disease, but 91.7% agreement on the year of secondary progression.

THE CLINICAL COURSE

It is customary to recognise that the course of multiple sclerosis may be remittent, remittent/progressive or progressive from the onset, but there is little agreement on how these categories should be defined. For example, Patzold et al[55] require full recovery from relapse for their 'intermittent' course, while Confavreux et al[56] define remittent disease as a stable condition between relapses. They draw a distinction, which must be difficult to establish in retrospect, between 'pure' relapses followed by complete remission and relapses with sequelae, the former comprising 36% of the entire series. It is not always possible to determine exactly what is implied by the remittent category. Poser[4] stated that the remitting group had 'full remissions' and yet, among other severe disabilities, 10% are listed as having lost the ability to walk. In therapeutic trials in relapsing/remitting disease it is evident that full recovery has not been demanded as most patients admitted have some degree of disability. It is noteworthy, however, that Weiner & Ellison[21] in their protocol for clinical trials define relapse, but do not define remission. Charcot[57] had spoken of 'intermissions complètes' that he distinguished from 'rémissions' and perhaps clarity would have been served had this separation been maintained.

There is further confusion concerning the relapsing/progressive category. Most authorities[4,56,58] define this as progression following an initial relapsing/remitting course, but Weinshenker et al[5] require disease progressive from the onset with acute episodes of worsening and the definition of Patzold et al[55] can be interpreted in this way. The term 'progressive cumulative' used by

Phadke[19] is a good description of the familiar course in which each relapse is followed by partial recovery and accumulating deficit. The definition of the progressive form often seems to be regarded as self-evident and yet, particularly in retrospect, there are obvious difficulties in identifying continued progression without relapse, remission or periods of stability. Except in treatment protocols, the duration of progression required may not be specified. There is also little acknowledgement that disability can remain unchanged over long periods. That prolonged clinical inactivity of the disease can occur in established cases is shown by Gudmundsson's[59] report that 59% of the surviving patients in the multiple sclerosis survey in Iceland had shown no progression over 14 years. Stazio et al[60] reported no progression in 34 of 128 patients over 11 years.

The relapse

The word 'relapse' has the slightly inconvenient connotation of excluding the first attack of the disease, and numerous other terms have been used, including bout, attack, exacerbation, episode and the expressive French poussée. When considering the natural history of the disease in broad terms it is not necessary to define a relapse as precisely as in the assessment of a therapeutic regime aimed at reducing the relapse rate. Indeed most epidemiological studies do not clearly define relapse or remission which would certainly present difficulties in retrospect.

McAlpine,[61] basing his criteria partly on those of Müller,[62] defined a relapse as the appearance of a new symptom or the reappearance of a previous symptom at any time after the initial attack. He rightly drew attention to the distinction between a relapse, with the implication of a fresh lesion, or reactivation of an old lesion, and a temporary exacerbation, defined as the reappearance of an old symptom for a short period of a few minutes, hours or days. The distinction is no doubt generally valid but may be difficult in application, particularly to the reappearance of former symptoms where the clinical differentiation is based solely on duration. For example, Matthews & Small[63] showed that a complaint of slight visual

blurring for a day or two might be accompanied by a permanent increase in latency in visual evoked potentials from the affected eye, indicating fresh damage to the optic nerve. As there is no routine laboratory method of determining activity of the disease process, the judgment of whether fleeting symptoms are indeed a relapse or the result of fatigue, temperature change, intercurrent infection or temporary decline in morale must be somewhat tenuously based on clinical experience.

Schumacher et al,[20] who were particularly concerned with assessing the effect of treatment, considered that changes in clinical state lasting for less than 24 hours should not be accepted either as relapse or remission. They faced the problem, so important in this particular context, of a change in clinical state, usually for the worse, *reported* to have occurred between two visits to the observing physician, with subsequent recovery. For their particular purpose it was correct to exclude as a relapse any phenomena not witnessed, but intelligent and trained observers who suffer from multiple sclerosis in an active phase will convincingly report brief episodes, usually involving the sensory system or the cranial nerves, that are strongly suggestive of the presence of fresh lesions.

There is little precise information on the usual duration of the initial attack or of relapses. This must in part be due to difficulty in defining progression during the phase encountered in many relapses in which some symptoms are improving or even recover while others are increasing in severity or appearing for the first time. The point of termination of a relapse can also present difficulties. McAlpine[61] defined a remission as the partial or complete disappearance of a symptom or symptoms. McAlpine & Compston[34] considered the length of relapse in patients recently diagnosed, but confined their study to the initial attack and first relapse. They recorded great variation from less than one day, which would have been excluded by many authors, to twelve months. No clear pattern emerged, although the relapse tended to last rather longer than the first attack. Confavreux et al[56] distinguished between 'pure' relapse where full recovery occurred and relapse with permanent sequelae but did not indicate the duration of either form. Müller[62] regarded as a remittent case one where symptoms improved or became stationary, a most difficult end-point. Broman et al,[17] in the early reports of the eagerly-awaited study from Gothenburg, realistically acknowledged the difficulties inherent in recognising a relapse but were reduced almost to incoherence in accepting 'bouts', 'minibouts' and 'periods' of progression, both 'distinct' and 'indistinct' without defining any of these terms.

It has been convenient to count all fresh symptoms occurring within a period of one month or sometimes three months as part of the same relapse. Some such definition is necessary if conclusions are to be drawn from the rate of relapse but the time scale is more related to the convenience of the follow-up than to the reality of the disease.

Relapse rate

There is much disagreement on the annual relapse rate but figures are sometimes reported differently. Some authors refer to the relapse rate in their whole series while others refer to the rates in remitting cases alone. It is not always clear whether the initial attack is counted as a relapse. Müller[62] in a large retrospective study found an annual relapse rate of 0.5 for the entire series collected from hospital records over 25 years. In contrast Thygesen[64] studied intensively 60 patients for a much shorter period of up to 18 months. Very disabled patients and monosymptomatic cases were excluded. An annual relapse rate of 1.15 was found. McAlpine & Compston[34] found a rate ranging from 0.42–0.2 according to the duration of the disease, the study being in part prospective. Alexander et al[65,66] in a large series personally examined, found a rate of 0.75 but their definition of a relapse may not have coincided with that of other authors. Gudmundsson[59] reported a rate of 0.14 in a series of patients, most of whom were examined annually. Millar et al[67] also found a very low rate of 0.104 in a group of 262 women of child-bearing age. Leibowitz et al[24,68] report two different rates, one of 0.28 for remitting cases during the whole course of the disease and one of 0.39 for the whole series in the first five years of the disease. Confavreux et al[56] reported a relapse rate of 0.85 for the remittent stage but 0.31 for the whole series.

There are certainly many factors operating to produce this marked disparity, perhaps including genuine differences in clinical pattern in different geographical areas. Methods of case ascertainment and selection, diagnostic criteria and presentation of data are probably more important. A number of reports confirm the clinical impression that relapse is more common in the first few years of the disease. Müller[62] found that relapse was much more common in the first five years and particularly in the first year after onset. McAlpine & Compston[34] documented a decline from a peak rate in the second year of the disease but even 25–30 years from the onset the relapse rate of 0.2 was double that in some series described above. Millar et al[67] showed a consistent decline in rate with duration of disease. Broman et al[17] also found a sharp decrease in relapse rate after the first five years. Confavreux et al[56] in contrast found that the interval between relapses tended to shorten with the passage of time. Lhermitte et al[69] found a rate of 0.51 (including the initial attack) in the first five years of the disease and 0.26 for each of the next two five-year periods. Additional factors can be identified, although less clearly. Fog & Linnemann[10] found a relapse rate of 0.3 in retrospective case studies but 0.56 prospectively. Lhermitte et al[69] found an even more remarkable difference, but in the reverse direction. In the whole group the rate was 0.83 retrospectively and 0.34 prospectively. Fog & Linnemann[10] also drew attention to the possible effect of frequency of examination. Thygesen[64] saw the patients every three weeks and the rate was 1.15, comparable figures being 3 months and 0.5;[61] 6 months and 0.3;[34] and one year and 0.14.[59] As already noted, patients with multiple sclerosis often forget symptoms and possible relapses not observed are in any case excluded.from consideration by many investigators.

Even during this particularly vulnerable period estimates of the frequency of relapse to be expected vary from one a year to one in four years. These average figures of course conceal patients who have very frequent relapses, several a year for a prolonged period.

The natural decline in relapse rate with increasing duration of disease is of great importance when assessing the effects of treatment and is discussed further in Chapter 9.

The outcome of relapse

The clinical features of an attack of multiple sclerosis may remit completely or in part, may remain stationary for a prolonged period or may progress. Thygesen[64] found almost complete remission in approximately one half of observed relapses, partial recovery in a quarter and failure of remission in a quarter. Such figures will be greatly influenced by many aspects of selection and observation. There are few detailed studies of factors associated with remission following the initial clinical attack or subsequent relapse. Reports that are available are unsatisfactory in being largely retrospective or confined to hospital in-patients. In general they have shown a strong positive correlation between rapidity of onset and degree of recovery with much less relation to the severity or nature of the symptoms. Thygesen[64] in a prospective study found that with an 'apoplectic' onset in which all symptoms of the relapse developed within 24 hours 70% of maximum disability recovered within a month. Rather less acute onset was also relatively favourable, some remission occurring in 98% of patients compared with 48% of those in whom the symptoms of the relapse had progressed for several weeks. Alexander et al[65] also found that rapid onset was more likely to be followed by remission. Kurtzke et al[70,71] assessed rapidity of onset by the duration of symptoms before admission to hospital, a measure that must also be compounded to some extent by the severity of disability. Improvement was judged, in retrospect, at the point of leaving hospital. Those whose symptoms had been present for less than a month before admission were far more likely to improve. These findings confirmed those reported by Kurtzke[72] in greater detail who found improvement rate of 86% of patients with symptoms for up to a week before admission: 64% for 8–14 days and 36% for 15–31 days.

Müller[62] was able to follow the relationship between duration of relapse and chance of remission for much longer. In a relapse of two months, duration up to 85% of symptoms remitted completely, falling to 30% at three months and 10% at six months. Only 6% of patients improved if symptoms had persisted for a year and remission never occurred after eight years of progressive or static disease. Kurtzke[72] found no remission of symptoms of more than two years' duration.

The severity of the symptoms of an attack has also been found to be related to immediate outcome. Kurtzke et al[71] found that severe symptoms were more likely to improve; 95% of those with severe symptoms of short duration improved. With severe symptoms but longer duration, only 29% improved. With milder symptoms and short duration, 40% improved and with longer duration, 12%. Alexander et al[65] had found that mild relapses recovered better, but there is, of course, an important distinction between the percentage of patients who improve and the degree of recovery attained. Partial recovery from a severe relapse may be more disabling than persistence of mild symptoms.

More difficult to assess is the effect of earlier events, in particular the stage and duration of the disease, on the prospects in a relapse. It is generally assumed, from common observation, that complete remission more frequently occurs following the initial attack than after relapses. The proportion of patients remitting after the initial attack is well documented, as already described, but there appear to be no reliable figures on the degree of recovery compared with that following relapse. Kurtzke et al[71] found improvement in some 29% of their cases in whom first attack was recorded and in 20% of those who had had previous episodes. Improvement was assessed from records at the point of discharge from hospital, which cannot be an entirely reliable end-point. It is possible to calculate from Brown & Putnam's[73] figures that 60% of initial symptoms recovered or greatly improved as opposed to 43% of symptoms in relapse, but their conclusions were apparently based on patients' reports rather than on observation. Alexander et al[65,66] found that failure to recover from relapse was more common in the first few years of the disease, while Kurtzke et al[71] reported that a short duration of disease before the relapse increased the chance of remission. Patients already severely disabled are less likely to remit.[73] A prolonged initial attack is more likely to be followed by failure to recover from the next relapse.[62] The greater the degree of recovery from a relapse the better the expectation of remission in the next relapse.[66] In contrast, Kurtzke[72] could not relate the outcome of an observed relapse to the duration or severity of the disease or to the outcome of previous relapses.

Although precise figures are not available, and not perhaps to be expected, the prognosis for full or substantial recovery is much better for symptoms that might reasonably be attributed to 'small' lesions — optic neuritis, diplopia, vertigo, facial palsy or cranial nerve lesions in general.[73] Symptoms of this kind become less frequent in later relapses while signs of long tract involvement become increasingly common. Cutaneous sensory loss is also unlikely to become permanent. The prognosis for recovery from such distressing but not usually incapacitating symptoms must be distinguished from that for improvement, which, as already noted, is relatively good with severe symptoms such as paraparesis when of acute onset. The prospects of complete recovery from such symptoms is, however, much less favourable. Unexpectedly, Kurtzke et al[71] did not find that the nature of the symptoms, apart from sensory loss, had any detectable influence on the outcome of an attack of multiple sclerosis, whether onset or relapse. Personal observation suggests that cerebellar ataxia recovers less frequently than other symptoms encountered in the relapsing phase of the disease.

The latent phase

This has been identified[61] as the interval between onset and first relapse or between relapses, during which fresh symptoms do not occur. Whether the disease process is indeed inactive must be uncertain. Nevertheless, periods more or less prolonged are often observed during which all clinical evidence of active disease is in complete abeyance.

Of McAlpine's[61] 586 cases, 525 were known to have relapsed. Over one quarter relapsed within a year of the onset and just over one half within the first three years. One patient in 20 did not relapse until 15 or more years after the onset. In four cases the latent period lasted over 30 years, the longest being 37 years. Of those in whom the latent phase lasted over 15 years, the presenting symptom in 65% had been optic neuritis. Müller's[62] figures are similar, with an initial latent phase of 15 years or more in 6% of patients followed for this period.

Adams et al[74] found that 8% of their 389 cases had a latent phase of this duration. The only symptoms followed by such a prolonged period of inactivity were paresis, optic neuritis and diplopia. Bonduelle & Albaranès[75] reported that of their 114 remittent cases, the latent period between the initial attack and first relapse was less than six months in 20, six to twelve months in 27, one to two years in 20, two to five years in 25, five to ten years in 13 and over ten years in nine, with a maximum of 17 years.

The latent phase between relapses has already been discussed in general terms when considering the relapse rate. McAlpine[61] voiced the general opinion that the interval between first and second relapse is usually less than that between onset and first relapse.

The chronic progressive stage

Primary progression. The proportion of patients reported to have disease progressive from the onset has varied greatly, in part because of the difficulties in definition described above. If all whose initial symptoms do not clear completely are regarded as having progressive disease, the proportion is high, but not all variations are explicable in this way. Population surveys in Iceland[59] and Finland[76] found respectively some 13% and 10% of patients with progressive onset, while in Israel[77] (37%), the Netherlands[54] (37%), Canada[5] (33%) and Scotland[23] (27%) the figures were much higher. Clinic figures are similarly scattered: Bonduelle & Albaranès[75] (9%); Poser[4] (12.7%); Müller[62] (13%); Lhermitte et al[69] (13%); Confavreux et al[56] (18%); a personal series of 546 cases (18%); Verjans et al[58] (26%). In patients seen 'from onset', a smaller proportion were found to have progressive disease.[5] This was attributed to easy recall of recent events but may have been due to selecting out those with slowly progressive spinal cord disease who often present after a longer interval from onset than patients with more immediately alarming acute symptoms.

Most observers have found a clear relationship between progressive presentation and late age of onset. Leibowitz et al[24] reported progression from the onset in 57% of those with onset after 40 and Cazzullo et al[78] found 49% progression in the same age group compared with 17% in those below this age. Weinshenker et al[5] found a steadily increasing proportion of patients with progressive onset with increasing age, reaching 63% in the fifth decade and 74.5% after the age of 49. In Shepherd's[23] series, the mean age at onset was 43 in progressive disease and 31 in the remittent form. Confavreux et al[56] reported a mean age of onset of 30 for the remittent form and 37.3 for those with progression from the onset, a highly significant difference.

Secondary progression. The disease may become progressive at any point after the onset. This appears not to have been generally appreciated until the detailed individual follow-up studies of Birley & Dudgeon[79] showed that the progressive and remitting forms were not distinct as had originally been believed. The proportion of patients with initially relapsing and remitting disease in whom the progressive stage eventually develops is difficult to estimate as it increases with the length of follow-up. Müller[62] found that 25% of cases had become progressive within two years of the onset and 50% within ten years. Here again the influence of age of onset was apparent. With onset at 35 or over 80% had become progressive within five years. Riser et al[3] described a series of 203 cases followed for over ten years. Of particular interest are the 29 cases in which severe or progressive disease developed between ten and fifteen years after the onset and the 14 in whom this occurred after more than 15 years. Confavreux et al[56] found that 30% of patients had entered the progressive phase by 5 years from the onset and 50% by 11 years.

These clinic series might be thought unduly pessimistic but in a population based survey Broman[80] found that between 5 and 10 years from onset 45% of patients had progressive disease and a further 10% had stepwise deterioration that he refers to as 'pseudoprogression'. Between 10 and 15 years over 60% were progressive. Weinshenker et al[5] found that of patients with remitting disease, 41% had become progressive by 6–10 years from onset and 58% by 11–15 years. Progression is not, however, inevitable. Of the comparatively small proportion of the series who could be reviewed 20–25 years from onset, Broman found that 25% had not progressed. (It must be remembered that Broman's diagnostic criteria are not easy to relate

to those usually employed.) Weinshenker et al[5] found that 11% of those surviving for over 26 years from onset had not developed progressive disease.

Confavreux et al[56] were particularly concerned with the change from remittent to progressive disease. There appeared to be no difference at the onset between those who were still in the remittent stage at the time of reporting and those who had entered the progressive stage. The mean age of onset of progression in these latter patients was 38, very similar to the age of onset in patients with primary progression. In a later analysis[81] the course of the disease was described through the movement of patients from one disease state to another, the states being defined as relapsing with full recovery, relapsing with sequelae and progressive. Minderhoud et al[54] also found an almost identical mean age of onset of primary (35.7 years) and secondary (37.5) progression. These results are in keeping with the suggestion of Fog & Linnemann[10] that primary progressive disease has been amputated from the normally preceding remittent 'prephase', that has perhaps, been overlooked or forgotten. Patzold & Pocklington,[82] however, were unable to identify an average year of disease progression. The important prognostic implications of entering the progressive phase are discussed below.

Fog & Linnemann[10] in their extensive serial study of 73 patients measured the rate of deterioration in the progressive stage. Several distinctive patterns were identified and the original work must be consulted for details. They concluded that once the nature of the curve was established the subsequent course of the disease could be foretold with some accuracy in three-quarters of their patients. This implies that in these patients the course of the disease was predetermined and not influenced by later events. The diversity of forms of curve is somewhat daunting and the patients were selected on their willingness to attend regularly but the investigation is an admirable example of the serial application of scoring methods of clinical evaluation. The numerical values obtained are, however, based on arbitrarily assigned numbers rather than measurements and are therefore not wholly suitable for statistical and mathematical manipulation. In the prospective study of Patzold & Pocklington[82] 102 patients were followed for at least two years. Of these, 33 steadily deteriorated. In 21 there was rapid initial deterioration with later slower progression, while in a further 21 the course was the reverse, accelerating deterioration. In 9 patients the clinical state oscillated and in 1, initial deterioration was followed by improvement. In 15 patients there was no significant change during the period of observation. They derived seven different formulae for the course of multiple sclerosis and a further form where the curve was flat, indicating no change. The course could not be predicted from such factors as age or severity of onset. They confirmed Fog & Linnemann's[10] concept of a predictable course once the pattern can be identified. Again, the variety of curves detracts from the ease of application, which also demands much more meticulous documentation than is usually available. These interesting findings are at present of more theoretical than practical value, particularly as quite prolonged observation is needed before the individual curves can be identified.

PROGNOSIS

Prognosis as to life

The effect of multiple sclerosis on life expectancy has frequently been examined by a variety of methods, all influenced by the usual hazards of retrospective data and difficulty of diagnosis and of case ascertainment. In this context, hospital series are particularly prone to bias towards severe cases with excess mortality.[83]

The duration of the disease at death provides essential but inadequate information and Gudmundsson[59] provides a useful table of such reports. The early estimates of Gowers[84] of a duration of 3–6 years and of Bramwell[85] of 7 years are of historical interest and have been much extended. In Bramwell's later series[86] the average duration in fatal cases was 12 years. Müller's[62] average figure was a duration of 10.4 years at death while in Allison's[87] smaller but closely observed series, the duration was 20 years. With few exceptions subsequent estimates of the average duration of the disease in fatal cases has been be-

tween 13 and 20 years: 17 (Leibowitz et al[88]); 14 (Lazarte[89]); 13 (Carter et al[7]); 20 (H R Müller[90]); 13 (Panelius[76]): 15 (Poeck & Markus[91]); 14 for men and 20 for women (Ipsen[33]) and 13 for women and 9 for men (Confavreux et al[56]). Despite the expected bias no difference between hospital and population based figures appeared in these results. Two large geographical surveys have, however, shown longer survival. Hyllested[35] in Denmark reported an average duration at death of 25–29 years. It is difficult to see how this can be accounted for by delay in diagnosis as suggested by McAlpine.[92] In the Grampian region of Scotland Phadke[19] found a mean duration of disease in fatal cases of 24.5 years: 25.7 for women and 23.5 for men.

Apart from the earliest reports there is no obvious trend towards longer survival in the last two decades as might be expected both from earlier diagnosis and better care of the disabled. Hyllested[35] found that in Denmark incidence had remained the same but prevalence had increased as a result of falling death rate. Dassel[93] examined reported deaths from multiple sclerosis in the Netherlands and found an increase in the mean age at death between 1950 and 1968 from 47.6 to 56.9 years in men and from 50.8 to 55.2 years in women.

Of greater interest are the chances of survival. Only 10 of Bramwell's 200 cases survived for more than twenty years and only 2 for more than thirty years. In contrast, Kurtzke et al[94] found that 76% of their male patients survived for twenty years and 69% for twenty five years. Bauer et al[95] in a large series found that no patients died within the first five years. Within 6–10 years of the onset 1.6% had died; from 11–15 years 16.7%; from 16–20 years 18.8%, and over 21 years 22.7%. Median (or average) survival has been calculated as over 21 years,[60] 21 years,[96] over 30 years,[97] 20–25 years,[91] 30 years,[35] 27 years,[98] and 35–42 years.[99]

These figures convey little unless compared with expected survival. Leibowitz et al[88] found the mean age at death in 47 patients in their series of 260 who died from multiple sclerosis-related causes in the decade of observation was 51.6 years compared with 63.3 years for the general population over the age of 14. The mean age at death with multiple sclerosis but dying of other causes was 59.8 years and the excess of deaths was therefore largely due to multiple sclerosis. Poskanzer et al[25] found that the life expectancy of men with multiple sclerosis was reduced by a mean of 9.5 years and that of women by 14.4 years. Percy et al[12] found the 25-year survival rate in multiple sclerosis to be 74% compared with an expected 86%. Kurtzke et al[94] found the risk of death even in their selected group of young men with early onset to be three times the expected level. Their cases experienced about four-fifths of normal survival after 20 years and about three quarters of normal after 25 years.

A large series[83] of patients seen in German hospitals between 1972 and 1980 was followed for a mean of 4.9 years by which time 263 had died. The excess death rate was calculated as the number of deaths in excess of natural mortality per 1000 subjects at risk per year. For the whole series this was found to be 19. This was not affected by sex and very little by age of onset but in progressive disease the excess rate was 27. Initial involvement of the motor system, intellectual loss or sphincter disturbance carried a poor prognosis, while sensory symptoms or double vision were associated with long survival. In a population survey,[99] survival was 60% of the expected figure after 35 years of illness.

The degree of disability at a given point in time is the strongest indicator of life expectancy. Hyllested[35] found a close relationship with the six points on the disability scale used as summarised in Table 5.1.

The survey carried out by Phadke[19] of death and survival of multiple sclerosis patients in the Grampian region of Scotland is of prime importance, being population based and covering a large number of deaths. Between 1970 and 1980, 216 patients died, the age at onset being known in 200.

Table 5.1 Effect of degree of disability on survival (Hyllested[35])

Disability	% Dying within 10 years
Walks unaided	7
Walks with one stick	21
Walks with two sticks	34
Can just stand	49
Able to sit	64
Bedridden	84

Mortality was compared with that in the Scottish population. Four adverse factors stand out inescapably: age at onset, duration of disease, progressive disease and severe disability. In the first ten years after onset, increased mortality, although present, was not marked except in those over 50 years old at onset, in whom survival was reduced by 44% in men and 22% in women. With longer duration of disease the difference between observed and expected survival widened. This was particularly marked in the group aged 40–49 at onset of whom only 5% of men and 26% of women were alive 30 years after the onset, compared with 60% and 70% respectively in the age-matched population. The probability of a man with onset of disease at the age of 25 reaching 65 years of age was only 4% and for women 6%, contrasted with 77% and 84% in controls. Of those with disease progressive from the onset, 30% survived for less than 10 years and only 3.3% survived 30 years and none for 40 years. For relapsing cumulative disease, 6% died in the ten years from onset while 23% survived for more than 40 years. The effect of severe disability on a given date is illustrated by the relative survival ten years from onset of those with no disability (94% survival) and those confined to chair or bed (28% survival).

The cause of death

Death from a direct effect of multiple sclerosis on the nervous system is uncommon and results either from respiratory paralysis or coma of uncertain origin or following status epilepticus. Death usually results from infective complications of the paralysed state, from unrelated disease or, occasionally, from suicide. In the survey conducted by Leibowitz et al,[88,100] 58% of deaths were related to multiple sclerosis but only one patient had died in acute relapse. Four patients had committed suicide. The causes of death in the remaining patients did not differ from those in the general population. In the Gothenburg prospective study[80] multiple sclerosis was the sole direct or indirect cause in 20 of 49 deaths. Of the remainder, malignant disease was responsible in 11, cardiac disease in 12, asthma in 2, uraemia in 1 and there were 3 suicides. In Phadke's[19] series of 216 deaths, the cause was unknown in 2 patients; 132 had died of complications of multiple sclerosis: broncho-pneumonia, septicaemia, inhalation asphyxia and pulmonary embolism; 25 had died of malignant disease, chiefly of the bronchus, and 41 of cardiovascular disease including stroke. Miscellaneous causes included 1 patient with pneumothorax.[101] In contrast to the other studies referred to, no patient is said to have committed suicide.

Prognosis as to disability

There are few reports of quantitative data relating disability to duration of disease.[1] The series of McAlpine & Compston[34] was, unfortunately, as the authors acknowledged, so heavily tilted in favour of mild cases as to be unrepresentative. The US Armed Forces series has the built-in disadvantage of referring only to previously fit young men but is prospective, with reasonable case ascertainment up to 15 years from onset. Data from this and from the retrospective clinic series of Confavreux et al[56] and the population study, also retrospective, of Panelius[76] are summarised in Table 5.2.

The most striking disparity is the relative lack of cases with mild disability at five years from the onset in both series from the US army. This is unlikely to be due to the different disability scales used as a considerable difference persists even if Kurtzke DSS 3 is included in mild disease. After 15 years about 25% of patients were still fully active and a slightly larger proportion were severely disabled. Confavreux et al[56] found that the mean interval from onset to moderate disability in all patients was 3.45 years. With progressive onset

this interval was only 0.34 years. The interval to severe disability was 9.5 years, again shorter in progressive disease. Weinshenker et al[5] reported a slower course with a median time to reach DSS 3 of 7.69 years and 15 years to reach DSS 6. Their figure of 46.39 years as the median time from onset to reach the bedridden stage has an air of unreality. In patients followed from the onset the recorded course was more rapid.

In these reports, progress is judged almost exclusively on ability to walk. The alternative criterion of the capacity to work is subject to many influences but must also reflect the patients' view of the impact of the disease. Müller,[62] in his pessimistic retrospective study, found that 40% of patients were incapacitated for work within five years, 50% within ten years and 66% within 15 years. Kolb's[103] figures were apparently even more depressing. Of patients, 75% had given up their position at work within a year of the initial symptoms but this clearly cannot mean that they were incapable of any work. Between six and ten years of the onset, only 10% were working at all although this proportion was maintained during the succeeding five-year period. Ipsen[33] reported that 50% of patients had to stop work within five years of the onset. H R Müller's[90] figures were little different. In the first five years 50% were able to work, falling to 42% in the next five years and to 27% from 11–15 years from onset. Lazarte[89] mentioned the effect on work in his study of the prognosis in ambulant and non-ambulant cases, but it is difficult to accept or interpret the figures. One patient regained the ability to walk and reported complete recovery at least 16 years after discharge from hospital in a non-ambulant state.

Table 5.2 Percentage of whole series (C and K, A and B) or of survivors (P) in different grades of disability at 5, 10 and 15 years from onset

Author	Mild				Moderate				Severe			
	C	K		P	C	K		P	C	K		P
Years from onset		A	B			A	B			A	B	
5	53	18	19	58	40	71	61	33	8	10	16	9
10	40	22	24	32	35	51	47	46	20	22	20	22
15	28	17	20	24	33	44	45	37	28	22	18	39

Mild disease is Kurtzke DSS 0–2, McAlpine & Compston 0–1[34] or Hyllested.[35] Moderate disease is K DSS 3–6 and grades 2–3 on the other two scales. Severe disease is Kurtzke DSS 7–9 and 4–6 on the other scales. C is Confavreux et al;[56] K is Kurtzke et al[102] and P is Panelius.[76]

Bauer et al[104] made a thorough study of a large group of patients with particular attention to working capacity. The sex distribution was not stated and the series contained a large but unspecified proportion of subjects claiming for the effect of wartime experiences in aggravating their condition. Thirty two per cent were in full work up to five years from the onset and a total of 71% were capable of some work. From 6–10 years, 23% were in full work, falling to 11.3% in the next five year period. Thereafter there was no further fall and from 12–16% of survivors remained in full work and up to 40% were capable of some useful activity. Numbers were of course smaller but these findings agree with those of Kolb[102] and indicate that a relatively constant proportion of long-term survivors had mild disease. Poser[4] also found that in those who survived for more than 20 years, the admittedly small proportion of those able to work normally showed a tendency to increase. Allison[87] found that of the 12 survivors of the 40 patients he had examined 20 years earlier, only 4 were severely disabled.

Some diagrammatic representations of the course of multiple sclerosis suggest that once the progressive stage has begun, acute relapse and remission no longer occur. This impression is not wholly justified.

A woman of 47 was investigated in hospital because of a five-year history of progressive left spastic hemiparesis, beginning in the leg and later involving the arm. Vibration sense was absent at both ankles. Her sister had multiple sclerosis. CSF examination, visual evoked potentials and a myelogram were normal. The right leg was later gradually involved and after two years was also moderately weak. She then suddenly developed paroxysmal symptoms consisting of pain spreading rapidly up the left arm from the hand without loss of use or change in posture. The pain would extend to the neck and head and she would be unable to speak clearly. Each attack lasted a few seconds but she had many attacks every day, not obviously triggered. They could not be induced by overbreathing and were not witnessed. Carbamazepine abolished the paroxysms. Six months later she rapidly developed loss of postural sense in the fingers of both hands, increased weakness in both legs and paraesthesiae in the left foot. These additional symptoms and signs subsided in the course of the next two months, leaving her with her original disability.

Certainly relapse becomes less common. Lher-mitte et al[69] found a relapse rate of 0.08 per annum in their group of patients with progressive disease in contrast to 0.75 for the remitting form. Without detailed assessment it is particularly difficult to make any convincing distinction between those cases where progression occurs between relapses and those in whom the clinical condition in remission is static.

The cause of disability

Bauer & Firnhaber[103] examined the clinical features responsible for the loss of the ability to work. Spastic paresis of the legs was a major cause of disability in over 60% of disabled patients, incoordination in 39% and sphincter disturbance in 23%, many patients having more than one severe disability. Larocca et al[105] investigated the reasons for the 77% unemployment in a series of 77 men and 233 women. Reasons given by the patients included poor vision in 7.4%, physical limitations in 27.5% and fatigue in 13.9%. Surprisingly, only 14% of the difference between employed and unemployed could be accounted for by factors that might be assumed to be important: degree of disability, sex, age, duration of disease and level of education. Occupation, marital status and the clinical syndrome appeared to make no contribution.

MALIGNANT AND BENIGN FORMS

The course of multiple sclerosis varies from death in the initial attack within a few weeks of the onset;[7,106] to imperceptible disease discovered accidentally at necropsy in extreme old age. It is therefore natural to consider whether there are indeed different forms of the disease of intrinsically different severity or whether malignant and benign cases are merely the extremes of a continuous variation.

The term 'malignant' has been rather loosely applied to cases dying within 5 years of the onset. Death in the first attack is the result of respiratory paralysis or of inappropriate surgery.[7,106] It is unlikely that these events are evidence of a separate 'form' of multiple sclerosis but merely indicate the lethal anatomical site of the initial lesions. Bonduelle & Albaranès[75] emphasised that their 'acute' form, while dangerous to life, might well remit. They did, however, describe a patient who died of disseminated disease, including transverse myelitis, within 18 days of the onset, although it is not stated whether the diagnosis was pathologically confirmed. Guillain & Alajouanine[107] reported death from bulbar paralysis 3 weeks from the onset. Autopsy showed three plaques, in the medulla, cervical spinal cord and pons. The most rapid fatality personally witnessed was in a young woman who died in coma 57 days after the onset of unilateral optic neuritis, the diagnosis being confirmed at autopsy. Death within the first 5 years is uncommon. McAlpine estimated that 1 in 22 patients died within this period. Similar figures were reported by Müller[62] and Kolb[103] but in a later series Bauer et al[95] reported no deaths within 5 years of the onset. Severe disability within this period, however, has been reported in up to 12% of patients[95] but Poser[4] found a figure of only 3%. Confavreux et al[56] recognised five forms of multiple sclerosis, ranging from hyperacute to benign, based on the duration of disease before the onset of severe disability. Of their cases, 8.3% fell into the first category, defined as severe disability, within 5 years. In these cases the disease was either progressive from the onset or characterised by severe relapses with clinical evidence of long tract involvement and without significant remission. It is tempting to speculate on absence of resistance to the disease process in these cases but the malignant course might equally be due to overwhelming exposure to some causative agent. In the complete absence of knowledge of either of these aspects it is not justifiable to regard these cases as a separate 'form' of the disease in the sense of being related to some difference in pathogenesis.

The benign form of multiple sclerosis has been the subject of much more detailed study, largely as the result of McAlpine's important observations.[2,61] In his series of 241 patients, 78 were unrestricted in their daily life after a minimum follow-up period of 10 years and a mean of 13 years. In practice they were able to walk half a mile without any form of assistance and were working away from or at home. The diagnostic categories of these patients were as follows: definite, 46 cases; probable, 20 cases, and possible, 12 cases, using McAlpine's own classification. This series of patients with apparently benign disease was followed at intervals, mostly by examination and a few by correspondence. After a minimum of 15 years' duration of disease (mean 18 years), 52 were still unrestricted and 12 had become disabled. Four years later a further eight patients had become disabled and 49 were still in the unrestricted category, of whom the diagnosis was regarded as definite in 33. These observations illustrate several important points. The original definition of a benign case was one where no disability had resulted 10 years from the onset. Inevitably such cases must include a significant proportion of patients in whom the diagnosis is uncertain, mainly because they have not developed the characteristic disabilities. These serial observations also demonstrated that disease that is benign after 10 or 15 years may eventually become disabling. McAlpine estimated that in any series of patients first seen relatively soon after the onset, approximately one third could be classified as benign at 10 years, but only one quarter of the total would still be without significant disability after 15 years and only one fifth after 20 years. Thompson et al[108] found that 47 (42%) of 111 patients with clinically definite multiple sclerosis who survived for 10 years had disability of Kurtzke DSS 3 or less, and the same proportion was maintained 15 years from onset.

The benign form has been differently defined by other authors. Poser[4] required 14 years from onset and disability of not more than 3 on Kurtzke's scale. Riser et al[3] chose 10 years with slight disability; Bauer et al[5] regarded continued ability to work after 20 years as the criterion; Bonduelle[109] originally regarded 10 years with slight disability as benign disease but in a later paper[110] required 15 years. Poeck & Markus[91] reported benign cases of at least 14 years' duration. It is not clear that Lehoczky & Halasy-Lehoczky[111] regarded duration of disease as an important element in the benign forms they described. Their material was drawn from cases admitted to hospital between 1952–62 and their report was in 1963. Kurtzke et al[102] defined their benign cases as being those with a score of 0–2 on the disability scale after 10 or 15 years. Confavreux et al[56] required no disability after 10 years or slight disability after 15 years. Fog & Linnemann[10] regarded the slope of the course of progression of the disease as recorded by their scoring system as the significant factor, an angle of less than 5° when plotted by this method indicating a benign case.

The proportion of patients satisfying these criteria can be expressed in different ways: either as the percentage of an entire series who eventually prove to have benign disease as defined, or the percentage of those who survive for the required period and have little or no disability. The latter figure is the more realistic but cannot be equated with the proportion of the total incidence that will behave in this way as patients dying before the qualifying period will be excluded. For example, Poser et al[112] reported 5% of benign cases, but this was with reference to the whole series with a mean duration of 11.2 years. From the data they present it is not possible to calculate the proportion of those with a 14-year duration who were not disabled. Similarly Confavreux et al[56] reported 14.3% of benign cases but the mean period of follow-up was 9 years with a mean delay of 4.7 years between onset and first examination. Riser et al[3] provide figures for patients followed for 10 years or more. Of 203 cases, 74 (36%) were benign at the chosen point of 10 years from the onset, but at the time of reporting only 31 were still without significant disability. Twenty three had been followed for 15–30 years from the onset. In this series all patients were in McAlpine's 'definite' (assuré) category. At 15 years, the duration required by most observers, 45 cases (22%) had mild disease. Poeck & Markus[91] reported that 17.5% of those surviving for more than 14 years were not disabled. In Bonduelle et al's[110] series of 175 definite or probable cases (McAlpine), the duration was more than 15 years at the time of reporting in 53, of whom 38 were classified as benign. It is not clear whether this figure refers to the clinical state at 15 years or at the time of reporting. Kurtzke et al[102] reported that at 10 and 15 years from onset about 20% of their exclusively male patients had mild disease.

These figures provide further confirmation that long duration may be associated with slight disability. This is not unexpected as those with severe disease would survive in much smaller numbers. For example, Bauer et al[95] found that the percentage of those able to work at all was higher in

survivors of more than 21 years (39.5%) than in those surviving 11–15 years (31.8%). Müller[62] found that although there were far fewer survivors at 15 years than at 10, the proportion of slightly disabled patients did not change, whereas in the first 10 years of the disease there was a steep decline. Percy et al[12] found that two thirds of those patients who survived for over 25 years were still ambulant but they did not give figures for earlier periods. Obviously most, but not all, such patients will be more affected than they were 25 years earlier but survival of such duration by definition excludes malignant cases and in practice many severe cases. Long survivors with benign disease are not, however, immune to relapse. Aggravation leading to disability occurred between 10 and 15 years in 29 of the 74 benign cases described by Riser et al[3] and in a further 14 after 15 years of disease. McAlpine's[61] study also showed a steady decline in the numbers of his original group of benign cases with the passage of time. In most of those in whom disability developed, it was the result of multiple sclerosis but other factors began to be important in patients over 60: arthritis and cardiac disease in particular. Whether patients with benign multiple sclerosis can legitimately be considered as having a different 'form' of the disease cannot be decided on clinical evidence. The existence of possibly 20% of benign cases has been amply demonstrated but the unreliability of any rigid classification is emphasised by Bonduelle's[109] patient in whom progressive paraparesis began after a latent period of 20 years which had included five pregnancies. As with the malignant form there has been speculation on different degrees of resistance to the disease process but nothing is known of this hypothetical mechanism.

Not unnaturally, there is little pathological evidence of the type of disease in benign cases. The accidental discovery of unsuspected multiple sclerosis at necropsy has already been mentioned.[14–16] Fog et al[113] reported an autopsy on a patient who had sustained sensory symptoms at the age of 20 and a further sensory episode with retrobulbar neuritis a year later. Thereafter she had experienced only vague paraesthesiae and died at 65 of other causes. Numerous small partially demyelinated plaques were present. Vuia[114] described autopsy findings in three benign cases and emphasised the isolated sharply defined nature of the plaques, sometimes only partially demyelinated. Changes in the blood vessel walls within the plaque, fibrous thickening of the media and fibrosed periadventitial space, were suggested· as possible factors in limiting spread of the disease process in the perivascular spaces. Vascular changes of this kind have not been noted in other necropsy studies of benign or clinically silent cases.

PROGNOSTIC INDICATORS

It would be of the utmost practical value to be able to predict the course of multiple sclerosis, in particular a benign course, at or near the onset of the disease. Although much evidence of a statistical nature has accumulated, this objective has not been achieved and it is still impossible to provide an individual patient with an accurate prognosis.

It has proved easier to identify indications of a bad prognosis. In virtually every series in which this aspect has been studied, disease progressive from the onset has been found to herald severe disability. It is, however, difficult to distinguish this from the effects of age at onset as most investigators have found the progressive form to be much more common with late onset. Cazzullo et al,[78] reported a progressive course in 49% of those with onset after 40 compared with 17% of those with earlier onset. Leibowitz et al[68] found progression in 17% of those with onset below 20, 32% between 20 and 29, and 57% with onset after 40. Shepherd[23] found the mean age of those with progressive onset to be 43 years in contrast to 31 for the relapsing type of disease. In Freidman and Davison's[27] patients with late onset, nearly all had progressive disease. Detels et al[115] and Clark et al[116] found that onset after the age of 40 and a rapid initial course were adverse factors but also believed that residence in a hot climate had an important contributory influence. Poser et al[99] agreed that onset after 40 and a progressive course indicated a bad prognosis. Leibowitz & Alter[77] concluded that it was the age of onset rather than the progression that was related to the severe disability and higher death rate as progressive onset in young patients did not indicate a bad prognosis. Poser[4] has criticised these results on the grounds

of selection of an undue proportion of mild cases although the survey was thought to include all patients with the disease in Israel and certainly contained a higher percentage of progressive cases. The figures in Poser's study showed virtually no difference in the ability to walk and work between patients with different age of onset but with the same type of disease, remittent or progressive, or with the same duration.

The findings of Riser et al[3] were different. All their cases progressive from the onset either died or became severely disabled within 10 years. The age range of their patients was not given but the mean age of onset of their severely disabled patients was 34, not greatly different from that expected. In addition, however, they detected an effect of advanced age of onset as, of the 50 patients in whom the first symptoms occurred after 35 years of age, 37 had severe disease. White & Whelan[117] in an epidemiological study could not detect any difference in severity that could not be attributed to longer duration of disease and discounted the effect of late age of onset. Panelius[76] and Gudmundsson[59] came to similar conclusions. These findings should not be allowed to conceal the small group of patients with late onset and mild course to which Hyllested[35] drew attention. These often approximate to a clinical picture of primary lateral sclerosis and are progressive but only over many years.

Published figures usually refer to the duration of disease at death or at the time of reporting, together with mean age of onset. The mean age at death is also stated in many reports but comparative ages at death between the progressive and relapsing forms are difficult to find. For example, Leibowitz et al[100] estimated death rates in those under and over 30 at onset and under and over 45 at the time of initial observation but did not give the mean age of onset in the group, nor the mean age of onset of those who died or the mean duration in the fatal cases, although the information must have been available. Confavreux et al[56] did not give the ages of their patients who died (or even the number of fatal cases) but only the mean duration of disease. The duration of the disease from onset to death or to severe disability is on average shorter in those with late rather than with early onset but these patients will have experienced at least 40 years of life without symptoms of multiple sclerosis. The prognosis with respect to early onset of severe disability is almost certainly better in young patients but prognosis for disruption of the pattern of life from an early age may indeed be worse. A man of 45 who develops multiple sclerosis may be quickly disabled and may even die before reaching 50 but he will have had 45 years without multiple sclerosis, will have experienced a normal family life and will have seen his children through their early years. This point is clearly illustrated by Confavreux et al[56] who showed that many patients with early onset and a prolonged interval before severe disability will nevertheless be dead before the age of onset in patients with more rapidly disabling and fatal disease. In autopsy proven cases, onset after the age of 45 was found to be associated with significantly shorter duration than in patients with earlier onset.[118] Progression from the onset and death within 5 years were also significantly more common in this group.

Visscher et al[119] found that onset after 40 was more likely to be followed by a malignant course and Thompson et al[108] showed that even onset in the fourth decade reduced the chances of a benign course compared with earlier onset. Noseworthy et al[26] in their study of multiple sclerosis after 50 years of age unfortunately did not analyse separately patients with onset and those presenting after this age.

The definition of a progressive onset is seldom attempted and must inevitably be based almost entirely on retrospection. Thygesen[120] considered that progression within the first year was the important prognostic sign. This author, however, also found that the prognosis was better in those older at onset in contrast to many of the reports already cited.

Relapse rate

There is no consistent relationship between the rate of relapse and the outcome of disease. McAlpine[2] emphasised the low relapse rate in his benign cases, particularly after the second year from onset, while Confavreux et al[56] found a highly significant increase in number of relapses in their least disabled group of cases. Bonduelle et al[110] found that in half the benign cases, the relapse rate was high, the relapses often being brief and followed by good remission.

In contrast, there is an unusual measure of agreement on the significance of the duration of the first remission. McAlpine[2] and Bonduelle & Albaranès[75] found that a prolonged first remission was a good prognostic sign. In the 31 benign cases in the series of Riser et al[3] the first relapse occurred within 5 years in 13, between 5–10 years in 10 and from 10–15 years in 5. Shepherd[23] reported a better prognosis if the first remission was longer than 4 years. The mean interval before the first relapse in 42 patients with benign disease in the series of Confavreux et al[56] was 6.2 years, much longer than in their more severe disease categories. The estimated hazard of moving from the state of relapsing disease with full remissions to that of relapses with sequelae and from either form of relapsing disease to the progressive stage decreased progressively with increasing length of the first remission.[81] Thompson et al[108] reported that initial remissions of more than 1 year and more than 5 years were more common in benign than in severe disease and Sanders et al[121] found a close relationship between length of remission following isolated optic neuritis and slow progression of disease. Phadke[19] reported an important influence on mortality. In all those with relapsing disease who died within 10 years of the onset, the duration of the first remission had been less than 2 years, and less than 6 months in one third. In 10 of the 23 patients who survived beyond 40 years, the duration of the first remission had been longer than 10 years.

Sex

It is probable that the sex of the patient has no consistent influence on the prognosis in multiple sclerosis. Several authors[34,62,76,115] have reported more severe disease in men while Leibowitz & Alter[77] found the reverse. Wolfson & Confavreux[81] estimated that men were at greater risk of passing from the stage of relapse with sequelae to that of progression. Others[56,57,99,108,119] have found no effect.

Onset symptoms

The relation of clinical symptoms at or near the

onset to subsequent course has been examined, again with conflicting results. Leibowitz & Alter[77,122] found that cerebellar or multiple system involvement at the onset was common in those with severe disease. Fog & Linnemann[10] regarded severe ataxia as the only initial symptom of prognostic importance, again indicating severe disease. Müller[90] thought that the outcome was to a great extent dependent on the initial symptoms, those with disturbance of mobility, including ataxia, being more rapidly disabled. Thygesen[120] also found tremor or inco-ordination in the first attack to indicate a poor prognosis. Others have found no relation of individual initial symptoms to the eventual outcome.[10,102] There has been much disagreement about the prognostic significance of an initial episode of optic neuritis. Some[62,89,91] have concluded that this is an indication of a bad prognosis but others[23] could detect no influence and McAlpine[34] included optic neuritis among the initial symptoms associated with a benign course.

Indications at the onset of a benign course have naturally been sought. McAlpine[2,34] found that in 50% of his benign cases the initial symptoms were sensory, paraesthesiae in particular, sometimes accompanied by weakness and in 36% optic neuritis occurred in the initial attack, as an isolated symptom in 25% of the total. Weakness without sensory loss was rare. Bonduelle[109] also found that monosymptomatic onset was common in benign cases, the most frequent sign being affection of one or more cranial nerves (it is not clear whether this included optic neuritis). This mode of onset occurred in 40% of benign cases and Bonduelle estimates that this compares with 35% in cases of usual severity — not a remarkable difference. Isolated sensory symptoms were also common (20%) and pyramidal weakness, either isolated or combined with sensory symptoms in 40%. Comparison between series is not easy as single or multiple cranial nerve palsies are not tabulated according to the number of patients involved, i.e. it is not stated in how many patients the palsies are multiple. Riser et al[3] confirmed the frequent occurrence of initial sensory symptoms in benign multiple sclerosis. Müller[62] found cranial nerve palsies more common at the onset in remittent cases (not necessarily benign). Thygesen[120] emphasised the good prognostic significance of mono-

or oliogosymptomatic onset. Shepherd[23] reported that sensory symptoms at the onset were significantly less common in patients in the severely disabled grades at the time of reporting. Poeck & Markus[91] also found that sensory loss due to spinal cord lesions and cranial nerve palsies, other than optic neuritis, were good prognostic signs at the onset.

Poser et al[53] found that optic neuritis as an initial sign was more commonly followed by a benign course. Kraft et al[123] reviewed published reports, conducted an enquiry among multiple sclerosis clinics and examined their own material. They concluded that indications at the onset of a benign course were: onset under 35, monosymptomatic onset, sudden onset, isolated optic neuritis or sensory symptoms and absence of motor or cerebellar signs or of an extensor plantar reflex at initial examination. The commonly but not universally held opinions have been largely confirmed in more recent series. Sensory symptoms at the onset, either alone or, inexplicably, when accompanying motor signs, are frequently followed by relatively mild disease.[119,121] Motor signs in isolation[108,119] and defects of co-ordination[119] more often lead to rapid disability. Riise et al[98] astonishingly found that onset with vertigo was an indicator of reduced life expectancy. Monosymptomatic onset does not appear to be of prognostic value[121] but this factor is sometimes ignored, all patients, whether with benign or severe disease, apparently presenting with a single symptom.[108] Wolfson & Confavreux[81] had conflicting results; for patients with relapses without sequelae, monosymptomatic onset increased the risk of entering the progressive stage, while the risk was reduced in those with relapses with sequelae. However sophisticated the statistics, results are dependent on the accuracy of patients' memories.

Only limited help in prognosis can therefore be obtained from the circumstances or symptoms of the initial attack. A sixth nerve palsy or an episode of numbness of the legs and trunk with complete remission may indeed be suspected as being the first attack of multiple sclerosis and in general heralding a mild course, but the uncertainties are plain enough and optimism is often disappointed. Much more can be learnt from the early course of disease. Alexander et al[40,65,66] using a scoring system, believed that a score below 125 points at five years from the onset identified benign cases, while a score of over 200 points indicated a severe case. A score at this level indicates moderate disability and the distinction between prognostic indicators and the actual state of the patient already becomes obscured. Alexander's interesting contention that the maximum rate of deterioration occurs in the first five years is not apparent from the charts of Fog & Linnemann[10] but received strong support from Kurtzke et al.[102] In this series, if there were no pyramidal or cerebellar signs at 5 years, the probability of little or no disability at 15 years was 72%. If moderate disability, especially involving several systems, was present at 5 years, the disease was severe at 15 years in 88%.

Bonduelle et al[110] felt that the status at 5 years was an uncertain guide to the future and concluded that if the 10 year stage could be gained without permanent disability, the further course would be benign in 9 out of 10 cases, although this could be interrupted at any point by the appearance of progressive spastic paraparesis. However, as they point out, to be able to say with certainty after 20 years of evolution that a case of multiple sclerosis is benign is not a prognostication but a conclusion. Detels et al[115] believed that patients likely to deteriorate over the following five years could be identified from the present level of disability, without reference to duration of disease or observed rate of progression. Of those needing help with walking, 50% became worse over this period.

Laboratory investigations

The results of laboratory investigations have so far contributed little to evaluation of the prognosis in individual patients. Examination of the CSF has been disappointing. The cell count and total protein levels are not related to outcome.[56] Stendahl-Brodin & Link[124] reported that absence of increased production of IgG and of oligoclonal banding was relatively frequent in benign disease, but others have failed to confirm this finding.[57,108] The absence of myelin basic protein from the CSF in patients in remission has been found to be re-

lated to a benign course[108] but this is of little practical value.

HLA

In 1973, Jerdsild et al[52] claimed that in patients carrying Dw2 (DR2) antigen, multiple sclerosis progressed more rapidly. This was supported by Stendahl-Brodin et al[125] but other investigators[126,127] found that the presence of DR2 exerted no influence on the course of the disease. DR2, both with and without B7 has been associated with mild disease[128,129] and B7 has been linked to severe multiple sclerosis.[130] It seems safe to conclude that any consistent association between HLA antigens and severity of disease that may exist has so far proved elusive.

Imaging

It is too early for extensive reports on the prognostic significance of symptomless lesions seen by MRI in patients presenting with clinical evidence of a single lesion but Miller et al[131] have shown that clinical relapse within a mean follow-up period of 12 months occurred significantly more frequently in those with such lesions than in those without.

Evoked potentials

Clinically silent lesions are more often detected by evoked potentials recorded on presentation with possible or suspected multiple sclerosis in patients who progress to definite disease within 3 years than in those who do not,[132] visual evoked potentials being the most valuable. There is little evidence that long-term outcome can be foretold. Nuwer et al[133] concluded that stabilisation or reduction of latency of visual and somatosensory evoked potentials on serial recording were predictive of arrest of disease progression, but it is difficult to apply these results based on mean values to individual patients.

The relevance of the clinical course

Despite the intermittent or remittent initial course

of the symptoms in the majority of patients there is growing evidence that the disease process is continuous.[134] It has long been known that the symptoms and signs of the disease may bear little apparent relationship to the site and extent of the lesions and this topic is discussed in detail in Chapter 8. Fluctuations in latency and amplitude of evoked potentials, unrelated to clinical change, are commonly found in patients with 'active' disease[135,136] but it has not been possible to relate these changes to the presence of new or expanding lesions. It is otherwise with imaging, either with CT scanning enhanced by large volumes of contrast medium or by MRI. Although the pathology of the acute and often transient abnormalities shown by the latter technique is uncertain, serial studies show that the frequency of appearance of new lesions, certainly some of which can be equated with plaques, greatly exceeds the number of clinical relapses (Chapter 8).

It might well be tempting to conclude that the course of multiple sclerosis, natural or as modified by treatment, should be traced entirely by imaging and clearly there is a great deal to be learnt from these methods, but patients will rightly remain more interested in their symptoms and disabilities than in shadows. The relapse rate has always been an uncertain guide to progress and is exposed to

further doubt by the clear demonstration of subclinical relapse. It is not, however, known why the majority of lesions shown on MRI do not produce symptoms. Judging from asymptomatic lesions found at autopsy[138] this is unlikely to be merely the result of their anatomical site. The presence of myelin basic protein in the CSF, an indication of myelin destruction, is closely linked to clinical relapse[139] and is not continuous as might be expected if demyelination was taking place at a constant rate. The overt relapse can scarcely be ignored as an indication of disease activity. The clinical indicators of prognosis are fallible and inconsistent but it remains true that a five year symptom-free first remission is likely to be followed by benign disease, while progressive cerebellar ataxia from the onset will soon lead to severe disability. It will be of great interest to learn whether during a prolonged 'latent period' the disease is indeed inactive or whether the onset of the progressive stage is the result of a change in the disease process or merely the effect of steadily accumulating damage during the remittent stage. There are important implications for attempted treatment. If the disease is indeed continuous it is immaterial when treatment is given; if intermittent it would be logical to treat active disease.

REFERENCES

1. Weinshenker B G, Ebers G C 1987 The natural history of multiple sclerosis. Canadian Journal of Neurological Sciences 14: 255–261
2. McAlpine D 1961 The benign form of multiple sclerosis: a study based on 241 cases seen within three years of onset and followed up until the tenth year or more of the disease. Brain 84: 186–203
3. Riser M, Geraud J, Rascol A, Benazet A M, Segria M G 1971 L'évolution de la sclérose en plaques (étude de 201 observations suivies au-delà de 10 ans. Revue Neurologique 124: 479–484
4. Poser S 1978 Multiple sclerosis: an analysis of 812 cases by means of electronic data processing. Springer, Berlin
5. Weinshenker B G, Bass B, Rice G P A et al 1989 The natural history of multiple sclerosis: a geographically based study. I. Clinical course and disability. Brain 112: 133–146
6. MacLean A R, Berkson J 1951 Mortality and morbidity in multiple sclerosis. Journal of the American Medical Association 146: 1367–1369
7. Carter D, Sciarra D, Merritt H H 1950 The course of

multiple sclerosis determined by autopsy proven cases. Research Publications of the Association for Research into Nervous and Mental Disease 28: 471–511
8. Poser C M, Presthus J, Hörsdal O 1966 Clinical features of autopsy-proven multiple sclerosis. Neurology 16: 791–798
9. Izquierdo G, Hauw J J, Lyon-Caen O et al 1985 Analyse clinique de 70 cas neuropathologiques de sclérose en plaques. Revue Neurologique 141: 546–552
10. Fog T, Linnemann F 1970 The course of multiple sclerosis in 73 cases with computer designed curves. Acta Neurologica Scandinavica 46 (suppl 47): 1–175
11. Nagler B, Beebe G W, Kurtzke J F, Kurland L T, Auth T L, Nefzger M D 1966 Studies on the natural history of multiple sclerosis: I: Design and diagnosis. Acta Neurologica Scandinavica 42 (suppl 19): 141–156
12. Percy A K, Nobrega F T, Ozaki H, Glattre E, Kurland L T 1971 Multiple sclerosis in Rochester, Minnesota: a 60-year appraisal. Archives of Neurology 25: 105–111
13. Poser S, Bauer H J, Poser W 1982 Prognosis of multiple sclerosis. Results from an epidemiological area in Germany. Acta Neurologica Scandinavica 65: 347–354
14. Georgi W 1961 Multiple Sklerose: pathologisch-anatomische Befund multipler Sklerose bei

klinisch nicht diagnostizierten Krankheiten.
Schweizerische medizinische Wochenschrift 91: 605–607

15. Phadke J G, Best P V 1983 Atypical and clinically silent multiple sclerosis: a report of 12 cases discovered unexpectedly at necropsy. Journal of Neurology, Neurosurgery and Psychiatry 46: 414–420

16. Gilbert J J, Sadler M 1983 Unsuspected multiple sclerosis. Archives of Neurology 40: 533–536

17. Broman T, Andersen O, Bergmann I 1981 Clinical studies on multiple sclerosis I: Presentation of an incidence material from Gothenburg. Acta Neurologica Scandinavica 63: 6–33

18. Shepherd D I, Downie A W 1980 A further prevalence study of multiple sclerosis in north-east Scotland. Journal of Neurology, Neurosurgery and Psychiatry 43: 310–315

19. Phadke J G 1987 Survival pattern and cause of death in patients with multiple sclerosis: results from an epidemiological survey in north east Scotland. Journal of Neurology, Neurosurgery and Psychiatry 50: 523–531

20. Schumacher G A, Beebe G, Kibler R F et al 1965 Problems of experimental trials of therapy in multiple sclerosis. Annals of the New York Academy of Sciences 122: 552–568

21. Weiner H L, Ellison G W 1983 A working protocol to be used as a guideline for trials in multiple sclerosis. Archives of Neurology 40: 704–710

22. Poser C M, Paty D W, Scheinberg L et al 1983 New diagnostic criteria for multiple sclerosis: guidelines for research protocols. Annals of Neurology 13: 227–231.

23. Shepherd D I 1979 Clinical features of multiple sclerosis in north-east Scotland. Acta Neurologica Scandinavica 60: 218–230

24. Leibowitz U, Alter M, Halpern L 1964 Clinical studies of multiple sclerosis in Israel III: Clinical course and prognosis related to age. Neurology 14: 926–932

25. Poskanzer D C, Schapira K, Miller H 1963 Epidemiology of multiple sclerosis in the counties of Northumberland and Durham. Journal of Neurology, Neurosurgery and Psychiatry 26: 368–376

26. Noseworthy J, Paty D W, Wonnacott T, Feasby T, Ebers G C 1983 Multiple sclerosis after 50. Neurology 33: 1537–1544

27. Freidman A P, Davison C 1945 Multiple sclerosis with late onset of symptoms. Archives of Neurology and Psychiatry 54: 348–360

28. Kurtzke J F 1970 Clinical manifestations of multiple sclerosis. In: Vinken P J, Bruyn G W (eds) Handbook of clinical neurology, Vol 9. North Holland, Amsterdam, pp. 161–216

29. Jéquier M 1957 Sclérose en plaques tardive (apparition après 50 ans). Encéphale 46: 603–611

30. Engell T 1989 A clinical patho-anatomical study of clinically silent multiple sclerosis. Acta Neurologica Scandinavica 79: 428–430

31. Mackay R P, Hirano A 1967 Forms of benign multiple sclerosis: report of two 'clinically silent' cases discovered at autopsy. Archives of Neurology 17: 588–600

32. Moriaru M, Klatzow W F 1976 Subclinical multiple sclerosis. Journal of Neurology 213: 71–76

33. Ipsen J 1950 Life expectancy and probable disability in multiple sclerosis. New England Journal of Medicine 242: 909–913

34. McAlpine D, Compston N D 1952 Some aspects of the natural history of disseminated sclerosis. Quarterly Journal of Medicine 21: 135–167

35. Hyllested K 1961 Lethality, duration and mortality of disseminated sclerosis in Denmark. Acta Psychiatrica et Neurologica Scandinavica 36: 553–563

36. Kurtzke J F 1961 Further notes on disability evaluation in multiple sclerosis with scale modifications. Neurology 15: 654–661

37. Kurtzke J F 1983 Rating neurologic impairment in multiple sclerosis. An expanded disability scale (EDSS). Neurology 33: 1444–1452

38. IFMSS minimal record of disability 1984 Acta Neurologica Scandinavica suppl 101: 169–207

39. Pedersen E 1965 A rating system for neurological impairment in multiple sclerosis. Acta Neurologica Scandinavica 41 (suppl 13): 557–558

40. Alexander L 1951 New concept of critical steps in course of chronic debilitating neurologic disease in evaluation of therapeutic response. Archives of Neurology and Psychiatry 66: 253–271

41. Fog T 1965 A scoring system for neurological impairment in multiple sclerosis. Acta Neurologica Scandinavica 41 (suppl 13): 551–555

42. Patzold U, Haller P, Deicher H 1978 Therapie der multiplen Seklerose mit Levamisole und Azathioprin. Nervenartz 49: 285–294

43. Poser C M 1979 A numerical scoring system for the classification of multiple sclerosis. Acta Neurologica Scandinavica 60: 100–111

44. Poser C M, Poser S, Paty D W 1984 A revised numerical scoring system for multiple sclerosis. In: Poser C M (ed) The diagnosis of multiple sclerosis. Thieme-Stratton, New York, pp 234–241

45. Sipe J C, Knobler R L, Braheny S L, Rice G P A, Panitch H S, Oldstone M B A 1984 A neurologic rating scale (NRS) in multiple sclerosis. Neurology 34: 1368–1371

46. Amato M P, Fratiglioni L, Groppi C, Siracusa G, Amaducci L 1988 Interrater reliability in assessing functional systems and disability on the Kurtzke scale in multiple sclerosis. Archives of Neurology 45: 746–748

47. Mickey M R, Ellison G W, Myers, L W 1984 An illness severity score for multiple sclerosis. Neurology 34: 1343–1347

48. Grynderup V 1969 A comparison of some rating systems in multiple sclerosis. Acta Neurologica Scandinavica 54: 611–622

49. Kuzma J W, Namerow N S, Tourtellotte W W et al 1969 An evaluation of the reliability of three methods used in evaluating the status of multiple sclerosis patients. Journal of Chronic Diseases 21: 803–814

50. Tourtellotte W W, Haerer A F, Simpson J F, Kuzma J W, Sikowski J 1965 Quantitative clinical neurological testing I: A battery of tests designed to evaluate in part the neurological function of patients with multiple sclerosis and its use in a therapeutic trial. Annals of the New York Academy of Sciences 122: 480–505

51. Kuzma J W, Tourtellotte W W, Remington R D 1965 Quantitative clinical neurological testing II: Some statistical considerations of a battery of tests. Journal of Chronic Diseases 18: 303–311

52. Jersild C, Fog T, Hansen G S, Thomsen M, Svejgaard A, Dupont B 1973 Histocompatability determinants in multiple sclerosis with special reference to clinical course. Lancet 2: 1221–1224

53. Poser S, Raun N E, Poser W 1982 Age at onset, initial

symptomatology and the course of multiple sclerosis. Acta Neurologica Scandinavica 66: 355–362

54. Minderhoud J M, van der Hoeven J H, Prange A J A 1988 Course and prognosis of chronic progressive multiple sclerosis. Acta Neurologica Scandinavica 78: 10–15

55. Patzold U, Hecker H, Pocklington P 1982 Azathioprine in treatment of multiple sclerosis: final results of a 4½ year controlled study of its effectiveness in 115 patients. Journal of the Neurological Sciences 54: 377–394

56. Confavreux C, Aimard G, Devic M 1980 Course and prognosis of multiple sclerosis assessed by the computerised data processing of 349 patients. Brain 103: 281–300

57. Charcot J–M 1875 Leçons sur les maladies du système nerveux, Tome 1. Bourneville, Paris, p 258

58. Verjans E, Theys P, Delmotte P, Carton H 1983 Clinical parameters and intrathecal IgG synthesis as prognostic factors in multiple sclerosis. Part I. Journal of Neurology 229: 155–165

59. Gudmundsson K R 1971 Clinical studies of multiple sclerosis in Iceland. Acta Neurologica Scandinavica 47 (suppl 48): 1–78

60. Stazio A, Kurland L T, Bell L G, Saunders M G, Rogot E 1964 Multiple sclerosis in Winnipeg, Manitoba: methodological considerations of epidemiological survey. Journal of Chronic Diseases 17: 415–442

61. McAlpine D 1972 In: Multiple sclerosis: a reappraisal, 2nd edn. Churchill Livingstone, Edinburgh, p 197

62. Müller R 1949 Studies in disseminated sclerosis. Acta Medica Scandinavica 133 (suppl 222): 1–214

63. Matthews W B, Small D G 1979 Serial recordings of visual and somatosensory evoked potentials in multiple sclerosis. Journal of the Neurological Sciences 40: 11–21

64. Thygesen P 1953 The course of multiple sclerosis: a close-up of 105 attacks. Rosenkilde and Bagger, Copenhagen

65. Alexander L, Berkeley A W, Alexander A M 1958 Prognosis and treatment of multiple sclerosis — quantitative nosometric study. Journal of the American Medical Association 166: 1943–1949

66. Alexander L, Berkeley A W, Alexander A M 1961 Multiple sclerosis: prognosis and treatment. Thomas, Springfield

67. Millar J H D, Allison R S, Cheeseman E A, Merrett J D 1959 Pregnancy as a factor influencing relapse in disseminated sclerosis. Brain 82: 417–426

68. Leibowitz U, Halpern L, Alter M 1964 Clinical studies of multiple sclerosis in Israel I: A clinical analysis based on a country-wide survey. Archives of Neurology 10: 502–512

69. Lhermitte F, Marteau R, Gazengel J, Dordain G, Deloche G 1973 The frequency of relapse in multiple sclerosis: a study based on 245 cases. Journal of Neurology 205: 47–59

70. Kurtzke J F, Beebe G W, Nagler B, Auth T L, Kurland L T, Nefzger M D 1968 Studies on the natural history of multiple sclerosis 4: Clinical features of the onset bout. Acta Neurologica Scandinavica 44: 467–494

71. Kurtzke J F, Beebe G W, Nagler B, Auth T L, Kurland L T, Nefzger M D 1973 Studies on the natural history of multiple sclerosis and correlates of

clinical change in an early bout. Acta Neurologica Scandinavica 49: 379–395

72. Kurtzke J F 1956 Course of exacerbations of multiple sclerosis in hospitalised patients. Archives of Neurology and Psychiatry 76: 175–183

73. Brown M R, Putnam T J 1939 Remissions in multiple sclerosis. Archives of Neurology and Psychiatry 41: 913–920

74. Adams D K, Sutherland J M, Fletcher W B 1950 Early clinical manifestations of disseminated sclerosis. British Medical Journal 2: 431–436

75. Bonduelle M, Albaranès R 1962 Etude statistique de 145 cas de la sclérose en plaques. Semaine des Hôpitaux de Paris 38: 3762–3773

76. Panelius M 1969 Studies on epidemiological, clinical and etiological aspects of multiple sclerosis. Acta Neurologica Scandinavica 45 (suppl 39): 1–82

77. Leibowitz U, Alter M 1973 Multiple sclerosis — clues to its cause. North Holland, Amsterdam

78. Cazzullo C L, Ghezzi A, Marforio S, Caputo D 1978 Clinical picture of multiple sclerosis with late onset. Acta Neurologica Scandinavica 58: 190–196

79. Birley J L, Dudgeon L S 1921 A clinical and experimental contribution to the pathogenesis of disseminated sclerosis. Brain 44: 150–212

80. Broman T 1963 Further studies concerning the natural history of multiple sclerosis. In: Pedersen E, Clausen J, Oades L (eds) Actual problems in multiple sclerosis research. FADL's Forlag, Copenhagen, pp 74–76

81. Wolfson C, Confavreux C 1987 Improvements to a simple Markov model of the natural history of multiple sclerosis. Neuroepidemiology 6: 101–115

82. Patzold U, Pocklington P R 1982 Course of multiple sclerosis. First results of a prospective study carried out on 102 MS patients from 1976–80. Acta Neurologica Scandinavica 65: 248–266

83. Poser S, Poser W, Schlaf G et al 1986 Prognostic factors in multiple sclerosis. Acta Neurologica Scandinavica 74: 387–392

84. Gowers W R (ed) 1893 A manual of diseases of the nervous system, 2nd edn, Vol 2. London, p 553

85. Bramwell B 1905 Clinical studies 3. Edinburgh, p 228. (Cited by Allison[87])

86. Bramwell B 1917 The prognosis of disseminated sclerosis: duration in 200 cases of disseminated sclerosis. Edinburgh Medical Journal 18: 16–23

87. Allison R S 1950 Survival in disseminated sclerosis: a clinical study of a series of cases first seen twenty years ago. Brain 73: 103–120

88. Leibowitz U, Kahana E, Jacobson S G, Alter M 1972 The cause of death in multiple sclerosis. In: Leibowitz U (ed) Progress in multiple sclerosis. Academic Press, New York, pp 196–209

89. Lazarte J A 1950 Multiple sclerosis: prognosis for ambulatory and nonambulatory patients. Research Publications of the Association for Research into Nervous and Mental Disease 28: 512–523

90. Müller H R 1966 Zur Frage von Krankheitzdauen und Invalidität bei der multipler Sklerose. Deutsche Medizinische Wochenschrift 91: 996–998

91. Poeck K, Markus P 1964 Gibt es ein gutartige Verlaufsform der multiplen Sklerose? Münchener Medizinischer Wochenschrift 106: 2190–2197

92. McAlpine D 1972 In: Multiple sclerosis: a reappraisal, 2nd edn. Churchill Livingstone, Edinburgh, p 216

93. Dassel H 1973 The mortality from multiple sclerosis in the Netherlands. Acta Neurologica Scandinavica 49: 659–674

94. Kurtzke J F, Beebe G W, Nagler B, Nefzger M D, Auth T L, Kurland L T 1970 Studies on the natural history of multiple sclerosis 5: Long-term survival in young men. Archives of Neurology 22: 215–225

95. Bauer H J, Firnhaber W, Winkler W 1965 Prognostic criteria in multiple sclerosis. Annals of the New York Academy of Sciences 122: 542–551

96. Kurland L T, Westland K B 1954 Epidemiological factors in the etiology and prognosis of multiple sclerosis. Annals of the New York Academy of Sciences 58: 682–701

97. Kurtzke J F, Auth T L, Beebe G W, Kurland L T, Nagler B, Nefzger M D 1969 Survival in multiple sclerosis. Transactions of the American Neurological Association 94: 134–139

98. Riise T, Grønning J A, Aarli J A, Nyland H, Larsen J P, Edland A 1988 Prognostic factors for life expectancy in multiple sclerosis analysed by Cox-models. Journal of Clinical Epidemiology 41: 1031–1036

99. Poser S, Kurtzke J F, Schlaf G 1989 Survival in multiple sclerosis. Journal of Clinical Epidemiology 42: 159–168

100. Leibowitz U, Kahana E, Alter M 1969 Survival and death in multiple sclerosis. Brain 92: 115–130

101. Melton L J, Bartleson J D 1980 Spontaneous pneumothorax and multiple sclerosis. Annals of Neurology 7: 492

102. Kurtzke J F, Beebe G W, Nagler B, Kurland L T, Auth T L 1977 Studies on the natural history of multiple sclerosis 8: Early prognostic features of the later course of the illness. Journal of Chronic Diseases 30: 819–830

103. Kolb L C 1950 The social significance of multiple sclerosis. Reseach Publications of the Association for Research into Nervous and Mental Disease 28: 28–38

104. Bauer H, Firnhaber W 1963 Zur Leistungsprognose Multiple-Sklerose-Kranker. Deutsche Medizinische Wochenschrift 88: 1357–1364

105. Larocca N, Kalb R, Scheinberg L, Kendall P 1985 Factors associated with unemployment of patients with multiple sclerosis. Journal of Chronic Diseases 38: 203–210

106. Zimmerman H M, Netsky M G 1950 The pathology of multiple sclerosis. Research Publications of the Association for Research into Nervous and Mental Disease 28: 271–312

107. Guillain G, Alajouanine T 1928 La forme aigue de la sclérose en plaques. Bulletin de l'Académie de Médicine (Paris) 99: 366–376

108. Thompson A J, Hutchinson M, Brazil J, Feighery C, Martin E A 1986 A clinical and laboratory study of benign multiple sclerosis. Quarterly Journal of Medicine 58: 680

109. Bonduelle M 1967 Les formes benignes de la sclérose en plaques. Presse Médicale 75: 2023–2026

110. Bonduelle M, Bouygues P, Degos C F, Gauthier C 1979 Les formes benignes de la sclérose en plaques — réévaluation. Revue Neurologique 135: 593–604

111. Lehoczky T, Halasy-Lehoczky M 1963 Forme 'benigne' de la sclérose en plaques. Presse Médicale 71: 2294–2296

112. Poser S, Wikström J, Bauer H J 1979 Clinical data and the identification of special forms of multiple sclerosis in 1271 cases studied with a standardised documentation system. Journal of the Neurological Sciences 40: 159–168

113. Fog T, Hyllested K, Andersen S R 1970 A case of benign multiple sclerosis with autopsy. Acta Neurologica Scandinavica 48 (suppl 51): 369–370

114. Vuia O 1977 The benign form of multiple sclerosis: anatomo-clinical aspects. Acta Neurologica Scandinavica 55: 289–298

115. Detels R, Clark V A, Valdiviezo N L, Visscher B R, Malmgren R M, Dudley J P 1982 Factors associated with a rapid course of multiple sclerosis. Archives of Neurology 39: 337–341

116. Clark V A, Detels R, Visscher B R, Valdiviezo N L, Malmgren R M, Dudley 1982 Factors associated with a malignant or benign course of multiple sclerosis. Journal of the American Medical Association 248: 856–860

117. White D N, Wheelan L 1959 Disseminated sclerosis: a survey of patients in the Kingston, Ontario area. Neurology 9: 256–272

118. Lyon-Caen O, Izquierdo G, Marteau R, Lhermitte F, Castaigne P, Hauw J J 1985 Late onset multiple sclerosis. A clinical study of 16 pathologically proven cases. Acta Neurologica Scandinavica 72: 56–60

119. Visscher B R, Kai-Shen Liu, Clark V A, Detels R, Malmgren R M, Dudley J P 1984 Onset symptoms as predictors of mortality and disability in multiple sclerosis. Acta Neurologica Scandinavica 70: 321–328

120. Thygesen P 1949 Prognosis in initial stage of disseminated primary demyelinating disease of central nervous system. Archives of Neurology and Psychiatry 61: 339–351

121. Sanders E A C M, Bollen E L E M, van der Velde E A 1986 Presenting signs and symptoms in multiple sclerosis. Acta Neurologica Scandinavica 73: 269–272

122. Leibowitz U, Alter M 1970 Clinical factors associated with increased disability in multiple sclerosis. Acta Neurologica Scandinavica 46: 53–70

123. Kraft G H, Freal J E, Coryell J K, Hana C L, Chitnis N 1981 Multiple sclerosis: early prognostic guidelines. Archives of Physical Medicine and Rehabilitation 62: 54–58

124. Stendahl-Brodin L, Link H 1980 Relation between benign course of multiple sclerosis and low-grade humoral immune response in cerebrospinal fluid. Journal of Neurology, Neurosurgery and Psychiatry 43: 102–105

125. Stendahl-Brodin L, Link H, Moller E, Norby E 1979 Genetic basis of multiple sclerosis: HLA antigens, disease progression and oligoclonal IgG in CSF. Acta Neurologica Scandinavica 59: 297–308

126. Paty D W, Dossetor J B, Stiller C R et al 1977 HLA in multiple sclerosis. Journal of the Neurological Sciences 32: 371–379

127. Dejaegher L, de Bruyere M, Ketelaer P, Carton H 1983 HLA antigens and prognosis of multiple sclerosis. Part II. Journal of Neurology 229: 167–174

128. Madigand M, Oger J F, Fauchet R, Sabouraud O, Genetet B 1982 HLA profiles in multiple sclerosis suggest two forms of disease and the existence of protective haplotypes. Journal of the Neurological Sciences 53: 519–529

129. Collins R C, Espinoza L R, Plank C R, Ebers G C, Rosenberg R A, Zabriskie J B 1978 A double blind trial of transfer factor vs placebo in multiple sclerosis patients. Clinical and Experimental Immunology 33: 1–11

130. Bertrams J, Höher P G, Kuwert E K 1974 HLA antigens in multiple sclerosis. Lancet 1: 1287

131. Miller D H, Ormerod J E C, McDonald W I et al 1988 The early risk of multiple sclerosis after optic neuritis. Journal of Neurology, Neurosurgery and Psychiatry 51: 1569–1571

132. Matthews W B, Wattam-Bell J R B, Pountney E 1982 Evoked potentials in the diagnosis of multiple sclerosis: a follow up study. Journal of Neurology, Neurosurgery and Psychiatry 45: 303–307

133. Nuwer E R, Packwood J W, Myers L W, Ellison G W 1987 Evoked potentials predict the clinical changes in a multiple sclerosis drug study. Neurology 37: 1754–1761

134. Poser C M 1985 The course of multiple sclerosis. Archives of Neurology 42: 1035

135. Robinson K, Rudge P 1978 The stability of the auditory evoked potentials in normal man and patients with multiple sclerosis. Journal of the Neurological Sciences 36: 147–156

136. Likosky W, Elmore R S 1982 Exacerbation detection in multiple sclerosis by clinical and evoked potential techniques: a preliminary report. In: Courjon M, Maugiere F, Revol M (eds) Clinical applications of evoked potentials in neurology. Raven Press, New York, pp 535–540

137. Paty D W 1986 Magnetic resonance imaging in the evaluation of disease activity in multiple sclerosis. IFMSS Meeting, Rome, II/1

138. Namerow N S, Thompson L R 1969 Plaques, symptoms and the remitting course of multiple sclerosis. Neurology 19: 765–774

139. Whitaker J N, Lisak R P, Bashir R M et al Immunoreactive myelin basic protein in the cerebrospinal fluid in neurological disorders. Annals of Neurology 7: 58–64

6. Differential diagnosis

The diversity of symptoms, signs and course of multiple sclerosis that continues to astonish even the most experienced physician, affords almost unlimited opportunities for misdiagnosis. Most of these can, with prudence, be rejected and only the more exacting problems need be considered here.

A mere catalogue of conditions that have been mistaken for multiple sclerosis and vice versa would be interminable and sources of diagnostic difficulty may be conveniently, if approximately, divided as follows:

1. Diseases capable of causing multiple lesions of the CNS, often with a relapsing and remitting course
2. Systematised CNS diseases, also often causing lesions in separate regions of the CNS but in a more orderly and usually symmetrical pattern and with a progressive course
3. Single lesions of the CNS with relapsing and remitting symptoms
4. Single lesions with a progressive course
5. Monosymptomatic onset
6. Non-organic symptoms.

These categories may be considered in more detail.

1. DISEASES CAUSING MULTIPLE LESIONS

In theory, and occasionally in practice, virtually any form of disease that can produce scattered lesions of the nervous system may be confused, at least temporarily, with multiple sclerosis.

Systemic lupus erythematosus

Clinically overt involvement of the nervous system occurs in a high proportion of cases, 37% and 42% in two series,[1,2] but in majority accompanied or preceded by unmistakable evidence of systemic disease and a diagnosis of multiple sclerosis is not likely to be considered. Systemic involvement may, however, be relatively unobtrusive or absent at the onset of neurological symptoms. Neurological or psychiatric symptoms occurring in isolation as the initial manifestation present far more diagnostic difficulty. Such cases are uncommon and in many the presentation would not suggest multiple sclerosis as the immediate diagnosis: chorea, psychosis, peripheral neuropathy, hemiplegia or pseudobulbar palsy.[1,34] In a few patients, however, the clinical picture is indistinguishable from that of multiple sclerosis. In the remarkable case described by Hutchinson & Bresnihan,[5] relapsing and remitting symptoms of disseminated lesions, indistinguishable from those of multiple sclerosis, were accompanied by a greatly raised ESR, a finding that led to the eventual diagnosis of SLE. Bilateral internuclear ophthalmoplegia,[6,7] even as an initial symptom,[8] and unilateral tonic seizures,[5] both characteristic features of multiple sclerosis, have been described in SLE.

A striking report of multiple scattered partially or wholly remitting symptoms is that of Allen et al.[9] Their patient had experienced double vision, with recovery, when aged about 30. When 62, the left leg became weak and numbness spread up to the waist on that side, followed by recovery within a few weeks. She then had an episode of vertigo and unilateral deafness, again with recovery. When 63 she became blind in one eye, thought to be due to retinal infarction. She again became weak and was admitted to hospital with chest pain. Signs of a spinal cord lesion were found. A greatly elevated ESR provided the essential clue to the eventual diagnosis of SLE. In case 1 of Penn & Rowan,[10] the disease also ran a relapsing and remitting course, although over a much shorter period, but again including both brainstem and spinal cord signs. The long preceding history of joint pains was probably relevant.

The commonest presentation that could be confused with multiple sclerosis is that of varying combinations of optic neuritis and myelopathy. Schwartzberg et al [11] reviewed optic neuritis in SLE, emphasising that it may be the presenting symptom, not differing in any distinctive way from optic neuritis at the onset of multiple sclerosis. Hackett et al [12] thought that recovery of vision was relatively poor in SLE. Optic neuropathy in SLE may take various forms; acute retrobulbar neuritis, ischaemic neuropathy or slowly progressive visual failure.[13]

Spinal cord symptoms may be steadily progressive over a number of years,[10,14] recurrent or, more commonly, rapid or sudden with little tendency to remission.[16,17,18] The association with optic neuritis, either preceding[11] or subsequently[19] has frequently been remarked[12] and may justify the title of Devic's syndrome.[19] Oppenheimer & Hoffbrand,[20] applying strict diagnostic criteria, rejected a number of reported cases. They regarded persistent visual field defects and low amplitude VEP without prolonged latency, characteristic findings in ischaemic optic neuropathy,[21] as features in favour of a diagnosis of SLE as opposed to multiple sclerosis. Prolonged latency of VEP has, however, been described.[13] The difficult distinction of autoimmune optic neuropathy from the optic neuritis of multiple sclerosis has important implications, as in the former, prolonged steroid treatment may be required to restore and maintain vision.[22] Patients with progressive or persistent visual loss should be investigated for collagen-vascular disease but laboratory tests may be inconclusive and the diagnosis only established by the appearance of characteristic clinical features of disseminated lupus.[23]

Before discussing how to distinguish SLE from multiple sclerosis it is important to consider whether, in the patients in whom this difficulty arises, the two diseases may co-exist. Demyelination has been reported in the spinal cord and optic nerves[16,19] but the more usual appearance is that of necrosis.[9] The areas of myelin loss described have been diffuse with indistinct edges and only one brief report describes plaques.[24] April & Vansonnenberg[16] reviewed 13 autopsy reports on myelopathy in SLE, of which 4 showed haemorrhage, 4 vasculitis, 5 massive necrosis, apparently unrelated to vascular change, and 2 in whom the lesion was predominantly demyelination. Allen et al[9] were not convinced that primary demyelination occurred and stressed the reported axonal loss. Certainly the demyelination illustrated by Ellis & Verity[25] is not primary but the result of infarction.

A possible relationship between the two diseases is suggested by the occurrence of multiple sclerosis in one identical twin and SLE, without CNS involvement, in the other.[26] In another family, a brother and sister had multiple sclerosis and the former had three children with SLE.[27] The patient described by Devos et al[28] almost certainly had both diseases. There appears to be no necessity to introduce the term 'lupoid sclerosis'.[14]

Once suspicion has been aroused, the diagnosis of SLE can be pursued by laboratory tests of immune function that need not be elaborated here. These must be interpreted with caution as antinuclear factor has been found in the serum of 25% of patients with multiple sclerosis[29] and, in low titre, in 81%.[30] O'Connor[31] found that the specificity of all laboratory methods of diagnosis were low and that 'other causes of nervous system dysfunction' must be ruled out: scarcely an easy task when attempting the distinction from multiple sclerosis. Of more relevance is to discuss the findings on routine neurological investigation that might arouse such suspicions. A raised ESR may be the alerting factor.[5,9] It is still the practice in many centres to perform routine serological tests for syphilis in organic nervous disease and these may be falsely positive in SLE. The CSF may be normal or contain a cell count and total protein well within the range found in multiple sclerosis. The proportion of IgG was found to be increased in 69% of cases in one series.[32] Oligoclonal IgG may be found [33] but Oppenheimer & Hoffbrand[20] considered its presence to be a strong point against the diagnosis of SLE. Features not found in multiple sclerosis are the occasional very high total protein[10] or, rather more frequently, a high cell count[1] including polymorphs.[6]

The CT scan in cerebral SLE is either normal or shows widening of the sulci or obvious vascular insults.[34] None of the cases reported, however, would have been mistaken clinically for multiple sclerosis. Cranial MRI shows white matter lesions, both periventricular and discrete, not immediately distinguishable from those of multiple sclerosis.[35,36]

Primary Sjögren's syndrome

Alexander et al[37,38] drew attention to the occurrence of central nervous system disease in primary Sjögren's syndrome and later emphasised a remarkable resemblance to multiple sclerosis. They described 20 patients, all of whom had been regarded as having multiple sclerosis. Sicca syndrome had been diagnosed before the onset of neurological disease in only 4. The clinical features included a relapsing and remitting course in the majority, signs of spinal cord and cerebellar disease, internuclear ophthalmoplegia in 3, and visual loss. No clear account of optic neuritis was given, the visual symptoms described more resembling those of ischaemia, but visual evoked potentials were frequently abnormal. Oligoclonal IgG was present in the CSF in nearly all cases examined. MRI showed small numbers of cerebral lesions resembling those seen in multiple sclerosis.[39] The pathology is, apparently, that of infarction and microhaemorrhage and not primary demyelination. Sjögren's syndrome is a relatively common condition and, although only in a minority of cases is the central nervous system involved, it must now be specifically excluded when making the diagnosis of multiple sclerosis, particularly as optic neuropathy has now been described as an initial isolated symptom.[40] It is reassuring that Metz et al[41] found no instance of Sjögren's syndrome in 42 consecutive patients diagnosed as multiple sclerosis — dry eyes and mouth, when encountered, being due to drugs. Noseworthy et al[42] similarly found no evidence of Sjögren's disease in a large population of multiple sclerosis. Steroid treatment of persisting symptoms of central nervous disease in Sjögren's syndrome may well prove to be more effective than in multiple sclerosis.

Polyarteritis nodosa

Polyarteritis nodosa, although affecting the nervous system in a high proportion of cases, poses less of a diagnostic problem.[43,44] Lesions are often multiple but occur relatively later in the disease so that even if the presenting symptoms are neurological, evidence of systemic disease is usually obvious. The brainstem syndromes that are occasionally seen might be mistaken for multiple sclerosis but remission is uncommon. Waisburg et al[45] claimed that the syndrome in their patient resembled multiple sclerosis and certainly the remitting course was remarkable, and unilateral internuclear ophthalmoplegia was observed in one episode. The onset was, however, at the age of 11 and no histological material was examined, the diagnosis being made on renal angiography.

Behçet's disease

Involvement of the CNS in Behçet's disease bears a variable resemblance to multiple sclerosis. The age range is similar but Behçet's is commoner in men.[46] The characteristic mucocutaneous ulceration of the mouth and perineum usually precedes or accompanies the neurological symptoms but may occasionally only occur later.[47] Neurological involvement has been reported in 4–42% of cases.[48]

Early reports of small numbers of affected patients[49–51] recognised three forms that the disease might take: a brainstem syndrome, meningomyelitis or encephalitis, or confusion and dementia. In many cases, the onset far more closely resembled acute encephalitis than multiple sclerosis. It has since become apparent that progressive pseudobulbar palsy is probably the commonest form of the disease in Europe[52] and Japan,[47] while in the Middle East intracranial hypertension without focal signs is the most frequent manifestation.[53,54]

Symptoms of disseminated lesions are comparatively uncommon, occurring in only 3 of 22 cases in one series[53] The course is usually progressive but partial remission may occur and, in particular, ocular palsies and other cranial nerve lesions may recover or show marked fluctuation.[46,47,55]

It is involvement of the optic nerve and spinal cord that is most likely to cause confusion with multiple sclerosis. Optic neuritis is uncommon[46] but retrobulbar neuritis has been described as the initial neurological symptom.[52] Paraplegia has been reported in 4 of 23 and 4 of 22 cases in the different series[47,53] and may be sudden in onset.[51]

The positive criteria for the clinical and laboratory diagnosis of Behçet's disease are succinctly reviewed by Haim & Gilhar.[56] It is generally believed that there is no specific test. Apart from the presence or history of mucocutaneous lesions and other systemic manifestations of the disease, certain clinical features should help to make the distinction from multiple sclerosis where doubt exists. Headache, fever, a raised ESR and, less commonly, signs of meningeal irritation, are present in acute attacks of Behçet's disease.[46,47,52,55,57] Dysarthria and organic mental symptoms are often early features. Lhermitte's sign and internuclear ophthalmoplegia have not been reported.[47] The total protein and cell count in the CSF may be within the range found in multiple sclerosis[46] but very high protein levels may sometimes be found[53] The cell count may sometimes be greatly in excess of that found in multiple sclerosis and polymorphs are often found even with low total counts.[47,52,55] Rather surprisingly the gamma globulin level has been found to be normal.[46,55] Oligoclonal IgG was not found in a single case-report, but may be present (E J Thompson, personal communication). High levels of myelin basic protein have been found in the CSF.[58] Focal brain lesions may be demonstrated by MRI,[59] the white matter lesions resembling those of multiple sclerosis.[60]

AIDS

AIDS-related vacuolar myelopathy presents as progressive spastic paraparesis and sensory ataxia.[61] Both clinically and pathologically it more closely resembles subacute combined degeneration than multiple sclerosis.[62,63] Confusion might arise, however, because the myelopathy is often associated with AIDS-related dementia — in 60% in one series.[61] The clinical evidence of multiple lesions may be supported by cerebral white matter

lesions displayed by MRI, indistinguishable from those of multiple sclerosis.[61] The total protein concentration and cell count in the CSF are usually increased, within the range acceptable for multiple sclerosis, but oligoclonal bands are uncommon.[61] Berger et al[64] have described seven men, seropositive for HIV 1, with clinical disease indistinguishable from relapsing and remitting multiple sclerosis. The histopathology at autopsy in one case and on brain biopsy in two was that of multiple sclerosis and it is probable that their neurologial disease was not due to the infection. The report raises several matters of interest, among them the fact that immunodeficiency did not ameliorate the course of multiple sclerosis.

Tropical spastic paraparesis

As its name implies, the endemic form of tropical spastic paraparesis is a disease predominantly of the spinal cord occurring in regions where multiple sclerosis is rare. The age incidence of the two conditions is similar, although late onset is more common in tropical paraparesis and in some series males are predominantly affected.[65,66] Pain in the back and distally in the legs is common at the onset and bladder symptoms occur early. Sensory symptoms in the lower limbs are constantly present The onset of spasticity may be unilateral but is eventually symmetrical. Tendon reflexes are increased in the upper limbs, but the ankle jerks are sometimes absent There are no remissions but after slow progression the condition may become arrested. There are no ocular symptoms, but visual and other modes of evoked potentials are often abnormal.[67,68] There is increased intrathecal production of IgG and oligoclonal bands may be present.[68] Periventricular lesions similar to those in multiple sclerosis, but of lesser extent, may be seen on MRI. Román & Sheremata[69] state that this syndrome could not be mistaken for multiple sclerosis and, indeed, it does not resemble the relapsing and remitting form of this disease, but is not immediately distinguishable from multiple sclerosis progressive from the onset.

Great interest has been aroused by the discovery that tropical spastic paraparesis is associated with, and no doubt directly or indirectly due to, infection with human lymphotropic virus type I (HTLV-I). This conclusion was originally based on the finding that the great majority of patients have a high titre of antibodies to this virus.[70–72] HTLV-I has been extracted from peripheral lymphocytes and from cells from the CSF.[73] A similar association (HTLV-I associated myelopathy: HAM) has been recorded in a temperate region of Japan where T-cell leukaemia, due to the same virus, is endemic.[74,75] Coexistence of T-cell leukaemia and myelopathy is, however, rare. The clinical features are described in detail by Shibasaki et al.[76] There is no doubt that the two forms of myelopathy are identical.[77] Isolated cases have been found in both black [67] and white[78,79] subjects who have not lived in the tropics or in Japan. In surveys in the UK[68] and USA,[67] a high proportion of black subjects with progressive spastic paraparesis for which no other cause could be found who have been born in the tropics have high antibody titres and, from some, the virus has been isolated.[68]

On rather more slender grounds HTLV-I had been incriminated in multiple sclerosis by Koprowski et al,[80,81] who reported raised antibody titres in a small number of patients. This association has not been confirmed. Hauser et al[82] found no HTLV sequences in tissue from active multiple sclerosis plaques and serum antibodies have not been detected.[83–86] At present it must be concluded that the two diseases are distinct.[87] The resemblance between tropical spastic paraparesis and chronic progressive multiple sclerosis must raise obstacles to the admission of certain patients to therapeutic trials. Chronic myelopathy in black subjects, particularly immigrants from the tropics, should not be accepted for such trials without a test for HTLV-I antibodies, not at present universally available. As knowledge increases it may be necessary to widen these grounds for exclusion.

Sarcoidosis

Sarcoidosis involves the nervous system in approximately 5% of cases.[88] This figure is heavily weighted by the inclusion of patients with an isolated VII cranial nerve palsy and the incidence of more diffuse and potentially more serious disease is much lower.

Diagnostic confusion with multiple sclerosis should only rarely arise. Solitary granulomatous intracranial masses mimic cerebral tumours. Meningeal involvement at the base of the brain may cause visual failure and optic atrophy, but often with manifestations not expected in multiple sclerosis, such as diabetes insipidus or obstructive hydrocephalus. The commonest presentation of sarcoid of the spinal cord is with progressive spastic paraparesis from compression, ischaemia or parenchymal disease[89] and the differential diagnosis naturally includes multiple sclerosis. The onset may occasionally be rapid or sudden, followed by spontaneous remission. Myelography often shows complete or partial obstruction from intramedullary, intradural or extradural mass lesions, but may be normal.[90] The course of the disease could not be distinguished on clinical grounds from that of progressive or static multiple sclerosis. In the case described by Nathan et al[91] with repeated relapse and remission, it was never possible to demonstrate that the proven systemic sarcoidosis was the cause of the spinal cord lesion.

Diffuse sarcoid meningoencephalitis naturally causes symptoms of multiple lesions and may present with mental symptoms,[92] epilepsy or signs of brainstem or cerebral hemisphere lesions. Features much more common in sarcoid than in multiple sclerosis include anosmia, facial palsy, deafness and progressive optic atrophy. Raised intracranial pressure may develop at any stage. There is seldom any evidence of peripheral nerve disease in this form of neurosarcoidosis. Remission from early or relatively insignificant symptoms is common but the spontaneous remission of severe symptoms seen in multiple sclerosis is not a common feature of sarcoidosis.

The characteristic cranial polyneuritis of sarcoidosis might well be confused with multiple sclerosis by those who have not encountered this remarkable syndrome.[93,94] Relapsing and remitting cranial nerve palsies, particularly of the facial nerve but also including bulbar palsy and such curiosities as unilateral accessory nerve lesions and anosmia, may occur over a period of several weeks or months. There is often some evidence of spinal nerve involvement but very seldom of multiple symmetrical peripheral neuropathy. Bizarre areas of cutaneous sensory loss on the trunk bear some resemblance to the sensory changes of multiple sclerosis. Of particular importance in the present context is the apparent involvement of the optic nerve in some patients.

It is clearly important to establish whether optic neuritis and, in particular, retrobulbar neuritis, occurs in sarcoidosis. The optic nerve may indeed be involved in a number of ways; the optic disc may be swollen during an attack of uveitis; papilloedema may result from raised intracranial pressure; optic atrophy may follow intracranial compression. The nerve may be invaded by sarcoid granulomata.[95] None of these conditions bears more than a superficial resemblance to the optic neuritis of multiple sclerosis but there are a few more convincing reports. In the patient described by Piéron et al[96] the only neurological manifestation was blurred vision and pain in one eye. Acuity deteriorated very rapidly to bare perception of light within two days. The optic disc was normal in appearance. On steroid treatment vision recovered fully in less than three weeks, more rapidly than usually expected in demyelinating retrobulbar neuritis of such severity. Beardsley et al[97] described three patients with known sarcoidosis who developed painless unilateral visual loss, in one case in the course of a week. Vision improved spontaneously or on steroids but the visual field defect had been that of enlargement of the blind spot and not a central scotoma. Rush[98] however, described acute but painless loss of vision in one eye with a dense central scotoma and a normal optic disc in a young woman with sarcoidosis. There was full recovery on steroids and the retrobulbar lesion was thought to have been a granuloma of the nerve. Graham et al[99] found that in sarcoid optic neuropathy, visual loss was usually much more gradual than in demyelinating optic neuritis and visual field changes more extensive. In two patients, improvement in vision could only be maintained by continued steroid treatment.

Findings on routine investigation of a patient with undiagnosed neurological disease that should arouse suspicion of sarcoidosis rather than multiple sclerosis are hypercalcaemia, hyperglobulinaemia and, in particular, a persistently raised level of total protein in the CSF. In personal experience this may remain elevated for many years in the presence of entirely static clinical signs.

Oligoclonal bands of IgG have been reported by Kinnman[100] but are unusual and there is little evidence of intrathecal synthesis of IgG.[101] High levels of angiotensin converting enzyme were found in the CSF in 11 of 20 cases of sarcoidosis of the central nervous system by Oksanen et al.[102] Visual evoked potentials do not distinguish demyelinating optic neuritis from acute sarcoid optic neuropathy. The CSF glucose has occasionally been found to be reduced.[103]

A positive diagnosis must depend on histological demonstration of the characteristic granulomata. A positive biopsy from a number of sites can readily be obtained in cases where the diagnosis presents little difficulty on clinical grounds, but when there is no detectable evidence of sarcoid outside the nervous system, biopsy is also usually negative. The Kveim test is negative more often than not in extra-thoracic sarcoid[104] and little help can be obtained from a negative tuberculin test.

In cerebral sarcoid the appearances on CT scanning are naturally often entirely different from those in multiple sclerosis, as involvement of the basal meninges by granulomatous tissue can be demonstrated, as well as high density intracranial lesions.[105-107] The periventricular distribution of such lesions is sometimes striking.[108] MRI is even more successful in demonstrating intracranial sarcoid,[37,109] but both periventricular and discrete white matter abnormalities may resemble those of multiple sclerosis.

Acute disseminated encephalomyelitis (ADEM)

It is by no means certain that ADEM is a disease entity separate from multiple sclerosis. The clinical presentation is very different. ADEM occurs predominantly, but not exclusively, in children, frequently preceded or accompanied by a clearly identifiable viral infection or following inoculation. In the acute form, the child rapidly develops headache, fever and a declining level of consciousness, often to the point of coma. Convulsions may occur but signs of meningeal irritation are uncommon and the cell count in the CSF may be normal. Neurological abnormalities usually indicate mulitple lesions of the brain and spinal cord, the optic nerves may be involved and sometimes also the peripheral nervous system. Mortality is high, up to 20% being reported[110] and permanent sequelae are common, particularly when the spinal cord has been severely affected. A slower form of progression has been described[111] but with essentially similar clinical features. It is in this form that a favourable response to corticosteroid treatment is most obvious.

Apart from the presence of multiple lesions of the CNS, the relation with multiple sclerosis is established by the pathology and by the occasional development of relapsing disease. In both multiple sclerosis and ADEM an essential feature of the pathological process is perivenous demyelination. Lumsden[112] wrote that he could find 'no meaningful pathological distinctions' between the two conditions.

Reports on recurrent ADEM are extremely difficult to interpret. In the frequently cited cases of Alcock & Hoffman,[113] a close relation to infection was seldom established and the later symptoms were often much more closely observed than the first episode of disease. For example, their case 4 is extremely suggestive of some continuing disease process. At the age of nine a boy had an acute illness with headache, vomiting, fever and some disturbance of visual acuity from which he made a complete recovery. At the age of 14, and again at 20, he sustained definite attacks of optic neuritis. The subsequent history of this young man would be of great interest with regard to the relationship of ADEM and multiple sclerosis. Alcock & Hoffman specifically stated that they excluded multiple sclerosis in their cases solely on the grounds that the disease was not thought to occur in children. In contrast, a patient described by Poser et al[114] had recurrent remitting very severe CNS disease but eventually developed acute polyneuritis. The relapses reported in cases of ADEM following influenza vaccination[115,116] could not be regarded as typical of multiple sclerosis. The question of whether such cases are relapsing ADEM or multiple sclerosis triggered by infection or vaccination could not be answered even if the histology was available in view of Lumsden's view of the indistinguishable nature of the changes.

The problem may be illustrated by a personal case.

One week after influenza vaccination a girl of 11 complained of headache that gradually increased for a week. In the next few days both legs became weak and she could not feel them normally. She was alert but irritable and had a mild paraparesis with partial loss of sensation below T7 segment. The temperature was 37.8°C. There was slight neck rigidity. The CSF contained 57 lymphocytes/mm^3 and the total protein was 0.65 g/l. Over the next ten days her condition continued to give rise to great anxiety as she developed bilateral swelling of the optic discs, without loss of acuity, nystagmus and inco-ordination of the upper limbs, while continuing febrile up to 39°C. After all attempts at finding an infective process had failed she was given prednisolone 30 mg a day with immediate benefit. Her headache resolved and she became afebrile. On a reducing dose of steroids all symptoms and signs cleared in the course of the next three months and she was completely well. Eleven months from the onset of her illness, without any preceding infection or inoculation, she developed left optic neuritis with severe visual loss, recovering in two months. Four months later she had a mild episode of right retrobulbar neuritis and again three years after her first symptoms, at the age of 14, the left optic nerve was again involved. Recovery was complete in a further two months. The optic discs were normal in colour and colour vision was intact. VEP were delayed bilaterally. At the age of 21 she remains well.

Neuromyelitis optica (Devic's syndrome)

As with other euphonious titles, that of neuromyelitis optica is deeply imprinted on the memory but what precisely it implies is in many respects obscure. A common concept is of some specific Devic's *disease* comprising, simultaneously or in succession, an acute transverse spinal cord lesion and bilateral optic or retrobulbar neuritis. This clear cut clinical syndrome, however, shades almost imperceptibly in published reports into subacute cases with perhaps uniocular visual loss and weakness of one lower limb. These difficulties of clinical definition, certainly not resolved in the original descriptions, are well reviewed by Cloys & Netsky.[117]

The supposedly classical syndrome can certainly result from diverse causes: Behçet's disease[47] SLE,[16] ADEM and multiple sclerosis included, but a number of authors have believed that an entity distinct from these conditions can be identified.[118]

A growing recognition of the modifying role of age and tempo on the process of demyelination has led a number of observers, notably Ferraro[119] and Lumsden[120] to regard neuromyelitis optica as a form of multiple sclerosis. The evidence for this conclusion comes from clinical and pathological sources. Recovery from the initial attack of myelitis may be followed sooner or later by the appearance of such signs as nystagmus, ocular or other cranial nerve palsies, tremor or ataxia, euphoria or mental changes. Sometimes these are associated with a fresh attack of myelitis or of optic neuritis. Rarely, such evidence of fresh damage may appear after a lapse of many years, as in a Japanese patient reported by Okinaka et al[121]: recovery from the initial attack of neuromyelitis optica at the age of 18 was followed by signs of multiple sclerosis 22 years later, no relapse having occurred in the interval.

From the pathological standpoint, areas of demyelination and, in more chronic cases, typical plaques may be observed in the brainstem or elsewhere in the brain. Stansbury[122] analysed the distribution of the lesions in 20 unselected cases from the literature: optic nerves (not obtained in four cases) 16; optic chiasm 5; optic tract 5; cerebral hemispheres 5; brainstem 12; spinal cord 19; cerebellum 13. In a statistical analysis of 40 autopsy reports of multiple sclerosis and neuromyelitis optica in Japanese subjects, Shibasaki & Kuroiwa[123] classified cases according to the nature and location of the pathological lesions: multiple sclerosis 18 cases; neuromyelitis optica 13 cases; intermediate 13 cases. In the neuromyelitis optica group, however, demyelinating lesions were also present in the brainstem (8 cases) and in the cerebrum (1 case) and in these sites in six of the 'intermediate' (optic-spinae) cases. In only seven of the 40 cases therefore, was demyelination limited to the optic nerves and spinal cord.

The following case, originally seen by Professor Ritchie Russell, illustrates the progression from 'pure' Devics's syndrome to classical multiple sclerosis.

A man of 18 developed blurred vision in both eyes, leading within two days to total blindness with swollen optic discs. He then immediately became paralysed in both lower limbs with dense sensory loss below T3 segment. He was mildly febrile. The CSF intially contained 8 lymphocytes/mm^3 and a total protein of 0.6 g/l but on a second examination there were 372 lymphocytes/mm^3 and a protein of 2.5 g/l, both values beyond those normally acceptable for multiple sclerosis. With corticotrophin treatment he improved, being left with 6/18 vision in both eyes and with· spastic paraparesis. Four years later he had transient double vision due to weakness of abduction of the right eye. A month later he developed paroxysmal ataxia and dysarthria, prevented by carbamazepine and remitting after six weeks. Nine months later he had right retrobulbar neuritis with little recovery of vision. This was followed by right sided tonic seizures and a single major fit. These symptoms were controlled and did not return when treatment was stopped some months later.

In the absence of histological examination there can be no certainty of diagnosis but the occurrence of four highly characteristic symptoms of multiple sclerosis subsequent to the Devic's syndrome strongly suggests that the initial drastic illness was the first episode of this disease.

Lyme Disease

Lyme disease, now known to be due to tick-borne infection with the spirochaete *Borrelia burgdorferi*, may closely mimic multiple sclerosis. The disease is endemic in many parts of the world, being especially prevalent in wooded areas where ticks and their usual hosts lurk. The initial acute manifestations characteristically occur in summer.

The tick bite often passes unremarked and the diagnostic skin lesion, erythema chronicum migrans, may not be recognised. It consists of a slowly spreading red ring surrounding the site of the bite. There is often an acute febrile reaction without specific features, followed by a second stage in which neurological involvement is common. Headache is severe but signs of meningism are minimal.[124] Facial palsy, often bilateral, is common and ocular palsies may occur.[124,125] Spinal radiculopathy and mononeuritis multiplex cause scattered sensory and motor signs. The localised paraesthesiae on the trunk or extremities combined with cranial nerve lesions might well arouse suspicion of multiple sclerosis,[126] but the constitutional disturbance is far more marked and the CSF cell count is often much higher than would be acceptable for multiple sclerosis. The central nervous system is occasionally severely involved at this early stage, acute transverse myelitis being described within a few days of the rash.[127]

Far more difficult diagnostic problems are posed when chronic progressive or exacerbating neurological disease develops in what is regarded as tertiary Lyme disease, apparently several years after infection or, indeed, with no clinical evidence of infection at all. Syndromes include progressive spastic paraparesis,[128] transverse myelitis,[129,130] cerebellar ataxia,[131] recurrent cranial nerve palsies[132] and hemiparesis.[128] Optic neuritis was mentioned, but not described, by Kohler et al,[128] the optic neuropathy in Schechter's[126] case being clearly ischaemic. The arthritis of chronic Lyme disease is a rare accompaniment.

Both CT scanning and MRI may show white matter and periventricular lesions.[128,132,134] The CSF may contain oligoclonal bands of IgG.[135,136] Even in these chronic cases, however, the CSF total protein and cell count are frequently far beyond the levels found in multiple sclerosis.[128,134] The diagnosis must rest on serological tests for antibodies,[137] but even when these are positive, some doubt may persist as to their relevance in endemic areas. Fumarola[138] described a patient with multiple sclerosis and a raised antibody titre that increased in relapse. Muhlemann et al,[139] who examined sera from 15 multiple sclerosis patients from an endemic area, found a low titre in a single case. In a much larger series of 106 patients from the Austrian Tyrol, abnormally high titres of antibody were found in 14.2%, but this figure was lower than the 20.1% found in matched controls.[140] Patients with the clinical and radiological features of chronic multiple sclerosis who are found to have slightly raised serum antibodies to *B. burgdorferi* are unlikely to have neuroborreliosis.[141]

The differential diagnosis from multiple sclerosis is of considerable importance as early cases of neurological involvement in Lyme disease may respond to penicillin[124] and other antibiotics may prove effective in late disease.[142]

Subacute myelo-optic neuritis (SMON)

A clear description of the clinical features of this condition in no less than 752 Japanese cases was given by Sobue et al.[143] The initial neurological symptoms were nearly always sensory, either acute or subacute in onset. Numbness and unpleasant paraesthesiae spread from the feet to the mid dorsal region in the great majority, with minor variations in distribution and mode of extension. Weakness was less common but blurred vision due to optic neuropathy occurred in 25%, in a few patients as the presenting symptom. Partial remission, especially of motor symptoms, was common and relapse also occurred. Paraesthesiae were persistent and distressing.

The association with intestinal disorders was immediately recognised and although still regarded by some as unproven there is no serious doubt that the syndrome resulted from the toxic effects of clioquinol, taken for real or imagined bowel complaints.[144] The Japanese appear to be peculiarly susceptible to the effects of clioquinol, but clinical cases, have been reported outside Japan, at least one with autopsy confirmation.[145] SMON should be included in the differential diagnosis of acute or subacute spinal cord disease with predominant sensory symptoms, with or without optic nerve involvement. In addition to a history of clioquinol ingestion, not always very prolonged, a further diagnostic hint is the excretion of green urine.

Cerebrovascular disease

Only rarely does diagnostic confusion arise between multiple sclerosis and CVD but occasionally the distinction may be extremely difficult. Subacute bacterial endocarditis presenting with emboli involving the CNS should be detected by all but the most highly specialised neurologist, but should be remembered as one cause of an acute spinal cord lesion in a young adult.[146,147] The cardiac lesion in myxoma of the left atrium may be clinically occult or diagnosed as mitral stenosis. The symptoms of scattered cerebral lesions sometimes with a remitting course may on occasion strongly suggest the diagnosis of multiple sclerosis, particularly if the visual system is involved (Davies-Jones, personal communication). The constitutional disturbance with fever, raised ESR and weight loss should indicate the need for cardiological investigations. Albers et al[148] described a patient in whom emboli from a tumour of the left ventricle, classified as cavernous angiectasia, resulted in a diagnosis of multiple sclerosis.

The most difficult problem is that of the young woman, taking an oral contraceptive, who presents with the rapid onset of focal neurological signs. If these are clearly attributable to a single lesion, for example, weakness and sensory loss in one upper limb, it may not be possible to distinguish the effects of a brainstem plaque from those of an infarct. The latter would probably not be seen on CT scanning, evoked potentials very seldom show abnormalities of diagnostic value in the initial episode of multiple sclerosis and oligoclonal bands of IgG have been found in the CSF in acute CVD.[149] In such circumstances it seems best to forbid the oral contraceptive and await events.

The 'apoplectic' onset of multiple sclerosis may easily be mistaken for a stroke.[150] As a personal impression, the onset with acute hemiplegia of what is subsequently revealed as multiple sclerosis is rare and usually affects men.

Meningovascular syphilis

Neurosyphilis is now a comparative rarity in countries where multiple sclerosis is prevalent, and is therefore the more likely to be overlooked. Oculomotor palsies, perhaps combined with hemiparesis, certainly bear a superficial resemblance to multiple sclerosis but headache is often prominent, epilepsy is common and pupillary abnormalities may be detected.

Syphilitic optic neuritis was carefully studied by Graveson.[151] Onset of unilateral visual loss is sudden but ocular pain is uncommon. Both optic discs are characteristically found to be hyperaemic and swollen. The visual field changes are those of an enlarged blind spot and peripheral constriction rather than central scotoma. Lorentzen[152] described unilateral optic neuritis in secondary syphilis. Again the visual field defects were not typically those of the optic neuritis of multiple sclerosis.

Remote effects of carcinoma

By far the commonest non-metastatic effect of carcinoma on the nervous system is peripheral neuropathy, bearing no resemblance to multiple sclerosis. The rare subacute cerebellar syndrome is accompanied by signs of much more widespread involvement, particularly dementia, pyramidal signs and diplopia. In a few personally observed examples, the rapid deterioration in a patient usually well beyond the peak age of onset of mul-

tiple sclerosis and the frequent accompaniment of signs of peripheral nervous or muscle disease, has allowed the distinction. More slowly developing forms have, however, been described, where the diagnosis is difficult,[153,154] particularly if accompanied by optic neuritis.[155] The CSF, on routine examination, may not be distinguishable from that of multiple sclerosis.

Migrant sensory neuritis

In 1958, Wartenberg[156] collected his previous experience and outlined the clinical features of what he termed migrant sensory neuritis. It might be thought that a purely peripheral condition could not closely mimic multiple sclerosis, but it is highly probable that in one of Wartenberg's own cases this was the correct diagnosis. The symptoms are, however, quite distinctive and apparently arise from stretch of cutaneous nerves.[157] The characteristic sequence is of a searing pain, clearly perceived as superficial, in a strictly localised area of an extremity, occurring during rapid movement of the limb. This is immediately followed by loss of cutaneous sensation in the area in which the brief pain was experienced. The sensory loss always involves the distribution of a cutaneous nerve and is never segmental as in lesions of the nerve roots, nor extensive as often found in acute relapses of multiple sclerosis. Nerves frequently involved are digital, sural, terminal radial and ulnar and the patellar plexus.

From these descriptions it might be thought that the syndrome would be instantly recognisable, but accounts of unfamiliar symptoms are all too easily moulded to fit recognised patterns. The initial pain and the character of the areas of sensory loss may be overlooked and the recovery within a few weeks reinforces the imagined resemblance to multiple sclerosis. Migrant sensory neuritis is a relapsing and remitting condition that may recur for a great many years but it is entirely benign and confusion with multiple sclerosis can be avoided by the attentive listener to the history.

2. SYSTEMATISED DISEASES

Hereditary spino-cerebellar ataxia

Multiple sclerosis should not be confused with

classical Friedreich's ataxia which develops in the first or second decade and is progressive. The physical signs are those of cerebellar ataxia, although nystagmus is sometimes unexpectedly absent, weakness of the lower limbs with extensor plantar reflexes and clear evidence of peripheral nerve involvement with absent tendon jerks. To this picture may be added, in some families, optic atrophy, early dementia or deafness. Cardiac myopathy is common and there is an undue tendency to diabetes. Inheritance is recessive, so cases in preceding generations will not be found.

This classical picture is distinctly rare, but, if fully developed, is sufficiently distinctive. Much more difficulty is presented by atypical cases of hereditary or sporadic cerebellar ataxia and in particular by hereditary spastic paraplegia. Of course, if it is possible to examine several members of a family, all showing an identical clinical syndrome, a diagnosis may be confidently pronounced, but in practice many obstacles arise. Genetically controlled diseases, particularly if recessively inherited, frequently present as single apparently sporadic cases. A vague history of 'difficulty in walking' in near relatives is often impossible to confirm as relevant. Certain clinical features are of diagnostic value.

Disease is never wholly symmetrical but marked asymmetry of physical signs is a strong indication of multiple sclerosis rather than a systematised degeneration. Pes cavus, absent ankle jerks and scoliosis are all features in favour of the latter diagnosis. I have not found the presence or absence of the abdominal reflexes to be of any value in this context. Moderately severe spastic weakness of the legs with no loss of vibration sense on stringent testing is more typical of hereditary spastic paraplegia than of multiple sclerosis. A pure cerebellar syndrome with a progressive course is highly likely to be some form of degeneration as this is not a feature of multiple sclerosis.

For a number of years I followed the progress of a middle-aged woman with a slowly progressive symmetrical cerebellar ataxia, nystagmus and dysarthria, with flexer plantar reflexes, normal tendon reflexes, no sensory loss and normal optic fundi. She told me that she had nursed her mother who had died of multiple sclerosis and that this diagnosis had been made by Sir Charles Symonds,

to whom I wrote. He found his notes in which he had recorded the diagnosis of hereditary cerebellar ataxia, at that time in the absence of a family history, on the grounds mentioned above — the pure cerebellar syndrome.

Diagnostic difficulty is notably increased by the presence of optic nerve involvement. Members of the family described by Ferguson & Critchley[158] were often diagnosed as having multiple sclerosis but visual involvement was confined to pallor of the discs without loss of acuity, a notoriously fallible sign. Suggestive or definite evidence of optic neuritis may, however, be present hereditary cerebellar or spinal cord disease.[159] In the large family with spastic paraplegia described by Bickerstaff,[160] some members had acute optic neuritis and an association with Leber's optic atrophy was suggested. Similarly, patients presenting with the classical bilateral optic neuritis of Leber's hereditary optic atrophy may subsequently develop signs of widespread neurological disease, including a progressive spinal cord syndrome.[161]

Evoked potential techniques are of limited value in distinguishing multiple sclerosis from hereditary ataxias as VEP are often abnormal in the latter.[162] Marked asymmetry of the response would favour multiple sclerosis. The CSF is normal in hereditary spastic paraplegia, the condition most difficult to distinguish, from multiple sclerosis, and oligoclonal IgG has not been described. MRI may show periventricular and, rarely, discrete white matter abnormalities in both sporadic and hereditary cerebellar degeneration.[36]

Subacute combined degeneration of the spinal cord (SACD)

SACD is seldom mistaken for multiple sclerosis. The condition is rare and usually occurs at an older age than multiple sclerosis. The onset with symmetrical, often very unpleasant paraesthesiae in the lower limbs, or very occasionally in the hands alone, and the absent ankle jerks at this stage should suggest some form of peripheral neuropathy rather than multiple sclerosis. On the few occasions where I have encountered an erroneous diagnosis of multiple sclerosis, the patient has been young, signs of peripheral neuropathy have been absent and the presentation has been that of spastic weakness of the lower limbs with impaired proprioception, developing in the course of a few weeks or months. Lhermitte's sign, so common in multiple sclerosis, may be present.[163] Asymmetry is minimal, sphincters are involved much later than in multiple sclerosis and there may, of course, be other evidence of vitamin B_{12} deficiency, anaemia and glossitis. Visual impairment, when this occurs, is usually independent of the spinal cord disease, and does not resemble that of acute optic neuritis, but VEP may be delayed even in the absence of visual symptoms.[164] Bilateral centro-coecal scotomata develop, followed by some pallor of the optic discs. Mild mental impairment is the rule in SACD.

Provided the diagnosis is considered at all, it can readily be confirmed by estimation of the level of vitamin B_{12} in the serum, normal values differing between laboratories. Only if B_{12} has been given prior to the establishment of the diagnosis, and it has been used without scientific basis as a form of 'tonic' in many diseases including multiple sclerosis, is it necessary to perform confirmatory tests of B_{12} absorption.

Leukodystrophy

Adrenoleukodystrophy in the form predominantly affecting the brain and adrenals is largely a disease of childhood and is unlikely to be mistaken for multiple sclerosis. Adrenomyeloneuropathy, however, usually presents in adult life with progressive spinal cord disease combined with some clinical evidence of peripheral neuropathy.[165] Disturbance of adrenal function may only be detected by a diminished response to ACTH. In the absence of a family history indicating sex-linked inheritance, a diagnosis of multiple sclerosis is naturally considered. Female heterozygotes may also present with spastic paraparesis[166] or with mild remitting neurological symptoms, the resemblance to multiple sclerosis being increased by the presence of oligoclonal IgG in the CSF.[167] The diagnosis can be established in both homozygous cases and in carriers by estimation of very long chain fatty acids in the plasma.

Dominantly inherited adult-onset leukodystrophy may resemble chronic progressive multiple sclerosis with signs of spinal cord and cerebellar disease.[168]

3. SINGLE LESIONS OF THE CNS WITH A RELAPSING AND REMITTING COURSE

The clinical course of many single progressive expanding lesions involving the CNS is marked by fluctuations, particularly sudden exacerbation and more rarely partial remission. In most such circumstances as, for example, the sudden onset or worsening of symptoms following haemorrhage into a cerebral tumour, no confusion with multiple sclerosis can arise. In some special circumstances a clinical diagnosis of multiple sclerosis may be so strongly suggested that investigations necessary to reveal the real cause may be omitted. A most remarkable example is the onset of symptoms due to an intracranial meningioma during pregnancy followed by remission in the weeks after delivery. This pattern has been thought to be characteristic of multiple sclerosis although relapse in the puerperium is, in fact, more common. Bickerstaff et al[169] described unilateral visual loss, with a central scotoma occurring during pregnancy, with subsequent complete recovery, due to a meningioma placed where it could exert pressure on the optic nerve. The influence of pregnancy is no doubt related to the presence of female hormone receptors in intracranial tumours, particularly in meningiomas.[170,171]

There is no obvious explanation for the occasional relapsing and remitting course of the symptoms of glioma of the brain stem.[172] The initial symptoms, such as ocular palsies and focal weakness may remit completely in a manner quite indistinguishable from multiple sclerosis. More important is the similarly fluctuating course of many extramedullary tumours in the region of the foramen magnum. Cohen & Macrae[173] described four such patients, all initially diagnosed as having multiple sclerosis. Remission in some patients had been complete and prolonged and the initial symptoms sometimes typical of multiple sclerosis, including paraesthesiae of both legs. In addition to prolonged remission marked day to day fluctuations may occur, as often observed in multiple sclerosis. Points that should arouse suspicion are headache, a Horner's syndrome and paralysis of the spinal accessory nerve.

Perhaps the most remarkable example of prolonged remission of severe symptoms, admittedly not always closely resembling those of multiple sclerosis, is the epidermoid of the IVth ventrical where a remission of no less than 20 years has been reported.[174] Primary cerebral lymphoma has been reported as causing cerebellar ataxia repeatedly remitting on treatment with ACTH and diagnosed as multiple sclerosis for several years.[175]

Arteriovenous malformations and other forms of 'angioma' involving the brainstem are usually diagnosed as multiple sclerosis, often for many years before subarachnoid haemorrhage reveals the true diagnosis.[176] Again, the fluctuating and sometimes remitting symptoms of brainstem disease are not to be distinguished from those of multiple sclerosis.[177,178] Large vessel malformations are readily detectable by radiology, including CT scanning, but capillary telangiectasis, that can cause similar symptoms, may be undetectable. In reported cases where diagnostic confusion has occurred, the resemblance to multiple sclerosis has been less remarkable. Dysphagia in the first attack and eventual persistent unilateral paresis of the tongue and palate scarcely suggest this diagnosis.[179]

Arachnoid cysts in the cisterna magna may present with remitting and relapsing symptoms, often difficult to attribute to the effects of a single lesion. In the case described by Lehman & Fieger,[180] there were repeated episodes of weakness of the right arm between the ages of 9 and 22 years, eventually followed by a left hemiparesis and diplopia. In reviewing published reports they found that pain was often a prominent symptom, as in their case. Arachnoid cysts involving the spinal cord may also cause intermittent symptoms.

The symptoms of tumours involving the spinal cord may also fluctuate or remit. Again vascular malformations provide the most striking examples. Progressive signs may be preceded by transient episodes of weakness, sensory loss or sphincter disturbance without accompanying pain.[180,181] The onset of paraplegia during pregnancy, sometimes in successive pregnancies, with full subsequent remission, is almost inevitably diagnosed as multiple sclerosis. Personal observation of one of the cases of spinal angioma described by Newman[183] has left an indelible impression.

The clinical signs of other spinal cord tumours may also remit, sometimes for a number of years. Such tumours may be intra- or extramedullary[184,185] and again relapse in pregnancy may occur.[186] It has been suggested that the recurrence of symptoms with the same localising indications in each attack should distinguish a spinal tumour from multiple sclerosis, but the majority of relapses of multiple sclerosis do not involve new regions of the CNS, but repeat earlier symptoms.

4. SINGLE LESIONS WITH A PROGRESSIVE COURSE

Tumours involving the cerebral hemispheres should now seldom be mistaken for multiple sclerosis. Slowly progressive spastic weakness of one leg presents a difficult problem of localisation as the responsible lesion may lie anywhere between the thoracic spinal cord and the opposite motor cortex. Multiple sclerosis may certainly begin in this way and weakness may eventually spread to the upper limb on the same side. Before the advent of reliable non-invasive radiology the management of such patients with no evidence of multiple lesions greatly depended on the detection of physical signs involving the opposite limbs. The decision whether to submit the patient to a myelogram or a carotid angiogram might be swayed by a dubious plantar reflex or variable blunting of pinprick sensation on the asymptomatic side. The CT scan now readily confirms or excludes, for example, a convexity or parasagittal meningioma. The theoretical possibility of paraplegia resulting from a tumour impinging on the leg area of the motor cortex on both sides is hardly ever encountered.

Tumours in the posterior fossa or foramen magnum may present greater difficulty as the combination of cerebellar signs, weakness and cranial nerve involvement is by no means dissimilar from that of multiple sclerosis. Shephard & Wadia[187] commented on the mistaken diagnosis of an acoustic neuroma, without hearing loss, as multiple sclerosis, but this source of error is now avoidable with modern diagnostic techniques. The patient with an intrinsic tumour of the medulla and cervical cord described by Leon-Sotomayor[188] was examined by several teams of experts but eventually died undiagnosed. Multiple sclerosis had been suspected because of brainstem signs, trigeminal neuralgia at the age of 19, Lhermitte's sign and an apparent response to ACTH. Some suspicion might have been aroused by the initial symptom of headache and subsequent unilateral wasting of the hand muscles. Extrinsic tumours in the posterior fossa may extend through the tentorium and produce bizarre clinical syndromes that might well be attributed to multiple lesions.

The distinction between progressive spinal multiple sclerosis and spinal cord compression is a common and highly important problem. As McAlpine[189] wrote: 'No more unfortunate mistake can be made than to give the label "multiple sclerosis" to a case of paraplegia which subsequently proves to be one of spinal cord compression.' In this age group many causes of compression are benign and potentially curable.

There must be few neurologists who have not 'missed' a spinal cord tumour. Such tumours are nearly always intramedullary and have not shown on myelography or raised the CSF protein level beyond that found in multiple sclerosis. Little harm results from such almost unavoidable mistakes, but to be told after ten years or more that the diagnosis is that of a glioma of the spinal cord may even bring some relief to a patient expecting eventually to lose vision and mental acuity from multiple sclerosis.

A benign tumour should not be missed. Poser et al[190] attempted to determine whether the spinal form of multiple sclerosis could be distinguished on clinical grounds from other forms of spinal cord disease, but were able to give little guidance. In practice, clinical features much more common in spinal cord compression than in multiple sclerosis include a persistent cutaneous sensory level, root pain and segmental muscle wasting. The patient described by Conrad & Mergner[191] had a high cervical neurinoma but was diagnosed as multiple sclerosis because of pain in the trigeminal distribution, interpreted as paroxysmal neuralgia, although it was not triggered and was accompanied by sensory loss. Most physicians are now so alert

to be possibility of mistaking spinal cord compression for multiple sclerosis that there is a tendency towards over-investigation. Fortunately, advances in imaging techniques have made this process both more precise and less arduous for the patient.

Cervical spondylotic myelopathy

The damage to the spinal cord in cervical spondylotic myelopathy is related to narrowing of the spinal canal by osteophytes and ligamentous thickening. The precise means by which this damage is produced, whether by direct pressure or ischaemia, is not fully known and perhaps varies between different patients. Spondylosis itself is almost universal in middle age and beyond and is responsible for many annoying symptoms of pain around the neck and shoulders and less often root pain, sensory loss and weakness in the arms. Such symptoms, although sometimes distressing, do not have the serious implications of myelopathy and indeed many patients with extravagantly abnormal radiographic appearances of the neck have no symptoms at all. A completely normal cervical spine on X-ray excludes spondylosis as the cause of spinal cord involvement. Spondylosis should not be held responsible for such symptoms unless the antero-posterior diameter of the cervical canal is reduced.

The cardinal feature of spondylotic myelopathy is spastic paraparesis not differing in any important respect from that of multiple sclerosis. The distinction is made even more difficult by the undoubted fact that the two conditions may coexist. This was shown conclusively by Brain & Wilkinson[192] who suggested that trauma to the cord favoured the formation and spread of plaques in that region. Oppenheimer[193] more specifically believed that traction through the denticulate ligaments was in some sense responsible for the localisation of plaques in the lateral columns of the spinal cord.

In the absence of post mortem evidence, seldom obtained, it is not therefore entirely realistic to list features characteristic of one or other condition. McAlpine[194] made such an attempt including some highly pertinent observations. The average age of onset in patients adjudged to have spondylotic myelopathy was 52, some ten years later than a group of patients with the spinal form of multiple sclerosis. A progressive hemiplegic onset was sometimes found in multiple sclerosis but not in myelopathy. Pain in the upper limbs was only slightly more common in the spondylotic group. Early disturbance of sphincter control was much more common in multiple sclerosis, a point emphasised by Brain & Wilkinson[192] and naturally segmental wasting in the upper limb, sometimes with fasciculation, is relatively common in myelopathy. McAlpine[194] could not confirm that loss or reduction of one or more of the tendon reflexes in the upper limbs was of any diagnostic value as suggested by Brain & Wilkinson.[192] Certainly in personal experience 'inversion' of the supinator jerk — finger flexion without elbow flexion on tapping the radius — considered a valuable sign of spondylotic myelopathy,[192] is not infrequent in multiple sclerosis. Obviously any evidence of lesions above the cervical spinal cord or earlier relapse and remission would strongly support a diagnosis of multiple sclerosis.

The practical importance of making the distinction, when this exists, lies in prognosis and treatment. Provided trauma to the neck can be avoided, the prognosis for escaping a wheelchair life is relatively good in myelopathy and in some patients can be improved by immobilisation of the neck by collar or fusion, or by decompression of the cervical canal. If the clinical criteria outlined above are all met, the canal is narrowed and the cord is shown by imaging techniques to be compressed, it is safe to proceed on the assumption that there is spondylotic myelopathy, although even so, a contribution from multiple sclerosis cannot be excluded. If there is suggestive evidence of multiple lesions, even if a narrowed canal and compressed cord can be demonstrated, little or no benefit can be obtained from surgery.

The Chiari malformation

It is well recognised that the Chiari malformation, in which ectopic cerebellar tissue passes through the foramen magnum into the cervical canal, may present with symptoms for the first time in adult life in the absence of skeletal deformities of the neck or skull.[195] In the majority of such patients the clinical syndrome does not resemble multiple sclerosis but is that of classical syringo-

myelia or more rarely of hydrocephalus. In a proportion of patients, however, the predominant signs are those of cerebellar ataxia, spastic weakness of the limbs and nystagmus and a diagnosis of multiple sclerosis may naturally be considered. Trigeminal neuralgia may also occur and increase the resemblance.[196] Lhermitte's sign may be positive. The CSF total protein may be moderately increased in the Chiari malformation[197] and there has been a report of delayed VEP.[198] There are, however, clinical features suggestive of the correct diagnosis. Pain in the upper limbs and trunk is an extremely common symptom, much more so than in multiple sclerosis.[197] The nystagmus is often vertical, either up or down beat. This may certainly be encountered in multiple sclerosis but persistent nystagmus of this nature should arouse suspicion.[199]

A woman of 44 had been diagnosed as having multiple sclerosis, the initial symptoms occurring at the age of 29, when she developed numbness at the back of the head and oscillopsia. These symptoms fluctuated and sometimes remitted completely. When she was 37 her walking became unsteady and her physician treated her with ACTH, apparently with temporary benefit. When seen she had nystagmus in all directions of gaze but most severely on looking down. In all positions the fast movement was downwards and she had persistent oscillopsia. There was cerebellar ataxia of the limbs and slight blunting of cutaneous sensation distally in the left arm. The Chiari malformation was shown radiologically. Decompression reduced the nystagmus and abolished the oscillopsia but her ataxia continued to deteriorate.

Definitive diagnosis has, until recently, depended on myelography with particular emphasis on filling the posterior aspect of the cervical canal and foramen magnum where the ectopic tissue is to be found. CT and MRI have greatly advanced ease of diagnosis.[200] There is some practical value in making the distinction from multiple sclerosis as although operative decompression will not result in complete resolution of symptoms, a high proportion of patients obtain some relief, particularly of pain and sometimes of troublesome oscillopsia.[199]

5. MONOSYMPTOMATIC PRESENTATION

In approximately 45% of patients the initial

symptoms and signs of multiple sclerosis can be attributed to the effects of a single lesion of the nervous system. Such symptoms are naturally extremely diverse and cannot be considered individually. Precise diagnosis may often be impossible with transient symptoms and, in the present state of the treatment of multiple sclerosis, perhaps even undesirable provided no alternative requiring different management is overlooked. Some such symptoms are much more evocative of multiple sclerosis than others. For example, an acute unilateral lower motor neurone facial palsy could conceivably be an initial symptom of the disease but other causes are far more likely, while acute retention of urine in a young man, without any other detectable cause, is highly suggestive. Trigeminal neuralgia as a symptom of multiple sclerosis cannot, in the absence of other symptoms, be distinguished from the idiopathic form, but an early age of onset will arouse suspicion.

Symptoms induced or greatly aggravated by exercise are common at the onset of multiple sclerosis. These may affect the strength of the limbs or vision but also the sensory system. Rapid fatigue of a weak limb is scarcely a specific symptom but, for example, severe weakness of one arm that is only apparent after two vigorous games of squash, with recovery over half an hour, is most likely to be due to multiple sclerosis.

Uhthoff's syndrome of loss of visual acuity on increasing body temperature or with exercise is well recognised in patients with established multiple sclerosis or with a history of optic neuritis, but may be the initial symptom in the absence of any other evidence of visual involvement.

A man of 34 became aware of an area of altered sensation on the right side of his scalp. At about the same time he noticed that on prolonged violent exertion the vision of the right eye became blurred. This only occurred after playing squash for about 20 minutes. Vision would not recover for about half an hour. At no other time did he have any visual symptoms and a hot bath had no adverse effect. Acuity, colour vision, visual fields and the appearance of the optic disc were normal but the VEP from that eye was greatly delayed. Apart from the area of blunted cutaneous sensation on the scalp there were no other abnormal signs.

Weakness of one or both limbs, a common mode of onset, may initially only be present after a long walk, no abnormality at all being detectable when examined at rest. In such circumstances there can be no certainty of diagnosis, but such a history should not be dismissed as that of natural fatigue or neurasthenia.

Visual failure

Optic neuritis is described in detail in Chapter 3 and rare causes have already been discussed under a number of diagnostic headings. The form most difficult to distinguish from that in multiple sclerosis is Leber's hereditary optic atrophy. The visual symptoms may be accompanied or followed by widespread signs of neurological disease or may occur in isolation.[201] The great majority of patients are young men and a family history may be obtained, the mode of inheritance not being fully understood.[202] The onset is often bilaterally synchronous with progressive visual failure for longer than usually encountered in multiple sclerosis. Variants occur such as sudden visual loss, unilateral involvement or onset in childhood. There is characteristically a centro-coecal scotoma[203] and specific fundal changes have been described.[204] Some recovery of vision may occur but the usual course is for the condition to become static. Apart from the absence of pain, the resemblance to the optic neuritis of multiple sclerosis may be close.

The clinical features of optic neuritis may be closely mimicked by central serous choroidoretinopathy. This condition affects young adults and causes the rapid onset of unilateral blurred vision. Loss of acuity is not severe. The changes at the fovea are likely to escape routine examination by a neurologist. However, there is no loss of colour vision and the pupillary light reflex is not affected. Vision recovers but recurrence is common. The cases reported by Krauscher & Miller[205] were wrongly diagnosed as having multiple sclerosis on the basis of presumed optic neuritis and dangerous 'soft' neurological signs.

The presentation of neuroretinitis resembles that of optic neuritis even more closely. Rapid visual loss is accompanied by pain in the eye or headache. The optic disc is swollen. Some patients report vague sensory or bladder symptoms. The clue to correct diagnosis is a macular star, either at the onset or within two weeks. This condition has not been shown to be related to multiple sclerosis.[206]

Ischaemic optic neuritis usually affects an older age group, although naturally there is some overlap, and is due to cranial arteritis or atherosclerosis. There is no pain in the eye although headache may be present in arteritis. Altitudinal field defects are common. In a small proportion of cases, sudden or rapid visual loss is accompanied by unilateral disc swelling and a central scotoma[207] and the distinction from optic neuritis is extremely difficult.

Vighetto et al[208] reported two disturbing examples of relapsing unilateral visual loss, responsive to steroid treatment, mistaken for optic neuritis, but in each case due to optic nerve compression by a craniopharyngioma. The visual field changes were not entirely typical of optic neuritis but the resemblance was close.

A far more important source of diagnostic error is progressive visual failure. This certainly occurs as a feature of multiple sclerosis[210] although detailed longitudinal studies on large groups of patients do not appear to have been reported.

Progressive visual loss as the initial and sole manifestation of multiple sclerosis should be accepted only with the greatest reserve.[210] In a patient seen personally, fluctuating but progressive asymmetrical visual failure had been reluctantly accepted as due to multiple sclerosis. She was thought to be slightly ataxic, the abdominal reflexes were absent (she had had 3 children), the left plantar reflex had been thought to be 'weakly extensor' and all symptoms were worse on exertion or in hot surroundings. CT scan was repeatedly normal as was the CSF. MRI was thought to show periventricular lesions compatible with multiple sclerosis. However, craniotomy revealed a meningioma *en plaque* compressing the chiasma. Even in retrospect, this could not even be suspected radiologically.

This case again illustrates the ease with which slight, dubious or irrelevant symptoms and signs can be misinterpreted.

Diplopia

The most probable cause of persistent double vision in an otherwise healthy young adult is multiple sclerosis. Other causes include myasthenia gravis, brainstem lesions including tumour, infarction, and, now rarely, neurosyphilis. If accompanied by other symptoms, notably headache, the differential diagnosis is, of course, greatly expanded. Where the diagnosis is subsequently shown to be multiple sclerosis, initial diplopia is usually due either to an isolated VIth nerve palsy or to internuclear ophthalmoplegia. Many patients referred as possibly having multiple sclerosis complain of fleeting double vision. This occurs with fatigue or on prolonged close work and rapidly clears with rest or even on blinking or rubbing the eyes. Paroxysmal diplopia can occur in multiple sclerosis[211] but has quite different characteristics. The fleeting diplopia described above appears to be due to the effects of fatigue on a latent strabismus.

Vertigo

Vertigo as the initial symptom of multiple sclerosis is indistinguishable from an attack of vestibular neuronitis. The onset is sudden, vertigo is prostrating, greatly aggravated by head movement and accompanied by vomiting. Hearing is not affected. The patient may be almost helpless for a few days. Improvement occurs over the succeeding few weeks and in multiple sclerosis is usually complete. In the more peripheral lesion of vestibular neuronitis, brief vertigo on rapid head movement may persist for many months. At that stage it is possible to demonstrate damage to the vestibular nerve as caloric reactions may be absent on that side, but this test cannot be done during the acute attack and is seldom contemplated after recovery.

Sensory symptoms

Despite the classifications of multiple sclerosis that do not permit the diagnosis on a single episode, to an experienced neurologist the common mode of onset with sensory symptoms is unmistakable. To the inexperienced, it is a frequent source of error.

The patient, usually a young woman, develops 'numbness' of one or both feet. In the course of a few days this spreads to involve the legs, buttocks and perineum and often rises to the waist. There is no disturbance of gait or of sphincter function, although the actual sensation of passing urine or passing a motion may be lost, and vaginal sensation is also abnormal. When examined there is no weakness or change in reflexes and indeed no complete loss of sensation. The patient, struggling to explain unfamiliar symptoms, may say that the doctor's pin feels 'distant' or as if there was something between the pin and her skin. It is not difficult to conclude that the young woman is 'hysterical' and the subsequent recovery, following reassurance and the prescription of a tranquilliser is thought to confirm this diagnosis. Unfortunately this sequence of events is almost pathognomonic of multiple sclerosis.

Surprisingly, it seems that the prodromal sensory symptoms of migraine, undoubtedly relapsing and remitting, can be mistaken for those of multiple sclerosis.[212]

6. NON-ORGANIC SYMPTOMS

Increasing numbers of young people are referred to neurological clinics because they fear that they have developed multiple sclerosis and their medical advisors, who will have had little experience of the disease, are also naturally uncertain of the exact significance of their symptoms. These are an almost stereotyped caricature of the genuine symptoms of multiple sclerosis. The patient, usually a young woman, will complain of 'numbness' or pins and needles, nearly always in the limbs on one side but sometimes bilaterally. These sensations are not, as in multiple sclerosis, persistent, but come and go throughout the day or may be absent for several days together. Accompanying complaints are of dizziness and blurring of vision. The former is not vertigo but a vague feeling of unsteadiness that is not apparent in any disturbance of gait. The visual disturbance is fleeting and relieved by rubbing the eyes. Naturally there are variants, some less easily recognised as the symptoms of anxiety. A complaint of clumsiness, leading to excessive breakage of crockery, is disturbing, but when not accompanied by demonstrable incoordination, does not herald the onset of multiple sclerosis.

The fears that in some way induce these symptoms are fostered by the spread of medical information via the radio, television and women's magazines. The intention is no doubt admirable although the temptation to heighten the interest with controversial statements is not always resisted. One result is that the recipients of this partial knowledge interpret banal symptoms as those of grave disease. Who has not experienced paraesthesiae, dizziness or momentary blurring of vision? To be told that such symptoms, particularly if transitory, are typical of multiple sclerosis, is indeed alarming. One girl when asked why she thought she had multiple sclerosis said that she had looked up pins and needles in her 'health book' and turned up this answer. Thorough examination and firm but understanding reassurance usually lay these anxieties to rest.

Conversion hysteria mimicking multiple sclerosis rather than the much more common paraplegia is rare.

A woman of 35 developed backache for which she was referred to a physiotherapy department, also attended by a number of patients with multiple sclerosis. In a few weeks she developed difficulty in walking that gradually increased until she was confined to a wheelchair. She became incontinent of urine. She was regarded as suffering from multiple sclerosis with particularly severe spasticity in the lower limbs. It was only when she developed total blindness in one eye with a normal pupillary reaction to light that the diagnosis was doubted and she was referred for neurological opinion. The lower limbs were 'paralysed' in the sense of having no useful movement, but were held rigidly extended until her attention was distracted, when they could be flexed with ease. Plantar reflexes were flexor and there were no signs of organic nervous disease.

The acceptance of such cases as hysterical is clouded by the well known hysterical elaboration of organic symptoms that is inexplicably so common in multiple sclerosis.

CONCLUSION

The differential diagnosis of multiple sclerosis obviously covers a large field in clinical neurology and cannot completely be covered in a brief chapter. This chapter has been devoted less to the positive diagnosis of multiple sclerosis than to the recognition of conditions, many with more hope from treatment, that have been mistaken for it. As recorded in Chapter 7, laboratory methods of

diagnosis, while highly sensitive, are not specific for multiple sclerosis and clinical knowledge and judgement are still required for their use and interpretation.

REFERENCES

1. Feinglass E J, Arnett F C, Dorsch C A, Zizic T M, Stevens M B 1976 Neuropsychiatric manifestations of systemic lupus erythematosus: diagnosis, clinical spectrum and the relationship to other features of the disease. Medicine (Baltimore) 55: 323–339
2. Abel T, Gladman D D, Urowitz M B 1980 Neuropsychiatric lupus. Journal of Rheumatology 7: 325–333
3. Johnson R T, Richardson E P 1968 The neurological manifestations of systemic lupus erythematosus. Medicine (Baltimore) 47: 337–369
4. Lim L, Ron M A, Ormerod I E C et al 1988 Psychiatric and neurological manifestations in systemic lupus erythematosus. Quarterly Journal of Medicine 66: 27–38
5. Hutchinson M, Bresnihan B 1983 Neurological lupus erythematosus with tonic seizures simulating multiple sclerosis. Journal of Neurology, Neurosurgery and Psychiatry 46: 583–585
6. Hammondeh M, Kahn M A 1982 Clinical variant of systemic lupus erythematosus resembling multiple sclerosis. Journal of Rheumatology 9: 336–337
7. Cogen M S, Kline L B, Duvall E R 1987 Bilateral internuclear ophthalmoplegia in systemic lupus erythematosus. Journal of Clinical Neuro-Ophthalmology 7: 69–73
8. Jackson G, Miller M, Littlejohn G, Helme R, King R 1986 Bilateral internuclear ophthalmoplegia in systemic lupus erythematosus. Journal of Rheumatology 13: 1151–1162
9. Allen I V, Millar J H D, Kirk J, Shillington R K A 1979 Systemic lupus erythematosus clinically resembling multiple sclerosis and with unusual pathological and ultrastructural features. Journal of Neurology, Neurosurgery and Psychiatry 42: 362–401
10. Penn A S, Rowan A J 1968 Myelopathy in systemic lupus erythematosus. Archives of Neurology 18: 337–376
11. Schwartzberg C, le Goff P, le Menn C 1981 Complications neuro-ophtalmologique de lupus erythémateux disséminé. Semaine des Hôpitaux 57: 1292–1300
12. Hackett E R, Martinez R D, Larson P F, Paddison R M 1974 Optic neuritis in systemic lupus erythematosus. Archives of Neurology 31: 9–11
13. Jabs D A, Mill N R, Newman S A, Johnson M A, Stevens M B 1986 Optic neuropathy in systemic lupus erythematosus. Archives of Ophthalmology 104: 564–568
14. Fulford K W M, Caterall R D, Delhanty J J, Doniach D, Kremer M 1972 A collagen disorder of the nervous system presenting as multiple sclerosis. Brain 95: 373–386
15. Yamamoto M 1986 Recurrent transverse myelitis associated with collagen disease. Journal of Neurology 233: 185–187
16. April R S, Vansonnenberg E 1976 A case of neuromyelitis optica (Devic's syndrome) in systemic lupus erythematosus. Neurology 26: 1066–1070
17. Siekert R G, Clark E C 1955 Neurologic signs and symptoms as early manifestations of systemic lupus erythematosus. Neurology 5: 84–88
18. Hachen H J, Chatraine A 1979 Spinal cord involvement in systemic lupus erythematosus. Paraplegia 17: 337–346
19. Kinney E L, Berdoff R L, Rao N S, Fox L M 1979 Devic's syndrome and systemic lupus erythematosus. A case report with necropsy. Archives of Neurology 36: 643–644
20. Oppenheimer S, Hoffbrand B I 1986 Optic neuritis and myelopathy in systemic lupus erythematosus. Canadian Journal of Neurological Sciences 13: 129–132
21. Wilson W B 1978 Visual-evoked response differentiation of ischaemic optic neuritis from the optic neuritis of multiple sclerosis. American Journal of Ophthalmology 86: 530–535
22. Dutton J J, Burde R M, Klingele T G 1982 Autoimmune retrobulbar optic neuritis. American Journal of Ophthalmology 94: 11–17
23. Kupersmith M J, Burde R M, Warren F A, Klingele T G, Frohman L P, Mitnick H 1988 Autoimmune optic neuropathy: evaluation and treatment. Journal of Neurology, Neurosurgery and Psychiatry 51: 1381–1386
24. Shepherd D I, Downie A W, Best P V 1974 Systemic lupus erythematosus and multiple sclerosis. Archives of Neurology 30: 423
25. Ellis S G, Verity M A 1979 Central nervous system involvement in systemic lupus erythematosus: a review of neuropathologic findings in 57 cases, 1955–1977. Seminars in Arthritis and Rheumatism 8: 212–221
26. Holmes F F, Stubbs D W, Larsen W E 1967 Systemic lupus erythematosus and multiple sclerosis in identical twins. Archives of Internal Medicine 119: 302–304
27. Sloan J B, Berk M A, Gebel H M, Fretzin D F 1987 Multiple sclerosis and systemic lupus erythematosus. Occurrence in two generations of the same family. Archives of Internal Medicine 147: 1317–1320
28. Devos P, Destée A, Prin L, Warot P 1984 Sclérose en plaques et maladie lupique. Revue Neurologique 140: 513–515
29. Singh V K 1962 Detection of antinuclear antibodies in the serum of patients with multiple sclerosis. Immunology Letters 4: 317–319
30. Dore-Duffy P, Donaldson J O, Rothman B L, Zurier R B 1982 Antinuclear antibodies in multiple sclerosis. Archives of Neurology 39: 504–506
31. O'Connor P 1988 Diagnosis of central nervous system lupus. Canadian Journal of Neurological Sciences 15: 257–260
32. Small P, Mass M F, Kohler P F, Harbeck R J 1977 Central nervous system involvement in SLE. Arthritis and Rheumatism 20: 869–878
33. Thompson E J, Johnson M H 1982 Electrophoresis of

CSF proteins. British Journal of Hospital Medicine 28: 600–608

34. Gonzalez-Scarano F, Lisak R P, Bilaniuk L T, Zimmerman R A, Atkins P C, Zweiman B 1978 Cranial computed tomography in the diagnosis of systemic lupus erythematosus. Annals of Neurology 5: 158–165

35. Aisen A M, Gabrielsen T O, McCune W J 1985 Magnetic resonance imaging of systemic lupus erythematosus involving the brain. American Journal of Roentgenology 144: 1027–1031

36. Ormerod I E C, Miller D H, MacDonald W I et al 1987 The role of NMR imaging in the assessment of multiple sclerosis and isolated neurological lesions. A quantitative study. Brain 110: 1579–1616

37. Alexander G/E, Provost T T, Stevens M B, Alexander E L 1981 Sjögren syndrome: central nervous system manifestations. Neurology 31: 1391–1396

38. Alexander E L, Malinow K, Lejewski J E, Jerdan M E, Provost T T, Alexander G E 1986 Primary Sjögren's syndrome with central nervous system disease mimicking multiple sclerosis. Annals of Internal Medicine 104: 323–330

39. Alexander E L, Beall S S, Gordon B et al 1988 Magnetic resonance imaging of cerebral lesions in patients with the Sjögren syndrome. Annals of Internal Medicine 108: 815–823

40. Wise C M, Agudelo C A 1988 Optic neuropathy as an initial manifestation of Sjögren's syndrome. Journal of Rheumatology 15: 799–802

41. Metz L M, Fritzler M J, Seland T P 1988 Sjögren's syndrome infrequently mimics multiple sclerosis. Canadian Journal of Neurological Sciences 15: 198

42. Noseworthy J H, Bass B H, Vandervoort M K et al 1989 The prevalence of primary Sjögren's syndrome in a multiple sclerosis population. Annals of Neurology 25: 195–198

43. Ford R G, Siekert R G 1965 Central nervous system manifestations of periarteritis nodosa. Neurology 15: 114–122

44. Sigal L H 1987 The neurologic presentation of vasculitic and rheumatologic syndromes. A review. Medicine (Baltimore) 66: 157–180

45. Waisburg H, Meloff K L, Buncic R 1974 Polyarteritis nodosa complicated by a multiple sclerosis-like syndrome. Canadian Journal of Neurological Sciences 1: 250–252

46. Schotland D L, Wolf S M, White H H, Dubin H V 1963 Neurologic aspects of Behçet's disease. American Journal of Medicine 34: 544–553

47. Motomura S, Tabira T, Kuroiwa Y 1980 A clinical comparative study of multiple sclerosis and neuro-Behçet's syndrome. Journal of Neurology, Neurosurgery and Psychiatry 43: 210–213

48. Chajek T, Fainaru M 1975 Behçet's disease. Report of 41 cases and review of literature. Medicine (Baltimore) 54: 179–196

49. Pallis C A, Fudge B J 1956 The neurological complications of Behçet's syndrome. Archives of Neurology and Psychiatry 75: 1–14

50. Wadia N, Williams C 1957 Behçet's syndrome with neurological complications. Brain 80: 59–71

51. Evans A D, Pallis C A, Spillane J D 1957 Involvement of the nervous system in Behçet's syndrome. Report of three cases and isolation of virus. Lancet 2: 349–353

52. Bergerin H, Bakouche P, Chaquat D, Nicolle M H, Reignier A, Nick J 1980 L'atteinte du système nerveux central au cours de la maladie de Behçet. Semaine des Hôpitaux 56: 533–538

53. Fadli M E, Yousef M M 1973 Neuro-Behçet's syndrome in the United Arab Republic. European Neurology 9: 76–89

54. Pamir M N, Kansu T, Erbengi A, Zileli T 1981 Papilloedema in Behçet syndrome. Archives of Neurology 38: 643–645

55. O'Duffy J D, Goldstein N P 1976 Neurologic involvement in seven patients with Behçet's syndrome. American Journal of Medicine 61: 170–178

56. Haim S, Gilhar A 1980 Clinical and laboratory criteria for the diagnosis of Behçet's disease. British Journal of Dermatology 102: 361–363

57. Kawakita H, Nishimura M, Satoh Y, Shibata N 1967 Neurological aspects of Behçet's disease. Journal of the Neurological Sciences 5: 417–439

58. Ohta M, Nishitani H, Matsubatra F, Inbe G 1980 Myelin basic protein in spinal fluid from patients with neuro-Behçet's disease. New England Journal of Medicine 302: 1093

59. Fukuyama H, Kameyama M, Nabatame H et al 1987 Magnetic resonance images of neuro-Behçet syndrome show precise brain stem lesions. Report of a case. Acta Neurologica Scandinavica 75: 70–73

60. Martinez J M, Barraquer-Bordas Ll, Ferrer I, Escartin A E, Rosich M, Barrequer-Feu M Ll 1988 Etude anatomo-clinique d'un syndrome de Behçet, avec atteinte du system nerveux central. Revue Neurologique 144: 130–135

61. McArthur J B 1987 Neurologic manifestations of AIDS. Medicine (Baltimore) 66: 407–437

62. Goldstick L, Mandubur T I, Bode R 1985 Spinal cord degeneration in AIDS. Neurology 35: 103–106

63. Petito C K, Navia B A, Cho E-S, Jordon B D, George D C, Price R W 1986 Vacuolar myelopathy pathologically resembling subacute combined degeneration in patients with acquired immunodeficiency syndrome. New England Journal of Medicine 312: 874–879

64. Berger J R, Sheremata W A, Resnick L, Atherton S, Fletcher M A, Norenberg M 1989 Multiple sclerosis-like illness occurring with human immunodeficiency virus infection. Neurology 39: 324–328

65. Vernant J C, Maurs L, Gessain A et al 1987 Endemic tropical spastic paraparesis associated with human T-lymphotropic virus type 1: A clinical and seroepidemiological study of 25 cases. Annals of Neurology 21: 123–130

66. Román G C, Román L N 1988 Tropical spastic paraparesis. A clinical study of 50 patients from Tumaco (Colombia) and review of the worldwide features of the syndrome. Journal of the Neurological Sciences 87: 121–138

67. Bhagavati S, Ehrlich G, Kula R W, Kwok S, Sninsky J, Udani V, Poiesz B J 1988 Detection of human T-cell lymphoma/leukaemia virus type 1 DNA and antigen in spinal fluid and blood of patients with chronic progressive myelopathy. New England Journal of Medicine 318: 1141–1147

68. Newton M, Cruikshank K K, Miller D et al 1987 Antibody to human T-lymphotropic virus type I in

West-Indian-born UK residents with spastic paraparesis. Lancet 1: 415–416

69. Román G C, Sheremata W A 1987 Multiple sclerosis (not tropical spastic paraparesis) in Key West, Florida. Lancet 1: 1199

70. Gessain A, Barin F, Vernant J et al 1985 Antibodies to human T-lymphotropic virus type I in patients with tropical spastic paraparesis. Lancet 2: 407–409

71. Rodgers-Johnson P, Gajdusek D C, Morgan O St C, Zaninovic V, Sarin P S, Graham D S 1985 HTLV-I and HTLV-III antibodies and tropical spastic paraparesis. Lancet 2: 1247–1248

72. Morgen O St C, Montgomery R D, Rodgers-Johnson P 1988 The myelopathies of Jamaica: an unfolding story. Quarterly Journal of Medicine 67: 273–281

73. Jacobson S, Raine C S, Mingioli E S, McFarlin D E 1988 Isolation of an HTLV-I-like retrovirus from patients with tropical spastic paraparesis. Nature 331: 540–543

74. Osame M, Usuka K, Izumo S et al 1986 HTLV-I associated myelopathy, a new clinical entity. Lancet 1: 1031–1032

75. Osame M, Matsumoto M, Usuku K et al 1987 Chronic progressive myelopathy associated with elevated antibodies to human T-lymphotropic virus type I and adult T-cell leukaemia-like cells. Annals of Neurology 21: 117–122

76. Shibasaki H, Endo C, Kuroda Y, Kakigi R, Oda K-I, Komine S-I 1988 Clinical picture of HTLV-I associated myelopathy. Journal of the Neurological Sciences 87: 15–24

77. Román G C, Osame M 1988 Identity of HTLV-I-associated tropical spastic paraparesis and HTLV-I-associated myelopathy. Lancet 1: 651

78. Annunziata P, Fanetti G, Giarratana M, Aucone A M, Guazzi G C 1987 HTLV-I-associated spastic paraparesis in an Italian woman. Lancet 2: 1393–1394

79. Johnson R T, Griffin D E, Aregui A et al 1988 Spastic paraparesis and HTLV-I infection in Peru. Annals of Neurology 23 (suppl): S151–S155

80. Koprowski H, Defreitas E C, Harper M E et al 1985 Multiple sclerosis and human T-cell lymphotropic retroviruses. Nature 318: 154–160

81. Koprowski H, DeFreitas E C 1988 HTLV-I and chronic nervous diseases: present status and a look into the future. Annals of Neurology 23 (suppl): S166–S170

82. Hauser S L, Aubert C, Burks J S et al 1986 Analysis of human T-lymphotropic virus sequences in multiple sclerosis tissue. Nature 322: 176–177

83. Gessain A, Abel L, de-Thé G, Vernant J C, Raverdy P, Guillard A 1986 Lack of HTLV-I and HIV antibodies in patients with multiple sclerosis from France and French West Indies. British Medical Journal 293: 424–425

84. Madden D L, Mundon F K, Tzan N R et al 1988 Antibody to human and simian retroviruses, HTLV-I, HTLV-II, HTLV-IV, STLV-III and SRV-I not increased in patients with multiple sclerosis. Annals of Neurology 23 (suppl): S171–S173

85. Epstein L, Blumberg B, Crowley J et al 1987 Serum antibodies to HTLV-I in human demyelinating disease. Acta Neurologica Scandinavica 75:231–233

86. Kuroda Y, Shibasaki H, Sato H, Okochi K 1987 Incidence of antibodies to HTLV-I is not increased in Japanese MS patients. Neurology 37: 156–158

87. Johnson R T 1987 Myelopathies and retrovirus infections. Annals of Neurology 21: 113–116

88. Delaney P 1977 Neurologic manifestations of sarcoidosis. Annals of Internal Medicine 87: 336–345

89. Day A L, Sypert G W 1976 Spinal cord sarcoidosis. Annals of Neurology 1: 79–85

90. Buge A, Escourolle R, Poisson M, Rancurel G, Gray F 1975 Sarcoidose medullaire. Observation anatomo-clinique. Annales de Médecine Interne (Paris) 126: 11–16

91. Nathan M P R, Chase P H, Elguezabal A, Weinstein M 1976 Spinal cord sarcoidosis. New York State Journal of Medicine 76: 748–752

92. Höök O 1954 Sarcoidosis with involvement of the nervous system. Archives of Neurology and Psychiatry 71: 554–575

93. Matthews W B 1959 Sarcoidosis of the nervous system. British Medical Journal 1: 267–270

94. Matthews W B 1965 Sarcoidosis of the nervous system. Journal of Neurology, Neurosurgery and Psychiatry 28: 23–29

95. Ingestad R, Stigmar G 1971 Sarcoidosis with ocular and hypothalamic pituitary manifestations. Acta Ophthalmologica 49: 1–19

96. Piéron R, Coulaud J M, Debure A, Mafart Y, Lesobre B 1979 Névrite optique et sarcoidose. Semaine des Hôpitaux 55: 137–139

97. Beardsley T L, Brown S V L, Sydnor C F, Grimson B S, Klintworth G K 1984 Eleven cases of sarcoidosis of the optic nerve. American Journal of Ophthalmology 97: 62–77

98. Rush J A 1980 Retrobulbar optic neuritis in sarcoidosis. Annals of Ophthalmology 12: 390–394

99. Graham E M, Ellis C J K, Sanders M D, McDonald W I 1986 Optic neuropathy in sarcoidosis. Journal of Neurology, Neurosurgery and Psychiatry 49: 756–763

100. Kinnman J, Link H 1984 Intrathecal production of oligoclonal IgM and IgG in CNS sarcoid. Acta Neurologica Scandinavica 69: 97–106

101. Christenson R H, Behlmer P, Howard J F, Winfield J B, Silverman L M 1983 Interpretation of cerebrospinal fluid protein assays in various neurologic diseases. Clinical Chemistry 29: 1028–1030

102. Oksanen V, Fyhrquist F, Somer H, Grönhagen-Riska C 1985 Angiotensin converting enzyme in cerebrospinal fluid: a new assay. Neurology 35: 1220–1223

103. Gaines J D, Eckman P B, Remington J S 1970 Low CSF glucose level in sarcoidosis involving the central nervous system. Archives of Internal Medicine 125: 333–336

104. Bradstreet C M P, Dighero M W, Mitchell D N 1976 The Kveim test: analysis of results using Colindale (K12) materials. Annals of the New York Academy of Science 278: 681–686

105. Kendall B E, Jatler G L F 1978 Radiological findings in neurosarcoidosis. British Journal of Radiology 51: 81–92

106. Ho S U, Berenberg R A, Kim K S, Dal Canto M C 1979 Sarcoid encephalopathy with diffuse inflammation and focal hydrocephalus shown by sequential CT. Neurology 29: 1161–1656

107. Post M J D, Quencer R M, Tabli S Z 1962 CT demonstration of sarcoid of the optic nerve, frontal lobes and falx cerebri: case report and literature review. American Journal of Neuroradiology 5: 523–529

108. Matthews W B 1986 Neurologic manifestations of sarcoidosis. In: Asbury A K, McKhann G M, McDonald W I (eds) Diseases of the nervous system. W B Saunders, Philadelphia, PP 1563–1570

109. Hayes W S, Sherman J L, Stern B J, Citrin C M, Pulaski P D 1987 MR and CT evaluation of intracranial sarcoidosis. American Journal of Roentgenology 149: 1043–1049

110. Miller H G, Stanton J B, Gibbons J L 1957 Acute disseminated encephalomyelitis and related syndromes. British Medical Journal 1: 668–672

111. Pasternak J F, de Vivo D C, Prensky A L 1980 Steroid-responsive encephalomyelitis in childhood. Neurology 30: 41–486

112. Lumsden C E, 1970 In: Vinken P J, Bruyn G W (eds) Handbook of clinical neurology, Vol 9. North Holland, Amsterdam, P 305

113. Alcock N S, Hoffman H L 1962 Recurrent encephalomyelitis in childhood. Archives of Disease in Childhood 37: 40–44

114. Poser C M, Roman G, Emery E S 1978 Recurrent disseminated vasculomyelinopathy. Archives of Neurology 35: 166–170

115. Yahr M D, Lobo-Antunes J 1972 Relapsing encephalomyelitis following the use of influenza vaccine. Archives of Neurology 27: 182–183

116. Saito H, Endo M, Takase S, Itahara K 1980 Acute disseminated encephalomyelitis after influenza vaccination. Archives of Neurology 37: 564–566

117. Cloys D E, Netsky M G 1970 Neuromyelitis optica. In: Vinken P J, Bruyn G W (eds) Handbook of clinical neurology, Vol 9. North Holland, Amsterdam, pp 426–436

118. McAlpine D 1938 Familial neuromyelitis optica: its occurrence in identical twins. Brain 61: 430–448

119. Ferraro A 1944 Pathology of demyelinating diseases as an allergic reaction of the brain. Archives of Neurology and Psychiatry 52: 443–483

120. Lumsden C E 1951 Fundamental problems in the pathology of multiple sclerosis and allied demyelinating diseases. British Medical Journal 1: 1035–1043

121. Okinaka S, McAlpine D, Miyagawa K et al 1960 Multiple sclerosis in northern and southern Japan. World Neurology 1: 22–42

122. Stansbury F C 1950 Neuromyelitis optica (Devic's disease). Archives of Ophthalmology 42: 292–335 and 465–501

123. Shibasaki H, Kuroiwa Y 1969 Statistical analysis of multiple sclerosis and neuromyelitis optica based on autopsied cases in Japan. Folia Psychiatrica et Neurologica Japonica 23: 1–10

124. Pachner A R, Steere A C 1985 The triad of neurologic manifestations of Lyme disease: meningitis, cranial neuritis and radiculoneuritis. Neurology 35: 47–53

125. Bateman D E, White J E, Elrington G, Lawton N F, Muhlemann M F, Greenwood R J 1987 Three Further cases of Lyme disease. British Medical Journal 294: 548–549

126. Schechter S L 1986 Lyme disease associated with optic neuropathy. American Journal of Medicine 81: 143–145

127. Rouseau J J, Lust C, Zangerle P F, Bigaignon G 1986 Acute transverse myelitis as presenting symptom of Lyme disease. Lancet 2: 1222–1223

128. Kohler J, Kasper J, Kern U, Thoden U, Rehse-Küpper B 1986 Borrelia encephalomyelitis. Lancet 2: 35

129. Weder B, Wiedersheim P, Matter L, Steck A, Otto F 1987 Chronic progressive neurological involvement in Borrelia burgdorferi infection. Journal of Neurology 234: 40–43

130. Reik L, Burgdorfer W, Donaldson J O 1986 Neurologic abnormalities in Lyme disease without erythema chronicum migrans. American Journal of Medicine 81: 73–78

131. Benoit P, Douron E, Destel A, Warot P 1986 Spirochaetes and Lyme disease. Lancet 2: 1223

132. Pachner A R, Steere A C 1986 CNS manifestations of third stage Lyme disease. Zentralblatt für Bakteriologie, Mikrobiologie und Hygiene. Series A. 263: 301–306

133. Reik L, Smith L, Khan A, Nelson W 1985 Demyelinating encephalopathy in Lyme disease. Neurology 35: 267–269

134. Kohler J, Kern U, Kasper J, Rhese-Küpper B, Thoden U 1988 Chronic central nervous system involvement in Lyme borreliosis. Neurology 38: 863–867

135. Henriksson A, Link H, Cruz M, Stiemstedt G 1986 Immunoglobulin abnormalities in the cerebrospinal fluid and blood over the course of lymphocytic meningoradiculitis (Bannwarth's syndrome) Annals of Neurology 20: 337–345

136. Depré A, Sindic C J M, Bukasa K, Bigaignon G, Laterre C 1988 Formes encéphalomyélitiques de l'infection à Borrelia burgdorferi. Revue Neurologique 144: 416–420

137. Muhlemann M F, Wright D J M 1987 The emerging pattern of Lyme disease in the United Kingdom and Irish Republic. Lancet 1: 260–262

138. Fumarola D 1986 Multiple sclerosis and Borrelia burgdorferi. Lancet 2: 575

139. Muhlemann M F, Markby D P, Wright D J M 1986 Multiple sclerosis associated with sinusitis. Lancet 1: 1097

140. Schmutzhardt E, Pohl P, Stanek G 1988 Borrelia burgdorferi antibodies in patients with relapsing/remitting form and chronic progressive form of multiple sclerosis. Journal of Neurology, Neurosurgery and Psychiatry 51: 1215–1218

141. Halperin J J, Luft B J, Anand A K et al 1989 Lyme neuroborreliosis: central nervous system manifestations. Neurology 39: 753–759

142. Dattwyler R J, Halperin J J, Volkman D J, Luft B J 1988 Treatment of late Lyme borreliosis — randomised comparison of ceftriaxone and penicillin. Lancet 1: 1191–1194

143. Sobue I, Ando K, Iida M, Takayanaki T, Yamamura Y, Matsuoka Y 1971 Myeloneuropathy with abdominal disorders in Japan. A clinical study of 752 cases. Neurology 21: 168–173

144. Tsubaki T, Honma Y, Hoshi M 1971 Neurological syndrome associated with clioquinol. Lancet 1: 696–697

145. Ricoy J R, Ortega A, Cabello A 1982 Subacute myelo-optic neuropathy (SMON) First neuro-pathological report outside Japan. Journal of the Neurological Sciences 53: 241–251

146. Pruitt A A, Rubin R H, Karchmer A W, Duncan G W 1978 Neurologic complications of bacterial endocarditis. Medicine (Baltimore) 57: 329–343

147. Wolman L, Bradshaw P 1967 Spinal cord embolism. Journal of Neurology, Neurosurgery and Psychiatry 30: 446–454

148. Albers G W, Avalos S M, Weinrich M 1987 Left ventricular tumour masquerading as multiple sclerosis. Archives of Neurology 44: 779–780

149. Roström B, Link H 1981 Oligoclonal immunoglobulins in cerebrospinal fIuid in acute cerebrovascular disease. Neurology 31: 590–596

150. Thygesen P (ed) 1953 The course of multiple sclerosis: a close-up of 105 attacks. Rosenkilde and Baggen, Copenhagen

151. Graveson G S 1950 Syphilitic optic neuritis. Journal of Neurology, Neurosurgery and Psychiatry 13: 216–224

152. Lorentzen S E 1967 Syphilitic optic neuritis. Acta Ophthalmologica 45: 769–772

153. Brain W R, Henson R A 1958 Neurological syndromes associated with carcinoma. The carcinomatous neuromyopathies. Lancet 2: 971–974

154. Brain W R, Wilkinson M 1965 Subacute cerebellar degeneration associated with neoplasms. Brain 88: 465–478

155. Boghen D, Sebag M, Michaud J 1988 Paraneoplastic optic neuritis and encephalomyelitis. Report of a case. Archives of Neurology 45: 353–356

156. Wartenberg R 1958 Neuritis, sensory neuritis, neuralgia. Oxford University Press, New York, pp 233–247

157. Matthews W B, Esiri M 1983 The migrant sensory neuritis of Wartenberg. Journal of Neurology, Neursurgery and Psychiatry 46: 1–4

158. Ferguson F R, Critchley M 1929 A clinical study of an heredo-familial disease resembling disseminated sclerosis. Brain 52: 203–225

159. Bruyn G W, Went L N 1964 A sex-linked heredo-degenerative neurological disorder, associated with Leber's optic atrophy. Journal of the Neurological Sciences 1: 59–80

160. Bickerstaff E R 1950 Hereditary spastic paraplegia. Journal of Neurology, Neurosurgery and Psychiatry 13: 134–145

161. Wilson J 1963 Leber's hereditary optic atrophy — some clinical and aetiological considerations. Brain 86: 347–362

162. Pedersen L, Trojaborg W 1981 Visual, auditory and somatosensory pathway involvement in hereditary cerebellar ataxia, Friedreich's ataxia and familial spastic paraplegia. Electroencephalography and Clinical Neurophysiology 52: 283–297

163. Gautier-Smith P C 1973 Lhermitte's sign in subacute combined degeneration of the spinal cord. Journal of Neurology, Neurosurgery and Psychiatry 36: 861–863

164. Fine E J, Hallett M 1980 Neurophysiological study of subacute combined degeneration. Journal of the Neurological Sciences 45: 331–336

165. Moser H W 1985 In: Vinken P J, Bruyn G W, Klawans H L, Koetsier J C (eds) Handbook of clinical neurology, Vol 47. Elsevier, Amsterdam, pp 583–604

166. Noetzel M J, Landau W M, Moser H W 1987 Adrenoleukodystrophy carrier state presenting as a chronic nonprogressive spinal cord disorder. Archives of Neurology 44: 566–567

167. Dooley J M, Wright B A 1985 Adrenoleukodystrophy mimicking multiple sclerosis. Canadian Journal of Neurological Sciences 12: 73–74

168. Eldridge R, Anayiotos C P, Schlesinger S et al 1984 Hereditary adult-onset leukodystrophy simulating chronic progressive multiple sclerosis. New England Journal of Medicine 311: 948–953

169. Bickerstaff E R, Small J M, Guest I A 1958 The relapsing course of certain meningiomas in relation to pregnancy and menstruation. Journal of Neurology, Neurosurgery and Psychiatry 21: 89–91

170. Martinez R, Marcos M L, Figueras A, Vaquiero J 1984 Estrogen and progesterone receptors in intracranial tumours. Clinical Neuropharmacology 7: 320–324

171. Poisson M 1984 Sex hormone receptors in human meningiomas. Clinical Neuropharmacology 7: 338–341

172. Sarkari N B S, Bickerstaff E R 1969 Relapses and remissions in brain stem tumours. British Medical Journal 2: 21–23

173. Cohen L, Macrae D 1962 Tumors in the region of the foramen magnum. Journal of Neurosurgery 19: 462–469

174. Rosenbluth P R, Lichtenstein B W 1960 Pearly tumor (epidermoid cholesteatoma) of the brain. Clinicopathological study of two cases. Journal of Neurosurgery 17: 35–42

175. Ruff R L, Petito C K, Rawlinson D G 1979 Primary cerebral lymphoma mimicking multiple sclerosis. Archives of Neurology 36: 598

176. Stahl S M, Johnson K P, Malamud N 1980 The clinical and pathological spectrum of brainstem vascular malformations. Long term course simulates multiple sclerosis. Archives of Neurology 37: 25–29

177. Heirons R 1953 Brain-stem angioma confirmed by arteriography. Relapsing symptoms and signs strongly suggestive of disseminated sclerosis. Proceedings of the Royal Society of Medicine 46: 195–196

178. Teilman K 1953 Hemangiomas of the pons. Archives of Neurology and Psychiatry 69: 208–223

179. Sadeh M, Shacked I, Rappaport Z H, Tadmor R 1982 Surgical extirpation of a venous angioma of the medulla oblongata simulating multiple sclerosis. Surgical Neurology 17: 334–335

180. Lehman R A W, Fieger H G 1978 Arachnoid cyst producing recurrent neurological disturbances. Surgical Neurology 10: 134–136

181. Aminoff M J, Logue V 1974 Clinical features of spinal vascular malformations. Brain 97: 197–210

182. Dhopesh V P, Weinstein J D 1977 Spinal arteriovenous malformation simulating multiple sclerosis: importance of early diagnosis. Disease of the Nervous System 38: 848–851

183. Newman N J D 1958 Spinal angioma with symptoms in pregnancy. Journal of Neurology, Neurosurgery and Psychiatry 21: 38–41

184. Schrader A, Weise H 1951 Kasuistiche Beitrag zur Differentialdiagnose zwischen spinaler Erscheinungsform der multiplen Sklerose und Rückensmarkstumor. Nervenarzt 22: 447–451

185. Hirschbiegel H 1967 Remittierende Verläufe bei Spinaltumoren. Deutsches Zeitschrift für Nervenheilkunde 190: 74–82

186. Reisner H 1962 Spinales Lipom unter dem Bild einen multiplen Sklerose. Wiener Zeitschrift für Nervenheilkunde 20: 157–162

187. Shephard R H, Wadia N H 1956 Some observations on atypical features in acoustic neuroma. Brain 79: 282–318

188. Leon-Sotomayor L A 1974 Posterior fossa tumor mimicking multiple sclerosis. Southern Medical Journal 67: 1485–1488

189. McAlpine D (ed) 1972 Multiple sclerosis: a reappraisal, 2nd edn. Churchill Livingstone, Edinburgh, p 234.

190. Poser S, Hermann–Gremmels I, Wikström J, Poser W 1978 Clinical features of the spinal form of multiple sclerosis. Acta Neurologica Scandinavica 57: 151–158

191. Conrad B, Mergner T 1979 High cervical neurinoma (C1/C2) diagnosed falsely as multiple sclerosis because of trigeminal neuralgia. Archiv für Psychiatrie und Nervenkrankheiten 227: 33–37

192. Brain W R, Wilkinson M 1957 The association of cervical spondylosis and disseminated sclerosis. Brain 80: 456–478

193. Oppenheimer D 1978 The cervical cord in multiple sclerosis. Neuropathology and Applied Neurobiology 4: 151–162

194. McAlpine D 1955 The clinician and the problem of multiple sclerosis. Lancet 1: 1033–1038

195. Spillane J D, Pallis C, Jones A M 1957 Developmental abnormalities in the region of the foramen magnum. Brain 80: 11–48

196. Banerji N K, Miller J H D 1974 Chiari malformation presenting in adult life. Brain 97: 157–168

197. Mohr P D, Strang F A, Sambrook M A, Boddie H G 1977 The clinical and surgical features in 40 patients with primary cerebellar ectopia (adult Chiari malformation). Quarterly Journal of Medicine 46: 85–96

198. McDonald W I, Halliday A M 1977 Diagnosis and classification of multiple sclerosis. British Medical Bulletin 33: 4–8

199. Pedersen R A, Troost B T, Abel L A, Zorub D 1980 Intermittent downbeat nystagmus and oscillopsia reversed by suboccipital craniectomy. Neurology 30: 1239–1242

200. Wolpert S M, Anderson M, Scott R M, Kwan E S K, Runge V M 1987 Chiari II malformation: MR imaging evaluation. American Journal of Roentgenology 149: 1033–1042

201. Perkin G D, Rose F C 1979 Optic neuritis and its differential diagnosis. Oxford University Press, Oxford

202. Stendahl-Brodin L, Möller E, Link H 1978 Hereditary optic atrophy with probable association with a specific haplotype. Journal of the Neurological Sciences 38: 11–21

203. Nikoskelainen E, Sogg R L, Rosenthal A R, Friberg T R, Dorfman L J 1977 The early phase in Leber hereditary optic atrophy. Archives of Ophthalmology 95: 969–978

204. Lawson-Smith J, Hoyt W F, Susac J D 1973 Ocular fundus in acute Leber optic neuropathy. Archives of Ophthalmology 90: 349–354

205. Krauscher M F, Miller E M 1982 Central serous choroidoretinopathy misdiagnosed as a manifestation of multiple sclerosis. Annals of Ophthalmology 14: 215–218

206. Parmley V C, Schiffman J S, Maitland C G, Miller N R, Dreyer R F, Hoyt W F 1987 Does neuroretinitis rule out multiple sclerosis? Archives of Neurology 44: 1045–1048

207. Bogen D R, Glaser J S 1975 Ischaemic optic neuropathy. The clinical profile and natural history. Brain 98: 689–708

208. Vighetto A, Davenas C, Bret P, Aimard G 1985 Pseudo-névrite optique révélatrice de craniopharyngiome (2 cas). Revue Neurologique 142: 490–492

209. Kahana E, Leibowitz U, Fishback N, Alter M 1973 Slowly progressive and acute visual impairment in multiple sclerosis. Neurology 23: 729–733

210. Ormerod I E C, McDonald W I 1984 Multiple sclerosis presenting with progressive visual failure. Journal of Neurology, Neurosurgery and Psychiatry 47: 943–946

211. Osterman P O Westerberg C-E 1975 Paroxysmal attacks in multiple sclerosis. Brain 98: 189–202

212. Murray T J, Murray S J 1984 Characteristics of patients found not to have multiple sclerosis. Canadian Medical Association Journal 131: 336–337

7. Laboratory diagnosis

Despite many recent advances in laboratory methods, the diagnosis of multiple sclerosis is made primarily on clinical grounds. At the very least suspicion must be aroused by suggestive symptoms or signs before the indication for sophisticated diagnostic methods is recognised. The astonishing variability of the course and symptomatology of the disease are potent causes of doubt and error and there is a clear need for diagnostic criteria. Before discussing the merits of the various schemes proposed it is useful to consider more precisely the purposes they were devised to serve.

Apart from the intrinsic desirability of knowing what is wrong with one's patients there are a number of reasons why diagnostic criteria may be useful. Tourtellotte[1] stated that there were seven 'goals' for the use of criteria:

1. dialogue with the patient
2. medical records
3. description of course of the disease
4. epidemiology
5. correlation with laboratory tests
6. the study of other diseases occurring with multiple sclerosis
7. the study of treatment.

The 'dialogue with the patient' may be taken to mean the clinical management of the individual case. Among the obvious reasons for establishing an assured diagnosis of multiple sclerosis is that of not overlooking some more tractable condition. For this purpose, tabulated criteria are less appropriate than Kurtzke's[2] 'multiple sclerosis is what a good clinician would call multiple sclerosis'.

Tourtellotte's goals 2 and 6, while certainly desirable, appear less intrinsically important.

Diagnostic criteria are, however, indispensible for epidemiological investigation and for following the course of the disease. For these purposes the recognition of different categories of diagnostic certainty is useful and even essential if early cases are to be included. The correlation with the results of laboratory investigations, Tourtellotte's fifth goal, also requires an established range of diagnostic categories.

The requirements for therapeutic trials are different as it is highly undesirable further to confuse this difficult field by treating patients in whom there is any doubt of the diagnosis.

DIAGNOSTIC CATEGORIES

The first scheme to receive wide acceptance was that of Allison and Millar.[3] Three categories were recognised.

1. Early disseminated sclerosis comprised patients with few or no physical signs but with a recent history of remitting symptoms of the kind commonly associated with the onset of the disease. Inclusion in this category would clearly be greatly dependent on the experience of the observer in interpreting a history of such symptoms as transient paraesthesiae, numbness, diplopia and urinary frequency in the absence of supporting physical signs. The number of relapses and remissions required was not stated.

2. Probable disseminated sclerosis. These patients had some physical disability, often a remitting course and physical signs indicating multiple lesions.

3. Possible disseminated sclerosis. Here the findings suggested the diagnosis and no other

cause could be found but the course was progressive or static and there was no definite evidence of multiple lesions. From the example given, this category included progressive spastic paraparesis.

This classification was later amplified and improved.[4] The first category was called 'early, probable and latent'. At least one physical sign 'typical of multiple sclerosis' was required but documentary evidence was accepted for the presence of such signs at an earlier stage in remitting disease. The probable category was unchanged except that an alteration in the colloidal gold curve or a negative myelogram was required in patients in whom the history was unreliable. The possible category remained essentially the same. This method was used unmodified in a number of epidemiological studies. In the survey in Iceland,[5] failure to find any abnormal physical signs or documentary evidence of such signs was held to exclude patients from the early, probable and latent class. Leibowitz & Alter[6] further elaborated this scheme. In the early, probable and latent category an important gloss was the acceptance of patients as probable multiple sclerosis after one attack provided that there was evidence of multiple lesions. The latent cases were those with a history suggesting scattered lesions confirmed by previous examination.

Although seldom mentioned, McAlpine, in previous editions of this book, described two schemes of diagnostic categorisation. The first[7] closely resembled that of Allison & Millar.[3] In the latent probable group he emphasised that the duration of the disease was irrelevant. It is not clear whether this implied that a single episode was sufficient for inclusion. The probable group was scarcely altered. In possible multiple sclerosis physical signs indicative of white matter disease were required.

This classification and its variants has retained its usefulness, particularly under field conditions[6] in which a large scale population survey is being undertaken. It realistically acknowledges the possibility of error by not accepting a definite diagnosis of multiple sclerosis on clinical grounds but only when confirmed at autopsy. This is of no importance as the probable category can readily be equated with the clinically definite group in other classifications. Little attention is paid to the results of laboratory investigation except in the possible group with progressive disease. The method has been found to be insufficiently precise for the detailed study of the course of the disease, the comparison with the results of laboratory diagnostic methods and, in particular, in therapeutic trials.

McAlpine's far better known classification[8] was derived from study of his own large series of patients. As these criteria have been very widely used, they are given here in full.

Definite

1. A history of an acute retrobulbar neuritis or of an episode of paraesthesiae, motor weakness, double vision, unsteadiness in walking or other symptom known to occur in multiple sclerosis which tended to improve or clear up, followed by one or more relapses during the course of years with, in addition, the presence of pyramidal and other signs indicative of multiple lesions in the central nervous system when the patient was first or subsequently seen. In mild cases these signs may remain minimal for many years.

2. A gradual onset of a paraplegia later followed by relapses and signs indicative of disease in brainstem, cerebrum or optic nerve.

Probable

1. During the original attack, clinical evidence of multiple lesions which, at the time, suggested the probability or possibility of multiple sclerosis, followed by a good recovery. During a lengthy follow-up, relative or complete absence of fresh symptoms after the first year but with a tendency to variability in pyramidal and other signs originally present or the occasional late appearance of an extensor plantar response, nystagmus, tremor or temporal pallor of a disc.

2. A history of one or more attacks of acute retrobulbar neuritis accompanied or followed by pyramidal or other signs, usually mild in degree. Subsequently no clinical evidence of relapse.

Possible

1. A history similar to that described under

Probable (1) but with unusual features or a paucity of signs, or insufficient follow-up information.

2. A history of a progressive paraplegia usually in early middle age without evidence of relapse or remission or of a lesion outside the spinal cord, appropriate investigations, including myelography, having excluded other causes of progressive paraplegia such as cervical spondylosis, spinal cord tumour and motor neurone disease.

Note: when doubt existed as to the diagnosis, attention was paid to the following:

1. the age of the patient
2. a history of the disease in another member of the family
3. the findings in the cerebrospinal fluid. No case of retrobulbar neuritis was included in this series, unless it was accompanied or followed by other neurological signs.

Careful perusal, which it may be doubted is universal, shows that there are a number of inevitable ambiguities. The 'minimal' signs permitted in mild but definite multiple sclerosis could be misinterpreted by the inexperienced. Every neurologist will be familiar with the failure to confirm reported signs such as slight inco-ordination, absent abdominal reflexes, impaired sensation and dubious plantar reflexes. It is the probable category as defined that presents the most difficulty. In both subtypes the pattern is that of a single attack with evidence of multiple lesions, followed by remission and virtual freedom from relapse during a 'lengthy' follow-up. Such cases are certainly encountered but are relatively infrequent and this is reflected by the small number of patients categorised as probable in most publications using this classification. The possible category includes very similar cases but with atypical features or insufficient follow-up. Progressive paraplegia without evidence of multiple lesions also comes under this heading. Factors such as the age of the patient, a positive family history and the findings in the CSF were considered if there was doubt on the history and physical signs.

This scheme was well suited to its original purpose as, from the nature of the study, follow-up confirmation, on which a great deal depended, was always available. It has proved rather less suitable for the assessment of the value of laboratory diagnostic methods or of therapeutic benefit. It may be suspected that many of those who have classified their patients 'according to McAlpine' in such trials have been tempted to interpret his criteria rather more liberally.

The diagnostic criteria laid down by Schumacher et al[9] were designed exclusively for use in therapeutic trials, although they have since been used in other contexts. They are concerned solely with identifying the clinically definite case. The six criteria may be summarised. Objective abnormalities on neurological examination are essential and symptoms alone are insufficient for diagnosis. There must be evidence on examination or in the history of two or more separate lesions of the CNS. This requirement is illustrated by the common problem of the pale optic disc. This should not be accepted as evidence of a separate lesion unless 'beyond the average range' and accompanied by visual impairment or a history of retrobulbar neuritis. The objective signs must be predominantly those of white matter involvement, i.e. the long motor and sensory tracts, particularly the posterior columns, the brainstem and cerebellum, with little evidence of lower motor neurone or peripheral nerve lesions. The requirement for cerebral and cerebellar 'sub-cortical' lesions might prove clinically taxing.

At least two episodes must have occurred separated by at least a month and lasting at least 24 hours. These arbitrary limits are a sensible attempt to exclude trivial variations in severity, not, it is thought, indicating a definite relapse. If the disease is progressive, deterioration must have persisted for at least six months. Age limits of onset are set as between 10 and 50 years. No better explanation for the symptoms and signs must be apparent to a physician 'competent in clinical neurology'. At the time (1965) it was not thought that any laboratory test was useful in the selection of cases for inclusion in a therapeutic trial, but minimum routine laboratory investigations were demanded, including examination of the CSF.

The authors of these relatively strict criteria recognised that some patients with evident multiple sclerosis would be excluded but insisted that for their purpose, definition should incline to a conservative view. The approval of this classification at the International Symposium at Göteborg in 1972[10] appeared to include its use in other contexts in which categories of less definite diagnostic grades might be essential. The Schumacher criteria are not adequate for studying the epidemiology or natural history of multiple sclerosis, nor were they designed for these purposes.

McDonald & Halliday[11] accepted the Schumacher criteria for clinically definite multiple sclerosis with the exception that progressive cases are excluded. They made an additional proviso that the history should extend for at least a year. The early probable or latent category included a single episode with evidence of multiple lesions, but excluded cases 'suggestive of acute disseminated encephalomyelitis'. A remitting and relapsing course with evidence of a single lesion was also included under this heading. The progressive probable category consisted of those with progressive paraplegia plus evidence of separate lesions, while in the progressive possible group there is evidence of only a single lesion. The suspected group is rather obscurely outlined but appears to include symptoms without physical signs and recurrent optic neuritis with one additional episode 'not involving the optic nerve but without evidence of lesions outside the eye'.

This classification has a number of advantages, particularly in a more rational handling of the case of progressive paraplegia that did not fit well into McAlpine's possible category. Exactly what comprises evidence of separate lesions, particularly with regard to the results of laboratory tests, will be referred to later.

Rose et al[12] proposed a simpler scheme. Clinically definite multiple sclerosis was as in Schumacher's criteria, including progression for six months or more. Probable multiple sclerosis consisted either of a relapsing and remitting history but with 'only one neurologic sign commonly associated with multiple sclerosis' or a single bout with multifocal signs and good recovery followed by 'variable symptoms and signs', thus closely resembling McAlpine's probable category.

Bauer,[13] in an attempt to resolve these difficulties, consulted many neurologists on desirable diagnostic criteria, and integrated their suggestions into a new classification. The clinically definite group is much as in the Schumacher criteria except that physical signs need only be documented rather than present when examined. Characteristic CSF changes are also required, including mononuclear pleocytosis, increase in gamma globulins or oligoclonal bands in the gamma globulin range and evidence of IgG synthesis within the central nervous system. It is not stated whether all these changes are obligatory for inclusion in the clinically definite category. If not, they should be used only as supportive evidence. If they are intended to be rigid criteria they cannot be complied with. For example, in many otherwise clinically definite and subsequently proven cases, pleocytosis in the CSF has not been found. Adherence to similar criteria leads to clinically definite cases being downgraded to the probable category.[14]

The clinically probable group closely resembles that of McAlpine but includes pathological changes in the CSF although the full profile as in the definite cases is not demanded. In the clinically possible group, again closely resembling McAlpine's scheme, no CSF changes are required. In both the latter categories, first attacks are included but are not clearly defined except that, for the first time in any classification, monosymptomatic retrobulbar neuritis is classified as multiple sclerosis, clinically possible.

The adoption of even generally agreed clinical criteria still appears remote. In the study of multiple sclerosis in Gothenburg[15] a fourstage multiple sclerosis grading was adopted:

1. possible but improbable
2. possible but doubtful
3. probable but not quite convincing
4. probable beyond doubt.

These were not closely defined and intermediate categories were recognised. In examples given, retrobulbar neuritis, acute reversible central vestibular syndromes and acute reversible myelopathy are graded 2–3. Eventually, three categories were accepted.

a. diagnosis convincing
b. at least probable
c. at least possible.

The frank acknowledgement that there is no sharp delineation between categories is refreshing and the classification eventually adopted closely approaches bedside diagnostic methods. As a result, however, it is difficult to compare the reports from Gothenburg with those in other investigations.

The elaboration of laboratory methods of diagnosis inevitably demanded revision of diagnostic categories to include the results. In what are some times referred to as the Washington criteria,[16] the attempt was made to combine clinical and laboratory findings into a coherent system. Evidence on earlier attacks was admitted if 'reliable'. Four main categories were defined, with a number of subdivisions. The 'clinically definite' category required two attacks, separated in time and location and signs on examination of two distinct lesions or (and here is the innovation) clinical signs of a single lesion and paraclinical evidence of the second. This evidence might be derived from a variety of sources: recording of evoked potentials, imaging, investigation of bladder function or even the hot bath test. A new category, for which oligoclonal IgG in the CSF or increased IgG synthesis was required, was defined as 'laboratory supported definite' multiple sclerosis, again divided into those with two attacks and signs of one lesion, one attack and signs of two lesions, or one attack and signs of one lesion and paraclinical evidence of a second. The 'clinically probable' categories were defined identically except that the CSF changes were not required. The 'laboratory supported probable' category required two attacks and characteristic CSF changes in the absence of clinical signs of disease. It is, of course, common enough to suspect the diagnosis of multiple sclerosis in the absence of physical signs and later to be proved correct, but as a diagnostic category this appears unsafe.

It is clear that much depends on the quality of evidence of paraclinical test abnormality that can be accepted. Kurtzke[17] in a wide-ranging critique of diagnostic criteria, in which he somehow avoided all mention of the still popular McAlpine system, emphasised the importance of the specificity of laboratory tests. In many instances this is incompletely known but is unlikely to approach 100% closely. Kurtzke was particularly disturbed by the suggestion of a separate category of MRI supported definite multiple sclerosis[18] and

preferred to describe the discrete lesions seen on scans as unidentified bright objects or UBOs in preference to their recent acceptance as plaques. The specificity of individual diagnostic tests is discussed below but it should be remembered that the CSF changes that form evidence of laboratory-supported definite multiple sclerosis may occur in a number of conditions easily mistaken for multiple sclerosis: tropical spastic paraparesis, Lyme disease, neurosyphilis, sarcoidosis and systemic lupus (see Ch 6).

Kurtzke[17] also drew attention to the artificiality inherent in claims that using a given diagnostic test increases the proportion of patients in the definite category, when abnormality in the test is used to define the category. This may be exemplified by a study[19] of 89 patients in various diagnostic categories of multiple sclerosis. Using McAlpine's criteria, 27% were classified as definite cases, while the acceptance of electrophysiological evidence of multiple lesions increased this proportion to 72%, but only because the definition of the category had been altered.

The value of diagnostic criteria would be greatly increased if it was known that they can be consistently applied. In descriptions of epidemiology it is sometimes stated that the clinicians involved discussed the cases and decided on the diagnostic category. It would have been illuminating if they had initially reached separate assessments and published the result as there seems to have been no systematic report on the reliability of the diagnostic criteria in action.

LABORATORY DIAGNOSTIC METHODS

The value of a laboratory or non-clinical diagnostic method in multiple sclerosis should be established by necessarily protracted stages. Sensitivity must be shown by a positive or abnormal result in a high proportion of clinically definite cases. Ideally this should be confirmed by histological proof but the course of multiple sclerosis is lengthy and the autopsy rate is low. Evaluation must therefore rest on clinical findings. A positive laboratory test in a clinically definite case is reassuring to the clinician but can scarcely be said to be of diagnostic value and the multiplication of reports all showing approximately the same proportion of abnormal results in the definite category is scarcely contributory. The test is then naturally used in patients in the less certain diagnostic categories and, in general, a smaller proportion of positive results is obtained. This may be interpreted as indicating either that the diagnosis is wrong in many of these patients or that the test in question is positive in a smaller proportion of early cases and is therefore of limited diagnostic use. It is, of course, in the probable, possible, latent and suspect categories that a diagnostic test is needed. The logical step is therefore to follow the patients in these categories to determine whether or not they develop clinically definite multiple sclerosis. Many reports include a reference to the necessity for such follow-up but few results are recorded. The patients in whom the outcome would be of particular interest are peculiarly difficult to follow. They are mostly young adults, far more mobile than their elders. Many will have had a single episode of neurological symptoms with full recovery and without any intimation that a diagnosis of multiple sclerosis has even been considered. The relapse rate, even in the first few years of the disease, averages around 0.5 per year, so that follow-up must be prolonged. Despite these difficulties, this type of investigation is essential if laboratory diagnostic methods are to be shown to be of value at the point where diagnostic help is needed. The specificity of a positive result, the proportion of all those reacting positively who actually have the disease, is more difficult to determine and, with increasing experience, estimates generally decline.

The cerebrospinal fluid

Changes in the CSF are described in Chapter 11.

EVOKED POTENTIALS

Electronic averaging has permitted the recording of low amplitude potentials evoked by many forms of sensory stimulus. The first application of these techniques in multiple sclerosis appears to have been that of Namerow[20] who examined the scalp-recorded somatosensory evoked potential (SEP) following electrical stimulation of nerve trunks and related prolonged latencies observed to differing degrees of sensory loss. The use of evoked potentials (EP) in diagnosis dates from the work of Halliday et al on visual EP (VEP).[21,22] They showed that the use of a form of stimulus different from the light flash that had been tried before would produce consistent results. The stimulus was the now familiar pattern reversal, a chequerboard of black and white that alternates the width of one square at regular intervals, usually two per second. The actual stimulus appears to be the edges of the squares. By this means they were able to show that the latency of the most conveniently measured component of the visual evoked potential was prolonged in patients who had experienced an attack of optic neuritis. This observation was of great intrinsic interest with regard to the pathophysiology of the symptoms of multiple sclerosis but was not of immediate diagnostic value as the visual system was known to be involved in these patients. In their next communication, however, the use of VEP in the diagnosis of multiple sclerosis was reported and a high degree of success was obtained.

Before detailed examination of methods and results, the rationale behind the use of EP in the diagnosis of multiple sclerosis should be considered. The objective is to demonstrate abnormalities in regions of the nervous system not known from the clinical manifestations to be involved in disease — silent lesions. The most obvious example is the finding of abnormal VEP in a patient with progressive paraparesis and no signs or previous symptoms of disease beyond the spinal cord. If achieved, this would demonstrate lesions, or at least abnormalities, at two sites both characteristic of multiple sclerosis, the spinal cord and optic nerves. The implication is that the optic nerves have been affected by subclinical or forgotten episodes of demyelination and that, in the absence of residual signs, abnormalities of VEP, presumed to be due to slowed or blocked conduction, have persisted. The same reasoning can be applied to other forms of EP in clinical diagnostic use, somatosensory (SEP) recording from the scalp and over the spinal cord, and auditory EP (AEP), usually of short latency, derived from the brainstem (BAEP).

Attention was quite rightly first centred on the demonstration that EP abnormalities were present in clinically definite multiple sclerosis, regardless of the presence or absence of overt clinical involvement of the systems examined. Clearly it was first necessary to show that these diagnostic tests were positive in known cases. The ideal of single or combined EP recordings 100% abnormal in definite multiple sclerosis has naturally not been achieved but a sufficiently high proportion of abnormalities was found to warrant the use of the techniques in patients in whom the diagnosis was in doubt. In such patients, in probable, possible or suspect categories, the proportion of abnormalities has understandably been lower. The interpretation of abnormalities of EP found, or not found, in such patients is not straight-forward. The immediate reaction is to accept that an abnormality unsuspected on clinical grounds does indeed indicate a silent lesion and confirms the presence of lesions at multiple sites. Abnormal EP have been used to 'transfer' patients from a dubious diagnostic category to one more definite, which was indeed the object of the investigation.[23] There is, however, remarkably little information on whether patients so transferred do indeed have multiple sclerosis or on the relation of abnormal EP to underlying lesions. The degree of specificity of abnormalities of EP for multiple sclerosis must also influence their interpretation.

The pattern of development of all three forms of diagnostic use of EP in multiple sclerosis has been similar. A large number of somewhat repetitive reports appear on the results in definite multiple sclerosis, with emphasis on the proportion of positive results — the 'take'. The stimulus is then elaborated or refined with the aim of increasing this proportion. Later reports are more critical, with emphasis on abnormalities of diagnostic value in showing clinically silent lesions. The task of determining by follow-up whether the diagnosis of multiple sclerosis indicated by such findings is correct has barely been attempted.

A further implication of abnormalities in EP presumed to be the result of subclinical relapse at some undetermined but possibly remote period is their persistence. An ephemeral abnormality would be of little value in diagnosis as the subclinical attack would soon leave no trace and would again be undetectable. This requirement for diagnostic use is, in general, met — the abnormalities usually do persist, certainly for long periods.

Visual evoked potentials

Technique

The great majority of reports have been concerned with pattern reversal VEP, although flash has been advocated and other forms of visual stimulus explored. In multiple sclerosis, uniocular full field stimulation has been the rule. Abnormalities have been judged from changes in latency, amplitude and symmetry of the P100, the most easily recordable potential. The method of stimulation has varied greatly in detail. Halliday,[24] reviewing 25 of the reports published up to 1979, remarked on the robustness of the technique in producing at least comparable results in such differing conditions. The size of field stimulated, the size of the squares of the pattern, the luminance of the white and black squares (not always stated), and the transition time of the pattern change, cannot be matched between any two reports. The mean normal latency of P100 in these studies varied from 93–120 ms.

Precisely which variables in the stimulus it is most important to control has not been fully established, but certainly reduction in luminance increases the latency.[25] Stimulating the fovea by using small squares or a single bright square[26] has been claimed to elicit a higher proportion of abnormal results than in the same patients when the stimulus consists of large squares. Conduction from the foveal region is of particular importance in multiple sclerosis but more peripheral visual defects can be overlooked and a method of demonstrating such abnormalities by stimulating a large area of retina and using large squares could also be useful. However, foveal stimulation has not been found to have any advantage in the detection of abnormalities compared with a larger target, although the two methods were supplementary.[27] Elaboration of technique to include stimulation with patterns of different check sizes[28,29] or with reversing sinusoidal grating patterns,[30,31] or stimulating half fields[32] will slightly increase the sensitivity of the test in clinically definite multiple sclerosis.

Regan et al [33,34] have used a variety of stimuli to induce a steady-state evoked response. Their reports are models of ingenuity and scientific method but in practical diagnostic terms the only advantage appears to be that the steady-state flicker response can be obtained when visual acuity has been much reduced. Celesia & Daly[35] also used flicker stimulation and measured the highest frequency of photic driving response in flashes per second. Fewer abnormalities were found by this method than by pattern reversal, but it was considered to be a useful adjunct.

Origin of the VEP

The component of the VEP commonly chosen for measurement, the P100 or P_1, as the first positive wave, is but one element of a complex response and is usually preceded by at least one wave of shorter latency, N_1. The P100 is therefore not the first indication that the stimulus to the retina has induced a cerebral response. The scalp topography of the response indicates an origin in the posterior part of the cerebral hemispheres but it is thought unlikely that the P100 is derived from the striate cortex. In the present context the precise generating site is less immediately relevant than the localisation of lesions that cause abnormalities. An abnormality to diffuse or central stimulation of the field of vision of one eye with a normal response from the other eye can scarcely be located other than in the retina or optic nerve, the latter being the more probable site in multiple sclerosis. If abnormalities are bilateral, however, it is not possible to exclude a contribution from lesions in the postchiasmal visual pathways. Stimulation localised to half-fields or smaller segments with an appropriate increase in recording electrodes can provide more detailed information but correlation between anatomically demonstrated lesions and abnormal VEP will be difficult to obtain in multiple sclerosis.

The inferences to be drawn from the effects of multiple sclerosis on EP with regard to the pathophysiology of multiple sclerosis are considered in Chapter 8. It is usual to equate delayed EP with delayed conduction, in this context the result of demyelination, and this is an adequate working hypothesis.

Standards of normality

The criterion in general use is the peak latency of P100. This is influenced by many factors: the method of stimulation, the sex and age of the subject, and by refractive errors and impaired visual acuity.[36] The latency is somewhat shorter in females and increases with age, although the latter effect is not pronounced until beyond the age of 60 when few patients will be suspected of having multiple sclerosis. A refractive error of more than 1 dioptre can significantly prolong latency.[36] A dilated pupil will shorten latency, apparently irrespective of acuity.[37] Certain important practical considerations stem from these findings. It is of the utmost importance that normal values are established for each laboratory and periodically checked. A film of dust over a projection bulb, for example, will affect the luminance of the stimulus and the latency of the response. Separate normal values should be established for each sex. Refractive errors should be corrected and spectacles should be worn during the test. Results when acuity is much reduced and uncorrected (6/18 or less) should be regarded as suspect.

Inevitably, reported normal values have varied over a considerable range, the term P100 being merely a convenient symbol indicating an approximate latency. It is necessary to set an upper limit of normal and probably the mean + 2.5 SD is the most realistic level. The more stringent criterion of mean + 3 SD will virtually exclude all normal eyes, but much reduce the proportion of 'abnormalities' in patients, the reverse of course being true if the mean + 2 SD is adopted. The distribution curve of latency values in known or suspected multiple sclerosis is such that a very slight shift of the accepted normal limit has a profound effect on the number of abnormalities detected.[38] It is therefore unwise to place great reliance on borderline abnormalities.

The symmetry of latency between the two eyes has also been used as a criterion. In normal subjects the difference in latency seldom exceeds 5 ms. More comprehensive latency measurements have included that of N_1, the first negative potential and Collins et al.[39] used an even more complex method of analysis.

It is less easy to place limits on acceptable normal values of the amplitude of P100. The mean amplitude is lower in males, no doubt because of the thicker skull. Gross asymmetry is not seen in normal subjects but is difficult to quantify. The range of normal values is large, approximately $4–35\mu V$.

Results in multiple sclerosis

The essential first step in the use of VEP in the diagnosis of multiple sclerosis was to show that abnormalities were present in overt optic nerve lesions. This was the essence of the initial report by Halliday et al[21] but it should be noted that even in acute optic neuritis, VEP were not invariably abnormal, a normal response being obtained from one of the 18 affected eyes examined. An important feature was the difference in latency between the affected and unaffected, presumably normal, eyes. In a slightly larger series, normal results were obtained in 6 out of 28 eyes observed to have been subject to optic neuritis within the previous three months.[38] Differences in latency between the affected and unaffected eyes were less impressive and, indeed, in one patient latency was more prolonged from the eye not known to have been involved. Shahrokhi et al[40] examined 51 patients without evidence of multiple lesions but with a history of optic neuritis at some time in the past, a notably different method of selection. Of 59 affected eyes no response was recordable from 8, in 4 latency was within the normal range but abnormally asymmetrical and one eye was regarded as abnormal because of asymmetry of amplitude of response. In the remainder, latency was increased in all but 3, from which a normal response was obtained.

The next stage was to record VEP in patients with clinically definite multiple sclerosis not suffering from recent optic neuritis. In the original series of Halliday et al,[22] abnormal VEP were found in 97% of such patients. This figure has been approached or even surpassed in a number of later studies [26,41,42] but somewhat lower proportions have more often been found. The number of confirmatory reports is now very great and only the larger series need be referred to.[23,38,39,40,43] In these series the proportion of definite cases with abnormal VEP has ranged from 75–97%.

These findings, while an essential preliminary, are of no diagnostic value, as the patients were already accepted as having multiple sclerosis. Of great significance for the use of the technique in patients merely suspected of having multiple sclerosis is the proportion of abnormalities in definite cases with no clinical evidence of involvement of the visual system. Most investigators have assessed such involvement by the usual clinical methods; a history of optic neuritis, loss of visual acuity and pallor of the optic discs. More elaborate examination would, no doubt, reveal further abnormalities in visual fields or colour vision but the use of simple clinical criteria is justifiable as it is in such circumstances that the test is normally employed. Not unexpectedly, a history of optic neuritis in patients with definite multiple sclerosis is associated with a much higher percentage of abnormal VEP than in patients with no such history. Nevertheless, percentage abnormalities in the latter group have ranged from 57–94[22,26] Even the presence of that notoriously unreliable sign, pallor of the optic disc in the absence of a history of optic neuritis, is associated with a higher incidence of abnormal VEP. The method is therefore capable of detecting clinically silent lesions and can legitimately be applied to the demonstration of multiple lesions in cases of otherwise doubtful multiple sclerosis.

In the original report abnormal VEP were found in 100% of patients in the category of probable multiple sclerosis and 92% of possible cases. The former figure has been repeated in one small series[41] but in most the percentage has been much lower, 33%;[35,44] 50%;[39] 58%;[38,42] — but also up to 83%.[43] Differences may be partly or wholly ascribed to the difficulties in strictly applying McAlpine's criteria for this category. The figure of 92% of abnormalities in patients in the possible group originally reported by Halliday et al has not been repeated or approached in any other series. The number of patients was perhaps unduly small, abnormalities being found in 11 of 12 patients in this category. By definition, very few patients graded as possible will have a convincing history of optic neuritis and therefore such abnormalities in VEP as are detected are likely to be of greater diagnostic value in demonstrating unsuspected lesions.

The numerous repetitive reports need not be reviewed in detail as they all confirm that in a widely variable proportion of patients in whom a diagnosis of multiple sclerosis is justifiably suspected, abnormal VEP are found in the absence of other evidence of visual involvement. In general, the stronger the suspicion the higher the percentage of abnormalities. In many reports it is possible to detect a slight uneasiness that the assumption that these abnormal VEP indicate without doubt the presence of unsuspected lesions, thus confirming the diagnosis of multiple sclerosis, has never actually been demonstrated. The intention to follow-up such patients to determine whether they do indeed develop clinically definite multiple sclerosis has often been expressed but seldom implemented. Other authors accept without hesitation that the basic assumption has been shown to be correct. Thus Lowitzsch[23] writes of 'proven dissemination of the demyelinating process' and, on these grounds, felt that the diagnostic category in 23% of probable and possible cases in the series examined could be advanced to clinically definite. This may well be correct but has not been shown to be so.

The diagnostic use of VEP in two common clinical problems may be considered. In the first, a young adult presents with an episode of neurological symptoms compatible with the onset of multiple sclerosis: diplopia or sensory symptoms in the limbs, for example. A single episode without evidence of multiple lesions does not enter into any category of McAlpine's diagnostic criteria, although McDonald & Halliday admit such cases as 'suspect'. How often will abnormal VEP suggest the presence of an unsuspected lesion in the visual system? This has seldom been specifically examined but in two series the proportion was small, 3 out of 39 and 2 out of 22 such patients.[37,45] A further question is whether even the small proportion of abnormalities found can be taken as reliably indicating that multiple lesions are already present and that overt multiple sclerosis will declare itself. This can only be answered by prolonged follow-up, a particularly difficult exercise in young adults who have recovered from their transient symptoms. The results of attempted follow-up are referred to when considering the use of multiple EP techniques.

Single modes of evoked potentials are now seldom used in the diagnosis of multiple sclerosis and the practical value of VEP in this context is discussed when considering the use of multiple techniques. The specificity of prolonged latency of P100 is obviously of great importance. Tartaglione et al[31] made the important comparison between patients in the probable and possible diagnostic categories, with no history or signs of optic nerve disease, and patients with other neurological diseases, not clinically involving the visual system. The chance of error in attributing prolonged latency of VEP to multiple sclerosis was over 30%. Recordings will also be abnormal in many conditions affecting the anterior visual pathways not likely to be mistaken for multiple sclerosis. Prolonged latencies may be found in hereditary ataxias,[46] hereditary spastic paraplegia,[47] neurosyphilis,[48] sarcoidosis,[49] vitamin B_{12} deficiency,[50] tropical spastic paraparesis[51] and systemic lupus.[52] The abnormality most helpful in the diagnosis of multiple sclerosis is of greatly prolonged, markedly asymmetrical latencies from eyes with normal vision and no history of optic neuritis.

Somatosensory evoked potentials (SEP)

SEP have usually been elicited by electrical stimulation of mixed nerve trunks, median, peroneal and posterior tibial. There are practical advantages in ease of location of the nerve and of evoking a response and theoretical difficulties in the complex nature of the structure stimulated. The possible effects of antidromic fibre stimulation or of afferent impulses from the contracting muscles have been little considered. There is, however, sufficient evidence that the results of purely sensory nerve stimulation are essentially similar.[53] The strength of stimulus has been related to the threshold of perception of the shock. Latency decreases and amplitude increases with stronger stimuli but there is little change beyond a strength of three times threshold and this is a convenient value to adopt.[54] Such a stimulus is above the twitch threshold for muscles innervated by the median nerve. Bipolar stimulation at this level is only mildly uncomfortable unless a cutaneous nerve twig happens to lie beneath the electrodes, when a more painful superficial sensation may be experienced. Square wave shocks of 0.3 ms duration, repeated twice a second have been routinely employed, with minor variations. In most contexts, averaging of 256 responses is adequate.

The siting of recording electrodes has been much more variable depending on the immediate purpose of the investigations. In the context of diagnostic use in multiple sclerosis electrodes over Erb's point, the lower and upper cervical spine and the hand area of the opposite parietal cortex referred to as a mid-frontal electrode give consistent results. Desmedt et al,[55] while accepting the practical usefulness of this array, have raised theoretical objections based on the presumed origins of the potentials to be recorded and recommended referral to the opposite hand. From personal experience this method is apt to produce uninterpretable results.

The recording of potentials over the lumbar roots and lower spinal cord evoked by stimulation of lower limb nerve trunks is relatively easy in normal young subjects,[52] but they may no longer be detectable beyond middle age (personal observation). The potentials are of small amplitude, easily obscured by muscle potentials in spastic patients, and subject to interference from EKG. An evoked potential can more reliably be recorded from the scalp.

The nomenclature of the potentials recorded from the scalp, neck and spine after stimulation of the median or posterior tibial nerve has been inconsistent. The polarity depends on the location and linkage of the recording electrodes. The normal latencies of recognisable components have varied between different laboratories. For the present purpose of detecting subclinical abnormalities in multiple sclerosis, the important potentials evoked by median nerve stimulation using a frontal reference electrode are: N9, recorded from Erb's point; N13, recorded from the cervical spine; N20, recorded from the scalp. A later scalp-recorded potential, P40, has received less attention.[56] N9 arises from the brachial plexus; N13 is probably derived from the posterior columns or their terminal nuclei; N20 is regarded as arising from the cerebral cortex.

From posterior tibial stimulation, the potential recordable over the 4th lumbar vertebra, thought to arise from the cauda equina, has been labelled N18.[57] A more prominent potential, N20, can usually be recorded over the first lumbar vertebra and is believed to arise from the terminal spinal cord. The most easily measurable scalp recorded potential has been designated P38.[58] To illustrate the degree of variation, in a personal investigation,[59] a potential recorded over the 1st lumbar vertebra with a reference electrode on the iliac crest had a normal mean latency of 21.8 ms (N21) and the scalp potential 39.5 ms (P40).

Standards of normality

Absolute latencies are greatly influenced by the length of peripheral nervous system involved and to a lesser degree by body height. The former difficulty is overcome by confining measurement as far as possible to conduction within the central nervous system. From median nerve stimulation, the differences in latency between N9 and N13 and between N13 and N20 are easily measured in normal subjects. Responses to lower limb stimulation are less reliable, but the difference in latency between the lumbar and scalp potentials can usually be determined. Normal values must be established for each laboratory. The mean values usually approximate closely to those implied by the nomenclature of the potentials, with small standard deviations. In personal experience, the mean N9–N13 as 4.0 ± 0.5 ms, but values of 3.7 ± 0.7 ms and 4.1 ± 0.5 ms have been reported. The mean duration of N13–N20 is close to 5.5 ± 0.5 ms.

The latency of the scalp potential evoked by posterior tibial nerve stimulation is more variable, 39.5 ± 2.35 ms,[59] perhaps because of the inconstant relationship of the termination of the spinal cord to the vertebral column.[60]

Asymmetry of latency of up to 5% for N13 and 8% for N20 is observed in normal subjects.[61]

Amplitude of the potentials is highly variable and cannot be used as an indication of abnormality. Potentials of less than 1 μV amplitude are unlikely to be repeatable on a second run. There is a considerable temptation to regard wave forms that show some departure from an accepted but unquantified 'normal' shape as indicative of disease. This should be resisted until aberrant patterns can be consistently linked with abnormal clinical findings.

Results in multiple sclerosis

Halliday & Wakefield[62] first examined scalp recorded SEP evoked by stimulation of nerve trunks in the lower limbs in patients with multiple sclerosis and attributed the abnormalities found to disease affecting the posterior columns of the spinal cord.

The first report of the use of SEP in the diagnosis of multiple sclerosis was that of Baker et al[63] in 1968, when abnormalities in the scalp potential were seen in 69 of 91 patients already diagnosed as having multiple sclerosis. The first such use of the cervical SEP was reported by Small et al at an international conference in Brussels in 1974, but full publication was unfortunately delayed until 1980.[64,65] Mastaglia et al[44] found abnormalities in 16 out of 17 definite cases but made no allowance for arm length which may have influenced their results. Small et al[66] reported abnormal cervical SEP in 69% of definite cases. N20 was very seldom abnormal in the presence of a normal cervical recording. In definite multiple sclerosis with severe disability, cervical SEP were always abnormal. Trojaborg & Petersen[42] recorded the scalp potential only but stimulated the peroneal as well as the median nerve in many of their patients. Abnormalities were found in 86% of definite cases. Other figures from studies using different degrees of sophistication of recording are 87%,[67] 96%,[68] 72%,[69] 77%.[70]

It was therefore abundantly demonstrated that this form of EP is also abnormal in a sufficiently high proportion of clinically definite cases to warrant extension of its diagnostic use to suspected multiple sclerosis. Before reviewing results, the definition of abnormalities of diagnostic value must be established. SEP, particularly the cervical potentials, are often abnormal in the absence of sensory loss detectable by careful routine clinical examination. At first there was a tendency to regard such findings as equivalent to abnormal VEP with normal vision, but this is not justifiable. Abnormal VEP in this context may be accepted as indicating involvement of an area of the CNS not otherwise known to be affected. In most patients

abnormal SEP cannot be regarded in the same light. Spastic weakness of the legs, with or without sensory loss, can be taken as evidence of spinal cord disease, and abnormal SEP cannot imply the presence of plaques in some other region of the CNS. Abnormalities should therefore only be accepted as of diagnostic value in the sense of indicating subclinical disseminated lesions when there is no clinical evidence of spinal cord disease.

In contrast to VEP, the abnormalities of SEP in multiple sclerosis more often consist of absence of recordable potentials rather than prolonged latency. This is particularly true of the low amplitude N13, recorded from the enck on median nerve stimulation. Even when this appears to be delayed, the form of the potential is distorted and it is by no means clear that this is the 'same' potential that is recorded in normal subjects. More convincing delays of N20 and P38 are not uncommon. In a recent small but thorough study[71] of a group of patients with multiple sclerosis of varying degrees of diagnostic certainty, N13 could not be evoked from 26% of arms stimulated and was thought to be delayed in 13%. N20 was absent in 20% and delayed in 37%. The scalp potential from stimulation of the peroneal nerve was recorded in 41% of attempts, the potential being delayed in 25%. Where distinct potentials can be recorded, the N9–N13 and N13–N20 intervals can be measured. The former has proved of little value. The mean value of N13–N20 has been found to be increased in definite cases of multiple sclerosis, but with many normal or inconclusive results. Mean values were not increased in probable and possible cases.[71]

In patients in whom the diagnosis of multiple sclerosis is less than clinically definite, abnormal SEP are commonly found. Mastaglia et al[44] found abnormal cervical responses in 4 out of 8 probable cases and 10 of 27 in the possible category. Small et al[66] reported abnormal SEP in 42% of probable and 52% of possible cases, the latter, of course, including progressive spastic paraparesis. In both series, abnormalities were often present without sensory loss but only a much smaller proportion had no evidence of spinal cord disease. In the latter series, 21% of patients with no sensory loss in the upper limbs and no signs of spinal cord disease had abnormal cervical SEP. In indefinite cases of multiple sclerosis, Khosbin & Hallett[70] found abnormal SEP in 5 out of 9 patients classified as asymptomatic with regard to the sensory system, but did not indicate the sites of the clinically overt lesions. The importance of the more rigid definition of the diagnostic help derived from the SEP is illustrated in the series of Green et al.[69] Of 15 indefinite cases of multiple sclerosis, SEP were abnormal in 8, but their table shows that there was clinical evidence of spinal cord or brainstem lesions in all these patients. Purves et al[72] considered that abnormal SEP could not be accounted of diagnostic value in the presence of either sensory loss or weakness in the arm examined. Using this stricter criterion, the number of abnormal SEP results judged to be of clinical value was approximately half that of the total abnormalities. In practice it is likely that even more strict limitations will be imposed. In a patient with weak and spastic lower limbs, an abnormal SEP derived from stimulation of an abnormal upper limb can scarcely be accepted as conclusive evidence of multiple lesions. False negative or paradoxical results occur more often than with VEP. Patients with appropriate loss of postural or vibration sense may have normal SEP.[72–74]

The ability to record SEP from several sites has led to attempts at measuring sensory conduction times or even velocities in the spinal cord. In slim co-operative normal subjects, using a very large number of stimuli to the posterior tibial nerve, potentials can be recorded over the spinal column with increasing latency from progressively more rostral sites. The potentials are of low amplitude but, on the reasonable assumption that they arise from the spinal cord, it is possible to demonstrate increased transit time in a proportion of patients with multiple sclerosis.[59] By this method, normal conduction velocity in the spinal cord is approximately 55 m/s. The technique is difficult and failure to record the potentials cannot be accepted as evidence of abnormality.

A number of ingenious indirect methods have been described, with findings of similar normal mean spinal sensory conduction velocities of 55 m/s[75] 61 m/s.[76] Application of these methods to multiple sclerosis has not been encouraging and it has been concluded that indirect measurements of this kind are far more laborious and no more useful than simply measuring the latencies of such SEP as can be recorded. Rossini et al[71] calculated sensory conduction velocity to the cortex by subtracting the latency of the lumbar potential from that of P38. The mean in normal subjects was 38.7 m/s and in a group of patients with multiple sclerosis, 34.5 m/s, mean values being slower in definite than in probable or possible cases. While these differences are significant, the values are too close to allow conclusions to be drawn from slight abnormalities.

Auditory evoked potentials

A click stimulus evokes a complex series of time locked responses recordable from the surface. Those of short latency, occurring within 10 ms of the stimulus, are believed to arise from a succession of sites on the auditory pathway in the acoustic nerve and brainstem. It is these potentials that have been mainly studied in multiple sclerosis but other components of longer latency and presumed cortical origin may also be disturbed.[77]

The potentials recorded are greatly influenced by many factors other than abnormalities of the nervous system.[78] The duration and loudness of the stimulus and the siting of the recording electrodes may affect the latency and amplitude of the response. For routine diagnostic work, clicks of 0.1 to 0.5 ms duration, delivered through earphones at 10 or 20 per second, produce consistent results in normal subjects. It is usual to adjust the strength of the stimulus by a fixed proportion above threshold; 512 or 1024 responses are averaged. Alternating polarity of the stimulus greatly reduces artefact. Stimulation should be monaural and binaural. The recording electrodes are placed over the mastoid processes referred to the vertex. In monaural recording, the non-stimulated ear should be masked with white noise. For complete examination, recording should be made both from the ipsilateral and contralateral mastoid. The sweep time must be adjusted to avoid recording the post-auricular muscle response as this is of much greater amplitude and can obscure the record. The longer latency components can be recorded from the same electrodes or from bipolar electrodes over the temporal lobe.

The stimulus naturally has to be given at a much slower rate.

Sites of origin

By analogy with findings in experimental animals, components I to V have been attributed to activity in or near the acoustic nerve, the cochlear nucleus, the superior olive, the ventral nucleus of the lateral lemniscus and the inferior colliculus respectively. Waves VI and VII are less constant and arise from subcortical or cortical structures. It is more realistic to regard I–III as a measure of conduction in more caudal and III–V in more rostal segments of the brainstem rather than to attempt too great precision of localisation that can only be presumptive.

Standards of normality

As with other EP techniques, each laboratory must establish normal values to allow for the possible effects of differences in technique. Separate normal values must be established for brainstem EP evoked by monaural stimulation and recorded from the ipsilateral and contralateral mastoid, as the latency from the ipsilateral recording is shorter.[79] Also, normal values must be established for each sex, as latency is shorter in females.[80]

It is not always possible to record all components even in normal subjects and when the response is abnormal, identification of individual waves may be problematic. Wave V is the most consistent feature and in the original study of BAEP in multiple sclerosis, abnormality was judged from the latency of this wave from the stimulus.[77] In most reports, the normal latency is around 5.7–6.0 ms, being some 0.2 ms shorter in women. The normal amplitude is more variable and more dependent on the recording and filtering techniques employed. More sophisticated measurement are now used. The latency of wave I from stimulus is subtracted from the latency of the other components with the aim of concentrating on abnormalities due to CNS involvement. A more useful compromise is to measure the latencies of the more prominent and consistent components I, III and V and the amplitude of V. The latency of I from stimulus is around 1.5 ms, I–III 2.3 ms and III–V 1.9 ms. These figures can be no more than

approximate guides to the order of latency expected and as already emphasised, precise values must be determined in every laboratory. Stockard et al[78] have emphasised the variation that may result from alterations in technique. The asymmetries normally present must not be misinterpreted as evidence of disease.

In the context of multiple sclerosis, comparatively little attention has been paid to longer latency auditory evoked potentials. P1 and P2, with latencies around 50 and 150 ms respectively, and N1 and N2 at 70 and 200 ms, can be consistently recorded from normal subjects. A series of components with latencies between 30 and 40 ms can also be detected.

Results in multiple sclerosis

Brainstem auditory evoked potentials were first recorded in patients with multiple sclerosis by Robinson & Rudge[81] and Starr & Achor.[82] The latter authors found potentials of reduced amplitude or loss of wave V in four patients with clear evidence of brainstem lesions. Robinson & Rudge examined a large series and were at first more impressed by reduction in amplitude than by prolongation of latency as evidence of abnormality. Later[77] they included examination of middle and late components although most subsequent investigations have been limited to BAEP.

They examined 88 cases of clinically definite multiple sclerosis and abnormalities of BAEP were found in 65%, the figure in those without clinical evidence of a brainstem lesion being 57%. Abnormalities of both amplitude and latency were considered, the latter being much more informative. Only the main component, wave V was examined systematically, but it was observed that if the latency of any of the other components was prolonged, that of wave V was prolonged also. Latency was measured from stimulus and not from wave I. Abnormalities of latency of middle and late components were less frequently found, but an additional 12% of abnormalities was detected by recording the former. Long latency potentials were seldom abnormal and never in isolation.

It was therefore established that abnormal AEP were present in a high proportion of cases of definite multiple sclerosis and that the lack of correlation between clinical and electrophysiological findings, necessary for their diagnostic use, was also satisfactorily displayed.

The proportion of abnormalities found in patients in the less definite diagnostic categories of multiple sclerosis has varied greatly between series, partly reflecting differences of stimulation and recording technique. Thus Kjaer[83] found 50% abnormal in probable and possible cases and Tackmann et al[84] using binaural stimuli found only 5 abnormalities in 31 such patients and indeed in only 6 of 23 definite cases. Prasher & Gibson[85] used both monaural and binaural stimulation and demonstrated the much higher proportion of abnormalities found by the former method. Barajas[86] confirmed that there are differences in latency between ipsilateral and contralateral recording, but found no cases of multiple sclerosis with an abnormality present with only one recording method. Robinson & Rudge[87] used binaural stimulation and found abnormal BAEP in 21 of 32 definite cases of multiple sclerosis. The use of paired stimuli may slightly increase the proportion of abnormalities detected in clinically definite multiple sclerosis.[88]

Chiappa et al[89] found a relatively low proportion of abnormal recordings, reaching only 57% in definite cases with clinical evidence of brainstem lesions and 20% in other diagnostic groups. In contrast, Stockard et al[90] reported 77% of abnormalities in probable and 35% in possible cases in whom no symptoms of brainstem disease had ever been recorded. Baum et al[91] wrote of the close relationship between clinical brainstem symptoms and BAEP, but this is far from being so. Although BAEP are abnormal when hearing is disturbed in multiple sclerosis,[92] the correlation with overt brainstem lesions is poor. Hutchinson et al[93] found normal BAEP in 24% of patients with clinically definite disease with signs of brainstem lesions and in 50% of patients with suspected multiple sclerosis. In another series,[94] only 7 of 25 patients with isolated brainstem lesions had abnormal BAEP. These results are not directly relevant to the diagnostic use of the technique in demonstrating abnormalities in the absence of abnormal signs, but BAEP have proved comparatively less useful in this respect. Chiappa[95] believes that they make an important contribution to diagnosis but some authorities have abandoned their use.[18]

The abnormalities in multiple sclerosis are in no sense specific for the disease and may result from other brainstem lesions. Absence of wave I, believed to arise from the acoustic nerve, should not be found in multiple sclerosis or in any other lesion confined to the central nervous system, but has been reported.[96] It should be remembered that the evidence for the sites of generation of BAEP is not conclusive. Waves that occur later in time do not necessarily arise successively from structures at increasing distances from the stimulus, which is the usual assumption. An event in the ear could generate a complex wave pattern that could be transmitted centrally.[97]

Multiple EP techniques

The use of two or more electrophysiological techniques in the attempt to demonstrate multiple clinically silent lesions was a logical extension. Mastaglia et al[44] used VEP and cervical and scalp recorded SEP. With this combination an abnormality was found in 16 of 17 definite cases, in 4 of 8 probable and 16 of 27 possible cases. Of those with abnormal VEP in whom the diagnosis was still in doubt, 66% had no history of optic neuritis and a similar proportion of those with abnormal SEP had no sensory loss at the time of examination but the diagnostic value of these findings is difficult to assess. Small et al[66] used the same combination and found abnormalities in 80% of probable and 69% of possible cases, and Trojaborg & Petersen[98] reported similar figures. The combined use of VEP, SEP by various techniques and BAEP have been described.[45,69,70,72,99–102] In some instances the blink reflex has also been examined[70,99,101,102] and nystagmography included.[102] The relative ability of the methods to detect abnormalities and to demonstrate unsuspected lesions has varied, but there is general agreement that the blink reflex is the least useful. The proportion of abnormal BAEP in probable and possible cases did not reach the high levels claimed in the original reports, and in general fewer abnormalities were found by this method than with VEP and SEP. A higher proportion of abnormal SEP was usually found, but abnormalities of diagnostic value in demonstrating silent lesions were relatively uncommon. VEP appeared to be the most useful of the tests. In a personal series,[45] VEP were abnormal in 10 of 15 probable cases, being diagnostic in 6; in 10 of 34 possible cases, diagnostic in 9; and in 2 of 22 cases with a single episode of neurological symptoms. In the whole series there were 13 patients with abnormal SEP of which only 3 were of diagnostic value, and 10 with abnormal BAEP of which no less than 9 indicated unsuspected lesions. A combination of all three methods detected at least one abnormality of diagnostic value in 6 of 15 probable cases, in 10 of 34 possible cases and in 4 of 22 patients with a single episode of symptoms.

It is now apparently customary in some centres to apply the whole battery of EP recordings in suspected, or even in clinically definite multiple sclerosis. The extent to which this 'multiple sclerosis workup' contributes significantly to diagnosis is not easy to establish. In definite multiple sclerosis some abnormality is recorded in the great majority of patients by this method.[72] In less certain diagnostic categories the proportion of abnormal findings naturally falls. Khosbin & Hallett[70] found some abnormality in 82% of 'indefinite' cases irrespective of whether overt lesions were present in the systems examined. This figure was compared with abnormalities in 58%, 55% and 31% for SEP, VEP and BAEP tested individually. The proportion of 'asymptomatic' patients in whom abnormalities were found was also analysed, asymptomatic being defined as being without clinical evidence of a lesion in the system tested. The criteria were not strict enough, as abnormal SEP were regarded as of diagnostic value if no sensory loss was present, without regard to evidence of spinal cord disease. The same difficulty is encountered in the small series presented by Green et al.[69] Of 15 patients in categories other than definite, some abnormality was found in 10. The findings, however, included abnormal SEP in 8 patients, all of whom had either spinal cord or brainstem disease. If these are ignored as being of no diagnostic value, 2 abnormalities were found using VEP alone and 2 by BAEP. Chiappa[100] examined 70 patients, including definite and suspected cases in unstated numbers, using all three modalities. A clinically unsuspected lesion was found by a single test alone in 27%, 21% and 14% by SEP, VEP and BAEP respectively. Absence of sensory loss was equated with absence of clinical evidence of a relevant lesion when assessing the value of SEP.

Recent advances in imaging have led to a spate of comparisons between the sensitivity of evoked potentials and MRI, the proponents of the former sometimes appearing to be on the defensive. Although the comparisons are interesting and, indeed, essential, the sensitivity of EP techniques naturally has not differed from the results of earlier studies. In a number of recent reports, the purpose of recording EP appears to have been overlooked.

As Kjaer[103] has re-emphasised, while the number of EP abnormalities is higher in definite multiple sclerosis, the number of abnormalities of diagnostic value is greater when the diagnosis is in doubt. The important distinction between EP abnormalities that indicate a silent lesion and those that merely confirm the obvious clinical findings is often not made. Apart from scientific curiosity there is little point in recording VEP in patients with optic neuritis or SEP in those with spinal cord disease.

Gebarski et al[104] compared the results of MRI and EP in 30 patients in whom the diagnosis of multiple sclerosis had been entertained. Lesions were seen on the scan in 26 patients. SEP were doubtfully abnormal in one patient with a normal scan and BAEP abnormal in another, but whether these EP abnormalities were of diagnostic value is not stated. Ormerod et al[94] examined patients with clinical evidence of a single lesion of the brainstem or spinal cord. Of the former, 11 of 37 patients examined had abnormal VEP and 5 of 31 abnormal SEP, all of these abnormalities naturally being of diagnostic significance. With isolated spinal cord disease, VEP were abnormal in only one of 23 patients and BAEP in 2. SEP would not, of course, be contributory in the context but were abnormal in only 4 patients. Of these patients, 12 with spinal cord lesions had changes on MRI of the brain typical of multiple sclerosis.

In contrast, Geisser et al[105] examined 23 patients with possible multiple sclerosis (McAlpine) by MRI and EP. In 14 patients, MRI was abnormal and there was at least one abnormality of EP. In

4, MRI was normal but EP abnormal, although again it is not stated whether the abnormalities indicated silent lesions. VEP revealed subclinical lesions in 10 patients, but these were not identified. The authors concluded that EP recording had a higher sensitivity than MRI in confirming a diagnosis of multiple sclerosis, a conclusion only justified if the EP changes were indeed diagnostic and the patients actually had multiple sclerosis.

The importance of distinguishing EP abnormalities of clinical significance is further illustrated by the report of Comi et al.[106] Of 60 patients with multiple sclerosis in different diagnostic categories, 10 had no abnormality on MRI. Of these, 4 had abnormal VEP, but all had optic neuritis: 2 had abnormal SEP but one had spastic paraplegia: 2 had abnormal BAEP but one had clinical signs of a brainstem lesion. The numbers of patients in whom each mode of EP showed asymptomatic lesions are given, but not the numbers in whom EP made a significant contribution to diagnosis. In a recent extremely detailed study[29] of the sensitivity of EP in clinically or laboratory supported definite multiple sclerosis, the practical diagnostic value of the investigation receives no mention.

Practical diagnostic use

The value of any diagnostic method must obviously be judged on its efficacy in the doubtful case. In multiple sclerosis, the most obvious applications are in the patient with clinical evidence of a single lesion, particularly acute or chronic myelopathy. MRI has already greatly influenced the approach to this common clinical problem,[107] but is neither universally available nor infallible. It is still important to consider the possible contribution of EP recording to the answers to two common questions:

1. Can myelography safely be avoided in isolated spinal cord disease?
2. Can multiple sclerosis be predicted at the time of monosymptomatic presentation?

Mastaglia et al specifically examined this aspect. They estimated how often the combined use of VEP recording and quantitative electrooculography[108] had or should have influenced the decision not to undertake invasive X-ray pro-cedures in patients suspected of having multiple sclerosis. From the condensed account of a retrospective study it is not easy to see why clinically definite cases were included nor at what stage they were investigated. Of 129 patients with probable or suspected multiple sclerosis, such procedures were avoided in 23 patients after taking account of electrophysiological findings and perhaps should have been avoided in a further 24. No follow-up was reported so it is not known whether the omission of radiology was always justified by the event. Blumhardt et al[109] have described the results in a large series of 131 cases of isolated spinal cord disease undiagnosed at the time of examination. In 31 the cord lesion developed acutely or subacutely; in 36 the clinical course was that of relapse and remission and in 64 there was chronic progressive paraparesis. Abnormal VEP were found in 38 patients, but the proportion of abnormal findings varied among different categories. Of the subacute cases 10% had abnormal VEP. In relapsing disease 33% were abnormal and in progressive cord disease 36%. The percentage of abnormalities was three times higher in those whose symptoms had been present for three years or more than in those of shorter duration.

Spinal cord compression was not excluded by myelography in all patients and it seems likely that the use of VEP influenced the clinicians' resort to radiology. The 77% abnormal VEP in chronic myelopathy in whom myelography was not done suggests that it was considered unnecessary to exclude cord compression because the diagnosis of multiple sclerosis had already been proven by abnormal VEP. Selection on these lines could scarcely have been avoided. The result was felt to be disappointing as it was calculated that no more than one third of those patients who would develop multiple sclerosis could be detected by this method within three years of the onset. There is, however, little information on the proportion of patients presenting with progressive paraparesis who can be proven to have multiple sclerosis and these calculations were based on a follow-up study published in 1955[110] and referring to a period when exclusion of spinal cord compression was much less effective. In a more recent series,[111] of 108 patients presenting with spastic paraparesis without sensory changes, 78 were diagnosed as having some condition other than multiple sclerosis.

Bynke et al[112] examined 25 patients with chronic myelopathy with VEP, detailed clinical examination of the eyes and CSF examination, including electrophoresis. Myelography had been carried out in 20 of the patients. VEP were abnormal in 19 and the CSF was also abnormal in 19, and eye examination in 9. In 4 patients all the tests were normal. Paty et al[113] investigated 72 patients, spinal cord compression being said to have been ruled out by appropriate methods. Oligoclonal banding was found in 44%, abnormal VEP in 35% (the reported figures are not wholly consistent), blink reflex surprisingly was abnormal in 50% and CT scan in 52%, nearly all showing diffuse atrophy. A high proportion of patients had at least one abnormality but in 12 all tests were normal. It was not thought that a clear distinction had been drawn between a group with multiple sclerosis and a group with other diseases.

The question of the predictive value of normal or abnormal EP in patients with acute neurological symptoms of the type encountered in multiple sclerosis can only be answered by prolonged follow-up of such patients. This has rarely been attempted. This may be in part because those who carry out the EP recordings usually do not have clinical charge of the patients. An additional difficulty is that it is ethically objectionable to cause alarm by recalling patients long recovered from a brief episode of, for example, paraesthesiae or vertigo.

Stockard et al[114] followed up patients with isolated optic neuritis or myelopathy in whom BAEP had been recorded. Results were abnormal in only 10% but all patients with abnormalities developed clinically definite multiple sclerosis within three years.

In a study[45] of 71 patients, 15 were classified as being probable and 34 as possible multiple sclerosis (McAlpine). Twenty two patients were assigned to a further category of 'acute not diagnosed' defined as a single episode of neurological symptoms of less than 3 months' duration. EP abnormalities were found as shown in Table 7.1

The patients were followed by enquiry from neurologists or general practitioners. In the following three years 34 patients had shown some clinical progression, 28 being classified as definite multiple sclerosis. In 14 of these patients, all later classified as definite cases, abnormal EP indicating silent lesions had been present at the initial investigation, a 50% detection rate. Clinical progression followed in 70% of those with such abnormalities. However, only 41% of those who progressed had EP evidence of silent lesions when first seen.

In a similar but larger study[115] that included patients with isolated optic neuritis, results were broadly the same. The distinction between abnormal EP and those of diagnostic value, designated positive EP, was emphasised. A positive EP result in a patient with suspected multiple sclerosis carried a 71% chance of clinical progression within approximately three years and a 48% chance of developing definite multiple sclerosis. If EP were initially normal, the chance of progression was 16% and of definite multiple sclerosis 4%.

Both of these studies showed that positive results were most frequent with VEP. Abnormal BAEP were relatively rare but a high proportion of abnormalities were positive and predictive of progression. The follow-up period was probably as long as practicable but was obviously insufficient

Table 7.1 Numbers of patients with EP abnormalities at presentation

	N	VEP	SEP	BAEP	Total
Probable	15	10(6)	3(1)	1(1)	10(6)
Possible	34	10(9)	9(2)	6(5)	13(10)
AND	22	2(2)	1	3(3)	4(4)
Total	71	22(17)	13(3)	10(9)	27(20)

Figures in parentheses indicate those in whom EP were of diagnostic value. Multiple abnormalities were found in some patients.
AND = Acute not diagnosed.

to establish even an approximate false positive rate.

A longer mean follow-up of almost 5 years was achieved by Deltenre et al.[116] 48 of the 56 patients who progressed to definite multiple sclerosis, had positive EP results at the beginning of the study. The number of patients with such findings who did not progress was not stated and it is not clear what was accepted as a positive EP result. In the two studies described above, abnormal SEP in a patient with spinal cord disease were regarded as confirmatory rather than positive.

Monitoring

The attempted use of EP in monitoring the course of multiple sclerosis and, in particular, the effect of treatment, is discussed in Chapter 9. As predicted,[117] here has been almost universal disappointment.[118,119] The essence of the use of EP in diagnosis is the persistence of abnormality in the absence of clinical evidence of disease. Persistence is not invariable as prolonged latencies may sometimes return to normal in remission[120] or rarely, after a long interval.[121] There is no evidence confirming the suggestion[122] that fluctuations in latency and amplitude, unaccompanied by clinical change, indicate subclinical relapse and remission. The only sustained claim that EP can monitor and indeed predict favourable response to treatment[56,123] is unconvincing, mainly because the evidence for clinical improvement was equivocal. As Anderson & Sherman[124] wrote: 'patients are not really interested in having their evoked potentials improved'.

Motor conduction

Measurement of conduction in motor pathways in the brain and spinal cord appears more promising in both diagnosis and monitoring than further elaboration of methods of examining the somatosensory system.

Experimental stimulation of the cerebral cortex in intact man was first achieved by Merton & Morton.[125] Single, brief high voltage shocks applied to the appropriate area of the scalp were found to induce contraction of the muscles of the opposite limbs. The amplitude of the compound action potential recorded from muscle is much increased by slight voluntary contraction. The same procedure applied to the neck at the level of the sixth cervical vertebra causes contraction of ipsilateral arm muscles.[126] The very high voltages originally used were found to be unnecessary and shocks of 'a few hundred volts' with a time constant of decay of 50 μs were found to be adequate. Discomfort from scalp stimulation is slight but stimulation over the spine causes 'a brisk jerk'. Variations of voltage and duration of current and of electrode placement were introduced later.

Abnormalities of conduction in patients with multiple sclerosis were reported by Cowan et al.[127] The latency of the response in biceps brachialis and thenar muscles from spinal stimulation was subtracted from that from the cortex to give a cortex to spine conduction time. To biceps the upper limit of normal (mean + 3 SD) was 5.9 ms and to thenar muscles 6.8 ms. The mean values in 8 subjects with multiple sclerosis were 10.8 and 16.2 ms respectively, some abnormality being present in every patient. The conduction time in some arms was more than four times the normal mean. Mills & Murray[128] used a similar technique except that the latency due to conduction in the peripheral nervous system was obtained by stimulation in the axilla. Slowing of central conduction of the same order was again demonstrated in multiple sclerosis.

Snooks & Swash[129] used electrical stimulation to measure motor conduction velocity in the spinal cord. Shocks were applied at the level of C6, L1 and L4 vertebrae, with recording from the muscles of the pelvic floor and from tibialis anterior. Conduction velocity in the spinal cord was calculated from the difference in latency of the responses of lower limb or pelvic muscles to cervical and upper lumbar stimulation and the distance between these two points. The difference in latency obtained by stimulation at L1 and L4 was used to calculate conduction velocity in the cauda equina, assuming the conventional anatomy of the termination of the spinal cord. In normal subjects spinal cord conduction velocity was 67.4 ± 9.1 m/s. In four patients with multiple sclerosis, all of whom had signs of disease of the corticospinal pathways, conduction was slowed to 24–43 m/s, but in a fifth patient velocity was 75 m/s.

Before the application of this method could be

thoroughly explored in multiple sclerosis and other diseases, it was superseded by magnetic stimulation, introduced by Baker et al.[130] The stimulus, which can be applied to the scalp, the neck and to peripheral nerves, appears to be free from adverse effects and causes little discomfort. Stimulating at the vertex, the lower cervical and lumbar spine, Ingram et al[131] examined conduction times in normal subjects and in patients with multiple sclerosis. Magnetic stimulation over the cervical spine did not excite descending motor pathways, in contrast to electrical stimulation, so motor conduction velocity could not be measured in the same way. Normal latencies from cortex to biceps brachialis and thenar muscles were similar to those obtained with electrical stimulation. Using a far from stringent upper limit of normal of mean + 2 SD, conduction times from cortex to leg muscles were increased in most patients. Abnormalities were closely correlated with the presence of an extensor plantar reflex. In the upper limb, the association of abnormal conduction with increased tendon reflexes was not constant. Conduction to muscles with normal strength in the upper limb was often slow.

In a large group of 83 patients with multiple sclerosis and 32 normal control subjects, Hess et al[132] examined motor conduction to the abductor muscle of the fifth finger. Magnetic stimulation was applied to the scalp and lower cervical cord and central conduction time calculated by subtraction. The normal mean cortex to cord time was 6.2 ± 0.86 ms. The upper limit of normal was taken as mean ± 2.5 SD, this value being exceeded in 72% of the patients. The amplitude of the compound muscle action potential induced by cortical stimulation was also measured and expressed as a percentage of the amplitude of the potential following stimulation at the wrist, but this was not found to be useful. Abnormalities of conduction were closely related to increased reflex activity in the arm, particularly the finger flexor stretch reflex. Conduction to strong muscles was sometimes delayed. Neurological examination was normal in 7 arms to which central motor conduction was delayed. Rather more patients had abnormal motor conduction and normal sensory evoked potentials than the reverse.

It is too early to know whether magnetic stimulation will prove to be of great assistance in the detection of silent lesions and in monitoring disease progress or whether it is an elaborate method of confirming an extensor plantar reflex or positive Hoffman's sign.

Long loop reflexes

The complex reflex response to ankle displacement has been shown to be disturbed in multiple sclerosis by Diener et al[133] who measured the M3 response in tibialis anterior induced by tilting the foot upwards. The response was delayed in 69% of patients, usually accompanied by abnormal SEP, although in isolation in 7% of 42 cases. Abnormalities were present in only one third of patients with possible multiple sclerosis. The long-latency reflex contraction of the thenar muscles induced by median or superficial radial nerve stimulation was examined by Deuschl et al.[134] Here again abnormalities usually paralleled those of SEP with only a small proportion of patients with definite or probable multiple sclerosis showing delayed reflex latency alone. These methods, while interesting, are unlikely to enter routine use.

PSYCHO-PHYSICAL VISUAL TESTS

Visual acuity

There is no question that abnormalities in the optic nerve can be detected more readily by recording VEP than by the Snellen test type. This is indeed the basis of the clinical value of the technique and the point is made in every report in which the visual acuity is mentioned. Thus Asselman et al[43] found acuity of 6/9 or better in 40 of the 57 eyes from which they recorded abnormal VEP. It is however a matter of common observation that the Snellen test can scarcely be regarded as a sensitive index of visual function. On recovery from optic neuritis, many patients who can read 6/5 with ease are aware that their vision is not normal. A number of psycho-physical tests of vision have been applied in order to explain this discrepancy. Some, although of great interest, are too complex to be applied as a routine diagnostic indication of occult optic nerve lesions, while others have been part of normal neurological or ophthalmological investigations.

Colour vision

A complaint of loss of brightness but not of failure to distinguish colours is common after recovery from optic neuritis. The results of examination of colour vision have been highly varied. Sloan[135] introduced the use of pseudo-isochromatic charts in the detection of central scotomata and Steinmetz & Kearns[136] showed that after recovery from optic neuritis defective colour vision, by this method of testing, might be the only detectable abnormality. Rosen[137] tested 272 definite cases of multiple sclerosis by this method and found defective colour vision in 67, being the only ocular abnormality in 56. Nearly all patients with one or more of the conventional signs of optic nerve lesion: a history of optic neuritis; reduction of acuity not corrected by lenses; optic atrophy; central scotoma; or abnormalities of pupillary reaction, had defective colour vision. It was not stated whether the defect involved both eyes. This is an important point as uniocular colour blindness with normal acuity must certainly be a significant abnormality indicating an acquired lesion.

Other reports have been less enthusiastic. Zeller,[138] using the Ishihara plates found that 68 of 123 (55%) patients with multiple sclerosis made errors of 15% or more of the charts, a smaller proportion than the 73% in whom visual field changes were found. Barde & Gallin[139] very thoroughly examined 9 patients who had recovered from optic neuritis. Colour vision was impaired on the 100 hue test in 3, a smaller proportion than in most of the tests employed, although these did not include VEP. Asselman et al[43] found normal colour vision on Ishihara plates in 25 of the 57 eyes from which abnormal VEP were recorded. They did not say, however, how often colour vision was abnormal with normal VEP. Regan et al[140] found that colour vision was not a sensitive indication of occult optic nerve damage, as in 48 patients the only abnormality detected was in one case with congenital colour blindness. Lowitzsch[23] compared defective colour vision with other indications of visual impairment in multiple sclerosis. Of 269 eyes tested, colour vision was impaired in 34%, acuity was reduced in 20% and an abnormality in visual field by the Friedmann method was found in 41%; 64% had abnormal VEP. Again, in this report, attention was centred on the VEP and it is not possible to determine how often examining colour vision would have assisted diagnosis when VEP were normal.

Harrison et al[141] used both the 100-Hue and Ishihara methods to examine 40 patients with multiple sclerosis. Abnormalities were found in 42.5% of eyes with the former and in 45% with Ishihara plates. Defective colour vision was detected by one or other test or by both in 65%. Surprisingly, abnormal results were not correlated with a history of optic neuritis or with delayed VEP. A past history of optic neuritis was found by Griffin & Wray[142] to be followed by defective colour vision on the 100-Hue test in 100% of eyes, the proportion with abnormal VEP being slightly less. In contrast, Engell et al[143] found that optic neuritis in the past made little difference to the incidence of defective colour vision with either test and that VEP abnormalities were more common. Frederiksen et al[144] found an abnormality of colour vision in 80% of eyes in 65 patients, Ishihara plates again proving the more useful. Colour vision was defective in 19 eyes from which normal VEP had been recorded.

In a carefully conducted investigation, rather awkwardly split between two populations of patients, MacFadyen et al[145] found VEP abnormalities to be more frequent than defects of colour vision but that the use of both examinations detected some abnormality in 75–85% of patients with definite or probable multiple sclerosis. Optic neuritis in the past increased the proportion of abnormalities. They also emphasised that colour vision was not affected solely on the red/green axis, as classically believed to occur in optic nerve lesions, but that blue/yellow vision was also often defective.

Monocular colour blindness in an eye with normal acuity should arouse suspicion of an optic nerve plaque, even when VEP are normal, but in personal experience defects in colour vision detectable in the clinic by the relatively rapid Ishihara or modified Farnsworth–Munsell test are infrequent in suspected multiple sclerosis.

Visual fields

Although charting the visual fields has long been

a part of routine neurological assessment, there have been remarkably few studies of the fields in patients with multiple sclerosis who do not have recent optic neuritis. The results obtained appear to depend critically on the method employed. Zeller[138] examined 123 patients with multiple sclerosis in remission, using a 2000 mm tangent screen and small objectives. The commonest abnormality, found in isolation in 52% of cases, was general depression or constriction of the field, defined quite carefully according to the size of objective used. In a further 21%, a central or paracentral scotoma was found, but always in association with general depression of the field. A low level of illumination was deliberately chosen with the aim of enhancing any field defects present, and as a result the normal field to a 1 mm or 2 mm objective was small.

Frisén & Hoyt[146] found quite different defects consisting of arcuate scotomata that they associated with lesions in the nerve fibre layer of the retina visible on ophthalmoscopy. Barde & Gallin[139] in their careful study of a small group of patients who had recovered from optic neuritis but who had persistent complaints about their vision, found that kinetic visual fields on the Goldman perimeter were normal but static field testing along the meridian 0–180° was abnormal in all affected eyes, showing parafoveal reduction in sensitivity. Asselman et al[43] examined the visual fields by a variety of methods in a large series of patients in whom VEP were also recorded. A field defect was found in only eight of the eyes from which a delayed VEP was obtained, but they did not indicate how often abnormal fields were found with normal VEP.

Patterson & Heron[147] in a most careful study found a very high proportion of field defects in patients with definite, probable or possible multiple sclerosis, the respective proportions in these categories being 100%, 94% and 81%. In patients with optic neuritis examined at least four weeks after the most recent visual symptoms, 92% were abnormal. Of the abnormalities found, 76% were arcuate scotomata, almost all beyond 20° from the fixation point. A paracentral scotoma accounted for 4%, localised depression for 14% and general depression of the field for 13%. The fields were examined on a 2000 mm tangent screen, using

5 mm or 2 mm objectives, but with bright illumination. Zeller[138] who deliberately used comparatively dim lighting, could not have detected these arcuate scotomata as the fields charted did not extend to 20°. From personal experience, these scotomata are difficult to detect and chart consistently. Patterson & Heron did not record VEP in the same patients, so that direct comparison of the two methods was not possible. The apparatus required for tangent visual field charting is simple and cheap and from these results the rate of detection of optic nerve lesions is at least as high as that obtained from VEP. The technique, using either the tangent screen or static perimetry, requires a higher degree of skill.

Other psycho-physical methods of examining visual function in multiple sclerosis do not form part of routine examination but have been especially devised. Great ingenuity has been displayed and the results are of particular interest in the relation of lesions in the visual system to symptoms, but these methods have not been widely accepted as practical diagnostic procedures. The topic has recently been reviewed by Regan[148] and with greater emphasis on disordered physiology by Hess & Plant[149] and by Foster[150] (see Ch. 8).

Flicker fusion

Above a certain frequency a flickering light is perceived as a continuous source of illumination. The topic has recently been reviewed by Regan[148] and with greater emphasis on disordered physiology by Hess & Plant[149] and by Foster[150]. The critical frequency can be determined either by increasing from a low rate of stimulation until flicker is no longer detected or by reducing from a rapid rate until flicker is perceptible. In normal subjects these values are not far apart and are closely repeatable provided the conditions of the test are kept constant. Early results indicated that the critical frequency was often reduced in multiple sclerosis. Titcombe & Willison[151] confirmed this in a more exacting study and found that flicker fusion was not closely related to visual acuity. Thorner & Berk[152] tested 60 patients with multiple sclerosis and 100 controls. All but 3 of the patients had a lowered flicker fusion frequency that deteriorated further on repeated testing, in contrast to normal subjects whose performance tended to improve. There appear to have been no recent attempts to use this technique as a diagnostic method in suspected multiple sclerosis, although the proportion of abnormalities found in definite cases is at least as high as that claimed for VEP recording. A modified technique in which the background illumination flickers rather than the point of fixation[153] produced comparable results with 78% abnormality, the proportion being related to the degree of disability and not to evidence of past or present visual involvement.

A further interesting example of the inability of the demyelinated nervous system to conduct trains of stimuli was the comparison of photic driving with VEP recording in the diagnosis of multiple sclerosis by Cohen et al.[154] They found that the failure of the evoked response to follow stimulus frequency beyond a limit well within the normal capacity was a more sensitive test than pattern reversal VEP. Romani et al,[155] however, found that the test provided poor discrimination from other diseases or from normal control.

The Pulfrich phenomenon

This is an optical illusion whereby the motion of a pendulum swinging at right angles to the line of vision appears to follow an elliptical path if the vision of one eye is dimmed by means of a dark glass. If this is due, as Pulfrich[156] thought, to prolonged latency of vision from the partially obscured eye in normal subjects, the illusion should also occur when latency is prolonged by disease, as in multiple sclerosis. This is indeed so, but the test does depend on the *difference* in latency between the two eyes so that bilateral abnormalities of conduction might not be detected. The use of the original pendulum method has proved far too difficult to quantify and more elaborate methods have been devised.

Rushton[157] used an ingenious technique whereby an oscillating spot of light was presented separately to each eye, forming a fused image. The patient could adjust the controls so as to produce a Pulfrich effect or to overcome this so that the spot appeared to move in a straight line. From the degree of adjustment needed to produce the latter effect, the difference in latency between the two

eyes could be calculated. The results were not impressive, as abnormal findings were recorded in 9 of 18 definite cases of multiple sclerosis, 3 of 9 probable and 2 of 8 with possible multiple sclerosis. In patients with no clinical evidence of optic nerve involvement, the important group from the diagnostic viewpoint, 3 out of 10 were abnormal. VEP were also recorded and were abnormal in a higher proportion of patients. There was a reasonably good correlation between abnormalities of the Pulfrich phenomenon and of VEP, but the size of interocular latency differences determined by the two techniques showed no correlation.

Wist et al[158] used quite a different technique whereby the stripes of a device for eliciting optokinetic nystagmus could be made to appear to be in front of or behind the screen on which they were actually projected. They claimed to find abnormalities in 93% of a small series of patients in different diagnostic categories of multiple sclerosis, 97% of whom had abnormal VEP. Their technique, they said, could be performed by a skilled technician (indeed what technique cannot?) but the correct assembling of the apparatus and the interpretation obviously required considerable skill. The Pulfrich phenomenon has not been generally adopted as a routine procedure.

Other visual methods

Heron et al[159] used a psycho-physical method to demonstrate delayed perception in eyes previously subject to an isolated episode of optic neuritis. The test involved one light being displayed to the right eye and one to the left. The interval between switching on the two lights was adjusted until the stimuli were judged by the patient to be simultaneous. In all 12 patients examined there was a difference in latency between the two eyes, greater than that in control subjects, the affected eye having the longer latency. The diagnostic value of this test was scarcely explored as all the patients had a clear history of optic neuritis and evident optic atrophy. The inadequacy of the Snellen test type as an indication of visual loss has already been emphasised. Regan et al[140] tested visual acuity by means of sine-wave gratings with varying degrees of contrast between dark and light areas of the stimulus and varying spatial frequency of the wave form. By this method they were able to test not only the ability to see fine detail at high contrast, as in the illuminated Snellen test card, but also coarse and medium detail with low degrees of contrast. They tested 48 patients and 29 matched controls by this method. In 20 patients an abnormality was found, and in 11 of these the visual sensitivity to detail of medium coarseness, and in a further three perception of coarse detail, was selectively impaired. These defects were not detectable by the Snellen test. The results are of great interest in exploring persistent symptoms in patients recovered from optic neuritis with 'normal' vision. Carter & Danta[160] found measuring spatial contrast sensitivity a useful complementary test, capable of demonstrating involvement of the visual system not revealed by VEP recording. Fahy et al,[161] however, reached the opposite conclusion and found the investigation much less sensitive than pattern reversal VEP.

The flight of colours is a phenomenon familiar to us all. After exposure to a bright light, fluctuating coloured after-images persist for several minutes. Swart & Millac[162] devised a practical standardised method of evaluating this effect. The eyes are dark adapted by wearing ultraviolet goggles and each eye is exposed separately, and at a suitable interval, to a bright light for 10 seconds. The subject reports the duration of the after-image and the number of colours seen, although the latter are not considered when assessing the results. The test was applied to 21 patients, mostly with clinically definite multiple sclerosis and pattern-shift VEP were recorded on the same patients. The results of these two tests, whether normal or abnormal, corresponded in 33 out of 36 eyes examined, the VEP being recorded without knowledge of the result of the other test. This method of detecting occult abnormalities in the visual system has great advantages in cheapness and simplicity. Quantification has not, however, proved to be as reliable as claimed.

BRAINSTEM FUNCTION

The latency of the blink reflex as an indication of conduction through the brainstem has been examined in multiple sclerosis in a number of studies. Its diagnostic value is relatively low compared with evoked potential techniques.[98,100,163] Khoshbin & Hallett[70] found the reflex abnormal in 9 of 22 definite cases of multiple sclerosis. In probable and possible cases it was abnormal in 3 of 23 patients without brainstem signs, comparable to the figures of 5 of 29 such patients with abnormal BAEP.

Kimura[164] examined the blink reflex, electrically induced by stimulating the supraorbital nerve, in 260 patients with definite or suspected multiple, sclerosis. The first (R1) component was delayed in 66% of definite cases, 56% of probable and 29% of possible cases. The proportion of abnormalities was much higher in those with clinical evidence of a pontine lesion. From a diagnostic viewpoint of course, the important figures are the number of abnormalities in suspected multiple sclerosis without signs of brainstem disease. The reflex was abnormal in 12 of 45 such cases.

The light stimulus evoked blink reflex[165] tests conduction in both the visual system and the brainstem. The reflex has a much longer latency than the R1 and is considerably affected by the intensity of the light stimulus. A high proportion (75%) of abnormalities was found in clinically definite multiple sclerosis, and the method was thought to be a sensitive detector of lesions of the visual system and brainstem. The diagnostic implications, that is to say the proportion of abnormalities found in the absence of clinical evidence of such lesions, were not reported.

It is unlikely that anyone's opinion on the diagnosis of multiple sclerosis would be swayed by the finding of an abnormal blink reflex.

Stapedius reflex

The crossed stapedius reflex in multiple sclerosis was examined in great detail by Hess[166] who paid particular attention to the shape of the reflex curve in addition to its latency. Some difficulty was encountered in establishing normal values. Abnormalities were detected in 10 of 30 patients with multiple sclerosis examined and of these, 9 had clinical evidence of brainstem lesions. Of those with a normal reflex, 70% had clinical brainstem lesions. The reflex as at present recorded is not therefore of diagnostic value in multiple sclerosis.

Ocular movements

Clinically overt disorders of ocular movement are so common that it is not surprising that clinically silent lesions can be detected by appropriate techniques. Nystagmography[167] notoriously detects 'abnormalities' in healthy subjects and this was confirmed in a controlled study on multiple sclerosis. Subjects over 44 without any evidence of disease might show directional preponderance of induced nystagmus, spontaneous nystagmus with eyes closed and some impairment of pursuit movements. Sixteen of 18 patients with multiple sclerosis showed more significant abnormalities, considered in context to indicate brainstem disease — horizontal and vertical gaze nystagmus, impaired optokinetic nystagmus and more pronounced defects in pursuit movement. The latter was also often found with defective saccadic movement by Solingen et al[168] in 13 of 16 patients said to have either little overt oculomotor disorder, although 6 had gaze nystagmus.

Saccadic and pursuit eye movements in definite and suspected cases of multiple sclerosis were systematically studied by Mastaglia et al[169] using quantitative electro-oculography. Not all of their patients were examined by the full array of tests but of those that were, in 15 of 29 suspected cases subclinical eye movement defects were detected. Similar abnormalities were found in all four progressive probable cases. Subclinical abnormalities, those of diagnostic significance, were naturally less common in definite multiple sclerosis where overt disorders of eye movement are to be expected. Saccadic and pursuit movements might be independently affected. Abnormal VEP were more frequent than eye movement disorders in definite multiple sclerosis, but less so in other diagnostic categories. As a result of these investigations 14 patients were reclassified to a category of higher diagnostic certainty on the presumption that clinically silent lesions had been displayed.

In a further study of 65 patients with suspected multiple sclerosis and normal eye movements, on clinical examination 23 were found to have saccadic abnormalities.[170] Ellenberger & Daroff[171]

stress the wide range of normal values and the effect of sedative drugs and inattention in producing bilateral abnormalities. Unilateral abnormalities of gaze can be accepted as pathological. In a study in which such factors were carefully controlled[172] the sensitivity of saccadic analysis was found to be similar to that of MRI but it is doubtful whether the abnormalities found can be accepted as revealing clinically silent lesions. There was a close correlation between abnormalities of peak saccadic velocity and signs of brainstem disease and a similar correlation of saccadic latency disturbances with visual signs.

Suppression of the vestibulo-ocular reflex is a normal mechanism that ensures that when a moving object is followed by turning the head, the eyes remain stationary in the orbits. This suppression has been shown to be deficient in 75% of clinically definite multiple sclerosis patients without signs of vestibular or oculomotor disease.[173] Here again the diagnostic value of this test has not been examined in early cases.

As far as these methods have been explored they appear to follow the pattern usual for diagnostic techniques in multiple sclerosis. A high, or relatively high, proportion of abnormalities is found in clinically definite cases where there is no diagnostic doubt, with a declining proportion of abnormalities, sometimes almost to vanishing point as with the stapedius reflex, in patients in whom a diagnostic test would be useful.

ELECTROENCEPHALOGRAPHY (EEG)

Even in the first flush of enthusiasm for the method it is doubtful whether the EEG has ever been claimed to be diagnostic of multiple sclerosis. The early literature was reviewed by Ashworth & Emery[174] who noted that the proportion of patients with abnormal records varied greatly between different series. The abnormalities observed are, of course, entirely non-specific and are often unrelated to clinical features. It is this point that might be of diagnostic value as the only indication of a cerebral lesion in a patient with clinical evidence of spinal cord disease or optic neuritis alone. This method of demonstrating multiple lesions has been suggested[174-176] but is less reliable than techniques developed subsequently. The point, originally of some diagnostic interest, that focal delta activity may disappear in serial records in multiple sclerosis as distinct from cerebral tumours, has also been overtaken by newer methods.

Danielczyk[177] found 26% of abnormalities in those with slight signs of multiple sclerosis and 85% in bedridden patients, irrespective of the length of history. The increase appeared to be related to the development of the organic brain syndrome, although an association with dementia has not always been found.[176] In contrast Levic[178] found a higher proportion of EEG abnormalities in patients with a benign course. The characteristic appearance was of high voltage 6–10 cps activity recorded from all areas of the scalp, with high voltage anterior sharp waves. These changes, if such they be, are quite different from the slow activity, often focal, seen in advanced disease.

THE HOT BATH TEST

The adverse effect of slight exposure to heat on certain symptoms of multiple sclerosis was noted by Simons[179] and attributed to localised vasocontriction by Brickner.[180] The phenomenon was investigated by Guthrie,[181] Namerow,[182] and Hopper et al[183] and this, and the related effect of exercise on visual acuity in optic neuritis are further considered in Chapter 5. The diagnostic use of inducing temporary deterioration in existing signs or the appearance of new signs has been suggested. Edmund & Fog[184] subjected 45 patients to dry heat for 10–15 minutes. Body temperature was not regularly monitored, but increases were small. In a high proportion of severe cases physical signs were aggravated but milder cases were not affected, suggesting that the method would have little application in early diagnosis. Nelson & McDowell[185] also examined patients in whom the diagnosis of multiple sclerosis was not in doubt, using immersion in hot water or radiant heat. An increase in physical signs was found to be related to the rise in body temperature and was much less pronounced in patients in remission.

A recent application of this technique was also confined to patients with clinically definite multiple sclerosis. Malhotra & Goren[186] immersed 20 patients in a hot bath and found an increase in physical signs in a high proportion. In 16 visual acuity was reduced, in 9 for the first time, and weakness occurred in 15. Nystagmus, usually not previously recorded, appeared in 7 and internuclear ophthalmoplegia in 6. Interestingly, dysarthria, aphasia, bilateral ptosis and athetosis were also noted in individual patients. The authors remarked on the difficulties inherent in conducting a detailed neurological examination of a patient immersed in hot water.

Rolak & Ashizawa[187] found this test to be positive in only 8 of 23 patients with definite multiple sclerosis and in only 4 of 27 patients with probable or possible disease. Sensitivity is evidently low. Nelson et al[188] examined specificity by submitting 72 patients with diagnoses other than multiple sclerosis to the same test and found induced abnormalities in no less than 40. These were in general less severe and less easily induced than in patients with multiple sclerosis, but it was evident that drugs, including anticonvulsants, might affect the result. Even normal subjects given barbiturates by injection developed nystagmus in a hot bath. Apart from a devoted band of adherents, few would now regard a positive hot bath test as strong evidence of multiple sclerosis where this diagnosis is in doubt.

Red cell cytopherometry

The diagnostic and predictive test devised by Field and colleagues,[189–191] based on the effect of linoleic acid on the migration of red cells in an electrical field, was extensively reviewed in the last edition of this book.[192] It was concluded that, whatever the theoretical implications, a test that does not work at all in the majority of laboratories that have reported results could not be of immediate value. There have been no further significant developments and it is unlikely that the test is used for the diagnosis of multiple sclerosis in any neurological centre.

IMAGING

Until the advent of computerised tomography (CT) the role of radiology in multiple sclerosis was largely confined to the exclusion of other diagnoses. Air encephalography had shown that cerebral atrophy was common in advanced disease.[193] Myelography, using a variety of contrast media, sometimes showed a swollen or shrunken spinal cord,[194] the former occasionally resulting in laminectomy on a mistaken diagnosis of an intrinsic tumour.[195] Results of radioisotope scanning at first appeared encouraging,[196] but even in patients in relapse with cerebral symptoms abnormalities were uncommon. The proportion of abnormalities in a large series was disappointingly small, only 3 of 160 patients having a positive scan.[197]

Computerised tomography

The first report of CT scanning in multiple sclerosis appears to have been that of Cala & Mastaglia,[198] closely followed by Warren et al.[199] These brief reports of positive findings were confirmed by Gyldensted[200,201] in a series of 110 patients. Of these, only 17% had normal scans, but the commonest abnormality was enlargement of the lateral ventricles, sometimes with widening of the cortical sulci, but with no evidence of focal lesions. In 37% of patients, however, low density areas were seen in the white matter around the anterior and posterior horns of the lateral ventricles, classical sites of multiple sclerosis plaques.

It was at first believed that the focal lesions seen in multiple sclerosis did not enhance with iodine contrast, but it was soon found that acute lesions that could often be related to symptoms of recent onset frequently enhanced[202–205] (Fig. 7.1a). The addition of techniques already developed for the detection of brain tumours — scanning delayed for one hour after contrast injection[206] and doubling the dose of contrast[207] — and high resolution scanners, much increased the number of lesions detected.[208] Vinuela et al[209] found that 20 of 39 patients with definite multiple sclerosis had an abnormal unenhanced scan, the number increasing to 25 with the conventional dose of contrast and to 32 with a double dose. Drayer & Barrett[210]

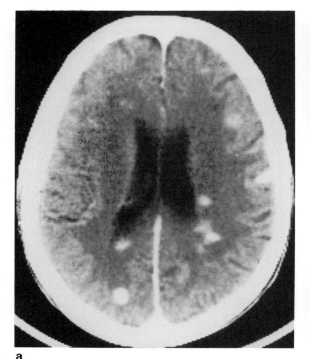
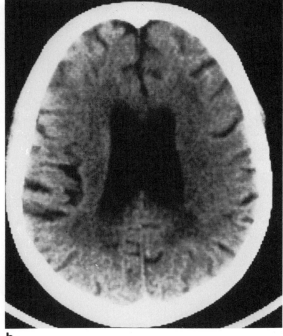

a　　　　　　　　　　　　　　　　　　**b**

Fig. 7.1　a. CT scan of a woman of 34 with clinically definite multiple sclerosis, showing numerous enhancing lesions. b. 17 months later there is considerable atrophy and diffuse white matter hypodensity. (Courtesy of Dr P. Anslow).

found enhancing lesions in 89% of patients within 8 weeks of relapse. Using these techniques 29 of 34 unselected patients with multiple sclerosis had abnormal scans, but again the commonest abnormality was non-specific cerebral atrophy[211] (Fig. 7.1b). Low density lesions were seen in 16 patients and enhancing lesions in 15. In this study a double dose of contrast did not significantly increase the number of lesions seen.

CT is relatively ineffective in showing lesions of the brainstem and cerebellum and plaques in the optic nerve can only doubtfully be detected. Lesions of multiple sclerosis have only occasionally been demonstrated in the spinal cord by CT.[212,213] In the cerebral hemispheres enhancement may occur in low density lesions but lesions isodense on the unenhanced scan may also be displayed (Fig. 7.2). In serial scans, enhancing lesions may become undetectable.[214] Many abnormalities seen by CT cannot be related to existing symptoms and symptoms often occur in the absence of relevant abnormalities on the scan.

The abnormalities seen in multiple sclerosis are not specific and the distinction from infarction or even cerebral tumour can sometimes be difficult. Multiple enhancing lesions can be interpreted as metastatic deposits that gratifyingly melt away on steroid treatment.[215] Diffuse low density of the white matter of the cerebral hemispheres, particularly marked in the immediate vicinity of the lateral ventricles, may be seen in multiple sclerosis, but also in subcortical arteriosclerotic encephalopathy or Binswanger's disease. As this condition can apparently present with non-specific symptoms, without dementia or focal neurological signs,[216–218] the CT appearances are often unexpected and can be mistaken for those of multiple sclerosis. Periventricular lucencies are also seen in normal pressure hydrocephalus, that may present with ataxia or apraxia of gait and urinary incontinence with mild dementia, all common features of multiple sclerosis. Indeed, periventricular CT hypodensity in multiple sclerosis has been attributed to hydrocephalus[219,220] on the strength of

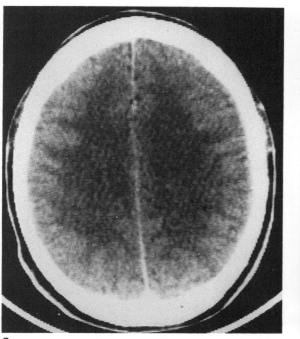
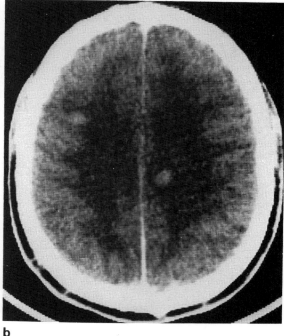

a   **b**

Fig. 7.2 a. Normal unenhanced CT scan of a man of 30 with suspected multiple sclerosis. b. After high dose contrast delayed scanning shows two lesions. (Courtesy of Dr A. Molyneux)

mildly disordered isotopic cisternographic patterns, although these findings have not yet been confirmed.[221]

There are comparatively few reports on the value of CT in the diagnosis of multiple sclerosis, no doubt because of the rapid development of magnetic resonance imaging (MRI). Even with the most advanced techniques the proportion of abnormalities found in suspected multiple sclerosis is not large. Jackson et al[222] included 7 patients in the probable or possible categories and in 5 of these both CT and MRI were normal. In 21 similar patients, the unenhanced scan was abnormal in 1, in 2 with conventional contrast and in 5 with a double dose.[209] Wright et al,[223] also using double dose contrast and delayed scanning, were more successful. Enhancing or low density lesions were found in 68% of 22 patients with clinically definite disease, in 72% of 25 probable cases and in 45% of 53 with possible multiple sclerosis. Paty et al[18] examined 200 patients with suspected multiple sclerosis. CT was abnormal in 50, in contrast to 131 using MRI. All lesions shown on CT were also shown by MRI. It is clear that where MRI is available, CT has little to offer in the diagnosis of multiple sclerosis.

Magnetic resonance imaging

The principles of MRI are not easy to grasp in detail and fortunately need not be expounded here. A lucid account for the non-physicist is provided by Kean & Smith.[224] In this chapter, the use of MRI in diagnosis and monitoring is described, the contribution to understanding pathophysiology being discussed in Chapter 8. Original articles should be consulted for details of field strength and pulse sequences.

The first application of MRI to multiple sclerosis was that of Young et al[225] in 1981. They examined 10 patients in whom CT had shown a total of 19 lesions. A further 112 focal abnormalities were shown by MRI. The brainstem was well shown using inversion recovery (IR). These remarkable results were followed by a pause, during which those who could afford it obtained the equipment. The superiority of MRI over high resolution CT was confirmed.[226] In 1984 Runge et al[227] established that cerebral lesions were best

shown by T_2 weighted spin-echo (SE) sequences and lesions in the brainstem by IR. That the abnormalities observed were related to actual lesions was shown by scanning an affected brain post mortem and comparing the results with the appearance of the cut surface.[228]

Abnormalities in the spinal cord were at first shown using the equipment designed for scanning the head, which confines the examination to the cervical region,[94,229] but body coils have also been used.[107,230] Lesions in the optic nerve can only be well visualised by using short inversion time IR sequences.[231]

The sensitivity of MRI in multiple sclerosis has been established by examining series of patients with clinically definite disease, the opportunity usually being taken to compare the results with those obtained with other diagnostic methods. With very few exceptions,[232] all abnormalities detected by CT are also seen by MRI. When assessing the results of MRI Paty et al[18] were careful to distinguish different grades of abnormality, depending on the number and site of the lesions shown. Not all authors have been so meticulous, Sheldon et al[233] accepting a single lesion as positive, but multiple lesions are the rule. Representative figures for abnormalities in definite multiple sclerosis are 16 of 19 patients,[234] 27 of 27,[235] 19 of 19,[29] 55 of 65,[233] 124 of 133, 117 with 3 or more lesions,[236] 113 of 114, the great majority with periventricular and discrete white matter lesions.[94] Most lesions demonstrated cannot be related to specific symptoms or signs, although what symptoms might be ascribed to periventricular lesions is unknown. Jacobs et al[237] found that the only lesions that could be directly related to symptoms were those in the brainstem or cerebellar peduncles. Conversely, many clinical features cannot be attributed to focal MRI abnormalities.[222]

These figures are clearly much more impressive than those cited above for CT. When direct comparisons are made, the difference remains wide. Thus, Kirshner et al[235] found MRI abnormalities in all of 35 patients but lesions were shown by CT in only 16, while a further 8 had cerebral atrophy without focal lesions. Jacobs et al[237] examined 27 patients with clinically definite multiple sclerosis. CT showed lesions in 12 and atrophy alone in 5, while MRI showed many more lesions in 21 patients. In 98 patients with multiple lesions typical of multiple sclerosis on MRI, the CT scan was abnormal in 36.[18] As described on p. 203, the comparison of the sensitivity of MRI with that of multimode EP recording is often obscured by uncritical acceptance of EP abnormalities that merely confirm clinical observation. In definite cases, particularly if there is severe disability, EP are as likely to be abnormal, as MRI and CSF oligoclonal bands of IgG are also usually present.[29]

Before considering the use of MRI in diagnosis of the doubtful case the specificity of the abnormalities seen in definite multiple sclerosis must be examined. These may be divided into periventricular abnormalities and focal abnormalities (Fig. 7.3) that may be seen anywhere in the cerebral hemispheres, brainstem, cerebellum and spinal cord. Neither the appearance nor the location of either type of lesion is specific for multiple sclerosis. The most thorough investigation of this problem is that of Ormerod et al[94] who

scanned patients with a variety of organic diseases of the brain, including 37 with non-vasculitic cerebral vascular disease. Of these, all had discrete lesions, as might be expected, but in 27 periventricular lesions were also present. In 7 patients with dementia, thought to have subcortical arteriosclerotic encephalopathy, the changes were indistinguishable from those of severe multiple sclerosis. Similar abnormalities were found in 18 patients with different forms of vasculitis involving the nervous system; in sarcoidosis; and in about one third of patients with degenerative cerebellar ataxia. In normal controls, discrete lesions were seen in 2 patients under the age of 60 and periventricular lesions in 2 over this age. One subject had widespread abnormalities resembling those of multiple sclerosis.

Although to expert eyes the periventricular lesions of cerebral vascular disease often differ from those in multiple sclerosis the possibility of confusion arises. The vascular lesions often form a

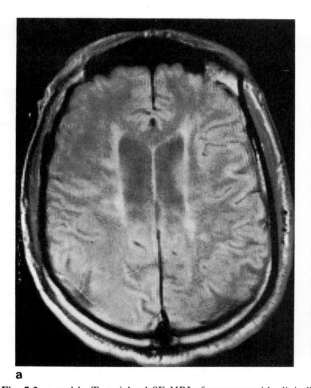
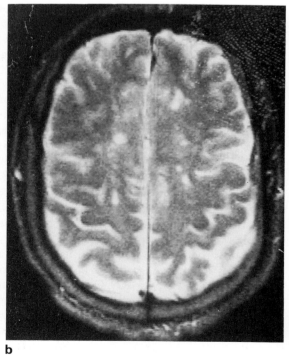

a   b

Fig. 7.3   a and b. T$_2$ weighted SE MRI of a woman with clinically definite multiple sclerosis, showing both periventricular and discrete white matter lesions. (Courtesy of Dr P. Anslow)

smooth line of increased signal around the ventricles on SE sequences, but irregular abnormalities, not to be distinguished from those of multiple sclerosis except in being less severe, are also frequent. Lesions confined to the distribution of a single cerebral artery are more easily distinguished, but discrete lacunar lesions occur in both vascular disease and multiple sclerosis. The clinical context is also, of course, highly relevant but it was naturally hoped that laboratory diagnostic techniques would elucidate the clinical state and not vice versa.

The introduction of enhancement with gadolinium DTPA[238] has probably not greatly increased the diagnostic power of MRI but, as with CT, enhancement appears to identify fresh lesions[239] and is therefore of great interest in following the course of the disease. Gadolinium passes through the broken blood-brain barrier in active plaques and greatly enhances the relaxation of the water hydrogen protons in what may be presumed to be oedema.

With increasing age, and particularly after 60, MRI becomes less reliable in the diagnosis of multiple sclerosis as asymptomatic lacunar and periventricular abnormalities become increasingly common, presumably the result of vascular disease. The age range of patients suspected of having multiple sclerosis by Paty et al[18] extended to 79, exceeded by the patient of 83 years included by Sheldon et al.[233] Fazekas et al[240] found three criteria valuable in identifying lesions of multiple sclerosis: lesions ≥6 mm in diameter; immediate proximity to the ventricles; location below the tentorium cerebelli.

Honig & Sheremata[230] examined 77 patients with clinically definite multiple sclerosis by MRI of the brain and spinal cord, although the thoracic cord was examined in only 34 cases. Areas of high T_2 signal were found in the cervical cord (Fig. 7.4) in 38 patients and in the thoracic cord in 16. Spinal cord atrophy was found in 14 patients and in 4 the cord was swollen. In 9 cases MRI abnormalities were found only in the cord; in 10 only in the brain and in 15 no lesions were seen at all. Spinal cord abnormalities were correlated with degree of disability but no attempt was made to relate them to specific signs. Swelling of the spinal cord may be mistaken for an intrinsic tumour.[241]

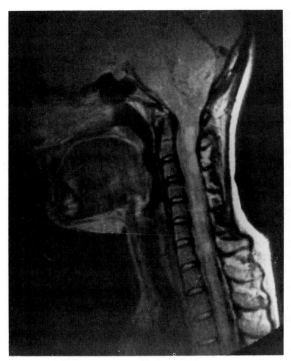

Fig. 7.4 SE MRI of the cervical spinal cord in a man with definite multiple sclerosis. Multiple lesions are present. (Courtesy of Professor W. I. McDonald).

MRI in suspected multiple sclerosis

Many reports of series of cases of clinically definite multiple sclerosis have included small numbers of patients in whom clinical diagnosis was less certain. The actual diagnostic categories and the degrees of MRI abnormality are variously defined, but by combining results[29,103,222,233,234,242] abnormalities were found in 85 of 108 patients. Twenty patients with chronic myelopathy were examined by cranial MRI by Miska et al[243] with results suggestive of multiple sclerosis in 13. MRI of the cranium and cervical spinal cord in 7 patients with progressive myelopathy enabled Ringelstein et al[244] to reach a diagnosis of multiple sclerosis in 4 and of spinal cord tumour in 3. MRI is unsurpassed in showing the anatomy of the cranio-cervical junction.

In a systematic evaluation of the diagnostic value of MRI in suspected multiple sclerosis Paty et al[18] investigated 200 such patients. Ninety eight showed the MRI abnormality described as 'strongly suggestive' of multiple sclerosis and defined as 4 lesions, or 3 lesions, one being periventricular. In these patients, there was a high rate of abnormality of EP and of oligoclonal CSF bands. Twenty six patients had MRI abnormalities of lesser degree and 69 had normal scans. Some MRI abnormality was found in 76% of patients with isolated optic neuritis; in 69% with chronic progressive myelopathy; in 59% of brainstem lesions and in 82% of those with cerebellar symptoms. In patients without physical signs 38% had abnormal scans. The figures for multiple MRI lesions strongly suggestive of multiple sclerosis were 66% for optic neuritis, 60% for chronic myelopathy, 26% for brainstem and 13% for cerebellar lesions. In the absence of physical signs 18% of patients had a scan strongly suggestive of multiple sclerosis.

These findings were related to those in other diagnostic tests, VEP, SEP and CSF examination. It was found that in isolated optic neuritis or chronic myelopathy a scheme of investigation beginning with MRI, followed by CSF examination and the recording of SEP or VEP as appropriate, identified all patients who could be classified as laboratory supported definite multiple sclerosis. No patient with these two clinical presentations who did not have a scan strongly suggestive of multiple sclerosis was found to have both oligoclonal bands and EP evidence of a separate lesion, the requirements for the laboratory supported definite category.

Whether the patients with 'strongly suggestive' MRI scans actually have multiple sclerosis will take some time to determine. During a follow-up period of less than one year, 19 patients progressed to clinically definite disease and in 18 of these, this had been predicted from the scan. Ormerod et al[94] found multiple MRI abnormalities of the brain in 29 (69%) of 42 patients with isolated optic neuritis; in 30 (75%) in brainstem lesions; but in only 14 of 23 with isolated chronic spinal cord disease and in 4 of 11 with acute myelopathy. They emphasised that multiple sclerosis could not be diagnosed on MRI evidence of multiple lesions in patients with a single episode of disease, as acute disseminated encephalomyelitis could not be excluded Repeat scans in 35 patients, however,

showed new lesions in 7 who were therefore thought to fulfil the Washington criteria for probable multiple sclerosis.

The most thorough examination of the contribution of MRI to the problem of isolated myelopathy is that of Miller et al.[107] One hundred and twenty one patients with symptoms and signs confined to the spinal cord and normal myelography were identified and examined by MRI of the head and, when possible, of the spinal cord. In acute myelopathy the head scan was abnormal in 18 of 32 patients, being typical of multiple sclerosis in 16. Of 50 patients with chronic progressive myelopathy, the head scan was abnormal in 42 and typical of multiple sclerosis in the great majority. Interestingly, all patients in this group over 50 years of age had multiple abnormalities. In chronic relapsing spinal cord disease, the proportion of scans suggestive of multiple sclerosis was equally high. MRI of the spinal cord, cervical or thoracic, was achieved in 98 patients and was abnormal in 47 of 73 with clinical evidence of a cervical cord lesion but in only 7 of 25 in whom the clinical signs indicated a lower lesion. Localised lesions often correlated well with the clinical findings. Swelling of the spinal cord was seen in six cases, intrinsic tumour being excluded by remission of acute symptoms. These results were compared with those of evoked potential recording and CSF examination that, with the exception of SEP in thoracic cord disease, produced a much smaller proportion of abnormalities.

The specificity of MRI in the diagnosis of multiple sclerosis is manifestly not high and the policy statement[245] on the interpretation of the findings should be heeded, despite some ambiguity of wording. It is recommended that single or multiple white matter lesions typical of multiple sclerosis can be used to satisfy the criterion of dissemination in space but that there must be independent clinical evidence of a second lesion. Presumably this means that there must be signs that could not be accounted for by any of the lesions seen on MRI. If MRI is to be used to establish dissemination in time, new lesions must be shown in later scans using the same sequences and precise repositioning.

The advantage of MRI over other methods of

demonstrating clinically silent lesions is that very often evidence of multiple lesions can actually be seen, measured and watched. Exactly what it is that is 'seen' is discussed in Chapter 8.

Monitoring

The lack of an objective method of monitoring progress of the disease has impeded the assessment of therapeutic measures in multiple sclerosis and the use of MRI for this purpose is highly promising. With present techniques it can never be applicable to all patients. Some find confinement in the machine intolerable and others are unable to keep still or submit to the meticulously exact repositioning necessary for comparable serial scans.

It would first be reassuring to know that the degree of MRI abnormality bore some relationship to clinical severity. A significant correlation has been reported[246,247] between the numbers and size of lesions and the degree of atrophy seen on MRI and the severity of disability, particularly that due to motor, cerebellar or brainstem involvement. Correlation with visual, mental or sphincter disorder was less marked. Huber et al[248] counted the number of lesions and graded from 1–5 the size of discrete lesions, the degree of generalised atrophy and of atrophy of the corpus callosum and the extent of periventricular abnormality. Although most of these criteria were based on measurements, general atrophy was related to age and simply judged against experience of the normal. The results of all these methods of MRI assessment were positively correlated with disability on the Kurtzke scale, but not with duration of disease.

Few results of serial MRI scanning have so far been published. Palo et al,[249] using very low field strength, scanned a series of patients at long intervals up to 2 years. The size of lesions had not changed in 55% of those rescanned after one year and in 64% after 2 years. The number of visible lesions was unchanged at one year in 72% and at 2 years in 60%. Fresh lesions could occur at any time, but more frequently in relapse. Ormerod et al[94] described the results of rescanning 17 patients after three months. In 7, new lesions were seen and in 2 lesions previously visible could no longer

be detected. Changes in size and signal intensity were common but difficult to evaluate.

Isaac et al,[250,251] by scanning at more frequent intervals, were able to follow the course of newly visible lesions. Comparatively large lesions reached maximum size within 2 months of detection. Over the following two months, lesions declined in size and some smaller lesions vanished completely. In a further study, nine patients with mild relapsing and remitting disease were scanned every two weeks for from six to nine months.[252] Six patients developed new lesions, none related to new symptoms. Serial MRI with gadolinium enhancement[253,254] has confirmed the often transient nature of acute lesions, at least as identified by MRI, whether or not associated with clinical relapse. Old lesions would sometimes enhance, often only at the edge.

At the time of writing, the use of MRI in monitoring the course of multiple sclerosis is clearly still in an exploratory stage. The application to clinical trials has so far been limited to serial scanning of patients with chronic multiple sclerosis treated with intravenous methylprednisolone.[255] Continued activity of the disease was observed. It is unlikely that simply measuring the area of unenhanced lesions will prove to be a useful indication of progress, as the extent of oedema shown in this way is greater than that of the inflammatory process[256] and a strong note of caution has been sounded.[257]

CONCLUSION

No test has been found to be consistently positive or abnormal in 100% of cases of clinically definite multiple sclerosis. This was not to be expected as there are few such diagnostic tests in medicine, but there is a significant gap in our knowledge concerning those patients in whom the tests are negative. For example, we do not know whether the 2–5% of clinically definite multiple sclerosis cases that do not have an oligoclonal IgG pattern in the CSF actually have multiple sclerosis. The pattern may be absent because the diagnosis is wrong or because oligoclonal IgG bands are not an essential feature of multiple sclerosis. The latter, the false negative, is the more likely explanation but the answer can only be obtained by continued clinical studies of these patients and eventual histological examination. It may be suspected that the authors of many reports of the diagnostic use of such methods may not be in clinical charge of the patients and do not have the opportunity for the necessary follow-up.

Patients in the less definite diagnostic categories almost invariably have a lower proportion of abnormal results in whatever test is examined. The question of the true diagnosis in patients with normal results is even more important as, by definition, the diagnosis at the time of the examination is in doubt. Follow-up is tedious and must be prolonged, but is essential.

The hope that the method under investigation will be of help in the *early* diagnosis of multiple sclerosis is frequently expressed. There are certainly some advantages in early diagnosis and these would be enormously increased if effective treatment was available. At present, however, the finding of an abnormal result, thought to be of diagnostic value, in a patient with, for example, a single remitting episode of neurological disease, can be more of an embarrassment than a scientific success. The patient may justifiably require

guidance or even wish to know what diagnosis has been arrived at by means of the elaborate tests. After recovery from an episode of sensory symptoms is a single 'diagnostic' test result sufficient evidence on which to 'transfer' a patient to a more definite diagnostic category, or even perhaps to establish a definite diagnosis? If not, what was the purpose of the test? No doubt more extended experience will answer these questions but the fruits of such experience are difficult to gather from the scanty published reports of the practical applications of the results of these methods to the management of the individual patient.

It must be remembered that the pronouncement of a diagnosis of multiple sclerosis, however early, carries significant disadvantages. Life and health insurance at once become more expensive or unobtainable and house purchase adversely affected. Job applications must either be falsified or carry the risk of automatic rejection. Immigration may be barred. Fiancé(e)s or spouses may depart. Child adoption is usually no longer possible. In the absence of clear clinical evidence, such dire effects should not depend on the results of a test of undetermined specificity.

REFERENCES

1. Tourtellotte W W 1974 International symposium on multiple sclerosis. Acta Neurologica Scandinavica 50 (suppl 58): 14
2. Kurtzke J 1974 International symposium on multiple sclerosis. Acta Neurologica Scandinavica 50 (suppl 58): 14
3. Allison R S, Millar J H D 1954 Prevalence and familial incidence of disseminated sclerosis. Report to Northern Ireland Hospital Authority on results of a 3-year survey. Ulster Medical Journal 23 (suppl 2): 1–92
4. Alter M, Allison R S, Talbert O R, Kurland L T 1960 Geographic distribution of multiple sclerosis. World Neurology 1: 55–66
5. Gudmundsson K R, Gudmundsson G 1962 Multiple sclerosis in Iceland. Acta Neurologica Scandinavica 38 (suppl 2): 1–63
6. Leibowitz U, Alter M 1973 Multiple sclerosis: clues to its cause. Elsevier, New York, pp 3–4
7. McAlpine D 1972 In: McAlpine D, Lumsden C E, Acheson E D Multiple sclerosis: a reappraisal. Churchill Livingstone, Edinburgh, p 225
8. McAlpine D 1972 In: McAlpine D, Lumsden C E, Acheson E D Multiple sclerosis: a reappraisal. Churchill Livingstone, Edinburgh, p 202
9. Schumacher G A, Beebe G, Kibler R F et al 1965 Problems of experimental trials of therapy in multiple sclerosis. Annals of the New York Academy of Sciences 122: 552–568
10. International Symposium on multiple sclerosis 1974. Acta Neurologica Scandinavica 50 (suppl 58)
11. McDonald W I, Halliday A M 1977 Diagnosis and classification of multiple sclerosis. British Medical Bulletin 33: 4–9
12. Rose A S, Ellison G W, Myers L W, Tourtellotte W W 1976 Criteria for the clinical diagnosis of multiple sclerosis. Neurology 26 (suppl 20): 22
13. Bauer H J 1980 IMAB-enquête concerning the diagnostic criteria for multiple sclerosis. In: Bauer H J, Poser S, Ritter G (eds) Progress in multiple sclerosis research. Springer, Berlin, pp 555–563
14. Lauer K, Firnhaber W 1986 An evaluation of laboratory investigations in patients with multiple sclerosis. Journal of Chronic Diseases 39: 767–774
15. Broman T, Andersen O, Bergmann L 1981 Clinical studies on multiple sclerosis I: presentation of an incidence material from Gothenburg. Acta Neurologica Scandinavica 63: 6–33
16. Poser C M, Paty D W, Scheinberg L et al 1983 New diagnostic criteria for multiple sclerosis: guidelines for research protocols. Annals of Neurology 13: 227–231
17. Kurtzke J F 1988 Multiple sclerosis: what's in a name? Neurology 38: 309–314
18. Paty D W, Oger J J F, Kastrukoff L F et al 1988 MRI in the diagnosis of MS: a prospective study with comparison of clinical evaluation, evoked potentials, oligoclonal banding, and CT. Neurology 38: 180–185
19. Sanders E A, Reulen J P, van der Velde E A, Hogenhuis L A 1986 The diagnosis of multiple

sclerosis. Contribution of non-clinical tests. Journal of the Neurological Sciences 72: 273–285

20. Namerow N S 1968 Somatosensory evoked responses in multiple sclerosis patients with varying sensory loss. Neurology 18: 1197–1204

21. Halliday A M, McDonald W I, Mushin J 1972 Delayed visual evoked response in optic neuritis. Lancet 1: 982–985

22. Halliday A M, McDonald W I, Mushin J 1973 Visual evoked response in diagnosis of multiple sclerosis. British Medical Journal 4: 661–664

23. Lowitzsch K 1980 Pattern-evoked visual potentials in 251 multiple sclerosis patients in relation to ophthalmological findings and diagnostic classification. In: Bauer H J, Poser S, Ritter G (eds) Progress in multiple sclerosis research. Springer, Berlin, pp 571–577

24. Halliday A M 1980 Event-related potentials and their diagnostic usefulness. In: Kornhuber H H, Deeke L (eds) Motivation, motor and sensory processes of the brain. Elsevier, Amsterdam, pp 469–485

25. Cant B R, Hume A L, Shaw N A 1978 Effects of luminance on the pattern visual evoked potential in multiple sclerosis. Electroencephalography and Clinical Neurophysiology 45: 496–504

26. Hennerici M, Wenzel D, Freund H J 1977 The comparison of small-size rectangle and checkerboard stimulation for the evaluation of delayed visual evoked responses in patients suspected of multiple sclerosis. Brain 100: 119–136

27. Oepen G, Brauer C, Doerr M, Thoden U 1981 Visual evoked potentials (VEP) elicited by checkerboard versus foveal stimulation in multiple sclerosis: a clinical study in 235 patients. Archiv für Psychiatrie und Nervenkrankheiten 229: 305–313

28. Oishi M, Yamada T, Dickins Q S, Kimura J 1985 Visual evoked potentials by different check sizes in patients with multiple sclerosis. Neurology 35: 1461–1465

29. Guérit J M, Argiles A M 1988 The sensitivity of multimodal evoked potentials in multiple sclerosis. A comparison with magnetic resonance imaging and cerebrospinal fluid examination. Electroencephalography and Clinical Neurophysiology 70: 230–238

30. Plant G T, Hess R F, Thomas S J 1986 The pattern evoked electroretinogram in optic neuritis. A combined psychophysical and electrophysiological study. Brain 109: 469–490

31. Tartaglione A, Oneto A, Bandini F, Spadavecchia L, Gandolfo E, Favale E 1987 Electrophysiological detection of 'silent' plaques in the optic pathways. Acta Neurologica Scandinavica 76: 246–250

32. Hammond S R, Yiannikas C 1986 Contribution of pattern reversal foveal and half-field stimulation to analysis of VEP abnormalities in multiple sclerosis. Electroencephalography and Clinical Neurophysiology 64: 101–118

33. Regan D, Milner B A, Heron J R 1976 Delayed visual perception and delayed visual evoked potentials in the spinal form of multiple sclerosis and in retrobulbar neuritis. Brain 99: 43–66

34. Regan D, Milner B A, Heron J R 1977 Slowing of visual signals in multiple sclerosis measured psychophysically and by steady-state evoked potentials. In: Desmedt J E (ed) Visual evoked potentials in man. Oxford University Press, London, pp 461–469

35. Celesia G G, Daly R F 1977 Visual electroencephalic computer analysis (VECA) — a new electrophysiological test for the diagnosis of optic nerve lesions. Neurology 27: 637–641

36. Collins D W K, Carroll W M, Black J L, Walsh M 1979 Effect of refractive error on the visual evoked response. British Medical Journal 1: 231–232

37. Hawkes C H, Stow B 1981 Pupil size and the pattern evoked visual response. Journal of Neurology, Neurosurgery and Psychiatry 44: 90–91

38. Matthews W B, Small D G, Small M, Pountney E 1977 Pattern reversal evoked visual potential in the diagnosis of multiple sclerosis. Journal of Neurology, Neurosurgery and Psychiatry 40: 1009–1014

39. Collins D W K, Black J L, Mastaglia F L 1978 Pattern-reversal visual evoked potentials: method of analysis and results in multiple sclerosis. Journal of the Neurological Sciences 36: 83–95

40. Shahrokhi F, Chiappa K H, Young R R 1979 Pattern shift visual evoked responses: two hundred patients with optic neuritis and/or multiple sclerosis. Archives of Neurology 35: 65–71

41. Chain F, Mallecourt J, Leblanc M, Lhermitte F 1977 Apport de l'enregistrement des potentiels évoqués visuels au diagnostic de la sclérose en plaques. Revue Neurologique 133: 81–88

42. Trojaborg W, Petersen E 1979 Visual and somatosensory evoked cortical potentials in multiple sclerosis. Journal of Neurology, Neurosurgery and Psychiatry 42: 323–330

43. Asselman P, Chadwick D W, Marsden C D 1975 Visual evoked responses in the diagnosis and management of patients suspected of multiple sclerosis. Brain 98: 261–282

44. Mastaglia F L, Black J L, Collins D W K 1976 Visual and spinal evoked potentials in diagnosis of multiple sclerosis. British Medical Journal 2: 732

45. Matthews W B, Wattam-Bell J R B, Pountney E 1982 Evoked potentials in the diagnosis of multiple sclerosis: a follow up study. Journal of Neurology, Neurosurgery and Psychiatry 45: 303–307

46. Carroll W M, Kriss A, Baraitser M, Barrett G, Halliday A M 1980 The incidence and nature of visual pathway involvement in Friedreich's ataxia. Brain 103: 413–434

47. Pedersen L, Trojaborg W 1981 Visual, auditory and somatosensory pathway involvement in hereditary cerebellar ataxia, Friedreich's ataxia and familial spastic paraplegia. Electroencephalography and Clinical Neurophysiology 52: 283–297

48. Conrad B, Benecke R, Müsers H, Prange H, Behrens-Baumann W 1983 Visual evoked potentials in neurosyphilis. Journal of Neurology, Neurosurgery and Psychiatry 46: 23–27

49. Streletz L J, Chambers R A, Sung H B, Israel H L 1981 Visual evoked potentials in sarcoidosis. Neurology 31: 1545–1551

50. Fine E J, Hallett M 1980 Neurophysiological study of subacute combined degeneration. Journal of the Neurological Sciences 45: 331–336

51 Newton M, Cruikshank K K, Miller D, Dalgleish A, Rudge P, Clayden S, Moseley I 1987 Antibody to human T-lymphotropic virus type 1 in West-Indian-born UK residents with spastic paraparesis. Lancet 1: 415–416

52. Jabs D A, Mill N R, Newmn S A, Johnson M A, Stevens M B 1986 Optic neuropathy in systemic lupus

erythematosus. Archives of Ophthalmology 104: 564–568

53. El-Negamy E, Sedgwick E M 1978 Properties of a spinal somatosensory evoked potential recorded in man. Journal of Neurology, Neurosurgery and Psychiatry 41: 762–768

54. Matthews W B, Beauchamp M, Small D G 1974 Cervical somatosensory responses in man. Nature 252: 230–232

55. Desmedt J E, Cheron G 1980 Central somatosensory conduction in man: neural generators and interpeak latencies of the far-field components recorded from the neck and right or left scalp and ear lobes. Electroencephalography and Clinical Neurophysiology 50: 382–403

56. Nuwer M R, Packwood J W, Myers L W, Ellison G W 1987 Evoked potentials predict the clinical changes in a multiple sclerosis drug study. Neurology 37: 1754–1761

57. Leuders H, Dinner D S, Lesser R P, Klem G 1983 Origin of far-field subcortical evoked potentials to posterior tibial and median nerve stimulation. A comparative study. Archives of Neurology 40: 93–97

58. Desmedt J E, Bourget M 1985 Color imaging of parietal and frontal somatosensory potentials evoked by stimulation of median or posterior tibial nerves in man. Electroencephalography and Clinical Neurophysiology 62: 1–17

59. Small M, Matthews W B 1984 A method of calculating spinal cord transit time from potentials evoked by tibial nerve stimulation in normal subjects and in patients with spinal cord disease. Electroencephalography and Clinical Neurophysiology 59: 156–164

60. Needles J H 1935 The caudal level of termination of the spinal cord in American whites and American negroes. Anatomical Record 63: 417–424

61. Strenge H, Tackmann W, Barth R, Sojka-Raytscheff A 1980 Central somatosensory conduction time in diagnosis of multiple sclerosis. European Neurology 19: 402–408

62. Halliday A M, Wakefield G S 1963 Cerebral evoked potentials in patients with dissociated sensory loss. Journal of Neurology, Neurosurgery and Psychiatry 26: 211–219

63. Baker J B, Larson S J, Sances A, White P T 1968 Evoked potentials as an aid to the diagnosis of multiple sclerosis. Neurology 18: 286

64. Small D G, Beauchamp M, Matthews W B 1980 Subcortical somatosensory evoked potentials in normal man and in patients with central nervous lesions. In: Desmedt J E (ed) Clinical uses of cerebral, brainstem and spinal somatosensory evoked potentials. Karger, Basel, pp 190–204

65. Small D G, Matthews W B, Small M 1977 Subcortical somatosensory evoked potentials in multiple sclerosis. Electroencephalography and Clinical Neurophysiology 43: 536

66. Small D G, Matthews W B, Small M 1978 The cervical somatosensory evoked potential (SEP) in the diagnosis of multiple sclerosis. Journal of the Neurological Sciences 35: 211–224

67. Eisen A, Stewart J, Nudleman K, Cosgrove 1979 Short-latency somatosensory responses in multiple sclerosis. Neurology 29: 827–834

68. Anziska B, Craco R, Cook A W, Feld E W 1978 Somatosensory far field potentials: studies in normal subjects and patients with multiple sclerosis. Electroencephalography and Clinical Neurophysiology 45: 602–610

69. Green J B, Price R, Woodbury S G 1980 Short-latency somatosensory evoked potentials in multiple sclerosis: comparison with auditory and visual potentials. Archives of Neurology 37: 630–633

70. Khosbin S, Hallett M 1981 Multiple evoked potentials and blink reflex in multiple sclerosis. Neurology 31: 138–144

71. Rossini P M, Basciani M, di Stefano E, Febro A, Mercuri N 1985 Short-latency scalp somatosensory evoked potentials and central spine to scalp propagation characteristics during peroneal and median nerve stimulation in multiple sclerosis. Electroencephalography and Clinical Neurophysiology 60: 197–206

72. Purves S J, Low M D, Galloway J, Reeves B 1981 A comparison of visual, brainstem auditory and somatosensory evoked potentials in multiple sclerosis. Canadian Journal of Neurological Sciences 8: 15–19

73. Kjaer M 1980 The value of brain stem auditory, visual and somatosensory evoked potentials and blink reflexes in the diagnosis of multiple sclerosis. Acta Neurologica Scandinavica 62: 220–236

74. Davis S L, Aminoff M J, Panitch H S 1985 Clinical correlations of serial somatosensory evoked potentials. Neurology 35: 359–365

75. Dorfman L J 1977 Indirect estimation of spinal cord conduction velocity in man. Electroencephalography and Clinical Neurophysiology 26: 26–34

76. Eisen A, Nudleman K 1979 Cord to cortex conduction in multiple sclerosis. Neurology 29: 189–193

77. Robinson K, Rudge P 1977 Abnormalities of the auditory evoked potentials in patients with multiple sclerosis. Brain 100: 19–40

78. Stockard J J, Stockard E J, Sharbrough F W 1979 Brain-stem auditory evoked potentials. Archives of Neurology 36: 597–598

79. Prasher D K, Gibson W P R 1980 Brain stem auditory evoked potentials — significant latency differences between ipsilateral and contralateral stimulation. Electroencephalography and Clinical Neurophysiology 50: 240–246

80. Beagley H A, Sheldrake J B 1978 Differences in brainstem response latency with age and sex. British Journal of Audiology 12: 69–77

81. Robinson K, Rudge P 1975 Auditory evoked responses in multiple sclerosis. Lancet 1: 1164–1166

82. Starr A, Achor L J 1975 Auditory brain stem responses in neurological disease. Archives of Neurology 32: 761–768

83. Kjaer M 1979 Evaluation and graduation of brain stem auditory evoked potentials in patients with neurological diseases. Acta Neurologica Scandinavica 60: 231–242

84. Tackmann W, Strenge H, Barth R, Sojika-Raytscheff A 1980 Auditory brain stem evoked potentials in patients with multiple sclerosis. European Neurology 19: 396–401

85. Prasher D K, Gibson W P R 1980 Brain stem auditory evoked potentials: a comparative study of monaural versus binaural stimulation in the detection of multiple sclerosis. Electroencephalography and Clinical Neurophysiology 50: 247–253

86. Barajas J J 1982 Evaluation of ipsilateral and contralateral brainstem auditory evoked potentials in multiple sclerosis patients. Journal of the Neurological Sciences 54: 69–78

87. Robinson K, Rudge P 1980 The use of the auditory evoked potential in the diagnosis of multiple sclerosis. Journal of the Neurological Sciences 45: 235–244

88. Zeitlhofer J, Hess C W, Ludin H P 1988 Brainstem auditory-evoked potentials studied with paired stimuli in multiple sclerosis. European Neurology 28: 131–134

89. Chiappa K H, Harrison J L, Brooks E B, Young R R 1980 Brainstem auditory evoked responses in 200 patients with multiple sclerosis. Annals of Neurology 7: 135–143

90. Stockard J J, Stockard E J, Sharbrough F W 1977 Detection and localisation of occult lesions with brainstem auditory responses. Mayo Clinic Proceedings 52: 761–769

91. Baum K, Scheuler W, Hegerl U, Girhe W, Schöner W 1988 Detection of brainstem lesions in multiple sclerosis: comparison of brainstem auditory evoked potentials with MRI. Acta Neurologica Scandinavica 77: 283–288

92. Fischer C, Joyeux O, Haguenauer J P, Maugière F, Schott B 1984 Surdité et acouphènes lors de poussées dans 10 cas de sclérose en plaques. Revue Neurologique 140: 117–125

93. Hutchinson M, Blandford S, Glynn D, Martin E A 1984 Clinical correlation of abnormal brain-stem auditory evoked potentials in multiple sclerosis. Acta Neurologica Scandinavica 70: 90–95

94. Ormerod I E C, Miller D H, McDonald W I et al 1987 The role of nuclear magnetic resonance imaging in the assessment of multiple sclerosis and isolated neurological lesions. A quantitative study. Brain 110: 1579–1616

95. Chiappa K H 1984 Pattern-shift visual, brainstem auditory and short-latency somatosensory evoked potentials in multiple sclerosis. Annals of the New York Academy of Sciences 436: 315–326

96. Hopf H C, Maurer K 1983 Wave 1 of early auditory evoked potentials in multiple sclerosis. Electroencephalography and Clinical Neurophysiology 56: 31–37

97. Ragi E F 1986 Analysis of brainstem auditory evoked potentials in neurological disease. Thesis, Oxford University

98. Trojaborg W, Petersen E 1979 Visual and somatosensory cortical potentials in multiple sclerosis. Journal of Neurology, Neurosurgery and Psychiatry 42: 323–330

99. Delterne P, Vercruysse A, van Nechel C et al 1979 Early diagnosis of multiple sclerosis by combined multimodal evoked potentials. Journal of Biochemical Engineering 1: 17–21

100. Chiappa K H 1980 Pattern shift visual, brainstem auditory, and short latency somatosensory evoked potentials in multiple sclerosis. Neurology 30 (7 pt 2): 110–123

101. Kjaer M 1980 The value of brainstem auditory, visual and somatosenory evoked potentials and blink reflexes in the diagnosis of multiple sclerosis. Acta Neurologica Scandinavica 62: 220–236

102. Tackmann W, Strenge H, Barth R, Sojka-Raytscheff A 1980 Evaluation of various brain structures in multiple sclerosis with multimodality evoked potentials, blink reflex and nystagmography. Journal of Neurology 224: 33–46

103. Kjaer M 1987 Evoked potentials in the diagnosis of multiple sclerosis. Electroencephalography and Clinical Neurophysiology (suppl) 39: 291–296

104. Gebarski S S, Gabrielson T O, Gilman S, Knake J E, Latack J T, Aisen A M 1985 The initial diagnosis of multiple sclerosis: clinical impact of magnetic resonance imaging. Annals of Neurology 17: 469–474

105. Geisser B S, Kurtzberg D, Vaughan H G et al 1987 Trimodal evoked potentials compared with magnetic resonance imaging in the diagnosis of multiple sclerosis. Archives of Neurology 44: 281–284

106. Comi G, Martinelli V, Medaglini S, Locatelli T, Filippi M, Canal N, Triulzi F, Delhaschio A 1989 Correlation between multimodal evoked potentials and magnetic resonance imaging in multiple sclerosis. Journal of Neurology 236: 4–8

107. Miller D H, McDonald W I, Blumhardt L D et al 1987 Magnetic resonance imaging in isolated spinal cord syndromes. Annals of Neurology 22: 714–723

108. Mastaglia F L, Black J L, Cala L A, Collins D W K 1980 Electrophysiology and avoidance of invasive neuroradiology in multiple sclerosis. British Medical Journal 1: 1315–1317

109. Blumhardt L D, Barrett G, Halliday A M 1982 The pattern visual evoked potential in the clinical assessment of undiagnosed spinal cord disease. Advances in Neurology 32: 463–471

110. Marshall J 1955 Spastic paraplegia of middle age: a clinicopathological study. Lancet 1: 643–646

111. Ungar-Sargon J Y, Lovelace R E, Brust J C M 1980 Spastic paraparesis, a reappraisal. Journal of the Neurological Sciences 46: 1–12

112. Bynke H, Olsson J-E, Rosén I 1977 Diagnostic value of visual evoked response, clinical eye examination and CSF analysis in chronic myelopathy. Acta Neurologica Scandinavica 56: 55–59

113. Paty D W, Blume W T, Brown W F, Jaatoul N, Kertesz A, McInnis W 1979 Chronic progressive myelopathy: investigation with CSF electrophoresis, evoked potentials and CT scan. Annals of Neurology 6: 419–424

114. Stockard J J, Stockard E J, Sharbrough F W 1986 Brainstem auditory evoked potentials in neurology: methodology, interpretation, clinical application. In: Aminoff M (ed) Electrodiagnosis in clinical neurology, 2nd edn. Churchill Livingstone, New York, pp 467–504

115. Hume A, Waxman S G 1988 Evoked potentials in suspected multiple sclerosis: diagnostic value and prediction of clinical course. Journal of the Neurological Sciences 83: 191–210

116. Delterne P, van Nechel C, Strul S, Ketelaer P 1984 A five-year prospective study on the value of multimodal evoked potentials and blink reflex as an aid to the diagnosis of suspected multiple sclerosis. In: Nodar R H, Barber C (eds) Evoked potentials II. Butterworth, Boston, pp 603–608

117. Matthews W B, Small D G 1979 Serial recordings of visual and somatosensory evoked potentials in multiple sclerosis. Journal of the Neurological Sciences 40: 11–21

118. Aminoff M J, Davis S L, Panitch H S 1984 Serial evoked potential studies in patients with definite

multiple sclerosis. Clinical relevance. Archives of Neurology 41: 1197–1202

119. Anderson D C, Slater G E, Sherman R, Ettinger M G 1987 Evoked potentials to test a treatment of chronic multiple sclerosis. Archives of Neurology 44: 1232–1236

120. Hely M A, McManis P G, Walsh J C, McLeod J G 1986 Visual evoked responses and ophthalmological examination in optic neuritis. A follow-up study. Journal of the Neurological Sciences 75: 275–283

121. Matthews W B, Small M 1983 Prolonged follow-up of abnormal visual evoked potentials in multiple sclerosis: evidence for delayed recovery. Journal of Neurology, Neurosurgery and Psychiatry 46: 639–642

122. Likosky W, Elmore R S 1981 Exacerbation detection in multiple sclerosis by clinical and evoked potential techniques: a preliminary report. In: Courjon J, Maugière F, Revol M (eds) Clinical applications of evoked potentials in neurology. Raven Press, New York, pp 535–540

123. Nuwer M R, Ellison G W, Myers L W 1989 Evoked potentials during multiple sclerosis therapeutic trials. Archives of Neurology 46: 11–12

124. Anderson D C, Sherman R 1989 Evoked potentials during multiple sclerosis therapeutic trials. Archives of Neurology 46: 12–13

125. Merton P A, Morton H B 1980 Electrical stimulation of the human motor and visual cortex. Journal of Physiology 305: 9P–10P

126. Merton P A, Hill D K, Morton H B, Marsden C D 1982 Scope of a technique for electrical stimulation of the human brain, spinal cord and muscle. Lancet 2: 597–600

127. Cowan J M A, Rothwell J C, Dick J P R, Thompson P D, Day B L, Marsden C D 1984 Abnormality in central motor pathway conduction in multiple sclerosis. Lancet 2: 304–306

128. Mills K R, Murray N M F 1985 Corticospinal tract conduction time in multiple sclerosis. Annals of Neurology 18: 601–605

129. Snooks S J, Swash M 1985 Motor conduction velocity in the human spinal cord: slowed conduction in multiple sclerosis and radiation myelopathy. Journal of Neurology, Neurosurgery and Psychiatry 48: 1135–1139

130. Barker A T, Jalinous R, Freestone I L 1985 Non-invasive magnetic stimulation of human motor cortex. Lancet 1: 1106–1107

131. Ingram D A, Thompson A J, Swash M 1988 Central motor conduction in multiple sclerosis: evaluation of abnormalities revealed by transcutaneous magnetic stimulation of the brain. Journal of Neurology, Neurosurgery and Psychiatry 51: 487–494

132. Hess C W, Mills K R, Murray N M F, Schreifer T N 1987 Magnetic brain stimulation: central motor conduction studies in multiple sclerosis. Annals of Neurology 22: 744–752

133. Diener H C, Dichgans J, Hülser P-J, Buettner U-W, Bacher M, Guschlbauer B 1984 The significance of delayed long-loop responses to ankle displacement for the diagnosis of multiple sclerosis. Electroencephalography and Clinical Neurophysiology 57: 336–342

134. Deuschl G, Strahl K, Schenk E, Lücking C H 1988 The diagnostic significance of long-latency reflexes in multiple sclerosis. Electroecephalography and Clinical Neurophysiology 70: 56–61

135. Sloan S L 1942 The use of pseudo-isochromatic charts in detecting central scotomas due to lesions of the conducting pathways. American Journal of Ophthalmology 25: 1352–1356

136. Steinmetz R D, Kearns T P 1956 H-R-R pseudo-isochromatic plates as a diagnostic aid in retrobulbar neuritis. American Journal of Ophthalmology 41: 833–837

137. Rosen J A 1965 Pseudo-isochromatic visual testing in the diagnosis of disseminated sclerosis. Transactions of the American Neurological Association 98: 283–284

138. Zeller R W 1967 Ocular findings in the remission phase of multiple sclerosis. American Journal of Ophthalmology 64: 767–772

139. Barde R M, Gallin P F 1975 Visual parameters associated with recovered retrobulbar neuritis. American Journal of Ophthalmology 79: 1034–1037

140. Regan D, Sliver R, Murray T J 1977 Visual acuity and contrast sensitivity in multiple sclerosis: hidden visual loss. Brain 100: 563–579

141. Harrison A C, Becker W J, Stell W K 1987 Colour vision abnormalities in multiple sclerosis. Canadian Journal of Neurological Sciences 14: 279–285

142. Griffin J F, Wray S H 1978 Acquired color vision defects in retrobulbar neuritis. American Journal of Ophthalmology 86: 193–201

143. Engell T, Trojaborg W, Rann N E 1987 Subclinical optic neuritis in multiple sclerosis. Acta Ophthalologica 65: 735–740

144. Frederiksen L, Larsson H, Olesen J, Stigsby B 1986 Evaluation of the visual system in multiple sclerosis. II. Colour vision. Acta Neurologica Scandinavica 74: 203–209

145. MacFadyen D J, Drance S M, Chisholm I A, Douglas G R, Kozak J F, Paty D W 1988 The Farnsworth–Munsell 100-Hue color vision score and visual evoked potentials in multiple sclerosis. Neuro-Ophthalmology 8: 289–298

146. Frisén L, Hoyt W F 1974 Insidious atrophy of retinal nerve fibres in multiple sclerosis. Archives of Ophthalmology 92: 91–97

147. Patterson V H, Heron J R 1980 Visual field abnormalities in multiple sclerosis. Journal of Neurology, Neurosurgery and Psychiatry 43: 205–208

148. Regan D 1964 Visual psychophysical tests in the diagnosis of multiple sclerosis. In: Poser C M (ed) The diagnosis of multiple sclerosis. Thieme-Stratton, New York, pp 94–102

149. Hess R F, Plant G T 1986 The psychophysical loss in optic neuritis: spatial and temporal aspects. In: Hess R F, Plant G T (eds) Optic neuritis. Cambridge University Press, pp 109–151

150. Foster D H 1986 Psychophysical loss in optic neuritis: luminance and colour aspects. In: Hess R F, Plant G T (eds) Optic neuritis. Cambridge University Press, pp 152–191

151. Titcombe A F, Willison R G 1961 Flicker fusion in multiple sclerosis. Journal of Neurology, Neurosurgery and Psychiatry 24: 260–265

152. Thorner M W, Berk M E 1964 Flicker fusion test I: In neuro-ophthalmologic conditions including multiple sclerosis. Archives of Ophthalmology 71: 807–815

153. Daley M L, Swank R L, Ellison C M 1979 Flicker fusion thresholds in multiple sclerosis: a functional

measure of neurological damage. Archives of Neurology 36: 292–295

154. Cohen S N, Syndulko K, Tourtellotte W W, Potvin A R 1980 Critical frequency of photic driving in the diagnosis of multiple sclerosis: a comparison to pattern evoked responses. Archives of Neurology 37: 80–83

155. Romani V, Torres F, Loewenson R 1984 Critical frequency of photic driving in multiple sclerosis. Archives of Neurology 41: 752–755

156. Pulfrich C 1922 Die Stereoskopie im Dienste der isochromen und heterochromen Photometrie. Naturwissenschaft 10: 553–564

157. Rushton D 1975 Use of the Pulfrich pendulum for detecting abnormal delay in the visual pathway in multiple sclerosis. Brain 98: 283–296

158. Wist E R, Hennerici M, Dichgans J 1978 The Pulfrich spatial frequency phenomenon: a psychophysical method competitive to visual evoked potentials in the diagnosis of multiple sclerosis. Journal of Neurology, Neurosurgery and Psychiatry 41: 1069–1077

159. Heron J R, Regan D, Milner B A 1974 Delay in visual perception in unilateral optic atrophy after retrobulbar neuritis. Brain 97: 69–78

160. Carter R, Danta G 1985 Spatial contrast sensitivity in patients with multiple sclerosis. Clinical and Experimental Neurology 21: 233–247

161. Fahy J, Glynn D, Hutchinson M 1989 Contrast sensitivity in multiple sclerosis measured by Cambridge low contrast gratings: a useful clinical test? Journal of Neurology, Neurosurgery and Psychiatry 52: 786–787

162. Swart S, Millac P 1980 A comparison of flight of colours with visually evoked responses in patients with multiple sclerosis. Journal of Neurology, Neurosurgery and Psychiatry 43: 550–551

163. Lacquaniti F, Benna P, Gilli M, Troni W, Bergamasco B 1979 Brain stem auditory evoked potentials and blink reflex in quiescent multiple sclerosis. Electroencephalography and Clinical Neurophysiology 47: 607–610

164. Kimura J 1975 Electrically elicited blink reflex in diagnosis of multiple sclerosis. Brain 98: 413–426

165. Yates S K, Brown W F 1981 Light-stimulus-evoked blink reflex: methods, normal values, relation to other 'blink' reflexes and observations in multiple sclerosis. Neurology 31: 272–281

166. Hess K 1979 Stapedius reflex in multiple sclerosis. Journal of Neurology, Neurosurgery and Psychiatry 42: 331–337

167. van Vliet A G M, van Lith G H M 1979 Nystagmography as a diagnostic tool in multiple sclerosis. Documenta Ophthalmologica 46: 334–344

168. Solingen L D, Baloh R W, Myers L, Ellison G 1977 Subclinical eye movement disorders in patients with multiple sclerosis. Neurology 27: 614–619

169. Mastaglia F L, Black J L, Collins D W K 1979 Quantitative studies of saccadic and pursuit eye movements in multiple sclerosis. Brain 102: 817–834

170. Mastaglia F L, Black J L, Thickbroom G, Collins D W K 1982 Saccadic eye movements in multiple sclerosis. Neuro–Ophthalmology 2: 255–260

171. Ellenberger C, Daroff R B 1984 Neuro-ophthalmic aspects of multiple sclerosis. In: Poser C M (ed) The diagnosis of multiple sclerosis. Thieme–Stratton, New York, pp 49–63

172. Tedeschi G, Allocca S, di Costanzo A, Diano A,

Bonavita V 1989 Role of saccadic analysis in the diagnosis of multiple sclerosis in the era of magnetic resonance imaging. Journal of Neurology, Neurosurgery and Psychiatry 52: 967–969

173. Sharpe J A, Goldberg H J, Lo A W, Herishanu Y O 1981 Visual-vestibular interaction in multiple sclerosis. Neurology 31: 427–433

174. Ashworth B, Emery V 1963 Cerebral dysrhythmia in disseminated sclerosis. Brain 86: 173–18

175. Macrae D, Aird R B 1954 The electroencephalogram in multiple sclerosis. Electroencephalography and Clinical Neurophysiology 6: 669–670

176. Goldstein N M, Satran R 1974 Serial electroencephalographic observations in chronic multiple sclerosis. Archives of Internal Medicine 134: 1055–1058

177. Danielczyk W 1978 Das EEG im Verlauf der multiplen Sklerose. Wiener Klinische Wochenschrift 90: 377–380

178. Levic Z M 1978 Electroencephalographic studies in multiple sclerosis: specific changes in benign multiple sclerosis. Electroencephalography and Clinical Neurophysiology 44: 471–478

179. Simons D J 1937 A note on the effect of heat and cold upon certain symptoms of multiple sclerosis. Bulletin of the Neurological Institute of New York 6: 385–386

180. Brickner R M 1948 The significance of localised vasoconstrictions in multiple sclerosis. Publications of the Association for Research into Nervous and Mental Diseases 28: 236–244

181. Guthrie T C 1951 Visual and motor changes in patients with multiple sclerosis: a result of induced changes in environmental temperature. Archives of Neurology and Psychiatry 65: 437–451

182. Namerow N S 1968 Circadian temperature rhythm and vision in multiple sclerosis. Neurology 18: 417–422

183. Hopper C L, Matthews C G, Cleeland C S 1972 Symptom instability and thermoregulation in multiple sclerosis. Neurology 22: 142–148

184. Edmund J, Fog T 1955 Visual and motor instability in multiple sclerosis. Archives of Neurology and Psychiatry 73: 316–323

185. Nelson D A, McDowell F 1959 The effects of induced hyperthermia on patients with multiple sclerosis. Journal of Neurology, Neurosurgery and Psychiatry 22: 113–116

186. Malhotra A S, Goren H 1981 The hot bath test in the diagnosis of multiple sclerosis. Journal of the American Medical Association 246: 1113–1114

187. Rolak L A, Ashizawa T 1985 The hot bath test in multiple sclerosis: comparison with visual evoked potentials and oligoclonal bands. Acta Neurologica Scandinavica 72: 65–67

188. Nelson D A, Jeffries W H, McDowell F 1958 Effects of induced hyperthermia on some neurological diseases. Archives of Neurology and Psychiatry 79: 31–39

189. Field E J, Shenton B K, Joyce G 1974 Specific laboratory test for multiple sclerosis. British Medical Journal 1: 412–414

190. Field E J, Joyce G 1976 Simplified laboratory test for multiple sclerosis. Lancet 2: 367–368

191. Field E J, Joyce G 1979 Multiple sclerosis: what can and cannot be done. British Medical Journal 2: 1571–1572

192. Matthews W B 1985 In: Matthews W B (ed) McAlpine's multiple sclerosis. Churchill Livingstone, Edinburgh, pp 199–201

193. Boudin G, Barbizet J 1954 Les données morphologiques de la pneumoencéphalographie au cours de la sclérose en plaques (dilatation ventriculaire et augmentation de l'air périhémisphérique). Revue Neurologique 90: 241–244 Physiology 305: 9P–10P

194. Haughton V M, Ho K-C, Boedecker R A 1979 The contracting cord sign of multiple sclerosis. Neuroradiology 17: 207–209

195. Feasby T E, Paty D W, Ebers G C, Fox A J 1981 Spinal cord swelling in multiple sclerosis. Canadian Journal of Neurological Sciences 8: 151–153

196. Gize R W, Mishkin F S 1970 Brain scans in multiple sclerosis. Radiology 97: 297–299

197. Antunes J L, Schlesinger E B, Michelsen W J 1974 The abnormal brain scan in demyelinating disease. Archives of Neurology 30: 269–271

198. Cala L A, Mastaglia F L 1976 Computerised axial tomography in multiple sclerosis. Lancet 1: 689

199. Warren R G, Ball M J, Paty D W, Banna M 1976 Computed tomography in disseminated sclerosis. Canadian Journal of Neurological Sciences 3: 211–216

200. Gyldenstedt C 1976 Computer tomography of the brain in multiple sclerosis. Acta Neurologica Scandinavica 53: 386–389

201. Gyldenstedt C 1976 Computer tomography of the cerebrum in multiple sclerosis. Neuroradiology 12: 33–42

202. Cole M, Ross R J 1977 Plaque of multiple sclerosis seen on computerised transaxial tomography. Neurology 27: 890–891

203. Harding A E, Radue E W, Whiteley A M 1978 Contrast enhanced lesions on computerised tomography in multiple sclerosis. Journal of Neurology, Neurosurgery and Psychiatry 41: 754–758

204. Sears E S, Tindall R S A, Zarnow H 1979 Active multiple sclerosis: enhanced computerised tomographic imaging of lesions and the effect of corticosteroids. Archives of Neurology 35: 426–434

205. Lebow S, Anderson D C, Mastri A, Larson D 1979 Active multiple sclerosis with contrast-enhancing plaques. Archives of Neurology 35: 435–439

206. Moriaru M A, Wilkins D E, Patel S 1980 Multiple sclerosis and serial computerised tomography. Delayed contrast enhancement of acute and early lesions. Archives of Neurology 37: 189–190

207. Davis J M, Davis K R, Newhouse J, Pfister R C 1979 Expanded high iodine dose in computerised cranial tomography: a preliminary report. Radiology 131: 373–380

208. Sears E S, McCammon A, Bigelow R, Hayman A L 1982 Maximising the harvest of contrast enhancing lesions in multiple sclerosis. Neurology 32: 815–820

209. Vinuela F V, Fox A J, Debran G M, Feasby T E, Ebers G C 1982 New perspectives in computed tomography of multiple sclerosis. American Journal of Neuroradiology 3: 227–281

210. Drayer B P, Barrett L 1984 Magnetic resonance imaging and CT scanning in multiple sclerosis. Annals of the New York Academy of Sciences 436: 294–314

211. Barrett L, Drayer B, Shin C 1985 High-resolution computerised tomography in multiple sclerosis. Annals of Neurology 17: 33–38

212. Coin C G, Hucks-Follis A 1979 Cervical computed tomography in multiple sclerosis with spinal cord involvement. Journal of Computer Assisted Tomography 3: 431–432

213. Latack J L, Gabrielsen T O, Knake J E, Gebarski S S, Dorovini-Zis K 1984 Computed tomography of spinal cord necrosis from multiple sclerosis. American Journal of Neuroradiology 8: 485–487

214. Weinstein M A, Lederman R J, Rothner A D, Duchesnau P M, Norman D 1978 Interval computed tomography in multiple sclerosis. Radiology 129: 689–694

215. Sagar H J, Warlow C P, Sheldon P W E, Esiri M M 1982 Multiple sclerosis with clinical and radiological features of cerebral tumour. Journal of Neurology, Neurosurgery and Psychiatry 45: 802–808

216. Rosenberg G A, Kornfeld M, Storring J, Bicknell J M 1979 Subcortical arteriosclerotic encephalopathy (Binswanger): computerised tomography. Neurology 29: 1102–1106

217. Goto K, Ishi N, Fukusawa H 1981 Diffuse white-matter disease in the geriatric population: a clinical and CT study. Radiology 141: 687–695

218. Kinkel W R, Jacobs L, Polachini I, Bates V, Heffner R R 1985 Subcortical arteriosclerotic encephalopathy (Binswanger's disease): computed tomographic, nuclear magnetic resonance, and clinical correlations. Archives of Neurology 42: 951–959

219. Bartolini S, Insitari D, Castagnoli A, Amaducci L 1982 Correlation of isotopic cisternographic patterns in multiple sclerosis with CSF IgG values. Annals of Neurology 12: 486–489

220. Volpi G, Insitari D, Fratiglioni L et al 1986 CT periventricular hypodensity in multiple sclerosis: isotopic cisternography and clinical correlations. Annals of Neurology 20: 146

221. Koopmans R A, Li D K B, Grochowski E, Cutler P J, Paty D W 1989 Benign versus chronic progressive multiple sclerosis. Magnetic resonance imaging features. Annals of Neurology 25: 74–81

222. Jackson J A, Leake D R, Schneider N J et al 1985 Magnetic resonance imaging in multiple sclerosis: results in 32 cases. American Journal of Neuroradiology 6: 1712–1716

223. Wright G D S, Anslow P, Davis C J F 1987 An evaluation of high-dose contrast delayed CT-scanning in multiple sclerosis. Journal of Neurology, Neurosurgery and Psychiatry 50: 952–953

224. Kean D M, Smith M A 1986 Magnetic resonance imaging. Principles and applications. Heinemann, London

225. Young I R, Hall A S, Pallis C A, Legg N J, Bydder G M, Steiner R E 1981 Nuclear magnetic resonance imaging of the brain in multiple sclerosis. Lancet 2: 1063–1066

226. Lukes S A, Crooks L E, Aminoff M J, Kaufman L, Panitch H, Mills C, Norman D 1983 Nuclear magnetic imaging in multiple sclerosis. Annals of Neurology 13: 592–601

227. Runge V M, Price A C, Kirshner H S, Allen J H, Partain C L, James A E 1984 Magnetic resonance imaging of multiple sclerosis: a study of pulse-technique efficacy. American Journal of Roentgenology 143: 1015–1026

228. Stewart W A, Hall L D, Berry K, Paty D W 1984 Correlation between NMR scan and brain slice data in multiple sclerosis. Lancet 2: 412

229. Maravilla K R, Weinreb J C, Suss R, Nunnally R L 1985 Magnetic resonance demonstration of multiple sclerosis plaques in the cervical cord. American Journal of Roentgenology 144: 381–385

230. Honing L S, Sheremata W A 1989 Magnetic resonance imaging of spinal cord lesions in multiple sclerosis. Journal of Neurology, Neurosurgery and Psychiatry 52: 459–466

231. Miller D H, Newton M R, van der Poel J C et al 1988 Magnetic resonance imaging of the optic nerve in optic neuritis. Neurology 38: 175–179

232. Poser C M 1985 MRI and CT scan in multiple sclerosis. Journal of the American Medical Association 253: 3250

233. Sheldon J J, Siddharthan R, Tobias J, Sheremata W A, Soila K, Viamonte M 1985 MR imaging of multiple sclerosis: comparison with clinical and CT examinations in 74 patients. American Journal of Roentgenology 145: 957–964

234. Cutler J R, Aminoff M J, Brant-Zawadzki M 1986 Evaluation of patients with multiple sclerosis by evoked potentials and magnetic resonance imaging: a comparative study. Annals of Neurology 20: 645–648

235. Kirshner H S, Tsai S I, Runge V M, Price A C 1985 Magnetic resonance imaging and other techniques in the diagnosis of multiple sclerosis. Archives of Neurology 42: 859–863

236. Robertson W D, Li D, Mayo J, Genton M, Paty D W 1985 MRI in the diagnosis of multiple sclerosis. Journal of Neurology 232 (suppl 1): 58

237. Jacobs L, Kinkel W R, Polachini I, Kinkel R P 1986 Correlations of nuclear magnetic resonance imaging, computerized tomography, and clinical profiles in multiple sclerosis. Neurology 36: 27–34

238. Grossman R I, Gonzalez–Scarano F, Atlas S W, Galetta S, Silberg D H 1986 Multiple sclerosis: gadolinium enhancement in MR imaging. Radiology 161: 721–725

239. Gonzalez-Scarano F, Grossman R I, Galetta S, Atlas S W, Silberberg D H 1987. Multiple sclerosis disease activity correlates with gadolinium enhanced magnetic resonance imaging. Annals of Neurology 21: 300–306

240. Fazekas F, Offenbacher H, Fuchs S et al 1988 Criteria for an increased specificity of MRI interpretation in elderly subjects. Neurology 38: 1822–1825

241. Lubetzki C, Dormont D, Debussche C et al 1989 Dilatation médullaire pseudo-tumorale au cours de la sclérose en plaques. Deux cas avec imagerie par résonance magnétique. Revue Neurologique 145: 239–242

242. Papadopoulos N M, McFarlin D E, Patronas N J, McFarland H F, Costel R 1987 A comparison between chemical analysis and MRI with the clinical diagnosis of multiple sclerosis. American Journal of Clinical Pathology 88: 365–368

243. Miska R M, Pojunas K W, McQuillen M P 1987 Cranial magnetic resonance imaging in the evaluation of myelopathy of undetermined etiology. Neurology 37: 840–843

244. Ringelstein E B, Krieger D, Hünermann B 1987 Evaluation by MRI of paraparesis and tetraparesis of undiagnosed aetiology. Journal of Neurology 234: 401–407

245. Paty D W, Asbury A K, Herndon R M et al 1986 Use of magnetic resonance imaging in the diagnosis of multiple sclerosis. Policy statement. Neurology 36: 1575

246. Stevens J C, Farlow M R, Edwards M K, Yu P 1986 Magnetic resonance imaging. Clinical correlation in 64 patients with multiple sclerosis. Archives of Neurology 43: 1145–1148

247. Edwards M K, Farlow M R, Stevens J C 1986 Multiple sclerosis: MRI and clinical correlation. American Journal of Roentgenology 147: 571–574

248. Huber S J, Paulson G W, Chakeres D et al 1988 Magnetic resonance imaging and clinical correlation in multiple sclerosis. Journal of the Neurological Sciences 86: 1–12

249. Palo J, Ketonen L, Wikström J 1988 A follow-up study of very low field MRI findings and clinical course in multiple sclerosis. Journal of the Neurological Sciences 84: 177–187

250. Isaac C, Li D K B, Genton M, Jardine C, Grochowski E, Palmer M, Low field MRI findings and clinical course in multiple sclerosis. Journal of the Neurological Sciences 84: 177–187

251. Isaac C, Li D K B, Genton M et al 1988 Multiple sclerosis: a serial study using MRI in relapsing patients. Neurology 38: 1511–1515

252. Willoughby E W, Grochowski E, Li D K B, Oger J, Kastrukoff L F, Paty D W 1989 Serial magnetic resonance scanning in multiple sclerosis: a second prospective study in relapsing patients. Annals of Neurology 25: 43–49

253. Miller D H, Rudge P, Johnson G et al 1988 Serial gadolinium enhanced magnetic resonance imaging in multiple sclerosis. Brain 111: 927–939

254. Grossman R I, Braffman B H, Brorson J R, Goldberg H I, Silberberg D H, Gonzalez-Scarano F 1988 Multiple sclerosis: serial study of gadolinium-enhanced MR imaging. Radiology 169: 117–122

255. Kesselring J, Miller D H, MacManus D G et al 1989 Quantitative magnetic resonance imaging in multiple sclerosis: the effect of high dose intravenous methylprednisolone. Journal of Neurology, Neurosurgery and Psychiatry 52: 14–17

256. Kermode A G, Tofts P S, Thompson A J et al 1990 Heterogeneity of blood–brain barrier changes in multiple sclerosis: an MRI study with gadolinium-DTPA enhancement. Neurology 40: 229–235

257. Thompson A J, Kermode A G, MacManus D G et al 1990 Patterns of disease activity in multiple sclerosis: clinical and magnetic resonance study. British Medical Journal 300: 631–634

8. Pathophysiology

At first sight understanding the pathophysiology of multiple sclerosis presents no difficulties. The symptoms and signs are all too evident and at autopsy there are massive demyelinated and gliotic lesions in appropriate regions of the nervous system. While these lesions undoubtedly play the major role in the disordered function of the nervous system in multiple sclerosis, the relationship between lesions and symptoms is unexpectedly complex. In addition to the obvious negative symptoms of the disease, any convincing theory of pathophysiology should account for the following common observations: the sometimes rapid or sudden onset of symptoms; temporary aggravation by heat and exercise; the frequent lack of correlation between symptoms and lesions demonstrated by imaging, electrophysiology or at autopsy; the occurrence of positive symptoms, paroxysmal or prolonged. Above all, the astonishing capacity for remission, apparently despite the persistence of lesions, must be explained.

DEMYELINATION

The effects of demyelination on axonal conduction are well understood but this information has not been obtained from the study of multiple sclerosis. Animal experiments and observations in man are both much more conveniently conducted on peripheral nerve, where the principles of saltatory conduction in myelinated fibres have been established and analysed in detail. The available evidence indicates that conduction in the CNS is normally saltatory, based on segmental myelination. Central and peripheral myelin are differently organised but it is reasonable to assume that the effects of demyelination observed in peripheral nerve can also be applied to central conduction and this assumption receives some experimental support. It is certainly not permissible, however, to extend the comparison to the processes of repair and restoration of function.

The mechanisms by which demyelination affects conduction have been extensively investigated. Their particular importance lies in the implications for restoration of function, assuming that the axons remain demyelinated. The experimental data are derived from peripheral nerve fibres but may be assumed to be applicable to the CNS. Only an abbreviated and simplified account need be given here, with particular reference to clinical relevance, and the interested reader is referred to the excellent reviews of Sears et al[1], Waxman[2], and Kocsis & Waxman.[3]

The axon of the internode, exposed by the destruction of its myelin sheath, is structurally and functionally different from the axon of the node or that of the normally unmyelinated fibre. An important and probably crucial difference is the absence of the sodium channels through which inward current passes at the nodes. There has been much debate on whether the demyelinated internodal axon is electrically excitable. The loss of the myelin sheath with its high impedance permits shunting of current. If demyelination is not complete but results in a thinner sheath, saltatory conduction is still possible but a longer time is required to build up sufficient current to pass to the succeeding node. Conduction is therefore slowed but may also be blocked, the response depending on many factors: the thickness of the myelin sheath, the length of fibre and number of internodes affected, the temperature and biochemical environment. If there is complete loss of myelin,

231

current can still pass over short gaps to a normal node but otherwise conduction block ensues.

Both from experimental work on peripheral nerve fibres and by inference in multiple sclerosis, conduction may be restored in demyelinated fibres. Interpretation of the results in some of the animal models is complicated by the rapid remyelination that occurs, but conduction returns before the appearance of myelin. How this is effected is of obvious relevance to multiple sclerosis although some reservations should be retained in view of the differences in the nature and site of the lesions.

Different views have been held on whether continued or restored conduction in demyelinated fibres remains saltatory or becomes continuous. These differences may well result from variations in technique and in methods of inducing demyelination. Rasminsky & Sears[4] using diphtheria toxin in the ventral spinal roots of the rat found persistence of delayed saltatory conduction. Later, Bostock & Sears[5] found continuous conduction in slowly conducting fibres, while Smith et al[6] using lysophosphatidyl choline in the same preparation found that restored conduction was always saltatory and was associated with the development of new foci of inward current. This was thought to indicate aggregation of sodium channels in demyelinated axolemma. The relevance to the restoration of function in multiple sclerosis must be doubtful as remyelination began three days later.

Waxman[2] considered in detail the properties necessary for conduction to occur in demyelinated fibres using a computer model. The data fed into the computer were, of course, derived from peripheral nerve. On this model conduction failed when only a single internode was demyelinated as the increased area of exposed membrane did not permit adequate current density. Possible adaptations to allow conduction to occur include a series of short internodes before the demyelinated segments. This would increase the safety factor: the ratio of current available to current necessary to effect conduction, and the demyelinated zone might be passed. In a number of physiological or pathological conditions, the existence of such short internodes has been shown, but there is no evidence from multiple sclerosis material. An alternative would be the transition to continuous conduction which would involve an increased density of sodium channels in the internodal membrane, either redistributed from the node or newly formed. Ritchie et al[7] could find no increase in total numbers of sodium channels in demyelinated mammalian nerve, although redistribution could not be excluded.

RELATION TO SYMPTOMS

Negative symptoms

In the peripheral nervous system experimental demyelination has been shown to cause slowed conduction in individual fibres, prolongation of, the relative refractory period, or conduction block.[8] Reduction of motor and sensory nerve conduction velocity is seen in human peripheral neuropathy of predominantly demyelinating type. Very similar results were obtained in the CNS following the injection of diphtheria toxin into the spinal cord of the cat.[9] This produces a discrete lesion with demyelination and some axonal degeneration. In the experiments, care was taken to demonstrate normal conduction above and below the lesions, indicating that the axons were not degenerating in the fibres examined. Large lesions blocked conduction while conduction velocity through small lesions was reduced. In single fibres conduction was slowed, the refractory period was increased and there was impaired ability to transmit trains of impulses at high frequencies. The histology of the lesion produced by diphtheria toxin resembles that of multiple sclerosis although of course it was not claimed to be identical. Demyelination, from whatever cause, may reasonably be held to have similar effects on axonal conduction.

Many features of the symptomatology of multiple sclerosis may be explained by these observed effects of demyelination. Conduction block will cause loss of function. It is uncertain whether slowed conduction will of itself cause symptoms. In the peripheral nervous system it is a common observation that in recovering peripheral neuropathy, restoration of normal conduction velocity lags far behind complete return of function.[10] Asynchronous arrival of impulses as a result of varying degrees of slowing of conduction in the fibres constituting a functional pathway is a possible cause of relative failure. McDonald & Sears[9] considered the possibility that the inability to conduct trains of impulses might contribute to the rapid fatigue with exercise seen in many patients with multiple sclerosis.

Direct evidence of the contribution of these observed effects of demyelination to the symptomatology of multiple sclerosis is difficult to obtain. The prolonged latency of evoked potentials, particularly of VEP, has plausibly been attributed to slowed conduction but, as indicated in Chapter 7, the diagnostic value of these techniques depends on the persistence of such delay in the absence of relevant symptoms. In any event it is not possible absolutely to equate prolonged latency with slowed conduction. McDonald[11] calculated that a 1 cm plaque in the optic nerve would introduce a 25 ms delay, a figure often observed in recording the P100 VEP in multiple sclerosis. There are experimental and theoretical reasons to suppose that conduction would still be possible even if conduction velocity was slowed up to 25 times. It was at first suggested that reduction in amplitude of the VEP, which may be restored as acuity improves, is the result of conduction block in a proportion of fibres, while increased latency, thought to persist 'indefinitely', is due to reduction of conduction velocity. Other possibilities, including conduction block in faster fibres and dispersion of the response due to unequal slowing in different fibres, must also be considered. No delay appears to be imposed at the retinal level,[12] but slowing of the cortical integrative process because of reduction of intensity of input from individual fibres has been suggested.[13] The peak latency of P100 is used simply for convenience as a readily identifiable wave. It is certainly not the earliest evoked potential, nor can it be regarded as the primary cortical response. Psychophysical tests of vision suggest that symptoms may arise from asymmetrical delay in conduction in the visual pathways,[14] but here also these abnormalities may be found in the absence of symptoms. Prolonged latency of the BAEP may also be the result of demyelination, although this has not been demonstrated directly. Again the basis of their use in diagnosis is the finding of

delay in the complete absence of signs or symptoms of a brainstem lesion. The latency of the cervical SEP is not often prolonged in multiple sclerosis, abnormalities usually taking the form of reduced amplitude or absence of response. If there is sensory loss in the arm tested, absence of the evoked response might be taken to indicate conduction block or, of course, axonal degeneration. If there is no sensory loss conduction block is still a possible explanation as methods of sensory testing are relatively crude, but asynchronous arrival of impulses from varied degrees of slowing of conduction could also be responsible. Serial recordings before, during and after a relapse causing profound loss of postural sense in the arm show no restoration of the cervical SEP on clinical recovery (personal observations).

The scalp recorded SEP, N20, does show changes in latency related to changes in sensory loss, as first described by Namerow.[15] Recovery from a sensory relapse may be accompanied by a reduction in latency of several ms. This observation, which I have repeatedly confirmed, does not, of course, demonstrate that the symptoms were due to slow conduction, the result of demyelination, but this is, at least, a reasonable assumption.

The failure to conduct rapid trains of stimuli has also been investigated,[16,17] by stimulating the median nerve and recording over the scalp. Using short trains of stimuli a potential with a one-to-one relation to each stimulus in the train could be demonstrated. In normal subjects this could be recorded up to the highest frequency used, 200 Hz. In patients with multiple sclerosis, with sensory loss in the arm stimulated this following response failed at quite low frequencies.[17] These results are not easy to interpret, as to exclude the longer latency responses to the first stimulus the recorded frequencies were confined to a very narrow band by filtering. It is also difficult to equate the recurrent response with the N20 as this is often absent in multiple sclerosis if there is sensory loss. There appears to be some confirmation of failure to conduct trains of stimuli, but no evidence that this is specifically related to symptoms.

Visual symptoms

The persisting visual disturbance following

recovery from acute optic neuritis has been minutely investigated. Many of the findings contribute to the understanding of normal vision but in the present context it is the defects that underlie visual symptoms despite restoration of acuity that are of interest. The symptom most commonly experienced is that objects appear less sharply defined when seen with the affected eye. Closer questioning sometimes reveals that the difficulty is only experienced with near vision, as in reading, or for middle distance. Vision is often worse in bright light. Colours are noted to be less vivid. When only one eye is affected such symptoms are easily ignored, but bilateral involvement is common.

The experimental work that has gone far to elucidate the cause of these symptoms is reviewed by Regan[18] and by Hess & Plant[19] and Foster[20] and only the findings and conclusions most closely relevant to causation of symptoms need be summarised. Visual acuity tested with the Snellen type measures the smallest object that can be seen with maximum contrast of black and white at a set distance and in good illumination, many other aspects of vision being ignored. Of the several relevant defects discovered probably the most important is elevation of the contrast threshold. This is measured by presenting sinusoidal grating patterns of light and dark, the threshold being the level of contrast at which the pattern is just discernible. Contrast sensitivity is the reciprocal of this value. Sensitivity also depends on the spatial characteristics of the grid, expressed as cycles of the sinusoidal pattern per degree of visual angle. Normally, sensitivity is maximal at intermediate frequencies. At low contrast levels, small objects (high spatial frequency) and also large objects (low frequency) are less easily detected. After optic neuritis sensitivity may be reduced at any point on the curve. A defect in low frequency sensitivity results in large objects being seen less clearly at short range as the visual angle is increased, the reverse of normal experience. A defect at high frequency is usually reflected in impaired acuity as normally measured. Impaired sensitivity for intermediate frequencies affects clarity of vision of the immediate environment and accounts for the complaint of indistinct vision at this distance.

The defects do not only affect contrast threshold but also perception of steady state and changing contrast.

A number of other defects no doubt contribute. The luminance threshold, the level of light just appreciated, may be raised and fluctuates according to the level of background illumination. The common complaint of poor vision in bright light has been variously explained, but is not now thought to be due to specific involvement of macular fibres. An alternative suggestion is that high illumination of the background gives rise to rapid trains of impulses that the demyelinated fibres of the optic nerve are unable to transmit, with resulting fluctuating conduction block.

Defects in temporal aspects of vision, that is to say the detection of changes over time, may also give rise to symptoms. Such defects can be demonstrated by elevation of the critical flicker fusion level[21-23] or the threshold of resolution of two flashes presented at brief intervals. Difficulties in timing visual events such as the movement of traffic or of a tennis ball are probably related although a specific connection does not seem to have been established. Plotting visual fields presents problems[24] as a moving object may be seen while a static object is invisible.

Impaired ability to discriminate between colours and in matching is closely related to elevation of luminance threshold.

Failure in these often complex tasks does not result from selective involvement of optic nerve fibres serving specific functions. A plaque in the optic nerve almost inevitably affects foveal fibres as these form a large proportion of the total and are centrally placed. Abnormalities are not, however, confined to central vision but affect retinal areas in random fashion. The psycho-physical defects can all be attributed to patchy demyelination in the optic nerve, with maximal effect on function of small diameter fibres, thus accounting for the common disturbance of colour vision. That persisting demyelination, rather than axonal loss, is at least partially responsible is shown by the adverse effect of a rise in environmental temperature[25] on psycho-physical functions and the transient beneficial effect of 4-aminopyridine[26]. (see below).

Positive symptoms

Symptoms due to excessive abnormal neural excitation are common in multiple sclerosis and their pathophysiology is comparatively well understood.

Paroxysmal symptoms

The clinical features of the paroxysmal symptoms of multiple sclerosis are described in detail in Chapter 2. In essence they consist of brief sensory and motor phenomena in varying combinations but stereotyped for the individual patient. They include trigeminal neuralgia, ataxia and dysarthria, tonic seizures, paraesthesiae, akinesia, diplopia and no doubt other forms yet to be recognised. Characteristically they last for no more than two minutes and are usually much more brief. They occur frequently, sometimes up to several hundred times in a day, and are often triggered by sensory stimuli or by voluntary movement of the limbs or trunk. They respond immediately to small doses of carbamazepine. Naturally variations in most of these characteristic features are encountered. They are remarkably different from the commonly accepted symptoms of multiple sclerosis.

The simpler forms of paroxysm such as isolated tonic spasm or trigeminal neuralgia afford no obvious clues to their pathophysiology. In more complex attacks it is often possible to recognise a pattern strongly suggesting spread of some form of abnormal excitation to contiguous anatomical structures in a manner quite different from the spread of epileptic discharges through anatomical and physiological connections. This is apparent in some earlier descriptions but was first emphasised by Ekbom et al[27] who described what they termed focal sensory-motor seizures of spinal origin. They postulated transversely spreading activation of 'damaged axons'[28] in fibre tracts of the spinal cord. The seizures began with unilateral burning paraesthesiae immediately followed by contralateral tonic muscle contraction, the interpretation being that of spread of activity from the spinothalamic to the corticospinal tract. This was thought to be effected by ephaptic transmission, a phenomenon that has been shown to occur in dysmyelinated fibres in the spinal roots of the dystrophic mouse, perhaps

a rather remote analogy. Prineas & Connell[29] have shown that in multiple sclerosis plaques, bared axons may be in close proximity without intervening glial tissue and commented that this might well allow lateral spread of excitation.

The theory was later elaborated to explain other forms of paroxysmal symptoms.[28] The pattern of spreading symptoms is often best exemplified by the combinations of paraesthesiae, dysarthria and ataxia. In a personally observed example,[30] an attack would begin with burning paraesthesiae in the left frontal region spreading to the cheek and to the second and third digits of the left hand. The right hand would then become clumsy and speech was slurred. These paroxysms lasted no more than ten seconds and were exceedingly frequent. At the time there were no abnormal neurological signs but later the patient developed clinically definite multiple sclerosis. Osterman & Westerberg[28] cite similar examples, but although the spread of abnormal activity through the pons can readily be envisaged it is necessary to assume that loss of normal function can result from excessive axonal excitation. It is not unreasonable to suppose that voluntary control of the limbs or articulation could be disturbed in this way but such symptoms are certainly less immediately acceptable as positive. This difficulty is even more pronounced in paroxysmal akinesia and it is necessary to postulate abnormal activation of an inhibitory pathway.[28]

Osterman & Westerberg[28] suggest that the origin of the initial activity that is permitted to spread transaxonally lies in some 'irritative lesion'. They pay little attention to a common feature of many paroxysmal symptoms, that of triggering. This is most obvious in trigeminal neuralgia, but is often observed in tonic seizures, sensory symptoms, ataxia and even akinesia, although many individual attacks may appear to be spontaneous. The commonest mode of triggering is voluntary movement, sometimes inseparable from the strong sensory stimulation implied by, for example, putting the foot to the ground. As an alternative to the 'irritative lesion' it may be suggested that normal activity is discharged along an anatomical pathway, as for example the corticospinal tract, as a necessary component of voluntary movement. On reaching a plaque, presumably in some specific state of demyelin-ation, normal conduction may be wholly or partially blocked but excitation may leak and spread to neighbouring demyelinated axons. Similar events could occur in sensory pathways following a triggering stimulus. The tonic dis-charge can be regarded as the result of simultaneous and repetitive firing of the axons of the corticospinal tract. If contralateral sensory symptoms are present they probably always precede the tonic spasm and, on this theory, the initiation of the spasm is from ephaptic spread of the normal sensory excitation on reaching the plaque.

The anatomical site of lesions apparently giving rise to paroxysmal symptoms are naturally dif-ficult to establish. Emphasis has been laid on the importance of spinal cord lesions in the genesis of tonic seizures[31-33] and, as originally claimed,[34] there is a strong association with elements of a Brown-Séquard syndrome. However, as Osterman & Westerberg point out, if tonic seizures are due to discharge of the axons of the corticospinal tract a spinal lesion is not essential. Watson[35] reported a patient with a hemiparesis and ipsilateral tonic seizures with a plaque demonstrated by CT scan in the internal capsule. Other lesions may, of course, have been undetected. In a personally ob-served example, the abnormal spread of excitation appears to have involved the cortex. The young man was demonstrating to me how his unilateral tonic seizures could be induced by using the hand in an intricate manner by tying his shoelace. The upper limb went into spasm as I watched, but on this single occasion, developed into a generalised epileptic fit. In general, paroxysmal symptoms are not associated with features usually regarded as epileptic and if their origin in axonal rather than neuronal discharge is accepted, would not be defined as epileptic.

Other theories of the cause of paroxysmal symptoms have been suggested, notably that of slight degrees of hypoxia acting on demyelinated axons.[36] This was suggested by the pronounced ef-fect of hyperventilation in precipitating attacks, thought possibly to act by reducing cerebral blood flow. The effect appears to be more probably re-lated to the improvement in negative symptoms

produced by overbreathing documented by Davis et al.[37] If, as suggested, this is the result of facilitating axonal conduction, paroxysms might well be exacerbated by an increase in activity reaching the plaque or by facilitating ephaptic transmission. A reduction of serum calcium also results in transient improvement in negative symptoms,[37] again apparently as a result of restora-tion of more normal axonal conduction. A comparison has been drawn between the posture adopted in many examples of tonic seizure and that of tetany.[34] Hemitetany of cerebral origin has been well recognised and indeed it is possible, al-though undesirable, to induce this in normal subjects by hyperventilation while one carotid artery is compressed (see ref. 34). It is not sug-gested that tonic seizures are caused by a fall in environmental calcium levels, merely that there is a state of abnormal axonal excitability perhaps similar to that in tetany.

Further circumstantial evidence for the axonal origin of paroxysmal symptoms is their response to treatment. Anticonvulsants were first used in tonic seizures because of their resemblance to focal epilepsy. In the first instance phenobaritone was remarkably successful but it has since become apparent that barbiturates, phenytoin and carbamazepine can be ranked in an ascending order of efficacy. Carbamazepine can be extra-ordinarily effective.[38] Paroxysmal dysarthria occurring 50 times a day may stop completely within an hour of the first dose of 100 mg. At first sight the beneficial effect of anticonvulsants might suggest that the paroxysms were indeed epilepsy due to excessive neuronal discharge. However, these drugs have diverse actions, among them a profound effect on the axonal membrane.[39] Carbamazepine levels comparable to those encountered in clinical use greatly reduce both sodium and potassium conductance and it is probably these properties that are responsible for its remarkable effect on paroxysms. Car-bamazepine also unfortunately has a profound effect on the negative symptoms of multiple sclerosis, particularly weakness. In treating paroxysms, particularly trigeminal neuralgia, the increased weakness of the legs may be a limiting factor. Moderate doses sufficient to prevent the neuralgia may also confine the patient to bed, not from ataxia but because of a profound increase in previously existing weakness of the legs.

A woman of 64 first developed symptoms of multiple sclerosis in 1962, at first intermittent but eventually slowly progressive with spastic weakness of the lower limbs as the main disability. In 1979 she developed trigeminal neuralgia which responded admirably to carbamazepine. Continued relief was obtained, although a rather higher dose became necessary. By December 1981 she found that if she took 400 mg of carbamazepine a day she was free from pain but was unable to walk at all. Following surgical treatment of the neuralgia she no longer required carbamazepine and again became mobile in the house. This effect of dose reduction had previously been noted on a number of occasions before surgical treatment.

This adverse effect may also plausibly be attributed to the action of the drug in impairing conduction in demyelinated fibres.

These contrasting effects of hyperventilation, possibly of calcium ions and of carbamazepine on paroxysms of all kinds, including akinesia, and on the usual negative symptoms of multiple sclerosis, provide supporting evidence for an abnormality in axonal conduction underlying these brief disorders of function.

Lhermitte's sign

This symptom occurs at some time in at least one third of patients with multiple sclerosis and has recently been reviewed by Kanchandani & Howe.[40] It consists of a brief unpleasant tingling 'electric' sensation induced by neck flexion or, less commonly, by other movements. The 'shock' usually passes rapidly down the spine to both legs but there are variants including involvement of the arms or unilateral sensations. It is not confined to multiple sclerosis, occurring in subacute combined degeneration, radiation myelopathy and, less certainly, in other forms of spinal cord disease. In the young adult, however, Lhermitte's sign is highly suggestive of multiple sclerosis.

Lhermitte's[41] suggestion that demyelinated fibres were unduly sensitive to mechanical deformation has received some experimental support.[42,43] Sensory fibres traversing the demyelinating lesion induced experimentally by lysophosphatidylcholine fire spontaneously and the rate of firing is increased by mechanical stimulation of the site of the lesion, resulting only in minute displacement. A similar mechanism in a multiple sclerosis plaque in the cervical spinal cord is a rational explanation for Lhermitte's sign.

It is seldom necessary to treat Lhermitte's sign. The response to carbamazepine reported by Ekbom[44] is far less consistent than that of paroxysmal symptoms but this may be due to lack of compliance because of the relative triviality of the symptoms. Consistent relief by carbamazepine would suggest that abnormal spread of excitations, rather than spontaneous firing of an 'irritative lesion' was responsible.

Movement phosphenes

A phenomenon probably related to Lhermitte's sign is the occurrence of brief flashes of light produced when the eye is moved, either in a dark room or with the eyes closed. This symptom was described by Earl.[45] and in more detail by Davis et al.[46] It appears to be most common shortly after recovery from optic neuritis but may precede the attack or be apparently unrelated to other visual symptoms. The optic nerve and the cervical spinal cord are the most mobile structures in the CNS. Whether this renders them peculiarly vulnerable to multiple sclerosis plaques, as has been suggested,[47] cannot be known, but they appear to be susceptible to movement-induced symptoms originating in demyelinated fibres. Phosphenes usually persist for approximately six weeks, a duration similar to that of many transient symptoms of multiple sclerosis.

Paraesthesiae

Paraesthesiae, tingling, 'pins and needles', are a familiar symptom of a great variety of conditions, serious or banal, affecting the peripheral or central nervous systems. In multiple sclerosis a common pattern is for these sensations to accompany other sensory phenomena — 'numbness' — of segmental distribution, spreading rapidly within the first few days of a relapse. In such circumstances they are not painful or paroxysmal but persist for a period, again of about six weeks. So universal are paraesthesiae in any form of sensory disturbance that thought is seldom devoted to how they are produced. The spontaneous discharges of sensory fibres in experimental demyelinating lesions[43] may well be paralleled by similar discharges from plaques in multiple sclerosis. The experimental discharges do not persist indefinitely but perhaps fortuitously for a period resembling that of a multiple sclerosis relapse.

Myokymia

The term myokymia wa first used by Schultze[48] to describe rapidly fluctuating benign fasciculation of the calf muscles, but has since been applied to other forms of involuntary movement. Like many such terms, it is difficult to define with any precision, but one form of myokymia is highly distinctive and characteristically, but not exclusively, occurs in multiple sclerosis. Although there had been earlier reports, the association of facial myokymia and multiple sclerosis was first emphasised by Andermann et al[49] and its relatively frequent occurrence was also recognised.[50] In multiple sclerosis, or as an isolated event that may that later prove to have been the initial symptom of multiple sclerosis, the onset is sudden. The complaint is of stiffness or tightening of one side of the face and observant patients may recognise the contractions. All the muscles of the affected side of the face appear to be in slight continuous contraction so that the palpebral fissure is narrowed and the naso-labial fold accentuated. Exceedingly rapid waves of flickering movement pass over the facial muscles in a pattern too fast for visual analysis. Remission is gradual over a period of from a few days to six months. In a personally observed case,[50] myokymia immediately appeared on the opposite side of the face. Nine years later the man developed spastic weakness of the legs.

Electromyography shows a characteristic pattern.[50] Motor units can be recognised as firing in brief runs, each with an individual rhythm (Fig. 8.1). In the illustration one unit can be seen to be firing in short bursts of from three to eight spikes approximately four times a second, while a second unit is firing longer bursts every 2.5 seconds. This pattern bears a remarkable resemblance to that of

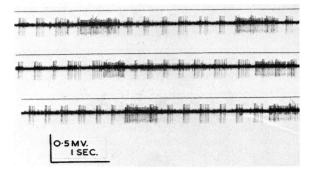

Fig. 8.1 EMG of facial myokymia. Recording from needle electrode, the three strips being continuous. At least three different motor units can be seen to be firing in short bursts at different frequencies (reproduced by permission from Journal of Neurology, Neurosurgery and Psychiatry 29: 35).

the spontaneous firing of sensory fibres in experimental demyelinating lesions recorded by Smith & McDonald[43] and these authors comment on the possibility of similar activity in motor fibres being the cause of myokymia.

If this is so, it might well be thought surprising that myokymia is confined to the facial muscles. These are, of course, far more exposed to view than the musculature of the limbs and even so facial myokymia almost completely eluded the observation of several generations of able clinicians. I have once observed myokymia in the muscles supplied by the trigeminal nerve.

A man of 37 developed persistent double vision and was found to have nystagmus and slight weakness of the right lateral rectus muscle. Four months later he had a transient right facial palsy. When seen five months later his wife remarked on 'rippling' on the right side of the face. Myokymia was present but appeared to be confined to the temporalis muscle with possibly some involvement of the masseter. Dr Geoffrey Rushworth carried out EMG at a time when the condition was subsiding but detected a motor unit in the temporalis muscle firing in bursts in a rapid rhythm. This unit participated in the jaw jerk.

A more minute examination of the muscles of the limbs and trunk might reveal more extensive involvement.

Facial myokymia may also occur in either intrinsic or extrinsic brainstem tumours[51] and in the Guillain-Barré syndrome. In an autopsied case[52] of the latter condition no lesion of the brainstem was found but there was extensive demyelination of the peripheral facial nerves.

Environmental effects

The observed effects of external agents on the symptoms of multiple sclerosis are also explicable by the known properties of demyelinated axons.

The most obvious influence is that of exercise and change in environmental temperature. Deterioration of vision induced by exercise was first described by Uhthoff[53] and is a common phenomenon. Perkin & Rose[54] found that 41 of 125 patients seen soon after the onset of optic neuritis experienced transient impairment of vision in response to external stimuli, exercise in 14 and an increase in temperature in 10. Other functions, particularly strength, are also commonly affected adversely by heat, such an effect being claimed by 93% of patients in one series.[55] Improved function in response to cold is less often observed but 50% of patients thought that a cold bath was beneficial[55] and this has been observed by Watson.[56] A small proportion of patients find that their symptoms deteriorate in cold weather and this has been objectively confirmed.[57,58]

Clinical investigation has repeatedly confirmed that in many patients the physical signs of malfunction of the nervous system in multiple sclerosis show a remarkable sensitivity to recorded or presumed changes in body temperature. Measurement of these changes has been largely confined to the visual system. Visual acuity and the visual fields may both be impaired by natural[59] or induced[60] increase in body temperature. The ability to detect double flashes of light can be improved or reduced by appropriate change in external temperature[25] and other forms of visual perception may be similarly affected. Namerow[61] demonstrated a remarkable effect of heat on critical flicker fusion threshold which was profoundly reduced by raising the temperature. Changes in VEP have been less convincing. Regan et al[62] using flicker stimulation found that change in EP latency with change in environmental temperature occurred less frequently than alteration in perception. Matthews et al[63] and Bajada et al[64] found that the amplitude of the P100 VEP was somewhat reduced by heating both in patients with multiple

sclerosis and in normal subjects. Persson & Sachs[65] found that exercise reduced the amplitude of the P100 only in patients with Uhthoff's symptom.

Other functions measured have included saccade velocities found to be reduced by heat[64] and blink reflex latency that was not significantly altered.[66] Alterations in the strength of limb and trunk muscles, particularly weakness on whole body heating, have often been observed but are less easy to quantify. The effect can be profound, Guthrie[67] describing patients requiring support to prevent them becoming totally submerged in the hot bath. Waxman & Geschwind[68] report a patient who sustained fatal burns because of inability to get out of a hot bath.

The effect of a change in environmental temperature begins very quickly, within 30 seconds of getting into a hot bath,[69] and may be sudden, leading to falling in a hot shower.[68] Hopper et al[70] reported that in one patient, visual acuity began to improve six minutes after drinking an ice emulsion before there had been any change in rectal or skin temperature. The change in acuity reversed while the temperature was still falling. Core temperature was not recorded in this case. It may not be possible to find any consistent change in body temperature despite obvious clinical effects. It is known from patients' descriptions that events that might be expected to have only trivial effects on body temperature — a hot drink or a hairdryer — can reduce visual acuity.[71] An increase of 0.15°C was associated with a 30% drop in flicker fusion threshold.[61] Recovery from the adverse effects of heat or exercise also begins rapidly but the period to full restoration to the previous level probably depends on the nature and severity of the environmental change. After bicycle exercise Persson & Sachs[65] found that recovery occurred within about seven minutes, while Namerow[61] illustrates recovery of flicker fusion over 30 minutes. Zweifach[69] found that the more rapid the increase in temperature the more severe the loss of function. Michael & Davis[60] examined the relation of visual acuity, measured with unusual precision, to oral temperature and found that acuity was better at a given temperature during the recovery phase than during heating. The lack of precise correlation between oral or even core temperature and change in function has already been noted. There is no way of measuring temperature in the optic nerve and profound conclusions can scarcely be based on the use of the ordinary clinical thermometer.

It was at first thought that the transient ill effects of a high external temperature were in some sense paradoxical in view of the known geographical distribution of multiple sclerosis and its relative rarity in the tropics.[71] An obvious possible explanation for such rapidly reversible phenomena was an effect of heat on the blood supply to the nervous system. Brickner[71] postulated localised vasoconstrictions in response to heat and claimed to have seen such constriction of the retinal vessels during heat induced visual loss. Guthrie,[67] however, detected no contraction of retinal vessels. A vascular cause has often been considered since, partly because of the difficulty in relating any rise in body temperature detected to the changes in function. Heckl[72] found that in a single case an injection of a vasodilator improved acuity that had been impaired by heat but that stellate ganglion block was without effect. Improvement was later shown to result from cooling caused by cutaneous vasodilatation (R W Heckl, personal communication). The injection of adrenalin has also been reported to improve acuity in these circumstances.[70]

A hormonal effect has also been suggested.[70] Certainly it is not necessary to heat or cool the whole body to produce clinical changes. Guthrie[67] demonstrated that heating one arm caused weakness of muscles of the other limbs and that this effect could be partially prevented by a venous tourniquet on the heated arm and entirely prevented by an arterial tourniquet. He naturally also considered the possibility that the humoral agent he had demonstrated was simply heated blood.

No change in blood chemistry or cortisol or urinary catecholamines has been found.[73] Zweifach[69] removed a large volume of blood at a time when heat-induced visual loss was maximal. When this was re-injected after vision had recovered, no further adverse effect was produced, again suggesting the absence of a humoral agent.

There is now little doubt that these experimental and clinical findings are due to the effect of temperature change on the capacity of demyelinated fibres to conduct. A rise in temperature increases the rate of ionic conductance at the node with resulting increase in speed of current build-up. With rise in temperature within physiological limits conduction velocity is increased in normally myelinated fibres, although conduction is abruptly blocked above 40°C. With loss of myelin, the short duration action potential spike will reduce the current density at the next active site along the axon and the safety factor is lowered. Conduction is therefore blocked at a lower temperature.[74] In a computer model, the thinner the myelin sheath the lower the temperature at which block occurred.[75] However, with slighter degrees of demyelination, the model shows that conduction velocity initially increases with rise in temperature and is reduced by cooling, as in the normal fibre. The occasional paradoxical effect of worsening of symptoms on cooling has been explained as due to the action of temperature change in initially adversely affecting conduction in partially demyelinated fibres.[58]

Calcium

It is known that lowering the concentration of ionic calcium in the environment lowers the excitation threshold of nerve fibre.[76] Theoretically this should assist conduction in demyelinated fibres as the amount of current required to maintain conduction would be reduced. A beneficial effect on the symptoms of multiple sclerosis might therefore be expected if a lowering of ionic calcium could be achieved. It has been suggested that the presence of Ca^{2+} ions reduces the surface negative charge of the axon membrane[3] and tends to repolarise the membrane, reduction of ionic calcium having the reverse effect.

Davis et al[37] demonstrated temporary improvement in nystagmus, in the size of scotomata and in visual acuity following measures designed to reduce ionic calcium concentration in the CNS. These included intravenous infusion of sodium bicarbonate, disodium edetate and hyperventilation. Improvements noted developed and receded gradually. All these measures also have effects other than that of lowering serum calcium but care was taken to avoid influences such as cooling induced by overbreathing. A further demonstration of a beneficial effect of lowering serum calcium was produced by giving a large oral dose of phosphate.[77] Again, disappearance of a scotoma and improved acuity accompanied the biochemical changes and the paraesthesiae induced by the 3 g of a mixture of sodium and potassium phosphate. A personal attempt in several subjects using an identical dose of phosphate did not lower serum calcium and had no effect on vision or on pattern reversal VEP.

The theoretical basis for an effect of lowering calcium concentration in improving conduction in partially demyelinated fibres has been examined in a computer model.[75] The interaction with the effects of change in temperature were also investigated. At a given temperature, lowering calcium concentration increases conduction velocity. At low calcium concentration the temperature required to block conduction is much higher than at high concentration.

These observations have not led to effective symptomatic treatment as persistent lowering of the serum calcium level is not feasible. It was rational to explore the use of calcium channel blocking agents. Verapamil by intravenous infusion was shown[78] to reduce abnormally prolonged latency of visual and brainstem auditory evoked potentials in patients with stable multiple sclerosis. The authors did not comment on any effect on visual function. Oral verapamil produced no objective or subjective improvement in 11 patients treated for 8 weeks.[79]

4-Aminopyridine. This agent has complex effects on synaptic transmission but its possible relevance to multiple sclerosis lies in its action in blocking voltage-dependent potassium channels. These channels appear to play little part in conduction in normally myelinated fibres and 4-aminopyridine consequently has no effect. In demyelinated fibres, however, 4-aminopyridine will reverse conduction block,[80] apparently by preventing the outward flow of current through potassium channels in the exposed internodal axon membrane. Attempts at treatment have concentrated on patients with heat or exercise labile symptom[26,81] and these, indeed, can be improved by oral or intravenous 4-aminopyridine. The agent is, however, toxic and may cause convulsions,[82] painful paraesthesiae and disorientation.[26] From personal observation a

small oral dose can cause a prolonged distressing state of mental excitation.

CORRELATION OF LESIONS AND SYMPTOMS

Although many of the symptoms of multiple sclerosis can be explained in terms of the properties of demyelinated axons there remain considerable difficulties in relating clinical features to the underlying lesions.

Evidence from autopsies is inevitably limited. The autopsy rate in multiple sclerosis is low and most patients die after many years of chronic disability during which detailed neurological examination is seldom recorded. Even if clinical data were available, the attribution of symptoms and signs to individual plaques is problematical, apart, of course, from such obvious associations as paraplegia and spinal cord disease. There are many reports of patients who died early in the course of the disease in whom most or all of the lesions found appear to have been symptomatic. In a personally observed example[83] a woman with multiple sclerosis died following rupture of an intracranial aneurysm. Chronic plaques were found in the left optic nerve and in restricted regions of the cervical spinal cord, precisely conforming to the distribution of the visual, motor and sensory symptoms she had experienced in the five episodes of multiple sclerosis she had sustained. As in most such cases, however, a number of small plaques, mostly less than 3 mm in diameter, were also present and not clearly related to symptoms.

It has long been known that multiple sclerosis plaques may be found at autopsy in subjects who have apparently not experienced any relevant symptoms.[84-86] In determining whether such lesions have in fact caused no clinical symptoms some regard must be paid to the eventual cause of death. Castaigne et al[87] described three cases in whom multiple small old plaques were found at autopsy and plausibly suggested that multiple sclerosis was never suspected because the visual system was not involved in any of the cases, and in the one case in whom it was examined the spinal cord was also normal. All three, however, had considerable impairment of higher cerebral functions from other causes and previous episodes of multiple sclerosis might well have been forgotten. Engell,[88] in 13 cases of clinically silent multiple sclerosis, found no lesions in the spinal cord and only one brainstem plaque, the great majority being periventricular.

There are, however, a number of remarkable reports of gross disparity between the site and extent of the lesions and the absence of expected symptoms. The patient described by Ghatak et al[89] was a man of 66 who complained of backache. A full neurological examination was normal. He died three weeks later of carcinoma of the bronchus. A large centrally situated demyelinated and gliotic plaque was found in the cervical spinal cord. Axons passing through the plaque appeared normal. At the age of 33 there had been an episode of diplopia and difficulty in walking, with full recovery. Wisniewski et al[90] briefly described persisting visual function in patients in whom autopsy a few days later showed complete demyelination of over 2 cm in both optic nerves.

The existence of multiple lesions, undetectable clinically, either because they are causing no disturbance of function or because the methods of clinical neurology are insufficiently refined, have often been described.[91] Perhaps the most remarkable example is that of Namerow & Thompson.[92] Their patient had been frequently examined during the course of her illness that had been characterised by numerous relapses. She died of an overdose some five years from the onset. She had been examined 19 days before death. A number of her earlier symptoms could be related to the numerous plaques found at autopsy, but many extensive lesions were almost or completely without recognisable clinical counterpart. For example, the posterior columns were almost completely demyelinated and yet position sense and vibration sense were only minimally disturbed in the toes. The pyramidal tracts were involved at many levels and almost totally in the cervical spinal cord but no signs attributable to this were present in the upper limbs. A plaque involving the nucleus and course of one VIth cranial nerve had caused no ocular palsy.

The use of evoked potentials in the diagnosis of multiple sclerosis is based on the persistence of defects of conduction in the absence of clinical evidence of disease. It may be true that after 'recovery' from optic neuritis some defect of visual function relative to the unaffected eye can always be demonstrated by refined methods of examination,[93] but nevertheless there is often a striking contrast between the absence of symptoms and the greatly prolonged latency of the VEP. Visible pallor of the optic disc may reinforce the evidence of a persistent lesion. SEP may be abnormal in the complete absence of sensory symptoms or signs, but routine clinical examination may not be sufficiently sensitive.

The frequent occurrence of asymptomatic lesions has been vividly illustrated by imaging techniques. Both CT and particularly MRI often show numerous abnormalities in apparently important functional regions of the brain in the complete absence of attributable symptoms.

A number of plausible explanations of these findings can be advanced. The lesions may be in 'silent' areas of the brain or may cause symptoms or signs not recognisable on routine neurological examination. This suggestion receives some support from the observation that in patients with symptoms of an isolated brainstem lesion, an abnormality in that region is usually demonstrable by MRI,[94] although the authors point out that lesions in the floor of the IVth ventricle are so commonly found in multiple sclerosis that their relevance to particular symptoms cannot be assumed. Symptoms would certainly be expected from lesions involving the long tracts of the spinal cord, but evidence from MRI is at present inadequate. That the site of the lesion cannot be the only factor in determining the presence or absence of symptoms is shown by the cases of Ghatak et al[89] and Namerow & Thompson[92] cited above.

The same objections can be raised to the possibility that the presence of symptoms depends on the size of the lesion. It is, of course, probable that lesions a few millimetres in diameter in the cerebral white matter would not cause detectable clinical effects, the relatively small number of fibres affected being insufficient to result in any deficit. Demyelination of short lengths of fibre might not block conduction and, as Gordon Holmes[95] pointed out, a number of such lesions in the course of a long tract might be necessary before symptoms result.

With chronic lesions, plasticity in the nervous

system may preserve function, but this explanation can scarcely be invoked in the optic nerve. It is more probable that sufficient conduction can be maintained or restored in demyelinated axons, as described above. Remyelination obviously cannot be claimed as the mechanism of preserving function in areas demonstrated histologically to be demyelinated.

MRI

The pathological basis of the abnormalities seen on MRI has attracted much discussion. It was established early that abnormalities shown by scanning the brain post mortem matched the chronic demyelinated gliotic plaques found on sectioning the brain.[96] It is obviously much more difficult to establish the pathology of the acute and often transient abnormalities seen in active disease. Although these appearances are more frequent in relapse, they are seldom related to the clinical features and frequently develop in the complete absence of any other evidence of activity.[97] Lesions may appear in previously unaffected areas or existing lesions may expand. Occasionally, several fresh lesions appear together but it is common for some to increase in size while others are fading.

T_1 and T_2 relaxation times depend on the concentration and behaviour of protons, almost exclusively those in the hydrogen of water. The responses can be modified by the chemical environment but, in general, the abnormalities seen on the scan indicate an excess of water, a highly non-specific finding. An increase in water content could result from an influx of cells or, much more probably, from oedema. Whether demyelination could produce an identical signal is unknown but considered unlikely.[94] Despite the similarity of the MRI signals, the histopathology of acute evanescent lesions would naturally be expected to differ from that of chronic gliotic plaques. The interesting possibility that the former are not, at least initially, plaques of demyelination but areas of inflammation and oedema has been raised.[98,99] Repeated episodes of asymptomatic breakdown of the blood-brain barrier are envisaged as eventually leading to demyelination and symptomatic relapse. Miller et al[100] also discuss the changes responsible for the MRI signals from acute and chronic

lesions. Excess water increases both T_1 and T_2 but the presence of protein shortens T_2 but not T_1. Vasogenic protein-rich oedema fluid might be expected in acute enhancing lesions and would result in a relatively high T_1/T_2 ratio. Their findings show very low ratios in some non-enhancing lesions, but the degree of overlap provides little support for their hope that relaxation time measurements would distinguish recent from chronic lesions or, indeed, throw much light on the nature of the pathology. The presence of excess water in chronic, non-enhancing lesions is not well understood. Even if the existence of a form of normal pressure hydrocephalus in multiple sclerosis[101,102] is accepted, this could not explain excess water in chronic lesions remote from the ventricles. A persistent defect in the blood-brain barrier is a possible explanation, but this is not indicated by gadolinium enhancement. In the original demonstration of breakdown of the barrier in multiple sclerosis by Broman,[103] trypan blue dye entered all types of plaque, both recent and chronic. Absence of enhancement in chronic lesions cannot with certainty be interpreted as indicating an intact blood-brain barrier. Quantitative MRI scanning[104] has shown excess water in normal-appearing white matter in multiple sclerosis, which was reduced by steroid treatment, although the signals from chronic lesions were not altered.

Oedema is a common feature of the acute plaque[105] and may be of such severity as to cause ventricular displacement[106] or swelling of the spinal cord.[107] Compression of nerve fibres leading to reversible conduction block is a highly probable consequence. The rapid effect of corticosteroids both in abolishing enhancement of lesions shown by CT[108] and in resolving symptoms of relapse has been attributed to repair of the blood-brain barrier and resulting relief of oedema. Corticosteroids are extremely effective in the relief of oedema around a cerebral tumour and consequent reversal of gross physical signs and a similar acute effect is probable in multiple sclerosis. Steroid treatment does not, however, appear to influence gadolinium enhancement of MRI[109] and, on this evidence, relief of oedema is not accompanied by restoration of the blood-brain barrier. To what extent natural remission extending over many weeks can be attributed to the clearing of oedema is unknown. In optic neuritis, the initial reduction of amplitude of the VEP has been ascribed to the effect of oedema in blocking a large proportion of optic nerve fibres,[110] the prolonged latency being attributed to demyelination. Serial MR imaging of symptomatic acute lesions, if such can be identified, might elucidate the role of oedema in the causation and remission of symptoms.

In serial scans in patients with relapsing or secondarily progressive disease, new lesions always enhance with gadolinium but in disease progressive from the onset they do not.[111] In experimental allergic encephalomyelitis, gadolinium enhancement occurs only at sites of inflammation.[112] The defect in the blood-brain barrier permitting the passage of gadolinium is probably not the result of opening of tight junctions but of increased cytoplasmic vesicular transport[112] and a similar effect in multiple sclerosis may be presumed. The lack of enhancement in new lesions in disease progressive from the onset is most easily explained by a lesser degree of inflammation and it is probably not necessary to postulate a distinctive pathogenesis. In relapsing disease, many of the abnormalities become undetectable after 4–6 weeks, while others shrink and no longer enhance.

Serial MRI scans in the few hours after gadolinium injection have shown that, initially, enhancement is often confined to a ring at the edge of a lesion identified on the unenhanced scan.[109] Enhancement then spreads to involve the lesion uniformly. Whether this pattern is the result of less severe inflammation in the centre of the lesion or of diffusion of the contrast is uncertain. Interestingly, lesions could sometimes be seen by enhancement before they became visible on the unenhanced scan, emphasising the possible primary role of breakdown of the blood-brain barrier.

Despite remarkable technical advances, there are still a number of obscurities in the relation of lesions to symptoms. Conduction block caused by oedema can be postulated as the cause of acute remitting symptoms, repeated damage eventually resulting in demyelination. Oedema in tightly packed regions such as the optic nerve, brainstem and spinal cord would be more likely to produce symptoms than lesions in the cerebral white matter. The observed lack of correlation between

demyelinated lesions and loss of function indicates that persistence of effective transmission through chronic plaques is possible. Other mechanisms may, however, be operating. Relapse of multiple sclerosis sometimes develops with startling rapidity. A man told me that his wife's severe paralysis came on 'in the time taken to turn round and close the door'. Remission, while never sudden, often occurs astonishingly quickly, particularly during intravenous steroid treatment. Changes on this time-scale have been attributed to blocking or unblocking of axonal conduction or synaptic transmission from causes other than oedema.

Neuroelectric blocking factors

The detection of factors in the blood of patients with multiple sclerosis with the property of blocking neuroelectric activity promised to be of great interest. Bornstein & Crain[113] found that serum from acute cases of multiple sclerosis exerted a rapid but reversible blocking action on synaptic responses of cultured cortex and spinal cord. The action was dependent on the presence of complement. An in vivo response was confirmed by Cerf & Carels[114] who showed that serum, again from patients with active multiple sclerosis, would reversibly block potentials transmitted through multineuronal pathways in an experimental spinal cord preparation. Bornstein[115] further examined the properties of this agent in cell cultures and concluded that it was distinct from a demyelinating effect also found to be present in multiple sclerosis serum.[116] Seil et al[117] found both myelination-inhibiting and neuroelectric blocking agents in the serum of animals with experimental allergic encephalomyelitis (EAE) but also in serum from controls. They confirmed the presence of a blocking agent in the serum of many patients with multiple sclerosis[118] but similar effects were produced by a high proportion of sera from normal subjects. The properties of the agents with respect to thermolability and complement-dependence showed great variation.

Schauf et al, in a series of reports and reviews [119–123] extended these observations. Using the frog spinal cord, multiple sclerosis and EAE serum reduced the ventral root response to dorsal root stimulation but the effect did not at first appear to be related to the activity of multiple sclerosis in the patients. Later they found that inhibition was more marked using serum from patients with active disease. The activity was thermolabile and was present in the serum IgG fraction, these properties suggesting that it was an antibody. The effect was not produced by normal serum or by serum from patients who had recently suffered a stroke as had been reported.[124] The site of action was shown to be on synaptic transmission and no effect was observed on conduction in myelinated or demyelinated fibres.

Serum neuroelectric blocking activity is not, however specific for multiple sclerosis, being present to a similar degree in motor neurone disease.[125] In both diseases, activity was higher than in controls but there was much overlap of individual values. The sudden onset of symptoms is by no means characteristic of motor neurone disease and these findings must throw considerable doubt on the relevance of neuroelectric blocking agents to the pathophysiology of multiple sclerosis.

REMYELINATION

It was long held as dogma that remyelination did not occur in the central nervous system[126] and therefore could not account for remission in multiple sclerosis. However in experimental animals remyelination occurs, often rapidly, after a great variety of physical, chemical and immunological insults to the central nervous system,[127] including chronic relapsing EAE, the supposed model of multiple sclerosis. These observations were made by examining batches of animals killed at increasing intervals from the event causing demyelination. An approximation of this method was achieved by Prineas et al[128,129] who examined lesions in patients with the acute form of the disease dying at intervals from clinical onset ranging from less than 3 months to 5 years. Within 3 months of onset there were many areas of obvious myelin breakdown, with depletion of oligodendrocytes. Such areas of active demyelination were less frequent in patients who had survived rather longer. Plaques in which all fibres were thinly myelinated to the same degree, with

short internodes, were increasingly common in patients dying 3–18 months from onset and were interpreted as showing remyelination. Shadow plaques, in which myelin sheaths stain poorly and are unduly thin, have usually been regarded as resulting from partial demyelination,[130] but both Lassmann[131,132] and Prineas[128] believe that they are remyelinating, although subject to reinvasion by disease.

Prineas' claim[128] that his observations are in temporal sequence in a manner comparable to animal experiments cannot be fully justified as it is increasingly apparent that onset of disease usually, or perhaps always, antedates onset of symptoms by an unknown period. Nevertheless, the findings provide support for the commonsense view that remission is the result of remyelination.

In chronic multiple sclerosis the picture is different, although shadow plaques may still be seen. A few fibres with thin myelin sheaths can be seen at the periphery of some chronic plaques[133] and it is probable that some remyelination occurs. Some degree of remyelination by Schwann cells also takes place, particularly in the spinal cord.[134] This strange phenomenon has been investigated experimentally[135,136] but it has not been shown that conduction can be restored in this way. The large areas of rapid remyelination by oligodendrocytes observed by Prineas et al,[129] if their interpretation is correct, are no longer present and, of course, clinical remission has usually long ceased. Progressive disease may therefore be attributed to failure of the remyelination that occurs in the relapsing and remitting stage. If this is so, the reason for this failure is obviously of great interest. It has been attributed to a variety of defects of function or proliferation of oligodendrocytes, but no conclusion has been reached. Gliotic scarring probably does not inhibit myelination, as Lassmann[131] found gliotic areas resembling plaques but fully myelinated and presumably remyelinated.

Axonal changes

It is characteristic of the early multiple sclerosis lesion that there is little or no axonal degeneration. The extent of axonal loss in long-established plaques has been a matter for controversy, to some extent because of difficulties with staining techniques. It is commonly presumed that permanent loss of function is due to axonal degeneration and is therefore irreversible. The evidence for this assumption is not compelling and even exhaustive accounts of the pathology of multiple sclerosis make little reference to the fate of the axons.[130] Using a staining technique for neurofibrils, Greenfield & King[137] found that only 10% of plaques showed severe reduction in numbers of nerve fibres. Peters[138] remarked on the relatively infrequent secondary ascending or descending degeneration of axons in tracts within the spinal cord, even in the presence of extensive demyelination, and that he had never found such axonal degeneration to be complete.

Using fundus photography, however, MacFadyen et al[139] have demonstrated extensive axonal loss in the retinal nerve fibre layer in a high proportion of patients with multiple sclerosis, indicating that the pathological changes in the optic nerve are not confined to demyelination. This finding may demand some reinterpretation of the pathophysiology of persistent visual defects after optic neuritis.

The glia

The glial reaction in multiple sclerosis, an obviously important component of the disease process, is described in Chapter 12. It is not known or at present conjectured that astrocytic proliferation has any direct role in the causation of symptoms.

Conclusion

The reinstatement of remyelination as a probable immediate cause of the remission of symptoms has done much to clarify ideas on the pathophysiology of multiple sclerosis. Much, however, remains to be explained and the evidence from MRI of ceaseless asymptomatic activity is disquieting.

REFERENCES

1. Sears T A, Bostock H, Sherratt M 1978 The pathophysiology of demyelination and its implications for the symptomatic treatment of multiple sclerosis. Neurology 28, 9(2): 21–26
2. Waxman S G 1978 Prerequisites for conduction in demyelinated fibres. Neurology 28, 9(2): 27–33
3. Kocsis J D, Waxman S G 1985 Demyelination: causes and mechanisms of clinical abnormality and functional recovery. In: Vinken P J, Bruyn G W, Klawans H L, Koetsier J C (eds) Handbook of clinical neurology., Vol 47. Elsevier, Amsterdam, pp. 29–47
4. Rasminsky M, Sears T A 1972 Internodal conduction in undissected demyelinated nerve fibres. Journal of Physiology 227: 323–350
5. Bostock H, Sears T A 1976 Continuous conduction in demyelinated mammalian nerve fibres. Nature 263: 786–787
6. Smith K J Bostock H, Hall S M 1982 Saltatory conduction precedes demyelination in axons demyelinated with lysophosphatidyl choline. Journal of the Neurological Sciences 54: 13–31
7. Ritchie J M, Rang, H P, Pellegrino R 1981 Sodium and potassium channels in demyelinated and remyelinated mammalian nerve. Nature 294: 257–259
8. McDonald W I, 1963 The effects of experimental demyelination on conduction in peripheral nerve: a histological and electrophysiological study. II: Electrophysiological observations. Brain 86: 501–524
9. McDonald W I, Sears T A 1970 The effects of experimental demyelination on conduction in the central nervous system. Brain 93: 583–598
10. Matthews W B, Howell D A, Hughes R C 1970 Relapsing corticosteroid-dependent polyneuritis. Journal of Neurology, Neurosurgery and Psychiatry 33: 330–337
11. McDonald W I 1977 Pathophysiology of conduction in central nerve fibres. In: Desmedt J E (ed) Visual evoked potentials in man. Clarendon Press, Oxford, pp 427–437
12. Plant G T, Hess R F, Thomas S J 1986 The pattern evoked electroretinogram in optic neuritis. Brain 109: 469–490
13. Plant G T, Hess R F 1986 The electrophysiological assessment of optic neuritis. In: Hess R F, Plant G T (eds) Optic neuritis. Cambridge University Press, pp 197–229
14. Heron J R, Regan D, Milner B A 1974 Delay in visual perception in unilateral optic atrophy after retrobulbar neuritis. Brain 97: 69–78
15. Namerow N S 1968 Somatosensory evoked responses in multiple sclerosis with varying sensory loss. Neurology 18: 1197–1204
16. Namerow N S, Sclabassi R J, Enns N F 1974 Somatosensory responses to stimulus trains: normative data. Electroencephalography and Clinical Neurophysiology 37: 11–21
17. Sclabassi R J, Namerow N S, Enns N F 1974 Somatosensory response to stimulus trains in patients with multiple sclerosis. Electroencephalography and Clinical Neurophysiology 37: 23–33
18. Regan D 1984 Visual psychophysical tests in the diagnosis of multiple sclerosis. In: Poser C M (ed) The

diagnosis of multiple sclerosis. Thieme–Stratton, New York, pp 64–75

19. Hess R F, Plant G T 1986 The psychophysical loss in optic neuritis: spatial and temporal aspects. In: Hess R F, Plant G T (eds) Optic neuritis. Cambridge University Press, pp 109–151

20. Foster D H 1986 Psychophysical loss in optic neuritis: luminance and colour aspects. In: Hess R F, Plant G T (eds) Optic neuritis. Cambridge University Press, pp 152–191

21. Titcome A F, Willison R G 1961 Flicker fusion in multiple sclerosis. Journal of Neurology, Neurosurgery and Psychiatry 24: 260–265

22. Thorner M W, Berk M E 1964 Flicker fusion test I: In neuro-ophthalmologic conditions including multiple sclerosis. Archives of Ophthalmology 71: 807—815

23. Daley M L, Swank R L, Ellison C M 1979 Flicker fusion thresholds in multiple sclerosis: a functional measure of neurological damage. Archives of Neurology 36: 292–295

24. Ellenberger C, Daroff R T B 1984 Neuro-ophthalmic aspects of multiple sclerosis. In: Poser C M (ed) The diagnosis of multiple sclerosis. Thieme–Stratton, New York, pp 49–63

25. Galvin R J, Regan D, Heron J R 1976 A possible means of monitoring the progress of demyelination in multiple sclerosis: Effect of body temperature on visual perception of double light flashes. Journal of Neurology, Neurosurgery and Psychiatry 39: 861–865

26. Jones R E, Heron J R, Foster D H, Snelger R S, Mader R J 1983 Effects of 4-aminopyridine on patients with multiple sclerosis. Journal of the Neurological Sciences 60: 353–362

27. Ekbom K A, Westerberg C-E, Osterman P O 1968 Focal sensory-motor seizures of spinal origin. Lancet 1: 67

28. Osterman P O, Westerberg C-E 1975 Paroxysmal attacks in multiple sclerosis. Brain 98: 189–202

29. Prineas J W, Connell F 1978 The fine structure of chronically active multiple sclerosis plaques. Neurology 28, 9(2): 68–75

30. Matthews W B 1968 The neurological complications of ankylosing spondylitis. Journal of the Neurological Sciences 6: 561–573

31. Kreindler A, Cardas M, Petresco A, Botez M I 1962 Considérations sur l'étiopathogénie des crises toniques dans l'encéphalomyelite disseminé. Revue Neurologique 107: 353–369

32. Kuroiwa Y, Araki S 1963 Lhermitte's sign and reflex tonic spasm in demyelinating diseases with special reference to their localising value. Kyushu Journal of Medical Science 14: 29–38

33. Castaigne P, Cambier J, Masson M et al 1970 Les manifestations motrices paroxystiques de la sclérose en plaques. Presse Médicale 78: 1921–1924

34. Matthews W B 1958 Tonic seizures in disseminated sclerosis.. Brain 81: 193–206

35. Watson C P 1979 Painful tonic seizures in multiple sclerosis: localisation of a lesion. Canadian Journal of Neurological Sciences 6: 359–361

36. Espir M L E, Watkins S M, Smith H V 1966 Paroxysmal dysarthria and other transient neurological disturbances in disseminated sclerosis. Journal of Neurology, Neurosurgery and Psychiatry 29: 323–330

37. Davis F A, Becker F O, Michael J A, Sorensen E 1970 Effect of intravenous sodium bicarbonate, disodium edetate (NA₂EDTA) and hyperventilation on visual and oculomotor signs in multiple sclerosis. Journal of Neurology, Neurosurgery and Psychiatry 33: 723–732

38. Espir M L E, Millac P 1970 Treatment of paroxysmal disorders in multiple sclerosis with carbamazepine. Journal of Neurology, Neurosurgery and Psychiatry 33: 528–531

39. Schauf C L, Davis F A, Mader J 1974 Effect of carbamazepine on the ionic conductances of myxicola giant axons. Journal of Pharmacology and Experimental Therapeutics 189: 538–543

40. Kanchandani R, Howe J G 1982 Lhermitte's sign in multiple sclerosis: a clinical survey and review of the literature. Journal of Neurology, Neurosurgery and Psychiatry 45: 308–312

41. Lhermitte J, Bollak, Nicholas M 1924 Les douleurs à type de décharge électrique consécutives à la flexion céphalique dans la sclérose en plaques. Revue Neurologique 42: 56–62

42. Smith K J, McDonald W I 1980 Spontaneous and mechanically evoked activity due to central demyelinating lesion. Nature 286: 154–155

43. Smith K J, McDonald W I 1982 Spontaneous and evoked electrical discharges from a central demyelinating lesion. Journal of the Neurological Sciences 55: 39–47

44. Ekbom K 1971 Carbamazepine: a new symptomatic treatment for the paraesthesiae associated with Lhermitte's sign. Zeitschrift für Neurologie 200: 341–344

45. Earl C J 1964 Some aspects of optic atrophy. Transactions of the Ophthalmological Society of the UK 84: 215–226

46. Davis F A, Bergen D, Schauf C, McDonald I, Deutsch W 1976 Movement phosphenes in optic neuritis: a new clinical sign. Neurology 26: 1100–1104

47. Oppenheimer D R 1978 The cervical cord in multiple sclerosis. Neuropathology and Applied Neurobiology 4: 151–162

48. Schultze F 1895 Beitage zur Muskelpathologie. I. Myokymie (Muskelwogen) besonders an den Unterextremitäten. Deutsche Zeitschrift für Nervenheilkunde 6: 65–70

49. Andermann F, Cosgrove J B R, Lloyd-Smith D L, Gloor P, McNaughton F L 1961 Facial myokymia in multiple sclerosis. Brain 84: 31–44

50. Matthews W B 1966 Facial myokymia. Journal of Neurology, Neurosurgery and Psychiatry 29: 35–39

51. Teuser R B, Corbett J J 1974 Myokymia and facial contraction in brainstem glioma. Archives of Neurology 30: 425

52. Van Zandyke M, Martin J-J, Vande Gaer L, Van den Heyning P 1982 Facial myokymia in the Guillain-Barré syndrome: a clinicopathologic study. Neurology 32: 744–748

53. Uhthoff W 1889 Untersuchen über die bei der multiplen Herdsklerose vorkommenden Augenstörungen. Archiv für Psychiatrie und Nervenkrankheiten 21: 55–116

54. Perkin G D, Rose F C 1976 Uhthoff's syndrome. British Journal of Ophthalmology 60: 60–63

55. Brenneis M, Harrer G, Seizer H 1979 Zur Temperaturempfindlichkeit von

Multiple-Sklerose-Kranken. Fortschritte der Neurologie-Psychiatrie 47: 320–325

56. Watson C V V 1959 Effect of lowering of body temperature on the symptoms and signs of multiple sclerosis. New England Journal of Medicine 261: 1253–1259

57. Geller M 1974 Appearance of signs and symptoms of multiple sclerosis in response to cold. Mount Sinai Journal of Medicine 41: 127–130

58. Honan W P, Heron J R, Foster D H, Snelgar R S 1987 Paradoxical effects of temperature in multiple sclerosis. Journal of Neurology, Neurosurgery and Psychiatry 50: 1160–1164

59. Namerow N S 1968 Circadian temperature rhythm and vision in multiple sclerosis. Neurology 18: 417–422

60. Michael J A, Davis F A 1973 Effects of induced hyperthermia in multiple sclerosis: differences in visual acuity during heating and recovery phases. Acta Neurologica Scandinavica 49: 141–151

61. Namerow N S 1971 Temperature effect on critical flicker fusion in multiple sclerosis. Archives of Neurology 25: 269–275

62. Regan D, Murray T J, Silver R 1977 Effects of body temperature on visual evoked potential delay and visual perception in multiple sclerosis. Journal of Neurology, Neurosurgery and Psychiatry 40: 1083–1091

63. Matthews W B, Read D J, Pountney E 1977 Effect of raising body temperature on visual and somatosensory evoked potentials in patients with multiple sclerosis. Journal of Neurology, Neurosurgery and Psychiatry 42: 250–255

64. Bajada S, Mastaglia F L, Black J L, Collins D W K 1980 Effect of induced hyperthermia on visual evoked potentials and saccade parameters in normal subjects and multiple sclerosis patients. Journal of Neurology, Neurosurgery and Psychiatry 43: 849–852

65. Persson H E, Sachs C 1981 Visual evoked potentials elicited by pattern reversal during provoked visual impairment in multiple sclerosis. Brain 104: 369–382

66. Rodnitzky R L, Kimura J 1978 The effect of induced hyperthermia on the blink reflex in multiple sclerosis. Neurology 28: 431–433

67. Guthrie T C 1951 Visual and motor changes in patients with multiple sclerosis. Archives of Neurology and Psychiatry 65: 437–451

68. Waxman S G, Geschwind N 1983 Major morbidity related to hyperthermia in multiple sclerosis. Annals of Neurology 13: 348

69. Zweifach P H 1978 Studies of hyperthermia in optic neuropathy. Archives of Ophthalmology 96: 1831–1834

70. Hopper C L, Matthews C G, Cleeland C S 1972 Symptom instability and thermoregulation in multiple sclerosis. Neurology 22: 142–148

71. Brickner R M 1950 The significance of localised vasoconstrictions in multiple sclerosis. Research Publications of the Association for Research in Nervous and Mental Diseases 28: 236–244

72. Heckl R W 1974 Das Phänomenon des inkonstanten Visus bei Multiplen Sklerose. Nervenarzt 45: 467–473

73. Symington G R, Mackay I R, Currie T T 1977 Improvement in multiple sclerosis during prolonged induced hypothermia. Neurology 27: 302–303

74. Rasminsky M 1973 The effects of temperature on conduction in demyelinated single nerve fibres. Archives of Neurology 28: 287–292

75. Schauf C L, Davis F A 1974 Impulse conduction in multiple sclerosis: a theoretical basis for modification by temperature and pharmacological agents. Journal of Neurology, Neurosurgery and Psychiatry 37: 152–161

76. Brink F, Bronk D W, Larrabee M D 1946 Chemical excitation of nerve. Annals of the New York Academy of Science 47: 457

77. Becker F O, Michael J A, Davis F A 1974 Acute effects of oral phosphate on visual function in multiple sclerosis. Neurology 24: 601–607

78. Gilmore R L, Kasarskis E J, McAllister R G 1985 Verapamil-induced changes in central conduction in patients with multiple sclerosis. Journal of Neurology, Neurosurgery and Psychiatry 48: 1140–1146

79. Komoly S, Jakab G, Fazekas A 1986 Multiple sclerosis: failure of treatment with verapamil in a pilot trial. Journal of Neurology 233: 59–60

80. Sherratt R M, Bostock H, Sears T A 1980 Effects of 4-aminopyridine on normal and demyelinated mammalian nerve fibres. Nature 274: 385–387

81. Stefoski D, Davis F A, Faut M, Schauf C L 1987 4-Aminopyridine improves clinical signs in multiple sclerosis. Annals of Neurology 21: 71–77

82. Sears T A, Bostock H 1981 Conduction failure in demyelination. Is it inevitable? Advances in Neurology 31: 357–375

83. Matthews W B, Esiri M 1979 Multiple sclerosis plaque related to abnormal somatosensory evoked potentials. Journal of Neurology, Neurosurgery and Psychiatry 42: 940–942

84. Georgi W 1961 Multiple Sklerose: pathologisch-anatomische Befund multipler Sklerose bei klinisch nicht diagnostizierten Krankheiten. Schweizerische Medizinische Wochenschrift 91: 605–607

85. Phadke J G, Best P V 1983 Atypical and clinically silent multiple sclerosis: a report of 12 cases discovered unexpectedly at necropsy. Journal of Neurology, Neurosurgery and Psychiatry 46: 414–420

86. Gilbert J J, Sadler M 1983 Unsuspected multiple sclerosis. Archives of Neurology 40: 533–536

87. Castaigne P, Lhermitte F, Escourolle R, Hauw J J, Gray F, Lyon-Caen O 1981 Les scléroses en plaques asymptomatiques. Revue Neurologique 137: 729–739

88. Engell T 1989 A clinical patho-anatomical study of clinically silent multiple sclerosis. Acta Neurologica Scandinavica 79: 428–430

89. Ghatak N R, Hirano A, Lijtmaer H, Zimmerman H M 1974 Asymptomatic plaque in the spinal cord. Archives of Neurology 30: 484–486

90. Wisniewski H M, Oppenheimer D, McDonald W I 1976 Relation between myelination and function in MS and EAE. Journal of Neuropathology and Experimental Neurology 35: 327

91. Mackay R P, Hirano A 1967 Forms of benign multiple sclerosis: report of two 'clinically silent' cases discovered at autopsy. Archives of Neurology 17: 588–600

92. Namerow N S, Thompson L R 1969 Plaques, symptoms and the remitting course of multiple sclerosis. Neurology 19: 765–774

93. Harding G F A, Wright C E 1986 Visual evoked potentials in acute optic neuritis. In: Hess R F, Plant G T (eds) Optic neuritis. Cambridge Unversity Press, Cambridge, pp 230–254

94. Ormerod I E C, Miller D H, McDonald W I et al 1987

The role of nuclear magnetic resonance imaging in the assessment of multiple sclerosis and isolated neurological lesions. A quantitative study. Brain 110: 1579–1616

95. Holmes G 1952 Introduction to clinical neurology, 2nd edn Livingstone, Edinburgh, p 8

96. Stewart W A, Hall L D, Berry K, Paty D W 1984 Correlation between NMR scan and brain slice data in multiple sclerosis. Lancet 2: 412

97. Isaac C, Li D K B, Genton M et al 1988 Multiple sclerosis: a serial study using MRI in relapsing patients. Neurology 38: 1511–1515

98. Willoughby E W, Grochowski E, Li D K B, Oger J, Kastrukoff L F, Paty D W 1989 Serial magnetic resonance scanning in multiple sclerosis: a second prospective study in relapsing patients. Annals of Neurology 25: 43–49

99. Koopmans R A, Li D K B, Oger J J F, Mayo J, Paty D W 1989 The lesion of multiple sclerosis: imaging of acute and chronic stages. Neurology 39: 959–963

100. Miller D H, Rudge P, Johnson G et al 1988 Serial gadolinium enhanced magnetic resonance imaging in multiple sclerosis. Brain 111: 927–93

101. Bartolini S, Insitari D, Castagnoli A, Amaducci L 1982 Correlation of isotopic cisternographic patterns in multiple sclerosis with CSF IgG values. Annals of Neurology 12: 486–489

102. Volpi G, Insitari D, Fratiglioni L et al 1986 CT periventricular hypodensity in multiple sclerosis: isotopic cisternography and clinical correlations. Annals of Neurology 20: 14

103. Broman T 1964 Blood-brain barrier damage in multiple sclerosis: supravital test-observations. Acta Neurologica Scandinavica 40 (suppl 10): 21–24

104. Kesselring J, Miller D H, MacManus D G et al: 1989 Quantitative magnetic resonance imaging in multiple sclerosis: the effect of high dose intravenous methylprednisolone. Journal of Neurology, Neurosurgery and Psychiatry 52: 14–17

105. Adams C W M 1977 Pathology of multiple sclerosis: progression of the lesion. British Medical Bulletin 33: 15–20

106. Sagar H J, Warlow C P, Sheldon P W E, Esiri M M 1982 Multiple sclerosis with clinical and radiological features of cerebral tumour. Journal of Neurology, Neurosurgery and Psychiatry 45: 802–808

107. Honig L S, Sheremata W A 1989 Magnetic resonance imaging of spinal cord lesions in multiple sclerosis. Journal of Neurology, Neurosurgery and Psychiatry 52: 459–466

108. Troiano R, Hafstein M, Ruderman M, Dowling P, Cook S 1984 Effect of high-dose intravenous steroid administration on contrast enhancing computed tomographic scan lesions in multiple sclerosis. Annals of Neurology 15: 257–263

109. Kermode A G, Tofts P S, Thompson A J et al. Heterogeneity of blood-brain barrier changes in multiple sclerosis: an MRI study. Neurology (in press)

110. Halliday A M, McDonald W I 1977 Pathophysiology of demyelinating disease. British Medical Bulletin 33: 21–27

111. Thompson A J, Kermode A G, MacManus D G et al 1989 Pathogenesis of progressive multiple sclerosis. Lancet 1: 1322–1323

112. Hawkins C P, Munro P M G, Mackenzie F et al.

Duration and selectivity of blood-brain barrier breakdown in chronic relapsing allergic encephalomyelitis studied using gadolinium-DTPA and protein markers. (Brain (in press)

113. Bornstein M B, Crain S M 1965 Functional studies of cultured brain tissues as related to 'demyelinative disorders'. Science 148: 1242–1244

114. Cerf J, Carels G 1966 Multiple sclerosis serum factors producing reversible alterations in bioelectric responses. Science 152: 1066–1068

115. Bornstein M B 1973 The immunopathology of demyelinative disorders examined by organotypic cultures of mammalian nervous tissues. In: Zimmerman H M (ed) Progress in neuropathology II. Grune and Stratton, New York, pp 69–90

116. Raine C S, Hummelgard A, Swanson E, Bornstein M B 1973 Multiple sclerosis-serum induced demyelination in vitro. Journal of the Neurological Sciences 20: 127–148

117. Seil F J, Smith M E, Leiman A L, Kelly J M 1975 Myelination inhibiting and neuroelectric blocking factors in experimental allergic encephalomyelitis. Science 187: 951–953

118. Seil F J, Leiman A L, Kelly J M 1976 Neuroelectric blocking factors in multiple sclerosis and normal human sera. Archives of Neurology 33: 418–422

119. Schauf C L, Davis F A, Sack D A, Reed B J, Kesler R L 1976 Neuroelectric blocking factors in human and animal sera evaluated using the isolated frog spinal cord. Journal of Neurology, Neurosurgery and Psychiatry 39: 680–685

120. Schauf C L, Schauf V, Davis F A, Strelkauskas A J, Mizen M R 1977 Lymphocyte subpopulations in multiple sclerosis: comparison with neuroelectric blocking activity. Neurology 27: 822–826

121. Schauf C L, Schauf V, Davis F A, Mizen M R 1978 Complement dependent serum neuroelectric blocking activity in multiple sclerosis. Neurology 28: 426–430

122. Schauf C L, Davis F A 1978 The occurrence, specificity and role of neuroelectric blocking factors in multiple sclerosis. Neurology 29, 9(2): 34–39

123. Schauf C L, Pencek T L, Davis F A, Rooney M W 1981 Physiologic basis for neuroelectric blocking activity in multiple sclerosis. Neurology 31: 1337–1340

124. Schmutz M, von Hahn H P, Honegger C G 1977 Effect of multiple sclerosis serum on ventral root responses in isolated frog spinal cord. European Neurology 15: 345–351

125. Schauf C L, Antel J P, Arnason B G W, Davis F A, Rooney M W 1980 Neuroelectric blocking activity and plasmapheresis in amyotrophic lateral sclerosis. Neurology 30: 1011–1013

126. Greenfield J G 1958 Demyelinating diseases. In: Greenfield J G, Blackwood W, McMenemey W H, Meyer A, Norman R M (eds) Neuropathology. Edward Arnold, London, pp 441–474

127. Ludwin S K 1987 Remyelination in demyelinating diseases of the central nervous system. Critical Reviews of Neurobiology 3: 1–28

128. Prineas J W 1985 The Neuropathology of multiple sclerosis. In: Vinken P J, Bruyn G W, Klawans H L, Koetsier J C (eds) Handbook of clinical neurology, Vol 47. Elsevier, Amsterdam, pp 213–257

129. Prineas J W, Kwon E E, Sharer L R, Cho E-S 1987

Massive early remyelination in acute multiple sclerosis. Neurology 37 (suppl 1): 109

130. Lumsden C E 1970 The neuropathology of multiple sclerosis. In: Vinken P J, Bruyn G W (eds) Handbook of clinical neurology, Vol 9. Elsevier, Amsterdam, pp 217–309

131. Lassmann H 1983 Comparative neuropathology of chronic experimental allergic encephalomyelitis and multiple sclerosis. Springer, Berlin

132. Seitelberger F, Lassmann H 1983 Comparative neuropathology and pathogenetic aspects of chronic relapsing experimental allergic encephalomyelitis and multiple sclerosis. In: Scarlato G, Matthews W B (eds) Multiple sclerosis: present and future. Plenum Press, London, pp 23–40

133. Prineas J W, Connell F 1979 Remyelination in multiple sclerosis. Annals of Neurology 5: 22–31

134. Feigin I, Ogata J 1971 Schwann cells and peripheral myelin within human central nervous tissues: the mesenchymal character of Schwann cells. Journal of Neuropathology and Experimental Neurology 30: 603–612

135. Harrison B M 1980 Remyelination by cells introduced into a stable demyelinating lesion in the central nervous system. Journal of the Neurological Sciences 46: 63–81

136. Gledhill R F, Harrison B M, McDonald W I 1973 Pattern of remyelination in the CNS. Nature 244: 443–444

137. Greenfield J G, King L S 1936 Observations on the histopathology of the cerebral lesions in disseminated sclerosis. Brain 59: 445–458

138 Peters G 1968 Multiple sclerosis. In: Minckler J (ed) Pathology of the nervous system. McGraw-Hill, New York, pp 821–843

139. MacFadyen D J, Drance S M, Douglas G R, Airaksinen P J, Mawson D K, Paty D W 1988 The retinal fiber layer, neuroretinal rim area, and visual evoked potentials in MS. Neurology 38: 1353–1358

9. Treatment

The treatment of multiple sclerosis is a highly emotive and controversial topic. The reasons are not far to seek. The disease imposes the threat of progressive severe disability in previously healthy young adults and personal involvement in their fate is difficult to avoid. The natural history of the disease is such that even experienced and level-headed neurologists have frequently been misled by the enthusiasm engendered in patients and observers alike by the trial of a new treatment. It is not easy to accept that after years of increasing endeavour there is no immediate prospect of any treatment that can be relied upon favourably to alter the course of the disease and the possibility of 'cure' still appears remote. The mostly well-conceived and admirably conducted therapeutic trials of recent years have been launched in the knowledge that the treatment under trial will do no more, at best, than retard the progress of the disease or alleviate symptoms of recent onset. This is not to deny the importance of such trials in attempting to trace the path ahead, but in such an atmosphere, optimism may sometimes outweigh scientific judgement.

The need for treatment

Recent advances in diagnostic techniques have emphasised the benign course of multiple sclerosis in many patients. Scheinberg & Van den Noort[1] advise that, apart from organised trials, the potentially hazardous forms of treatment of problematical value at present available should only be used in rapidly worsening disease, perhaps 5% of patients. There is little evidence that in this group any benefit would result, but it is difficult to resist the cry that 'something must be done'.

Nobody could doubt that if an even partially effective and harmless treatment were to be developed it should be used preferentially in early or even minimal disease, as the threat of progression is always present.

THE DESIGN OF THERAPEUTIC TRIALS

Increasing realisation that prolonged and costly efforts might fail to produce conclusive results because of faulty design of the trial led to thorough appraisal of methods and firm recommendations.[2,3] Most of these do not differ from the requirements of a therapeutic trial in any disease, but the chronic and often remitting course undoubtedly poses additional problems. Although the original should certainly be read in detail by anyone contemplating a trial it may be useful to comment on the protocol suggested by Weiner & Ellison.[4]

They propose that the rationale for the treatment under trial should be described and fully documented. This reasonable suggestion is usually complied with in published reports but sometimes amounts to little more than the hope that a powerful agent, shown to influence other diseases or to be active in regard to some possible pathogenetic factor, might alter the course of multiple sclerosis. For example, interferon has both an antiviral action and complex effects on immune mechanisms. Repeated unsuccessful attempts have been made to incriminate a virus in multiple sclerosis and it has often been regarded as an autoimmune disease. In the absence of knowledge of the causation of the disease, such a rationale for a trial of interferon is perfectly adequate. With other forms of treatment, notably with polyunsaturated fatty acids, the suggested rationale has been subject to, repeated radical change.

The goal or objective of the trial must be determined. Trials limited to treatment of the acute relapse are clearly quite different from those in which it is hoped to alter the course of the disease. A relapse has, however, several indices of severity: duration and degrees of disability and of recovery, and it must be stated which of these it is intended to influence. The definition of a relapse (exacerbation seems to be the fashionable term) for the purposes of a therapeutic trial is unexpectedly difficult. It is usually required that new symptoms and signs or an increase in existing signs should occur after the patient's state had been static or improving for a period of at least one month. No improvement should have occurred before instituting the treatment under trial, but Weiner & Ellison rather confusingly state that they would accept a patient 'whose condition had been improving minimally in one or a few areas as long as the overall neurologic condition was not one of improvement'. Exactly where this places the patient whose sensory loss is clearing from the legs but increasing on the face is not obvious.

The recommended time limits for an eligible relapse are given as less than 8 weeks and more than 5 days duration. The latter reasonably excludes fluctuations due to infection, fatigue or depression, but accepting relapses of up to 8 weeks duration is probably due to the relative difficulty in obtaining adequate numbers of patients seen nearer to the time of onset of the relapse. The duration of relapse has a distinct effect on the natural outcome, full remission being much more frequent after brief relapses.[5,6] Some studies have insisted on a shorter maximum duration of 4 weeks.[7]

Severity of relapse must be defined as a stated change in whatever assessment scale is used. Reduction in duration of relapse has been the aim of a number of recent trials. Brown et al[3] described wholly unrealistic methods of measuring this variable but in practice patients are assessed at stated intervals from the beginning of *treatment* rather than from onset of relapse.[7,8]

The aim of treatment of progressive disease is obviously to slow, halt or reverse deterioration. A problem that has not been overcome is that patients admitted to trials are often simply stated to have had progressive disease for a given number of years. Following treatment their condition is carefully assessed but there are no comparable assessments before treatment. Clearly the disease had progressed since the onset but if a change in course is to be shown, the previous course, at least for the year before treatment, must be charted in the same degree of detail. This is an excellent reason for regularly assessing in a quantitative way patients attending follow-up clinics, regardless of whether they are taking part in a clinical trial. Similar difficulties arise in assessing treatment in reportedly static disease. Valid comparison of disability before and after treatment demands a statement, not always provided, that the patients were not in relapse when treatment was begun.

Therapeutic trials in patients with relapsing/remitting disease are usually concerned both with change in clinical state and in the rate and severity of relapse. Comparison of relapse rate before and after treatment is still regarded as a legitimate method of judging its effect, but, even when compared to controls, is subject to a number of sources of error. Relapses before treatment are often said to be 'documented' but whether they fulfil reasonable criteria such as being accompanied by objective neurological signs cannot be determined. It is probable that in most patients relapse rate declines with the passage of time.[9] In prospective studies Patzold & Pocklington[10] found that the annual rate fell from 1.8 in the first year to 1.0 by the fifth year and Weinshenker & Ebers[11] reported a more rapid fall from 1.8 to 0.55 in the second year. The inclusion of a few patients with many relapses a year, a not uncommon pattern, may greatly distort the figures.

It is mandatory that in patients admitted to a trial, the diagnosis of multiple sclerosis is as certain as possible. Weiner & Ellison[4] give criteria for acceptance, and demand clinical evidence of two or more distinct lesions. They rightly emphasise that reliance should not be placed on temporal pallor of the optic disc as evidence of a second lesion and that motor and sensory abnormalities of spinal cord origin should not be counted as two distinct lesions. To these may be added the classical 'soft' signs beloved of non-neurologists: nystagmus at extremes of lateral gaze and slight inco-ordination of the non-dominant hand. The definition fits well with the 'clinically definite 1' category of Poser et al.[12] Problems arise as to what extent paraclinical evidence should be permitted to support a diagnosis of definite multiple sclerosis in this context, in the absence of conclusive clinical evidence. The 'clinically definite 2' category, with a history of 2 attacks, clinical signs of a single lesion, but laboratory evidence of a second lesion should be acceptable. The most common example would be the patient with evident spinal cord disease, a history of optic neuritis and unilateral prolonged latency of the visual evoked potential. The categories of 'laboratory supported definite multiple sclerosis' require less convincing clinical evidence, supported by paraclinical investigation and oligoclonal bands in the CSF. A deliberate stated decision must be taken on whether such patients may be included. A decision to accept evidence from imaging techniques as confirming the diagnosis for purposes of clinical trials, in the absence of sufficient clinical evidence, does not yet appear to have been taken. It must also be remembered that a number of diseases can exactly mimic the criteria of clinically definite multiple sclerosis.[13]

Patients may be excluded on grounds of age: limits of 18–59 years are often imposed. Severely disabled patients, in whom a therapeutic response may justifiably be considered improbable, may be deliberately excluded, but this would be inappropriate in a trial of, for example, an anti-spastic agent. Ambulant patients with persistent but not disabling symptoms are most suitable for investigation of an agent designed to alter the course of the disease.[14] Sometimes patients with frequent relapses or with rapidly progressive disease are deliberately selected in the hope that a change in pattern as the result of treatment will be immediately obvious. Such selection probably distorts results and to little purpose, as the future course of the disease cannot be foretold with sufficient accuracy. Intellectual function must be adequate for understanding what the patient is agreeing to and why. This is often stated to be so but is very seldom actually tested. The fallibility of clinical judgement of mental capacity is described on p. 57.

Advice from a statistician is essential when planning a trial, in particular to determine the size of population needed in order to reach a correct conclusion that the figures show that the desired effect has or has not been achieved. This will depend on what is expected or hoped from the treatment: significant reduction in relapse rate or severity, improvement by a certain minimum defined degree, or prevention of deterioration, for example. Brown et al[3] and Weiss & Dambrosia[15] give some examples of the numbers required to show that the desired objective has been achieved or that a positive result has not been overlooked. The greater the effect looked for, the smaller the number of subjects required. Unfortunately, most of the results actually claimed have required large numbers. There are many other aspects needing advice and careful planning. Weiss & Dambrosia[15] wrote that: 'Even experienced clinical researchers sometimes undertake investigations that are textbook examples of weakness in study design . . . . . .' The treatment of multiple sclerosis is a notorious minefield.

There is now little dispute that concurrent controls are essential in any but the most preliminary trial from which it is hoped to draw conclusions. This realisation is, however, comparatively recent, as it was not long ago that I was rebuked for making the 'unethical' suggestion that controls should be used in trials of immunosuppressive treatment as it was already proven that the treatment was successful. Matching is usually achieved by randomisation, particularly in large studies. Stratification before randomisation is an alternative adopted in many trials. Ideally, trials should be double-blind. This involves some alternative treatment for the controls, either placebo or some other therapeutic regime in common use. There can be no valid ethical argument against the use of placebo in the absence of any known effective treatment, but naturally, patients must be fully aware that they may not be receiving the agent under trial. The placebo effect in the treatment of multiple sclerosis is remarkably strong and frequent reference will be made to arrest or slowing of disease or great reduction in relapse rate in placebo-treated controls. It must also be recognised that relapse rates and progression in untreated multiple sclerosis have been less closely observed than in patients taking part in therapeutic trials.

The formidable difficulties of selecting and recruiting patients for a full randomised controlled trial have led to reconsideration of the possibility of using historical controls. As used in the past, no convincing results could be obtained. Ellison et al[16] discuss the construction of plots of the mean course of the untreated disease, derived from standardised scoring methods, and used in a manner similar to that of a 'growth curve'. A treated patient more than 3 standard deviations better than the mean for a given duration of disease would be counted a success. The course of multiple sclerosis is, unfortunately, far more erratic than the growth of a child and it was concluded that such methods could only be used in preliminary trials to determine whether a full trial might possibly be rewarding.

It is exceedingly difficult to maintain blinding of patients and observers when using an agent with pronounced side effects. For example, cyclophosphamide makes the hair fall out and patients know this. Supposedly blinded assessors are likely to suspect the truth whatever precautions are taken. At the other extreme is transfer factor, involving a single injection once a month, producing no side effects. Great ingenuity has been displayed in blinding trials of hyperbaric oxygen, intrathecal interferon and intravenous steroids, for example, but complete success must always remain difficult to guarantee.

Three types of trial are recommended.[3,4] A preliminary trial is largely concerned with establishing the appropriate dosage or other aspects of the agent or regime it is desired to test, and also, no doubt, to ensure that there is no immediately obvious adverse effect. Controls are not used. It is not legitimate to draw conclusions on the efficacy of the treatment from such trials, although this is still sometimes done.[17,18]

The pilot trial, as described, appears to have major disadvantages. Controls are not necessary; if used, patients may act as their own controls or historical controls accepted. Numbers are far too small to show anything but a massive benefit. It is difficult to see how such a trial, in which all the essential precautions are ignored, could; 'test the potential efficacy of a new treatment regime'.[4]

The history of the treatment of multiple sclerosis, until very recently, surely consists largely of pilot trials of this nature being taken far more seriously than the evidence warrants. The difficulties and cost of mounting a full therapeutic trial from which reliable conclusions can be drawn are indeed so formidable that few would make the attempt without a reasonable hope of success. The difficulties must be overcome as, apart from the unlikely discovery of an immediate universal cure, the properly conducted trial provides the only means of demonstrating convincing therapeutic benefit. It must also be recognised that, in the absence of deeper knowledge of the causation of multiple sclerosis, there is no way in which it can be established or denied that an individual patient has improved as the result of treatment.

ASSESSMENT

The assessment of the results of treatment must necessarily be based almost entirely on the objective and subjective clinical state of the patients, recognising that the 'objectivity' of clinical examination is relative and exposed to observer bias. It has long been known that changes in activity of the disease, as judged by clinical criteria, sometimes appear to be quite unrelated to activity indicated by other means: morbid anatomy, evoked potentials and imaging techniques, which may be presumed to provide a truer insight to the disease process. A completely effective treatment should extinguish all evidence of active disease, but no such success has yet been attained. The uncertain relationship between laboratory data and clinical state has not yet permitted monitoring of the effects of treatment by any means other than clinical assessment, although there have been many attempts to do so.

The Kurtzke disability status scale (DSS), either in its original[19,20] or extended[21] form (EDSS) has been extensively and, indeed, recently almost universally used for this purpose, for which it was specifically designed. In the extended system the original 9 grades between normal (0) and dead (10) have each been divided in two with the aim of making the scale more sensitive. Grading on the scale is to a considerable degree dependent on the neurological examination of functional systems

(FS): pyramidal, cerebellar, brainstem, sensory, bladder and bowel, visual and mental, all graded from 0 to 5 or 6. There is a separate category for defects in 'other functions' but these are simply noted and not graded. The lower points on the full scale, up to 3.5, are defined in terms of FS scores. In the higher grades, disability, with particular regard to mobility, is the main deciding factor, with FS scores indicated as those usually found at this level. In general the system works well but there are naturally imperfections. Bauer et al[22] pointed out that some important causes of disability: tremor, spasticity and mental disorder other than mood change or dementia, do not contribute to the FS scores. Significant relapse does not necessarily affect the grading. For example, if a patient with mild paraparesis (pyramidal FS 3) develops a weak arm, this important event does not warrant a change to FS 4 and therefore would not affect the DSS grade. It is also difficult to know where to place the patient severely disabled by vertigo. Willoughby & Paty[23] have additionally criticised the DSS as grading neurological impairment on a mixture of signs and symptoms rather than disability. They also object that the scale does not measure the pathological extent of the disease but it is not clear how this could be demanded from any clinical grading system. Kurtzke[24] has conducted a spirited defence of his scale and certainly his critics have not yet devised a more acceptable method of assessment.

Despite minor defects the system is an effective method of documenting improvement or deterioration but in therapeutic trials it is still necessary to insist that significant change is defined as at least one full grade on the scale. In practice, it is surely important that grading should be done without reference to earlier scores, although this is only occasionally stated as a requirement.[25] Kurtzke[26] states that the DSS approximates closely to a numerical scale and that for statistical purposes it might be legitimate to regard the grades as actual measurements, although he does not advocate this. It would certainly be difficult to maintain that grade 7 (essentially confined to a wheelchair) is only twice as 'bad' as 3.5 (fully mobile but with moderate disability in some FS). It has been generally recognised that non-parametric statistical methods should be used. Statistical comparisons of mean changes in EDSS grade between treated and untreated patients can certainly be made, but a difference of 0.18 of a grade[27] is difficult to envisage except as something unlikely to be of clinical importance. Results are probably best expressed as numbers of patients improved, unchanged or worse, with, if relevant, numbers of those who changed by different numbers of grades on the scale.

There have been remarkably few attempts at examining the reliability of the Kurtzke scales. Kuzma et al[28] reported good agreement between five examiners but did not state the actual grades awarded either on the DSS or FS. Amato et al[29] also found good agreement between observers when a patient was examined by one neurologist in the presence of three others. In a much more pertinent study,[30] however, in which 4 neurologists conducted separate examinations, agreement was far less complete. Of the 24 paired examinations, an identical DSS grade was scored on only 12 occasions. In 6, scores differed by 0.5 grade, in 5 by 1 grade and in one by 1.5 grades. Differences were more common at the lower end of the scales where grading is dependent on FS scores. There was most disagreement on scoring mental and sensory functions. The implications of this study are very considerable, as in virtually all therapeutic trials a difference of 1 DSS grade is regarded as significant change. Intra-observer variation, of even greater relevance to assessing the results of treatment, is much more difficult to test. With a short interval between examinations the observer will remember the previous score, while with a longer interval the clinical condition might well have changed.

In many therapeutic trials more than one clinical method of assessment has been used, although the purpose of doing so and how the results should be handled are seldom explained. If one method shows benefit and another does not which should be believed? It is not uncommon for the results of only one method to be given, the other being said to be in agreement.[31] In the Co-operative ACTH trial[32] multiple assessment methods were deliberately used experimentally in order to gain knowledge of reliability and comparability. The standardised neurological examination comprised

38 variables, separately graded. The 7-day symptom score recorded the presence and severity of 20 different symptoms in the preceding week. Quantitative measures of some 12 tests of ability or strength were recorded. The Kurtzke DSS and FS were used, and, finally, the estimated overall condition (EOC); better, the same or worse, as assessed by the physician. Comparability between the methods was relatively good and even the EOC performed surprisingly well. It was concluded that the Kurtzke scales were the most reliable index of change. The quantitative tests developed by Tourtellotte and colleagues[33] have disappointingly seldom been used.

A popular scale is the Ambulation Index[34] based on timed ability to walk with or without aids. In personal experience some intervals on the scale seem too wide. This is particularly so with respect to Grade 3: 'walks independently, able to walk 25 feet in 20 seconds or less' and Grade 4: 'requires unilateral support to walk'. The latter must imply that walking is not possible without support, a profound deterioration. The illness severity score of Mickey et al[35] derives a single figure from the Kurtzke DSS and FS and marks for duration and activity of the disease. Sipe et al[36] published a very detailed rating scale based on grading the results of examination. Given the same data, 4 physicians obtained close grouping of scores but they were not tested on examining patients, where errors would certainly have been greater. These scales approach in complexity the laborious Alexander[37] method of assessment.

There have been justified objections[1] that assessment based almost exclusively on the results of examination and ability to walk are not necessarily closely related to what individual patients hope to obtain from treatment. Short of cure, this must surely amount to some easing of the burdens of everyday life. Realisation of this has led to the proliferation of scales recording the ability to perform activities of daily living, of which Feinstein et al[38] reviewed no less than 43, many in contexts other than multiple sclerosis. Such scales have been used to a limited extent in trials, sometimes ad hoc versions[39] or with a label but no traceable description[31] (the references given unexpectedly lead back to a numerical scale for the neurological examination devised by Henry Miller). The Incapacity Status Scale that forms part of the International Federation of Multiple Sclerosis Societies' minimal record of disability,[40] grades 16 items on a scale of 0 to 4. It is probably too minutely divided to be suitable for use in trials and the scale of Cook et al[39] has much to recommend it. A plea for more input from the subjective views of the patients[41] is a welcome change, but intrinsically difficult to implement because of the pronounced placebo effect. The trial of amantadine in fatigue[42] was, however, necessarily based wholly on the opinions of the patients.

Laboratory methods of assessment have been frequently used but are seldom claimed to have made any important contribution to the results. Recording of evoked potentials is an obvious choice, being atraumatic, standardised and readily repeatable. However, the method is far from ideal as the diagnostic use of evoked potentials in multiple sclerosis depends on the persistence of abnormalities revealing clinically silent lesions. It is true that there is a general tendency for abnormalities to increase with the passage of time.[43–45] Mean changes in latency can be related to mean increase in disability, but correlation of evoked potentials and clinical changes in individual patients is far from precise.

When evoked potentials have been recorded as an element in monitoring response to treatment, the results have made little contribution. 'Improved' responses may accompany appropriate clinical changes[31,46,47] or may be no different from control even when the treated group has been thought to benefit.[48] Lack of therapeutic effect may be accompanied by absence of any consistent alteration in evoked potentials.[49] Nuwer at al[50] claimed that comparative lack of increase, or even reduction, in latency of pattern reversal visual and middle-latency somatosensory responses was predictive of significant arrest of progression in patients treated with azathioprine and steroids. The statistical significance of the difference between mean values for evoked potential latencies in the 3 treatment groups at 2 and 3 years was much greater than the difference in clinical status. It would have been of interest to have seen the correlation of evoked potentials and clinical change in individual patients. Whether evoked potential data can be accepted as *independent* evidence that the disease process has been favourably influenced, irrespective of clinical change (for this is what the claim of prediction must imply) requires further evaluation.

Not unexpectedly, if agents suppressing or otherwise affecting immune functions are given, disturbances of these functions will result.[51–54] As there is no conclusive evidence that such changes are related to the activity of the disease process, no legitimate conclusions as to the possible benefits of treatment can be drawn. It may, however, be permissible to conclude that if synthesis of IgG within the blood–brain barrier is not reduced by treatment under trial, the treatment is not affecting the disease process.[55] Apart from examining the peripheral blood lymphocytes, appropriate investigations require repeated lumbar puncture, permissible in a closely defined experimental context, but quite unsuitable for general use.

The use of imaging techniques for systematic monitoring of the effects of treatment has been infrequently described. CT scanning has shown rapid changes with steroid treatment in acute relapse[56] but was not found to be helpful in monitoring treatment of chronic disease. Magnetic resonance imaging promises to be of immense value in assessing the results of treatment, but is expensive and not well tolerated by some patients. The first report[57] of the use of this technique in monitoring treatment showed continued disease activity, not clinically detectable. It is already obvious that the events seen by MRI greatly outnumber clinical relapses and that, provided standardised methods of assessing the results can be agreed, MRI will supersede other methods of determining the effects of treatment. It must be hoped that in the process of counting shadows we do not neglect to ask the patients how they feel.

FORMS OF TREATMENT

Many of the early attempts at treatment have been excellently reviewed by Sibley[58] and Liversedge[59] described a few unconventional forms of therapy that have probably not spread to the USA. These methods, although extremely varied in detail, have several characteristics in common. They are based

either on some pre-conceived but ephemeral theory, or on chance observation, subsequently supported by theory based on the assumption that the treatment is effective. Occasionally the need for any theoretical basis is dispensed with altogether. Trials, however extended, never pass the stage of the preliminary trial as defined earlier. Controls, if used at all, are simply the undocumented previous state of the patients. Enthusiasm and the remitting nature of the disease result in a brief flowering of hope but in no lasting benefit. Morale is improved by any attempt at treatment, but the atmosphere of therapeutic optimism, however desirable, can undoubtedly influence assessment.[60]

A logical subdivision would be between treatment designed to modify the disease process and treatment directed to the alleviation of specific symptoms. The distinction is, however, far from absolute. The activity of the disease can only be judged from the symptoms and many forms of symptomatic treatment have been claimed by their proponents to be curative.

Corticosteroids and corticotrophin (ACTH)

Rationale

Although later reports refer to the anti-inflammatory and immunosuppressive actions of corticosteroids and ACTH it is probable that the earliest attempts to use these agents in the treatment of multiple sclerosis were based on the natural wish to observe the effect of a powerful new form of therapy on an intractable disease. These early reports, summarised by Miller et al[61] claimed some success, but were quite uncontrolled. It is not now easy to discern why controlled trials have largely concentrated on the use of ACTH rather than the far more readily managed oral steroids. The sequence of events probably began with Miller's[62] use of ACTH in acute disseminated encephalomyelitis extended in a later paper to multiple sclerosis.[63] No reason for the preference for ACTH was given but the choice was probably related to the hope of obtaining a more rapid effect by the injection of ACTH than by the use of oral cortisone. Once success was claimed for ACTH in serious trials it was natural to attempt to confirm these findings rather than to embark on an entirely new venture with all the difficulties of determining optimum steroid dosage.

Trials in acute relapse

Early uncontrolled preliminary trials were naturally inconclusive but suggested some value of ACTH in acute relapse. Alexander et al[64] were enthusiastic but their trial was inadequate in many respects. Miller et al[61] essayed a randomised single-blind trial but ran into insuperable difficulties of case selection and assessment of results. Nevertheless, the benefit claimed in this report, that of increasing the chance of patients making a substantial improvement within three weeks, was influential in popularising this form of treatment.

The Co-operative Study[32] of ACTH in acute relapse carried out in the USA was not the first multicentre randomised double-blind placebo-controlled trial in multiple sclerosis[65] but was, nevertheless, something of a landmark in therapeutic trials in this disease in its scale and organisation. Patient selection and methods of assessment were fully established from the outset. Unfortunately, the dose of ACTH gel was a good deal smaller than that usually employed, being only 40 units twice a day for a week, 20 units twice a day for 4 days, followed by 20 units daily for 3 days. Assessment was not followed for longer than 4 weeks from the beginning of treatment. Patients in whom recovery from relapse had begun were admitted to the trial. The results can be interpreted differently according to which method of assessment is used. The overall estimate of whether the patients were better, the same, or worse at the end of the course of treatment showed significant initial benefit over control, but this was no longer present at 4 weeks, suggesting that recovery had been accelerated but not otherwise influenced. Applying the Kurtzke DSS, however, shows persistent and increasing benefit of treatment over placebo at all examinations, at least according to Kurtzke.[26]

Hoogstraten et al[66] reported an interesting comparison of bed rest alone versus bed rest and synthetic ACTH in the management of acute relapse. No difference in result was found, but un-fortunately the study was retrospective and biased by differences in age, duration of disease and of relapse. ACTH became the standard treatment of acute relapse. It was usual to give the initial dose used in the Co-operative Study, 40 units of the gel twice a day by intramuscular injection for a week, or the synthetic equivalent, but to continue with reducing doses for a further 2 weeks or even longer. Steroid side effects, particularly weight gain and acne, were common and acute psychosis was occasional. As with untreated relapse, recovery was often rapid, but no more trials were undertaken, except in optic neuritis. Rawson et al[67] in a single-blind randomised trial of ACTH 40 units daily for 30 days, versus placebo, found that a much higher proportion of treated patients had normal visual acuity at the end of the course. A year later[68] there was no significant difference between the two groups, again suggesting accelerated recovery with no long-term effect. An immediate effect of treatment had been cessation of pain within 48 hours. These beneficial results could not be confirmed by Bowden et al,[69] but their patients began treatment considerably later so that less effect of treatment might be expected.

ACTH has, however, been largely superseded in the treatment of relapse by the use of high-dose intravenous methylprednisolone. This treatment was initiated by Dowling et al[70] who gave frequent infusions of methylprednisolone, amounting to some 2 g over $2\frac{1}{2}$ days, followed by high oral doses of prednisolone. Of the 7 patients treated, 5 rapidly improved and the patient described in detail recovered almost normal vision within 48 h, after being threatened with blindness.

Variants on this theme were eagerly adopted and enthusiastic reports of uncontrolled preliminary studies soon appeared.[71-73] Milligan et al,[8] however, compared methylprednisolone 500 mg intravenously for 5 days with placebo in a double-blind study. Patients were accepted up to 8 weeks from the onset of relapse. One week after entry 8 of the 13 patients given methylprednisolone had improved, sometimes by several grades on the Kurtzke DSS, and at 4 weeks 10 had improved by at least 1 grade. No patient was worse than at entry. Of the placebo group of 9 patients, 3 had improved at one week and at 4 weeks 2 had improved, 4 were unchanged and 2 were worse. One control patient was withdrawn because of psychosis. Durelli et al,[74] also in a double-blind trial, compared methylprednisolone 15 mg/kg daily, reducing to 1 mg/kg over 15 days, with placebo. The intravenous treatment was followed by oral steroids in an initially high dose, reducing over 4 months. Improvement was much more rapid in the treated group, particularly in the first 3–6 days. There was, however, no difference in the number of patients in the two groups who eventually improved. Side effects were minimal during intravenous therapy but became much more marked with oral prednisolone.

The efficacy of bolus methylprednisolone in inducing rapid improvement in acute relapse was established by these trials, but not whether this treatment was superior to ACTH. Barnes et al[7] conducted a randomised controlled study, with blind assessment. Patients were admitted within 4 weeks of relapse. Methylprednisolone 1 g by slow intravenous infusion daily for 7 days was compared with intramuscular ACTH 80 units a day for 1 week, followed by daily doses of 60, 40, and 20 units, each for 1 week. The patients treated with methylprednisolone were significantly less disabled than the ACTH group at 3 and 28 days after beginning treatment, but by 3 months the difference was no longer significant. Abbruzzese et al[75] compared the effect of methylprednisolone 20 mg/kg a day for 3 days, tapered over the succeeding 15 days, with that of intravenous synthetic ACTH 1 mg daily and found more rapid improvement with the former. In contrast, Thompson et al[76] conducted a double-blind trial of 1 g of methylprednisolone daily for 3 days versus ACTH 80 units daily for 7 days, reducing over a further 9 days. Placebo intravenous and intramuscular injections were given as appropriate. Both groups improved but no significant difference was found in rate of improvement or degree of recovery after 3 months. It was concluded that methylprednisolone was as effective as ACTH, but not superior, and more convenient to use, but it must be noted that methylprednisolone was given for only 3 days.

The optimum dose of methylprednisolone has not been determined, personal preference being for 500 mg daily for 5 days. A single dose of 1 g has been shown not to be followed by the benefit obtained from 1 g daily for 5 days.[77] Lyons et al[78] reviewed the adverse effects of this schedule, followed by reducing oral steroids for 10 days: 350 courses of treatment were given to 164 patients. Serious ill-effects were not seen. Infection was negligible. One patient had an epileptic fit during treatment and 2 patients had a subsequent fit. Eleven developed transient hyperglycaemia and 5 had gastric discomfort. Acne occurred in 3 patients. Euphoria was observed on 4 occasions and depression twice. Weight gain was mild. Most patients, if asked, mention an unpleasant taste during the infusion. The psychiatric effects at this dose level have not proved to be alarming but a sharp decline in mood after the course is not uncommon. An acute anaphylactic reaction has been described in one patient.[79] With larger doses, much more serious adverse effects will occur. Warren et al[80] using 2 g of methylprednisolone a day for 10 days recorded acute psychosis, attempted suicide, hair loss, withdrawal rash, cataract and necrosis of the femoral head.

There is now no doubt that a short course of high-dose intravenous methylprednisolone is the treatment of choice for acute relapse of multiple sclerosis. The necessity for prolonged tapering with oral steroids has not been demonstrated although favoured by some authorities.[81] In personal practice I do not treat purely sensory relapse with steroids. The prognosis in isolated optic neuritis is usually excellent, but steroid treatment is valuable if pain is severe and should also be used if acuity in the other eye has been previously permanently reduced. Reported results in optic neuritis are impressive but uncontrolled.[82] I have given bolus steroids without ill-effect to a patient who had suffered an epileptic fit while being treated with ACTH in an earlier relapse, but recurrent epilepsy might be regarded as a contraindication. An acute relapse can be disabling and frightening and even if there is no suggestion of a better recovery with treatment, more rapid recovery is certainly welcomed by the patient. The course can be repeated in subsequent relapses. Treatment can easily be given as an outpatient with little inconvenience and there is little obvious advantage in convenience in exploring the use of intramuscular dexamethasone.[83] As might be expected, bolus steroid treatment is not always successful.

The mode of action of methylprednisolone in acute relapse is uncertain. A single dose may result in rapid disappearance of enhancing lesions on CT scanning,[56] suggesting restoration of the blood–brain barrier. Warren et al,[80] however, examining the CSF albumen content could detect no such effect. Intrathecal synthesis of IgG is reduced for a few days and levels of myelin basic protein and anti-myelin basic protein are also reduced.[80] The latencies of visual,[84] somatosensory and brainstem auditory evoked potentials are not acutely altered.[85]

Chronic treatment

It has been common practice to give oral prednisolone or dexamethasone in acute relapse and also to use chronic low dose steroid treatment in chronic disease. There is no evidence to suggest that such treatment is effective. Miller et al[86] found that patients on aspirin fared better than those on 15 mg of prednisolone a day. Fog[87] could detect no effect of long-term steroids on the course of the disease in 77 patients. Tourtellotte & Haerer[88] reported a double-blind trial of 10–12 mg of oral methylprednisolone a day versus oral cyanocobalamine over 18 months. They felt that the patients on steroids did rather better but were unable to substantiate any clinically or statistically significant improvement. The effect of ACTH 15–25 units a day by intramuscular injection has been assessed in a large randomised single-blind trial against placebo.[89] Disability was assessed on the Kurtzke DSS. Relapses were defined, counted and scored for severity. The patients were seen every three months. The result was conclusive; no benefit resulted from this dose of ACTH. The incidence of side effects, including hypomania, osteoporosis, hypertension and a pathological fracture, was high enough to suggest that the dose could not be increased with safety. Rinne et al[90] tried two dosage schemes, 30 or 90 units of ACTH a day for 35 days. The chronic features of multiple sclerosis improved on both regimes, but did not differ from the effects of placebo.

Milligan et al,[8] as part of their double-blind trial of bolus methylprednisolone, examined the effect on 28 patients with chronic progressive disease. Of those receiving treatment 6 improved, while there was no improvement in the placebo group. Improvement may have been due to relief of severe spasticity.[91] In a larger series of patients with chronic multiple sclerosis Kesselring et al[57] found no benefit from bolus corticosteroid treatment. Poser et al[92] have suggested that restoring the blood–brain barrier with steroid treatment in acute relapse may prevent subsequent progress of disease. A patient with innumerable enhancing lesions on CT scanning was treated with ACTH. The radiological appearances steadily improved over the succeeding year and even with MRI only a single lesion was detected. The case is of great interest but the conclusion was probably over-optimistic. Patients successfully treated with intravenous prednisolone unfortunately frequently relapse or progress subsequently.

There is no scientific support for chronic oral steroid treatment that carries additional risks for the disabled patient: intractable pressure sores; weight gain; osteoporosis, and absorption of the femoral heads. A few patients so treated become in some way steroid dependent in that any attempt to reduce dosage leads to increased disability, only restored on returning to the customary dose, but, of course, with grave risk of dangerous toxicity. It is better not to begin such treatment.

Intrathecal methylprednisolone given by lumbar puncture enjoyed a brief localised vogue[93,94] but probably the only benefit was short-lived improvement in spasticity and sometimes in bladder function after each injection.[95,96] The occurrence of intractable adhesive arachnoiditis and pachymeningitis,[97,98] leading to paraplegia has, I believe, caused the abandonment of this form of treatment.

IMMUNOTHERAPY

Rationale

Evidence of disordered immunity in multiple sclerosis is discussed in detail in Chapter 11. While there is uncertainty as to the role that this plays in the pathogenesis of the disease, the concept opens several promising lines of treatment. Autoimmunity might be suppressed. Circulating antibodies or immune complexes might be removed. Desensitisation to an allergen might be attempted. Defective immunity to infective agents might be fortified. There are formidable difficulties in attempting immunotherapy when no responsible antigen has been identified and Lisak[99] has recently commented on the sharp contrast between progress in understanding in myasthenia gravis, where the antigen has been demonstrated, and multiple sclerosis where it has not.

Immunosuppression

Cytotoxic agents

Cyclophosphamide

The use of cyclophosphamide in the treatment of multiple sclerosis in open uncontrolled trials was first reported from Lyon.[100,101] The regime adopted was that of repeated intravenous infusion over a period of up to 6 weeks. In a $2\frac{1}{2}$ year follow-up no patient was said to have deteriorated and 17 out of 30 had improved. Despite this encouraging result this group of workers soon transferred their attention to azathioprine. Millac & Miller[102] attempted an open but controlled trial of oral cyclophosphamide but only 8 of 18 patients completed the one-year course. Toxic effects, including nausea, rashes, infections, alopecia and cystitis enforced the withdrawal of 5 patients. Three treated patients improved, none 'dramatically'. There was no improvement in controls but the trial was not regarded as successful. Drachman et al[103] tried to arrest acute relapse by a short course of high dose cyclophophamide, but did not succeed.

Short intensive courses of cyclophosphamide have been used extensively in large, open, uncontrolled trials, both orally, combined with steroids,[104,105] or by intravenous infusion.[106,107] Great reduction in rate and severity of relapse and arrest of progression were claimed. These trials were initiated comparatively early but it is disappointing to see an uncontrolled trial published as recently as 1980.[108] A retrospective study of 21 patients with both relapsing and progressive disease, who had been treated in this way, showed no alteration in the course of the disease over the succeeding 2 years compared with controls matched for disability.[109]

Fresh ground was broken by Hauser et al[34] who carried out an elaborate open three-armed controlled trial in progressive multiple sclerosis. All patients received intravenous synthetic ACTH. One group had high-dose cyclophosphamide; the second had low-dose cyclophosphamide and plasma exchange and the third had ACTH alone. In the first group after 6 months, of 20 patients, 8 had improved and 2 were worse. In the second group 5 of 18 had improved and 12 were worse. With ACTH alone only 1 of 20 had improved and 12 were worse. Morbidity from cyclophosphamide was limited to alopecia in those on high doses.

The results are at first sight impressive, but the trial was not perfectly designed (a criticism that might be levelled at virtually any trial reported). It is difficult to understand why a straightforward comparison of high-dose cyclophosphamide versus placebo was not organised, the use of three forms of treatment being unnecessarily confusing.[110] A double-blind trial of a drug that causes alopecia is scarcely feasible, but blind assessment might have been possible. By a quirk of chance, the age of onset of the disease was significantly lower in the high dose group, early age of onset being a relatively good prognostic sign. Any beneficial effect of treatment appeared to be transient as patients who had improved began to deteriorate within 1–3 years.

A rather similar trial has been carried out by Trouillas et al.[111] The trial was open and concerned three groups of 10 patients with progressive disease, the majority with severe disability. One group received high-dose cyclophosphamide, the second group was treated with a series of plasma exchanges followed by the same dose of cyclophosphamide, while the third group consisted of matched controls selected from patients who did not want to undergo the treatment. After six months, 8 of the cyclophosphamide group had improved as well as 7 of those receiving the combined treatment, but none of the controls had improved. The mean improvement for both groups was 1 grade on the Kurtzke DSS. Follow-up extended for three years and the degree of improvement gradually declined. Apart from the open nature of this trial a major problem is the lack of evidence of rate of progression before treatment. All patients were said to have progressed in the preceding six months but this was not documented or shown on the charts.

It was logical to explore other methods of using cyclophosphamide. Goodkin et al[112] examined the value of maintenance infusions. They organised a non-randomised open trial of cyclophosphamide in chronic progressive disease. Fifty one suitable patients were asked to take part; 27 agreed and the remaining 24 acted as controls. The 27 participants were randomly allocated to an intensive induction course alone or to a similar course followed by bimonthly maintenance infusions for two years. Different regimes of induction were used for in- and outpatients. At one year, 59% of treated and 17% of control subjects were stable. Change in status was, however, unusually minutely scored, half a grade on the Kurtzke EDSS being held to be sufficient, particularly inappropriate in an open study. Indeed, a number of patients were shown as 'worse' with no change in DSS or ambulatory index but deterioration in a test of manual dexterity. Assessment was by a neurologist, a physiotherapist and an occupational therapist, and repeated if not unanimous. Maintenance treatment was not shown to have any advantage over a single intensive course.

Myers et al[113] treated 14 patients with progressive disease with monthly intravenous infusions of cyclophosphamide, beginning with 400 mg/m^2 and increasing, if possible, to 2000 mg/m^2, monitored by checking blood B-lymphocytes and CD4 T-cells. The number of infusions varied from 5 to 13. The regime proved intolerable. Toxic effects included severe vomiting, amenorrhoea and frequent bacterial, viral and fungal infections. On the Kurtzke DSS, 3 patients improved, 9 were static and 2 worse. On the illness severity scale, 3 were better, 6 static and 5 worse.

The first controlled trial of cyclophosphamide in relapsing/remitting disease[114] unfortunately only recruited 14 patients, 8 given placebo and 6 the active agent, in a randomised double-blind study. Relapses were scored for duration but not for severity. Treatment consisted of cyclophosphamide 750 mg/m^2 monthly for 12 months, or dextrose saline. In both groups there was a fall in relapse rate and duration compared with pretreatment levels, the fall being greater in the cyclophosphamide group. The differences did not reach statistical significance. Patients in the placebo group subsequently treated openly with cyclophosphamide showed a further reduction in relapse rate. The pretreatment relapse rate was higher in the controls and disability greater in the treated group, both factors of possible relevance to the subsequent course of the disease.

Cyclophosphamide is still under trial but has also been extensively used in treatment. Carter et al[115] have reported results in 164 patients in an open uncontrolled trial and are convinced that a short course of high-dose cyclophosphamide combined with ACTH will stabilise the course of progressive multiple sclerosis for at least 1 year in most patients and that this response can be repeated, although with diminishing effect. What is clearly lacking is a placebo-controlled double-blind trial, preferably uncluttered by inclusion of other forms of treatment. Likosky[116] has described preliminary results of a single-blinded trial of cylcophosphamide versus folic acid. No significant benefit had been found at the time of reporting. This trial is naturally open to criticism on the grounds that ACTH was *not* given, but there appears to be no convincing evidence of a synergistic action and the original claims were of benefit from cyclophosphamide alone.

Azathioprine

Azathioprine, in effective immunosuppressant dosage, is somewhat easier to handle than cyclophosphamide, as gastrointestinal effects are less pronounced. Probably on this account it has been the subject of extended trials in multiple sclerosis over many years. Early reports cannot be seriously considered because of insufficient numbers or defects in reporting such essential details as the length of follow-up. Results varied from improvement in all cases[117] to improvement in few or none.[118,119] Silberberg et al[120] reported a well-conducted open pilot study of 3 mg/kg in a single daily dose for up to 15 months initially in 15 patients, 5 with progressive and 10 with relapsing disease. It was aimed to hold the white cell count to between 3500 and 4000/mm^3. One patient committed suicide and three withdrew. Deterioration or relapse continued in the great majority of those completing the course. It was concluded that evidence of immunosuppression was not linked to the clinical state.

In a larger pilot trial in both progressive and remittent disease Mertens and Dommasch[121] considered that the results were unsatisfactory. The patients were observed for at least six months before treatment and were given azathioprine 100–200 mg/day, regulated according to the leucocyte count, for at least six months. It is not easy to interpret their results, but it seems that after six months' treatment only 14% of 101 patients were thought to have improved, certainly a disappointing figure. Reduction in relapse rate and slowing of progression compared with the pre-treatment course were claimed, but significant benefit only in the relapsing form of disease. The difficulties of comparing pretreatment with subsequent relapse rates have frequently been mentioned. Rosen[122] reported arrest of progressive disease in the great majority of 35 ambulatory cases on long-term continuous azathioprine.

At this point a randomised double-blind trial against placebo would have been highly appropriate. However, large numbers of patients in France had already begun prolonged treatment with daily azathioprine. The experience gained was valuable but results were conflicting and, in the absence of concurrent controls, impossible to interpret.

Aimard et al[123] reported the results of long-term azathioprine in an average daily dose of 150 mg in 77 patients of whom 12 withdrew because of intolerance of the drug. Treatment in the remaining 65 patients was continued for an average period of five years, monitored by the blood count. No benefit was observed in the 27 patients with progressive disease although it is emphasised that many of them were already severely disabled. The course in the 38 relapsing cases was compared with that in 78 patients with relapsing disease not receiving this treatment. These were apparently matched with the treated group only in the mean duration of the disease and were not concurrently observed but extracted from a study of case notes. In the treated group the relapse rate fell from 0.73 before treatment to 0.14 and 18 patients (50%) had no relapse over a period of 76 patient-years. In the untreated group 13% had no relapse in 77 patient-years but in the remainder the mean inter-

val between relapses progressively shortened. A number of other benefits were noted, in particular the disease became progressive in 8% of treated cases and in 35% of those untreated. In a further report[124] extended to 213 cases similar benefits were noted, but again concurrent controls were not used in this open trial.

Sabouraud et al[125] reported the results in 67 of their patients who had taken azathioprine for more than 5 years. It is stated that only severe progressive cases were accepted, but this is not confirmed by the Kurtzke DSS scores and duration of disease before treatment. In all 40 patients with relapsing/remitting disease, the disability status remained stable for the duration of treatment. Some deteriorated on stopping treatment and improved again on restarting. In 27 patients with progressive disease, no benefit was observed. In another series Lhermitte et al[126] reported results in 145 patients who had taken azathioprine for more than one year. 97 patients had relapsing disease. In a mean observation period of 120 months since the start of treatment, 21 had no further relapse, 42 had further relapses with remission, and 34 had deteriorated, 14 of them entering the progressive stage. Patients with progressive disease fared much worse, with continued deterioration in 31 of 48. The absence of controls in these large trials is occasion for regret.

The first controlled trial was that of Swinburn & Liversedge[127] who compared 19 treated male patients with 25 controls in a single-blind study. Treatment consisted of 2.5 mg/kg versus ascorbic acid, monitored by the white blood count, and continued for 2 years. No significant difference between the groups was detected. In contrast, Rosen,[122] using much more prolonged treatment in an open trial in progressive disease, found that after 6 years (although this is difficult to reconcile with the average period of follow-up given as 4.5 years) 65% of the controls were in wheelchairs, as opposed to 9% of treated patients.

Patzold has conducted a prolonged controlled trial of azathioprine in patients with different clinical forms of multiple sclerosis. In most respects the trial was admirably conducted, with randomised concurrent controls. It is difficult to conduct a blind trial of such an active agent and this was not attempted. Selection of patients, dosage and clinical assessment were comparable to those in other trials. In the first report[128] on 56 cases and 51 controls, no difference in relapse rate was found between the two groups, but the authors believe that this, in any case, is a poor indication of therapeutic benefit. There was no effect on the rate of progression in patients with symptoms for more than two years, but a significant reduction in rate of decline in those with a shorter history. In a later report,[129] benefit was only seen in patients with an intermittent-progressive course, that is relapse without full remission. Remitting disease and steadily progressive disease showed no significant benefit. The course of the disease prior to treatment, the basis of the classification, was established solely on the statements of the patients. It was only by subsequent statistical analsysis of these insecure subdivisions that any benefit of azathioprine could be detected.

A randomised double-blind placebo-controlled trial was carried out by Milanese et al[130] but only 38 patients were included, of whom 17 dropped out. No effect on relapse rate was observed but the progression rate was significantly slower in the treated group at three years. This rate was defined as the ratio of the EDSS grade at the end of the period less the score at the beginning of treatment, to the duration of treatment expressed in months. Numbers were small and the groups were not well matched. A much larger trial was organised in Britain and the Netherlands.[27] One hundred and seventy four patients were treated with 2.5 mg/kg, adjusted as necessary, and 180 received inert tablets. Treatment was continued for 3 years. There was no significant difference between the rate of deterioration in the two groups as judged by change in the EDSS. The ambulation index declined in both groups but significantly slightly less in those on azathioprine. Relapses were also somewhat less frequent on treatment. The results indicate, at best, a very small beneficial effect. The difference between treated and placebo groups increased over the three years but as significant changes in EDSS were not achieved it is not legitimate to interpret this as a trend that might have increased to significant levels with more prolonged treatment.

After a scarcely encouraging pilot trial,[131] azathioprine combined with methylprednisolone has been compared with azathioprine and sham methylprednisolone and with sham azathioprine and sham methylprednisolone combined[50,132] Intravenous methylprednisolone or placebo was given by infusion for 3 days a month for 3 months, followed by oral steroids for a further 3 months. Azathioprine or, of course, placebo, was continued for 3 years. The results have not been published in full but there is a trend for the treated patients to fare better than those on double placebo. The results illustrate the advantages, or difficulties, of using multiple modes of clinical assessment. The Illness Severity Score and the Kurtzke DSS showed no benefit over control, while a significant slowing of deterioration on treatment was demonstrated using the Standard Neurological Examination and evoked potentials were stabilised. Relapse rate in the treated group was half that in those on placebo but the disease was not arrested. The authors believe that a trial of treatment with continuous steroids and azathioprine in early disease should be undertaken, but emphasise that they do not recommend the routine use of this regime. After so many trials of azathioprine it is likely that any worthwhile benefit would already have been clearly demonstrated.

Cyclosporin

A large double-blind trial of cyclosporin versus azathioprine has been published.[133] Patients were randomised to the two treatment groups, 85 receiving cyclosporin 5 mg/kg/day and 82 azathioprine 2.5 mg/kg/day for 24–32 months. There was no placebo group. No significant differences in relapse rate or progress of disability was found between the two groups, probably meaning that both treatments were equally ineffective. Rudge et al[134] conducted a double-blind randomised placebo-controlled trial. They reported that cyclosporin 8 mg/kg/day for 2 years produced minor degrees of benefit, but at the cost of severe toxicity. A lower dose of 5 mg/kg/day was less toxic but ineffective as treatment. Cyclosporin is nephrotoxic and has the further disadvantage of failure to penetrate the normal blood–brain barrier. It is a powerful immunosuppressant but does not seem to have any future in the treatment of multiple sclerosis.

Monoclonal antibody

Although there is considerable activity in this field[135] little beyond a pilot study,[136] mostly concerned with immunological responses, has been published. The ability to produce monoclonal antibodies does not help to decide on the most appropriate target. The one chosen was an anti-T-cell antibody derived from mice. The T-12 lymphocytes against which the antibody was directed, disappeared from the blood between days 1 and 7 of the 10-day course. No antibody appeared in the CSF. The patients developed anti-mouse antibodies. Clinical results resembled those familiar from many open trials: at three months, 3 patients were worse, 6 were improved and 2 stable; at six months, 8 were worse, 1 improved and 2 stable.

Antilymphocytic globulin

A number of attempts have been made to assess antilymphocytic globulin (ALG), antithymocyte globulin (ATC) and antilymphocytic serum (ALS) in the treatment of different forms of multiple sclerosis, nearly always in combination with other agents. Most of these trials have been inadequately conducted, leading to negative or uninterpretable results.[137–139] Lhermitte and colleagues[140,141] have conducted a prolonged investigation into the use of ALS derived from the horse. In their pilot study a 6-week course of ALS by intravenous infusion was given to patients with severe progressive disease, not in a terminal state. Treatment was combined with prednisone and azathioprine intended to prevent reaction to the foreign protein of the serum. Nevertheless, serum sickness interrupted treatment in 12% of cases. It proved possible to review the clinical course for four years in 32 patients. An attempt was made to compare the results with those in 18 patients not given ALS but receiving steroids, with or without azathioprine. Of those given ALS 45% had

deteriorated two years later and 16% had improved, while of those treated by other means 55% had deteriorated and none had improved. The unmatched nature of the control series prevented any valid comparison.

In a later study ALS was given daily in an initial intensive course, followed by less frequent infusions over the succeeding year, to patients with relapsing/remitting and progressive disease. Oral steroids and azathioprine, originally used to counter reactions to horse serum, were also given, the latter for three years. A similar group of patients receiving the same regime of steroids and azathioprine was used for comparison. The only significant finding was that at the end of the first year the number of patients improved was greater in the ALS group, and in the third year the number of improved and stable patients combined was also greater in that group. All other comparisons were not significantly different and the relapse rate in the two groups was identical. Despite these disappointing results, the authors believed that 'une impression favorable' persisted.

Combined treatment

In a number of trials already alluded to more than one agent has been used, not always in the interests of clarity. A number of deliberate attempts have been made to induce maximal immunosuppression by all available means. This was first attempted by Frick et al[142] and Brendel et al[143] consolidated results being reported in 1974[144]. Twenty patients with progressive disease not influenced by steroids or azathioprine were treated with intravenous ALG or thoracic duct drainage or a combination of both, together with azathioprine and steroids. In some patients an attempt was made to induce unresponsiveness to horse IgG. The clinical state of the patients was carefully assessed and eleven were thought to have shown significant improvement. All those that improved had the relapsing and remitting form of the disease but it is not stated whether they were in acute relapse when the treatment was begun, a factor that would have a profound influence on the immediate prognosis. There was some correlation between the degree of immunosuppression achieved and the clinical improvement. This elaborate trial was conducted without controls and the use of the patients as their own controls was unsatisfactory as the clinical condition was measured only at the point the trial was begun, without earlier documentation.

The use of a similar regime was described by Lance et al[145] who found that side effects were controllable and that in no patient was multiple sclerosis apparently aggravated. An idiosyncratic method of scoring the clinical condition was adopted although well tried and validated methods are available. After one year, 9 patients were thought to have improved, 3 were unchanged and 2 were worse. The relapse rate was lower after treatment. There were again no controls. Lance's[146] interpretation of the results of Ring et al was overoptimistic as the latter only claimed that disease activity was stopped in 4 patients and not that a halt in progression was achieved in all but one.

These trials had shown that intensive immunosuppression was possible and tolerable and did not exacerbate the disease, but the claims of benefit were uncontrolled and intrinsically unsatisfactory. The publication of the results of a double-blind controlled trial was therefore particularly welcome. The regime adopted was similar to that used by others except that thoracic duct drainage was not employed. The results in the first 30 patients (15 treated and 15 placebo) showed a significant excess in the treated group of patients having no relapse during the period of observation of 15 months. In women, but not in men, there was a barely significant retardation of the disease judged by disability scores. In the final report of this trial,[147] results in a somewhat larger series observed for a longer period were described but were not impressive from the viewpoint of attempted cure of the disease. Deterioration was marginally greater in the controls and the interval between relapses in the period of observation following treatment was prolonged in those receiving the regime. Some effect of intensive immunosuppression is probable but the benefit seems scarcely commensurate with the severity of the treatment. It is clear that the disease process remains active.

Total lymphoid irradiation

This method of immunosuppression was introduced as treatment of multiple sclerosis by Cook et al.[148] The method involves irradiation of the trunk from the level of the thyroid cartilage down to the first lumbar vertebra, with shielding of the spinal cord and lungs. This is given in 11 sessions to a total dose of 1980 cGy. A randomised double-blind comparison against sham irradiation was carried out in 40 patients with progressive disease, with 20 patients in each group. Assessment was on a disability scale and on a functional scale with much wider steps than the Kurtzke DSS. Particular attention was paid to the time from treatment at which the first evidence of deterioration was observed. This occurred earlier in the sham treated group and there was significantly less deterioration in the irradiated group after a mean follow-up of 21 months. Side effects were minimal. Patients in whom the total blood lymphocyte count fell persistently below 900/mm^3 were significantly less likely to deteriorate during the period of observation. Even in this group, however, some patients continued to deteriorate, presumably indicating continued disease activity. Myers et al[149] treated two patients by this method, although in one the spinal cord was not shielded, and, disappointingly, in both treatment was followed or accompanied by severe relapse. In another small series[150] unpleasant side effects and continued deterioration of progressive disease have been described.

Thymectomy

Thymectomy has been carried out in a large number of patients with multiple sclerosis in Argentina, with claims of benefit.[151] This has not been confirmed in an open controlled trial in both relapsing and progressive disease.[152] Thirty four patients were matched for disability and relapse rate with controls. Treatment was thymectomy or thymectomy and azathioprine for one year. Compared with controls, operated cases of relapsing disease did as well or slightly better, while progressive cases fared worse. It was concluded that no further investigation of this method of treatment was justified. The halving of the relapse rate in the untreated controls is worth noting.

Toxicity

All immunosuppressant agents have toxic effects that limit their use. Nausea and vomiting are commonly caused by azathioprine, cyclophosphamide and cyclosporin. Cyclophosphamide in high dosage causes alopecia, although this is not permanent, and cyclosporin causes hypertrichosis and, more importantly, renal damage. A particular problem with cyclophosphamide is haemorrhagic cystitis and liver function must be monitored when using any of these drugs. There is a constant risk of marrow depression and pancytopenia. All immunosuppressed patients are unduly prone to infections: bacterial, viral or fungal. Reactivation of apparently healed tuberculosis may occur and disseminated herpes zoster can be very troublesome. Occasional fatalities from such causes are recorded in a number of trials but, with vigilance, can be avoided, although often at the cost of abandoning the treatment. Patients of both sexes on prolonged immunosuppressant treatment must be warned to avoid procreation.

It is probable that the risk of cancer is increased, although the degree of risk is difficult to assess. Lhermitte et al[126] reported that 10 of 131 patients who had completed more than one year of azathioprine, with no other immunosuppressant drug, had developed cancer. All occurred more than 5 years after beginning treatment. The tumours were of epithelial tissues: 5 breast, 1 uterine cervix, 1 skin, 1 ovary and 1 sigmoid colon. Sabouraud et al[125] reported 8 known malignant tumours in 240 patients treated with azathioprine, including 2 breast, 2 uterus, 1 gastric, 1 skin and 1 bone marrow. In 131 patients with multiple sclerosis who were not given azathioprine, 4 cancers occurred. The possible carcinogenic action of cyclophosphamide in patients with multiple sclerosis has not been analysed in large series. Chlorambucil appears to have been used in the treatment of multiple sclerosis, but this is clearly undesirable as there have been 9 reported cases of associated leukaemia.[153] The reports of cancer in patients on azathioprine are disturbing.

The incidence has not been shown to differ significantly from that in controls but appears to be high. All patients in whom it is proposed to use this agent must be informed that some risk exists.

Conclusion

When contemplating the results of elaborate, expensive and enormously demanding trials, showing no more at best than minor, sometimes disputable and evidently transient benefit from immunosuppression, there is an increasing tendency to express a belief that *some* patients with multiple sclerosis are helped by such treatment.[154] This, indeed, may be so but there is no way of determining this from trials specifically designed to smooth out individual results and demonstrate an effect by comparing one group with another. It has not proved possible to detect any specific marker for patients who appear to do well or badly on treatment, apart from factors known to influence prognosis in untreated patients; young patients with early mild disease often remain well for a long time, while older patients with progressive disease usually do not.

Plasmapheresis

The attempt to remove any of the considerable number of putative noxious agents from the plasma is a rational method of treatment. There is no lack of candidates for removal although few have been consistently confirmed and none has been shown to be responsible either for the symptoms or for the lesions of the disease. Autoantibodies to myelin basic protein or oligodendrocytes, immune complexes, demyelinating activity of unknown origin and neuroelectric blocking agents have all been described and are potentially removable by plasmapheresis.

Trials

Dau et al[46] treated 8 patients in the progressive stage with weekly or biweekly plasma exchange, combined with azathioprine and intermittent prednisone. The results were unimpressive. Seven patients were thought to have improved during treatment, although 3 actually relapsed during the course. The methods of clinical assessment were not stated and it seems that no substantial benefit resulted. CSF IgG levels fell during treatment, but not serum demyelinating activity. Three patients treated during acute severe relapse showed marked improvement. In 2, somatosensory evoked potentials recorded on the scalp showed a return towards normality. The significance of this must be doubtful as the amplitude of the response recorded at Erb's point and derived from the brachial plexus also increased.

Weiner & Dawson[155] used a similar combined treatment regime in 8 patients with progressive disease and claimed some improvement in 6. The results in these two trials were thought to warrant controlled trials of plasmapheresis, although it is apparent that no important benefit had resulted. The occurrence of relapse in three out of eight patients with the progressive form of the disease, where relapse is relatively uncommon, was scarcely encouraging.

These preliminary studies, combined with unpublished results were not thought to be impressive.[156] This opinion received support from a controlled open trial of plasma exchange and azathioprine versus azathioprine alone.[157] After an initial course, plasma exchange was performed approximately monthly for 12 months. Azathioprine dosage began with 50 mg/day, increasing to 3 mg/kg/day. Seven patients in each group completed the course. No significant difference in mean degree of deterioration or in numbers of patients improved or worse was found, and one patient receiving plasma exchange became rapidly worse. Such a small trial could only have detected a massive effect. Trouillas et al[158] found that 4 of 12 severely disabled patients improved rapidly but briefly following a course of six plasma exchanges. Stefoski et al[159] found that serum neuroelectric blocking activity was briefly reduced following plasma exchange in 5 of 7 patients. Two patients showed clinical improvement but this was not related to the changes in serum activity.

In contrast to these discouraging findings Khatri et al[160] reported a pilot trial of plasmapheresis and oral cyclophosphamide in progressive multiple sclerosis. Of 45 patients, 28 improved significantly, 14 improved slightly and 3 remained the same: none deteriorated and 14 patients improved by at least 3 grades of Kurtzke DSS. Even more remarkably a patient with multiple sclerosis for $1\frac{1}{2}$ years, already in a helpless state (grade 9), returned to normal (grade 0) after treatment. Another patient recovered from grade 8 to grade 1 (abnormal signs but no disability). These results were described by Scheinberg[161] as 'miraculous' and by Weiner[156] as likely to be thought 'too good to be true'.

The double-blind controlled trial[31] by the same group was organised with great attention to detail. All patients were given oral cyclophosphamide 1.5 mg/kg/day and prednisone 1 mg/kg on alternate days. Twenty six patients received plasmapheresis weekly for 20 weeks, while 29 were allocated to have a sham procedure in which they were given back their own plasma. Each treatment was followed by 4 injections of human immune serum globulin. Considerable pains had been taken to ensure that the patients genuinely had progressive disease before entry, although this was not always reflected in the DSS grades recorded. The results were less remarkable than those of the pilot trial, but at 5 months from the beginning of treatment those receiving plasmapheresis had fared substantially better. The most impressive difference was that 5 patients had improved by 3 DSS grades or more while none of those receiving sham treatment had done so. Fourteen 'treated' patients had improved but also 8 of those on immunosuppressant alone. Improvement was not observed before 10 weeks of treatment, except in 2 patients who deteriorated on sham plasmapheresis but showed 'immediate' improvement when switched to genuine treatment. The 10-week interval is most unlike the effect of plasmapheresis in myasthenia gravis where a known antibody is removed from the circulation.

Weiner[156] reviewed this important work and pointed out that the results at 5 months, i.e. at the end of treatment, had received far more emphasis than the less encouraging state of affairs 6 months later. During this period, for example, 10 of the 14 patients improved at 5 months had begun to deteriorate. Of the 13 patients in the treatment group originally unable to walk, 9 were ambulant at 5 months, but only 2 of the 12 similarly disabled patients in the sham plasma exchange group. Six months later the figures were 4 of 13 and 3 of 12. The degree of improvement, by 3 DSS grades or more, is more suggestive of a relapsing than of a progressive course and this receives some support from the rapid deterioration in 2 of these patients in the year before treatment. Treatment was not assessed against placebo. With such a complex regime this might well have been unacceptable, but a simpler protocol could surely have been used. Khatri et al[31] gave some reasons for combining plasmapheresis with immunosuppression, including unpublished work showing that plasmapheresis alone is ineffective. It is possible that unless some 'accepted' form of treatment was given to all patients the hospital costs would have been prohibitive.

Gordon et al[25] in a small but very carefully executed double-blind trial against sham plasmapharesis found transient minor improvements in 7 treated patients and 3 controls but no other benefit. Unusually, they examined patients at the same time of day, without reference to earlier scores. They determined reasonable treatment goals for individual patients: these were not attained.

Lymphocytapheresis

The rationale is to induce immunosuppression by removing circulating lymphocytes.

Maida et al[162] used this method of treatment in 9 patients with frequently relapsing multiple sclerosis. The intention was to carry out the procedure 4 times in 8 days at 6–8 week intervals for at least a year. Four patients could not complete the course: two because of venous thrombosis, one patient developed chicken pox and in one, multiple sclerosis rapidly progressed. Three patients became worse, 3 were static and 3 improved. Relapses were much less frequent than before treatment. Lymphocytapheresis was recommended as treatment for relapsing multiple sclerosis. Not unexpectedly, Hauser et al[163] and Medaer et al[164] did not detect any significant benefit

Interferon

Rationale

Interferon is not a single substance with known and fixed properties. There are at least three main forms and many subtypes of which the actions and natural functions are incompletely known. Interferons influence the immune system and have an antiviral action that, in theory, might be of value in multiple sclerosis. There is conflicting evidence that interferon production may be deficient in multiple sclerosis.[165–168] McFarlin[169] indicated some of the dangers inherent in the use of such powerful agents. Panitch et al[170] using natural alpha interferon produced immunological effects that might be thought to be the opposite of those desired; for example, an increase in CSF IgG. Some patients developed antibodies to a protein contaminant and had symptoms of immune-complex disease. Recombinant interferon should be free of some of these ill-effects.

Trials

The first systematic use of interferon in multiple sclerosis was in a small open controlled trial.[171,172] Interferon β was given intrathecally because of failure to penetrate the blood–brain barrier. Ten patients were treated and the course of the disease compared with that in ten randomly-selected controls. Matching between the groups showed some discrepancies, in particular the relapse rate being very much higher in the treated group. The authors believe that this high rate would have continued had interferon not been given and that the observed fall is therefore even more impressive evidence of a therapeutic effect. This is scarcely acceptable as high relapse rates do not persist indefinitely and regression towards a mean value is to be expected. It is to be hoped that in future trials randomisation will be more even handed. Toxic effects consisted of headaches and a meningeal reaction. After some two years, 5 treated patients and 2 controls had improved and 4 cases and 2 controls had deteriorated. The number of patients relapsing and the number of relapses were both lower in the treated group. These patients have been followed up[173] and in the treated cases a continued fall in relapse rate was observed. Two years after the six months' course of treatment, the control cases were treated with interferon. Their relapse rate, previously stable, fell from 0.68 to

0.30. No claim was made that clinical status had improved with treatment.

The unavoidable defects of this trial, its open nature and the accidental mismatching of the controls, fed the scepticism that greets any claim of therapeutic benefit in multiple sclerosis. It was followed by a multicentre, double-blind, placebo-controlled trial.[174,175] Patients were stratified according to relapse rate and randomised to intrathecal interferon or sham lumbar puncture, both groups being given indomethacin to counter side effects of the active agent. Mean relapse rates before treatment were nearly identical. In the treated group, the mean rate fell by 57% and in the controls by 26%, a significant difference. However, the numbers of patients in whom the relapse rate was reduced were similar in the two groups: 28 of 34 treated and 25 of 35 controls. Five treated patients had more relapses after treatment and 9 or 10 (the text is at variance with the illustration) controls. The difficulties of assessing results by relapse rate, an essential method, are illustrated by the surprising suggestion that the 26% reduction in the control group was a placebo effect of sham lumbar puncture.[176] If a sham procedure can have such a profound effect what might be expected from real lumbar puncture? There appears to be some reluctance to accept a natural decline in relapse rate. There was no significant difference in clinical status between the two groups at the end of the trial.

A preliminary report of a trial using the same treatment schedule[177] disturbingly shows that the treated group sustained more relapses than controls and that CSF levels of myelin basic protein increased during the first month of treatment. A pilot study[178] of intravenous natural interferon β showed no benefit on clinical or MRI assessment and one patient entered a severe relapse soon after an infusion. Further trials of systemic interferon β are in progress.[135]

Difficulties of interpretation were encountered in a randomised, double-blind placebo-controlled crossover trial of intramuscular interferon α.[179] Relapse rates fell in both the active and placebo treatment periods, more so when interferon followed placebo. Lessening of frequency and severity of relapse could be detected in patients with strictly relapsing and remitting disease, but those with relapsing/progressive disease continued to deteriorate. Camenga et al,[180] using recombinant α-2 interferon in a different regime of systemic injection, found no benefit from treatment. As usual, mean relapse rate fell in both treated and control groups, but to an almost identical degree. The fall of 31% in the placebo group is another indication of the pitfalls of this method of assessment. Preliminary results of a large trial of subcutaneous interferon α in Australia[181] have also failed to show any benefit.

A pilot trial of intravenous γ interferon,[182] twice a week for 4 weeks, showed the risks of using powerful agents with incompletely known effects. Seven of 18 patients relapsed. This was attributed to activation of the immune system, predicted by Lisak.[183] Side effects, mainly resembling the systemic symptoms of influenza, were pronounced with high doses and it was suggested that release of interferon might be related to relapse of multiple sclerosis associated with infection.

Jacobs and colleagues[175] remain optimistic that intrathecal β interferon, perhaps in shorter courses than they tried or combined with some other agent, will prove effective treatment for relapsing multiple sclerosis. Side effects are largely controllable with indomethacin. It is clear, however, that the treatment protocol used does not inactivate the disease.

A more oblique approach has been a preliminary trial of an inducer of α and β interferon[184] in 18 patients with progressive multiple sclerosis. Similar side effects occurred and the clinical response was disappointing. Four patients withdrew, 3 became worse, 4 improved and 7 remained static.

Immunosupportive treatment

Levamisole has a complex effect on immune systems among which can be recognised the enhancement of cell-mediated immunity.[185] Its use in multiple sclerosis was reported by Dau et al[186] who gave 50 mg thrice daily for three days on alternate weeks to 7 patients. Three months from beginning treatment 1 patient had improved and 5 had deteriorated, despite a return towards normality of immunological defects. Cendrowski & Czlonkowska[187] conducted an open uncontrolled trial in 19 patients. After one month of 150 mg a day by mouth there had been no clinically significant (one grade on the Kurtzke disability scale) change in 15, 2 had improved and 2 were worse. After more prolonged but intermittent treatment no patient was found to have improved. Immunological indicators examined during the trial also showed no change. Double-blind controlled trials[188] using relatively high doses hvae also failed to show any benefit.

Derivatives of inosine have been used in small open trials[189,190] from which unjustified claims of resulting clinical improvement or reduction of relapse rate have been drawn. In neither report was it stated whether the patients were in relapse or not when treatment was begun. Confavreux et al[191] found that isoprinosine did not alter the course of multiple sclerosis in 12 patients.

Transfer factor, an extract from human leucocytes, particularly T lymphocytes, has the property of passive transfer of delayed type hypersensitivity, persisting for a prolonged period. The regime of treatment is peculiarly suited to the double-blind controlled trial as it consists of single injections, usually at monthly intervals, and there are no side effects apparent either to the observer or to the patient. No doubt partly because of these properties most therapeutic trials of this agent have been exemplary.

Early double-blind trials over one year failed to show any benefit.[192,193] In a two-year trial, using transfer factor obtained from the patients' spouses, and therefore possibly of particular relevance to their exposure to viruses, some significant benefit was obtained.[48] Treated and control patients were closely matched in clinical features and in HLA grouping. The benefit observed was limited to slowing the rate of progression in patients with mild to moderate disability. Relapses continued to occur in the treated group. If the trial had been stopped after a year no benefit would have been detected, an important observation in view of the earlier negative results. The interpretation of the results inevitably depends on the application of statistical methods to arbitrary scores on a disability scale and on this basis the treated patients fared rather better. The number of patients improving was the same in both groups but the number deteriorating was somewhat smaller in the treated group. These figures were not further analysed but are not statistically significant. After completion of the trial, transfer factor was offered to all participants.[194] Progress of disease in those who switched from placebo was observed to slow, apparently when treatment was begun rather than after 18 months as in the original trial. A further trial of transfer factor in Australia[181] failed to show any benefit after two years and Van Haver et al,[195] in a similar study, also using transfer factor derived from relatives, were unable to show any benefit after 3 years.

Desensitisation

Rationale

Experimental allergic encephalomyelitis (EAE) has long been regarded as a promising animal model of multiple sclerosis. It is an inflammatory and demyelinating disease that can readily be produced in many animal species by the injection of very small quantities of an extract of homologous or heterologous central nervous tissue, together with Freund's adjuvant. This agent, when complete, contains mineral oil and killed tubercle bacilli and has the property of enhancing many immune reactions. The component of CNS tissue essential for the production of this autoimmune disease has been identified as myelin basic protein and even fractions of this protein are encephalitogenic. The resemblance to multiple sclerosis is sufficiently obvious and has been greatly enhanced by the production of naturally relapsing and remitting forms of EAE[196] with a distribution of lesions remarkably similar to that in the human disease.[197] It cannot be claimed that the two diseases are identical, one important difference being that the encephalitogenic agent in multiple sclerosis has not been identified. EAE, particularly in its chronic form, clearly presents opportunities for the laboratory investigation of means of modifying the disease process that might be applicable to multiple sclerosis.

Of immediate interest is the effect of the injection of large doses of the encephalitogenic agent on the subsequent development or course of EAE. There is great species and strain variation, but with appropriate dosage of agent and adjuvant, prior treatment can prevent the appearance of EAE on subsequent challenge[198] or can suppress all activity of the already developed disease.[199] The mechanism of this effect is not fully known but does not appear closely to resemble that of the 'desensitisation' to common allergens in the prevention of, for example, hay fever. The prophylactic and curative effects may not be identical. It has been presumed that delayed hypersensitivity, the reaction responsible for the lesions in EAE, is inhibited by the destruction of sensitised cells or by the removal of antibodies by the massive dose of antigen.

An impediment to the immediate adoption of such attempted 'desensitisation' in multiple sclerosis is that the therapeutic agent is identical with that causing allergic encephalomyelitis with the attendant risk of inducing an acute relapse of multiple sclerosis, or, if it should prove to be a different disease, of causing EAE in man.

Therapeutic trials

For reasons outlined above therapeutic trials have been cautious. Campbell et al[200] treated a series of patients with chronic multiple sclerosis, originally 64, many evidently with severe disease. Many patients defaulted and the dose of human myelin basic protein was in most cases 5 mg/week. A complex regime of blind comparison with placebo was adopted. The patients conducted their own assessment and a number claimed to be able to distinguish myelin basic protein from placebo by the 'uplift' induced by the former. Some benefit from treatment was claimed but cannot be seriously substantiated. Gonsette et al[201] used bovine myelin basic protein in the same dose in 35 patients with relapsing disease, without controls. The relapse rate did not change and disability scores did not improve.

Alvord et al[202] have insisted that these trials bear little relationship to the animal experiments it was hoped to duplicate. The dose used in patients was approximately 0.07 mg/kg/week while the effective suppressant dose in the monkey is 67 mg/kg/week without adjuvant. It is unlikely that any investigator would find it ethical to administer Freund's adjuvant to patients but the beneficial effect of myelin basic protein on EAE in monkeys is greatly enhanced by simultaneous use of an antibiotic or

steroids, both acceptable in patients. Alvord recommended that if myelin basic protein is to be used in multiple sclerosis it is necessary to abandon the familiar idea of gradual desensitisation by means of increasing from infinitesimal doses and to use quantities larger by a factor of 1000, accompanied by an adjuvant.

Salk et al[203] have used larger doses than in previous trials but not approaching those suggested by Alvord. Patients with relapsing or rapidly progressing disease were given 75–300 mg of porcine myelin basic protein initially in two week courses but subsequently indefinitely. An impression of some initial improvement was gained in some patients but severe progressive disease was not halted in others. Alvord considered that these doses were based on animal experiments designed to prevent the next relapse rather than to reverse clinical features already present so that the lack of any evident curative effect was not surprising. Continued observation has failed to confirm any convincing effect.[204]

A much more promising agent is COP 1 (copolymer 1), a synthetic peptide with some cross-reactivity with myelin basic protein. It is non-encephalitogenic in animals but has the property of suppressing EAE. Preliminary trials[205,206] in multiple sclerosis showed no adverse effect, that had been a distinct possibility, and the results of an extensive pilot trial have been published.[207,208] Fifty patients with relapsing and remitting disease were enrolled in a double-blind, randomised, placebo-controlled trial. Patients and controls were matched in pairs. Treatment was daily subcutaneous injection of COP 1 or saline for two years.

Results were at first sight promising. There were significantly fewer relapses in the treated group and a greater tendency towards improvement of clinical status. As usual, however, doubts immediately creep in. The relapse figures are much influenced by frequent relapse in a few control patients in the first year. The natural tendency for relapse rate to decrease with time was again shown as the number of relapses in the placebo group in the second year was almost halved. Patients with minimal disability (Kurtzke DSS 0–2) fared better in the treated group, but numbers were small and room for improvement naturally limited. The only patient who improved by 3 grades was taking placebo. No important side effects were observed, but reaction at the site of injection was much more common with COP 1. It was not thought that this affected the blinding but that patients who were doing well believed they were on the active agent. It is difficult to feel sure that the reaction was not also important.

In a small preliminary trial in 5 disabled patients[55] no clinical benefit was observed, although this was scarcely to be expected after treatment for only two months. There was also no reduction in rate of synthesis of intra-blood–brain barrier IgG, leading to the conclusion that COP 1 had not reduced inflammatory demyelinaton in the central nervous system. There is, however, obviously sufficient encouragement from the reported clinical results to warrant further trials but these have been impeded by difficulties in obtaining a consistent product.

Hyperbaric oxygen

Rationale

It is probable that the original reason for treating multiple sclerosis with hyperbaric oxygen, first reported in 1970 from Czechoslovakia according to Bates,[209] was simply an empirical trial of a method that had proved helpful in other conditions. In 1978 it was reported[210] that hyperbaric oxygen would prevent or delay the onset of EAE in rodents. This immunosuppressant action is not notably different from that of a number of other agents. James[211] then introduced an entirely different theory of the causation of multiple sclerosis and reasons why treatment with hyperbaric oxygen might be successful. He proposed that the lesions of multiple sclerosis were the result of fat embolism, causing obstruction of venules, ischaemia and demyelination. A toxic factor from the fat was also thought to be deleterious. There is a long and continuing interest in a vascular component in the pathogenesis of multiple sclerosis and it is by no means improbable that some 'toxic' agent enters the central nervous system from vascular channels or from the CSF. There is, however, no evidence that fat embolism is involved. Lesions in known examples of such embolism do not show primary demyelination, but Wallerian axonal degeneration with inevitable loss of myelin. Evaluation of the role of the vascular system in multiple sclerosis will be of great interest, but of more immediate relevance is the question whether treatment based on this hypothesis is effective. There would be little point in controversy over the explanation of a phenomenon shown not to exist.

Neubauer[212,213] published large uncontrolled series of patients treated with oxygen at two atmospheres pressure and claimed improvement to some degree, often substantial, in a very high proportion. The necessity for controlled studies was obvious. Fischer et al[214] carried out a randomised, blind, placebo-controlled trial of hyperbaric oxygen versus 90% nitrogen plus 10% oxygen at the same pressure of 2 atmospheres in patients with advanced multiple sclerosis. Treatment was given for 90 minutes once a day for 5 days a week to a total of 20 exposures. The details of the treatment regime were decided arbitrarily. Seventeen patients completed the oxygen course and at the end of treatment 12 had improved and 5 had not changed. One of the control group had improved and the remainder had not changed. Improvement in the treated group persisted for a year in 5 patients. The degree of improvement was not great and the patients remained disabled.

Without waiting for further confirmation, patients were encouraged to establish centres where this treatment could be undertaken. With reasonable precautions there are few risks. An epileptic fit in a chamber has been described.[215] Mild barotrauma to the ears, amounting to no more than discomfort, is common.[216] There appears to be a reversible adverse effect on the retina, reflected in reduction of amplitude of visual evoked potentials.[217] Regrettably, there is no further acceptable evidence that hyperbaric oxygen has any useful role in the treatment of patients with multiple sclerosis.

Further fully described double-blind, placebo-controlled trials have been reported from England,[217,49] Sweden,[218] Australia,[219] Canada,[220] France[221] and Italy.[222] The only benefit statistically significantly different from control has been subjective improvement in mild bladder symptoms[217] and slowing of deterioration in cerebellar function. The former was no more than could be achieved using an anticholinergic drug and was not confirmed by urological assessment.[217] Anyone with experience of grading the Kurtzke cerebellar FS will recognise that some variation is not unlikely.

Three trials have been reported only in abstract.[223–225] No significant differences were found between treated and placebo groups except that in one trial[223] mildly affected patients fared better on treatment, although no details are available.

It is probable that no other suggested treatment for multiple sclerosis has been subjected to such thorough and expert investigation. The results have been almost uniformly negative and Bates' conclusion that: 'hyperbaric oxygen has no part to play in the management of the patient with MS' must surely be correct. This is not accepted by the enthusiasts who are, however, in some confusion as to the aims of treatment. Neubauer[226] claims benefit in chronic disease while James[227] believes that it is a travesty of the scientific method to assess the treatment in such patients at all and that hyperbaric oxygen should be used in acute relapse. If this had been the original claim quite different trials would have been necessary but the advocates of hyperbaric oxygen continue to treat chronic cases. The controlled trials have been attacked on various grounds, including possible contamination of the oxygen supply![228] Two atmospheres of pressures are now said to be possibly harmful and lower pressures are recommended. The effective pressure in one negative trial was 1.5–1.6 atmospheres[209] and in another 1.75 atmospheres.[220] The suggestion that treatment should be adjusted according to the response is impossible to follow if no response occurs. It is disappointing that after so much expenditure of effort by many departments and patients, the clear-cut conclusion cannot be accepted. Emotional involvement with theories of causation and treatment of multiple sclerosis is understandable and has a long history.

Dorsal column stimulation

Rationale

This form of treatment was introduced as the result of a chance observation and originally no theoretical basis for its possible efficacy was suggested. Cook[229, 230] used spinal cord stimulation in the treatment of otherwise intractable pain in a patient with multiple sclerosis and observed improvement in neurological function. As subsequent trials appeared to confirm that improvement in the symptoms of chronic multiple sclerosis could sometimes be achieved, possible mechanisms have been suggested. It now appears unlikely that any change observed is due to the development of new synaptic pathways under the influence of prolonged stimulation[231] and an effect on reflex activity is more probable.[232] Increased descending inhibition of spinal reflex activity would account for those effects that have been objectively demonstrated.

Method

Stimulation is applied through electrodes inserted percutaneously into the epidural space over the dorsal cord. The wires lead out to a radio receiver that may either be strapped to the skin if the electrode insertion is to be temporary, or embedded subcutaneously. The receiver picks up the stimulus from a loop antenna. The pulse width and frequency used in recent trials have been $200\mu s$ and 33 Hz respectively. If the electrodes are 'correctly' placed the patient experiences paraesthesiae in the lower limbs and trunk below the level of stimulation and the degree of discomfort can be regulated by the patient. Percutaneous electrodes can be left in situ for many weeks without infection. Technical difficulties are common, particularly shifting of the electrodes, broken wires and even electrode disintegration. For details the original papers must be consulted.

Results

The original results were reported in what must be called an uncritical manner. There is no a priori reason why electrical stimulation of the spinal cord could not improve symptoms but claims of 'substantial improvement' in at least 90% of 'more than 70' patients[229] with no particulars of disabilities or methods of assessment could only arouse the deepest scepticism in those familiar with multiple sclerosis. A similar lack of attention to any of the details demanded by a trial of treatment of multiple sclerosis was displayed in many of the communications to a symposium on the topic in 1978.[233] Illis et al[231] reported enthusiastically, but only on two cases. Following a series of largely negative results[234-236] it can be concluded that stimulation exerts an unpredictable effect on spinal reflex activity whereby spasticity and contractions of the detrusor may be influenced. It is not, however, a practicable or reliable method of symptomatic treatment and there is no evidence that it might alter the course of the disease.

DIETARY TREATMENT

Rationale

Dietary treatment of multiple sclerosis has been almost exclusively concerned with manipulation of the intake of fat. The original attempts were not, as might be supposed, related to presumed abnormalities in the lipid content of myelin, but were based on clinical and epidemiological observations. Swank[237] drew attention to an apparent fall in incidence of multiple sclerosis in Norway during the German occupation and an immediate increase after the Second World War, and suggested that these trends were due to changes in diet, in particular to reduction in dietary fat during the war. It was then reported[238] that over a prolonged period the incidence of multiple sclerosis in inland farming communities in Norway was, in general, about four times that in coastal fishing villages. This pattern was not absolutely constant and in some districts was not detected. A restricted dietary survey showed, as might be expected, that the farmers ate more butter than the fishermen, who consumed more fish liver oil, but the difference was not statistically significant. The theory was advanced that butter fat was a more potent precipitating agent of multiple sclerosis than fish liver oil. It is of interest that the emphasis was placed on the harmful effects of dairy fats rather than on any protective influence of fish oils. The suggested mechanism by which ingestion of fat might produce multiple sclerosis plaques was that of hypoxaemia resulting from occlusion of small blood vessels by aggregation of platelets, erythrocytes and chylomicrons. In a sense this was

a revival of the vascular aetiology of multiple sclerosis proposed by Putnam.[239]

Attention was then directed to the possible influence of diet on the lipid constitution of myelin. Sinclair[240] suggested that a deficiency of essential fatty acids might result in defective formation of myelin in multiple sclerosis but the subsequent 35 years have not sufficed to demonstrate whether this is true. On this theory, deficient delivery to the CNS of fatty acids from whatever cause would result in the formation of myelin of abnormal lipid content, vulnerable to agents that do not damage normal myelin. The lipid content of white matter known to contain multiple sclerosis plaques is inevitably abnormal but the theory demands that myelin in white matter not apparently affected by disease should also be chemically abnormal. It has not been possible to reach agreement on whether this is so, almost certainly because the presence of at least partial demyelination cannot be excluded.[241] A reduction in the proportion of elements of the lecithin fraction, including arachidonic acid $(20:4)$[242] and linoleic acid $(18:2)$[243] has been reported and also a reduction of the total amount of polyunsaturated fatty acids in apparently unaffected brain from patients with multiple sclerosis compared to normal brain. Others[244] have found no consistent difference. The wide variations between individual multiple sclerosis brain[245] certainly suggest that 'unaffected' white matter has already been subjected to some degradation of myelin.

The theory of a generalised abnormality of lipid metabolism was, however, obviously attractive and received strong support from the report of abnormal levels of blood lipids, notably a reduction of linoleate compared with controls.[246] The reduction was more obvious in active disease and, in fact, was not detectable in patients in whom there had been no evidence of clinical activity in the preceding month. The same group of workers have repeatedly confirmed these findings[247] and some independent confirmation is also available.[248] The significance and reality of these changes have, however, been questioned. Love et al[249] confirmed the reduced linoleate level in multiple sclerosis but found that this was not different from that found in other neurological diseases or, indeed, in other forms of acute disease. Other reports have indicated no difference between non-fasting levels in multiple sclerosis and normal subjects.[250,251] A decrease in linoleate concentration has been reported in the phospholipids of platelets and erythrocytes in multiple sclerosis.[252]

Thompson[253] advanced the theory of an inborn error of metabolism leading to insufficient delivery of essential fatty acids to the CNS and therefore faulty formation of myelin, that subsequently breaks down. Any metabolic defect dose not appear to include malabsorption, as low serum levels of linoleate are rapidly restored by oral supplementation[254] and evidence of a relevant abnormality of jejunal mucosa[255] has not been confirmed.[256]

More recently, interest has again shifted to a further possible function of PUFA in the control of multiple sclerosis, that of immunosuppression.[257] Essential fatty acids can inhibit EAE. The precise mechanism is unknown but arachidonic acid, formed from linoleic acid via linolenic acid, is a precursor of prostaglandins with recognised immunosuppressant effects. It is not, of course, known that any agent active in EAE will similarly influence multiple sclerosis, nor is it certain that essential fatty acids exert a prolonged immunosuppressant action.

Linoleic is the most obvious choice of therapeutic agent but γ-linolenic acid is more readily incorporated in the nervous system, at least in immature animals, and is a more efficient precursor of longer-chain fatty acids. What is needed, however, is firm evidence that manipulation of dietary fatty acids has any influence on the clinical course of the disease.

Therapeutic trials

Swank,[258] having long advocated dietary fat restriction, has published the results of this regime in 146 patients observed over a prolonged period.[259] The level of daily fat intake eventually recommended was 10–15 g and a diet book is available.[260] Claims of benefit include a reduction in the expected disability and in the death rate and a marked reduction in relapse rate with those relapses that occurred seldom affecting previously uninvolved regions of the nervous system. When this enterprise was begun the organisation of therapeutic trials in multiple sclerosis was relatively unsophisticated and no controls were used. All apparent benefits are judged against either published accounts of the natural history of multiple sclerosis or the course of the disease in individual patients before treatment. The possible fallacies of this method have already been discussed. The absence of a concurrently observed randomised control series must unfortunately render difficult the full acceptance of these results.

An admirably devised double-blind randomised controlled trial has, however, been conducted to determine whether linoleic acid dietary supplementation is beneficial.[261] The trial, conducted in Belfast and London, extended over two years and originally involved 87 patients of whom 75 completed the course. Thirty six patients took a daily dose of sunflower seed oil providing 8.6 g of linoleic acid and 39 controls took olive oil containing 3.8 g of oleic acid and 0.2 g of linoleic acid, the oils being suitably disguised. The interpretation of the results reflects the difficulties inseparable from therapeutic trials in multiple sclerosis. For example, the number of relapses in the control group was 62 and in the treated group 41, but this difference is not statistically significant and arose largely because a few patients on oleic acid had frequent relapses. No difference in the increase in disability could be detected between the two groups. Significant differences were found in the severity of relapse scored on a disability scale, which was reduced ($p < 0.01$) in the patients on linoleic acid. In the patients in Belfast, comprising two thirds of the total, this difference was not significant. The number of patients in whom relapse lasted for longer than ten weeks was significantly higher in those receiving oleic acid. The acknowledged difficulty in determining the duration of relapse would have been the same for both groups.

These results certainly provided some encouragement to the use of linoleic acid supplements in the treatment of multiple sclerosis, although the lack of any overall benefit was disappointing. Very large numbers of patients, naturally eager to follow any hopeful line, adapted their diet to exclude as far as possible the usual sources of animal fat and many have taken dietary supplements of PUFA in the form of sunflower seed oil or evening primrose oil. The possible advantage of the latter is its content of linolenic acid.

Further trials were clearly necessary and a large scale endeavour was mounted in Newcastle-upon-Tyne. The first results published[262] were those of a double-blind randomised controlled trial in non-relapsing disease. One hundred and fifty two patients were allocated to four groups: A, receiving Naudicelle (360 mg of linolenic and 3.42 g of linoleic acid per day); B, identical capsules containing oleic acid; C, linoleic acid 11.5 g in the form of a spread; and D, 4 g of oleic acid in the same medium. Results reported after two years' treatment showed no significant difference between the groups. Despite the title of the paper, some patients did relapse during the course of treatment, the number being slightly and insignificantly greater in the group on the larger dose of linoleic acid. This result was perhaps not unexpected as the original controlled trial had not shown any benefit with regard to disability states and in chronic progressive disease improvement must be considered unlikely.

More disappointing was the trial in Canada.[263] The methods were deliberately based on those of the previous controlled trial and the number completing the course was almost identical. No significant difference in disability status or in any aspect of relapse was found between treated and control groups.

The results of the Newcastle trial in acute remitting disease were published soon afterwards.[264] Again there were four groups — Naudicelle, low dose oleic acid, high dose linoleic acid and high dose oleic acid, with 29 patients in each group. Those taking Naudicelle deteriorated to a significantly greater degree than those in other groups and a larger number of patients deteriorated. No change in relapse rate was observed between treated and control groups. In those on 23 g of linoleic acid daily there was a marginally significant reduction in duration and severity of relapse. This last result was very similar to that found by Millar et al[261] but again no overall benefit could be detected.

The combined data from the three double-blind trials in relapsing disease have been re-analysed with rather more encouraging results.[265] Treated patients with little or no disability deteriorated significantly less than controls. The mean severity and duration, but not the frequency, of relapse were reduced in the treated group at all levels of disability. One is again left with contemplating the clinical significance of a mean difference of a fraction of a grade (0.71) on the Kurtzke DSS.

There are some theoretical grounds for exploring whether n-3 polyunsaturated fatty acids, of which α-linolenic acid is the parent, might exert a more definite effect on multiple sclerosis. A large controlled trial[266] of fish oil, rich in long chain n-3 polyunsaturated acids, versus olive oil, was organised, both groups being given the same advice about dietary fats. Although there appeared to be a trend in favour of the treated group, no significant benefit was obtained.

Conclusions

Despite the attractive theoretical background and the immense expenditure of effort in laboratory and clinic, the practical results of therapeutic trials of dietary supplementation with PUFA have been disappointing. In humanitarian terms, dietary treatment has much to commend it provided it is known to be harmless. Patients often ask 'Is there nothing *I* can do?' and it is reasonable to suggest that some benefit might be gained by the substitution of liquid vegetable fats and unsaturated margarine for animal fat solid at room temperature. The author does not personally advise the use of specific supplements of sunflower seed or evening primrose oil. There is no evidence that high doses of PUFA that have been used in the attempted treatment of multiple sclerosis are harmful but this possibility must not be neglected.

Gluten-free diet

Rationale

Although Shattin[267] had suggested an association between a diet high in gluten-rich cereals and the geographical distribution of multiple sclerosis, the vogue for treatment of the disease with a gluten-free diet was not based on theoretical considerations but on the clinical recovery of a single patient.[268,269] The adoption of a complex dietary regime of which the exclusion of gluten was one feature was accompanied by a remarkable degree of sustained improvement. While intensely gratifying to the individual concerned, no serious student of multiple sclerosis could be convinced by the results in a single case. Many other patients naturally seized on the hope of relief or even cure from a treatment apparently without risk that they could undertake themselves at home.

Thompson[253] had suggested the possibility of an intestinal disorder resulting in malabsorption of fatty acids and many neurologists carried out jejunal biopsies on small numbers of patients without significant findings. However, Lange & Shiner[255] found partial villous atrophy in one out of 12 patients examined, subtotal villous atrophy in one and increased inflammatory cell infiltration in 3. More subtle changes were found on electron-microscopy in 6 out of 8 specimens. A single case report of fulminating malabsorption developing in a patient with established multiple sclerosis[270] was severely criticised on grounds of incorrect preparation of the histology of the jejunum. In a large series of 52 patients, no instance of villous atrophy was found[271] but an inflammatory exudate was seen in seven. Abnormalities of absorption of fat, d-xylose and vitamin B_{12} were found in a proportion of these patients. In a controlled study, however, Bateson et al[256] found no abnormality of the mucosa and no increase in inflammatory cells. As already noted, the low levels of linoleic acid in the serum reported in some series of patients can be rapidly corrected by dietary supplementation rendering malabsorption an unlikely cause.

Therapeutic trials

The trial of a regime that involves the rigid exclusion of any common item of diet is always open to the objection that a minor indiscretion or accidental exposure to the food substance in question might invalidate the results. A double-blind trial of a gluten-free diet is impossible but blind assessment has not been attempted. Two open pilot trials have been reported. Jellinek[272] treated 6

patients of whom 3 sustained major relapses while on the regime. Liversedge[273] treated 42 patients of whom 5 found the diet intolerable. The remainder were followed for a mean of 23 months. The relapse rate in these patients was 0.5, a figure found in many series of untreated patients, and measured disability increased. A beneficial effect cannot be ruled out in such preliminary trials but it is plain that patients attempting to adhere to a gluten-free diet continue to sustain relapses.

TREATMENT OF URINARY SYMPTOMS

Symptoms arising from imperfect control of the urinary bladder are common and often peculiarly distressing. Of 297 cases examined by Miller et al,[274] 78% had experienced such symptoms at some time and in 52% they had persisted for more than six months at the time of examination; 60% had urgency of micturition and 50% frequency; 10% had been incontinent and 2% had suffered from recurrent retention. In the terminal stages of severe multiple sclerosis, bladder dysfunction is invariable and the resulting infection accounts for a proportion of deaths.

There can be no dispute that treatment has been unsatisfactory and laudable attempts have been made to improve results by exploring the underlying disorders of physiology with the aim of providing a scientific basis for therapy. The innervation of the bladder and urethra is, unfortunately, remarkably complex,[275] but the act of micturition is essentially the expulsion of urine by contraction of the detrusor accompanied by simultaneous relaxation of the bladder neck and urethra. Detrusor contraction is elicited reflexly by distention of the bladder but can, within reason, be voluntarily inhibited or initiated. Voluntary control is influenced by the familiar sensation of bladder fullness, apparently conveyed within the spinal cord in close relation to the lateral spino-thalamic pathway. The reflex arc is not, as at first thought, confined to the sacral segments of the spinal cord but involves connections to a centre in the pons, itself receiving input from the frontal lobe and other sources.

In multiple sclerosis urinary symptoms can therefore be caused by lesions at a variety of sites, but especially by interruption, in the spinal cord, of connections between the pontine centre and the conus medullaris. Symptoms may be conveniently divided into difficulties in storing urine or in emptying the bladder.[276] The former comprise urgency, frequency, nocturia and incontinence of different types. The latter include hesitancy and retention of urine. Combinations of symptoms from the two groups is common: an urgent call to pass water may be followed by inability to do so for several minutes.

The most usual cause of failure to store urine is an 'irritative' phenomenon, in fact increased spinal reflex activity leading to uninhibited detrusor contractions in response to minor degrees of bladder distension. Incomplete bladder emptying is due to failure of the internal sphincter at the bladder neck, or occasionally of the external sphincter, to relax appropriately; to weak or absent detrusor contractions; or to interruption of the afferent side of the reflex arc in the sacral segments of the spinal cord. Defects seldom occur singly and the commonest combination is of increased detrusor contractions with failure of synergistic sphincter opening; sphincter dyssynergia. Patients with symptoms apparently indicating isolated failure to store or to empty are frequently found on investigation to have more complex disorders of function.

The assumption that the familiar clinical symptoms could be related to obviously relevant disorders of function has also proved to be naive. Blaivas et al[278] found that of 28 patients with urgency and frequency, only 11 showed the expected isolated inability to retain urine in the bladder; 12 were also unable to empty the bladder; one had this defect in isolation, and 2 had normal bladder function as tested. There was similar lack of consistent matching of symptoms and findings in patients in whom the obvious clinical disability was failure to empty the bladder.

A remarkable finding that does not seem to correlate with any clinical symptom is the frequent occurrence of an 'areflexic' bladder.[227,278] Under test conditions detrusor contractions are not induced. This has been attributed to the effect of plaques in the conus. This is unlikely as comparable loss of reflex activity in the lower limbs is most uncommon. Serial studies show remarkable fluctuations in the test results in that 'areflexic'

bladders are soon found to be hyperreflexic.[279] A possible explanation of these findings is that they are nothing to do with the course of the disease but related to the absence of detrusor contractions under test conditions in 50% of normal women.[280]

Management

The regime of investigation and treatment advocated by Blaivas[278,281] appears eminently sensible. Initial investigation of patients with urinary symptoms is limited to determining bladder capacity and residual urine and the exclusion of infection. The well-hydrated patient passes water when the bladder feels full. The residual urine is obtained by catheter and the capacity is the sum of the two volumes. Treatment is given on the basis of symptoms and of evidence of retention.

Failure to store is treated with anticholinergic drugs, of which propantheline is favoured. Both this agent and emepromium bromide have been shown to be superior to placebo.[282,283] The former causes dryness of the mouth and the latter may irritate the oesophagus. Neither may be tolerated and, of course, they are not always successful. In ambulant patients it is usually possible to alleviate urgency and frequency and, much less commonly, urge incontinence, but effective doses sometimes cause retention. Imipramine is also sometimes helpful when taken at bedtime. Adrenergic drugs such as ephedrine have been disappointing. Nocturia is a particularly troublesome complaint in the disabled and can sometimes be overcome by an evening dose of antidiuretic hormone. Desmopressin, 20 mg by intranasal spray, has been shown to be much more effective than placebo in a crossover trial.[284]

Symptoms of failure to empty or an excessive residual urine volume are best treated by intermittent catheterisation. Clean, non-sterile, intermittent self-catheterisation, introduced by Lapides et al[285,286] should be more widely practised. Reasonable manual dexterity and adequate motivation are necessary and also expert instruction, particularly in the female. In favourable cases, the use of this technique can revolutionise the patient's life, bringing relief from the constant fear of moving too far from a lavatory and from the uncomfortable and undesirable restriction of fluid intake resorted to by many. Urinary infection may, of course, occur, but is uncommon. Blaivas et al[281] recommend continuous urinary antisepsis with methenamine (hexamine), and acidification of the urine with ascorbic acid. The proportion of patients for whom this treatment is appropriate naturally varies with the severity of disability. In a series of 67 patients with bladder symptoms, 14 were treated in this way.[276]

Intermittent catheterisation by hospital staff is also essential in the attempt to restore tolerable bladder function when this has recently been disturbed. Emptying the bladder at regular and later increasing intervals, combined with the eradication of infection, may allow a reasonable response to anticholinergic drugs.

Continued application to the details of the treatment outlined above, aided, perhaps by the remittent nature of the disease, can lead to considerable improvement in extremely distressing symptoms. Persistent urinary symptoms are regarded as an indication for full urodynamic studies, including cystometry, electromyography of the sphincters and radiologically controlled flow studies. Structural problems such as bladder neck obstruction or vesical stones can be recognised and treated. As with the neurological problem, it seems that sophistication of investigation has outstripped advances in therapeutic measures. The results may certainly clarify the nature of the defect but do not lead to fundamentally different treatment.

Appliances

The range of available appliances will not be considered in detail. In the male a urinal of the condom type is often successful and acceptable although there is some risk of skin sensitivity to latex developing. Firm constriction of the penis, either with a urinal constructed of hard material or a penile clamp can lead to pressure sores and infection although a few patients find the clamp helpful. At night a condom appliance can also be used or a bottle made of relatively soft material.

No satisfactory urinal has been devised for the female. Pants that allow the passage of urine outwards only, surrounded by padding, avoid much of the discomfort of incontinence but not that infallible and distressing sign of chronic disease, the smell of stale urine.

The urinary symptoms of multiple sclerosis, however distressing, have little effect on health. The upper urinary tract complications formerly reported in multiple sclerosis and commonly encountered in traumatic paraplegia do not occur provided infection is avoided. The mean time to the development of infection following insertion of an indwelling catheter with open drainage is four days, and with a closed system 30 days.[287] Other complications include local sepsis and fistulae, a very small capacity bladder, vesical stones and inability to retain the catheter. An indwelling catheter should therefore be a last resort. Chronic retention of urine is uncommon in multiple sclerosis and the usual reason for permanent catheterisation is uncontrollable incontinence. It is generally believed, perhaps correctly, that in the disabled patient a constantly wet bed increases the risk of bedsores, but the usual purpose of the catheter is to ease the strain of nursing, particularly in the home. In the helpless and perhaps demented patient with terminal multiple sclerosis an indwelling catheter is often the only practicable course, but before this stage is reached other solutions should at least be considered.

Surgery

The obvious rationale for bladder neck resection is difficulty in emptying the bladder, but Jakobsen et al[288] also recommended this operation in some patients with urge incontinence. In a large series, many with severe disability, they reported improvement in 60% of those with partial retention and what was judged to be a flaccid bladder. A high proportion of those with urge incontinence also improved and more than 30% became continent. Stress incontinence did not develop in a single patient but bladder function sometimes deteriorated and stricture was an unpleasant complication. They regarded the indications for bladder neck resection to be difficulty in emptying, not related to acute relapse, and urge incontinence unrelieved by drugs. In the latter group they believed that operation reduced detrusor activity but most surgeons have restricted this treatment to patients with partial or recurrent retention. Patients with multiple sclerosis are not immune to other causes of urinary obstruction and prostatectomy is sometimes necessary and beneficial.

Urinary diversion is less commonly employed in multiple sclerosis than in other, static, forms of neurological disability. Desmond & Shuttleworth[289] reported the results in the 12 patients on whom they operated out of 78 referred. They formed an ileal conduit and regarded the indication as uncontrolled incontinence with inability to tolerate a catheter. The post-operative complication rate was very high, particularly pyelitis and paralytic ileus, but the end result was rated a great success by most of the patients and their relatives. Bedsores were found to be an absolute contraindication to operating. Diversion through a suprapubic catheter has few, if any, advantages over urethral drainage in terms of ease of management.

Destructive operations on the nerve supply of the bladder to reduce reflex activity have been more commonly used in conditions other than multiple sclerosis. Selective sacral rootlet rhizotomy[290] is reported to produce only temporary improvement. Torrens & Griffith[291] selected patients and the site of operation by nerve root block and found that bilateral section of S3 root was the most effective procedure. Two of their nine cases had multiple sclerosis, and although results are encouraging it is not clear how much symptomatic improvement was obtained in these patients. The operation was remarkably free from undesirable effects and did not produce impotence in the male.

Stimulation

The effect of dorsal column stimulation on bladder function has already been described. Bradley et al[292] reviewed the results of implantable prosthetic devices designed to stimulate the impaired micturition reflex and concluded that little advance had been made. They believed that ignorance of many factors in smooth muscle function impeded progress. A simple device, successful in some patients with retention of urine, is the application of a vibrator to the abdominal wall overlying the bladder.[293,294]

Rectal symptoms

Disordered control of bowel action is much less commonly a cause of distress and, with a few exceptions, is more easily dealt with. Urgency of defaecation and occasional incontinence may accompany corresponding urinary symptoms. The response to anticholinergic drugs is variable and unpredictable but often apparently satisfactory. Unformed stools are obviously less easy to control and laxatives are contraindicated.

At a later stage of the disease constipation may be troublesome. Some patients find distension of the rectum and colon uncomfortable but of greater importance is the tendency for liquid faeces to pass round the obstructing mass with resulting incontinence. Severe constipation may also induce retention of urine. Severe constipation should therefore be avoided and here mild laxatives, such as senna, can be used. Bisacodyl, either orally or as a suppository, is also suitable. If distension of the lower bowel is allowed to develop it may be very difficult to correct, and repeated manual removal of faeces may be required before a reasonable bowel habit is restored.

These problems are well understood in the patient with traumatic paraplegia. There has been no recently published report relating specifically to multiple sclerosis.

Sexual symptoms

Erectile impotence is a common and often early symptom in multiple sclerosis.[295,296] When it occurs as a symptom of acute relapse, full recovery is possible. As the disease advances, interest in sex often declines and in severely disabled men and women spasticity, particularly adductor spasm, presents mechanical problems and advice on modification of techniques may be required. Investigation,[297] not unexpectedly, confirms the neurogenic nature of the problem in the great majority. The bulbo-cavernosus reflex and pudendal evoked potentials may be abnormal even when nocturnal erections are still present. There is no obvious advantage in performing these tests routinely in men asking for treatment as they do not predict the response.

Penile prostheses are sometimes successful. An inflatable implanted prosthesis has been used in a small number of patients,[298] but the very much cheaper permanently rigid prosthesis[299] is easier to insert. It is probable that treatment will be transformed by the use of intracavernous self-injection with papaverine. This is highly effective in producing erection in neurogenic impotence, but hypersensitivity may be encountered and small doses must be used initially. This method reliably produces erection in patients with multiple sclerosis.[297,300] The safety of long continued use of this method has yet to be assessed.

In women, the complaint of lack of lubrication can easily be overcome by artificial means but relative lack of sensation is intractable. Relief of spasticity is often the most important help that can be attempted.

TREMOR

The tremor commonly associated with multiple sclerosis is the familiar intention tremor on voluntary movement attributed to lesions of the cerebellum or cerebellar connections, in severe cases accompanied by tremor on sustaining any posture of the limbs or head. This can result in considerable disability and in a small proportion of patients, tremor of the upper limbs and head on any attempted movement can be virtually incapacitating. It may even be hazardous to approach the patient's bedside lest the lifting of an arm result in violent movement. Symptomatic treatment is therefore often required but has proved difficult.

Sabra et al[301] report encouraging results on treatment of action tremor with large doses of isoniazid (600–1200 mg/day) accompanied by pyridoxine 100 mg. Tremor was reduced or abolished but other evidence of cerebellar disease was not affected. The postulated mechanism was inhibition of GABA-aminotransferase and increased concentrations of GABA. Further trials have shown that with very large doses some reduction in postural tremor can be achieved in a few patients, but at the risk of unpleasant side effects and without improvement in function.[302–305] In

personal experience this treatment is useless. There is a favourable report[306] on the effect of a daily dose of carbamazepine 600 mg but this is not universally successful.

Hewer et al[307] investigated the effect of attaching lead weights to the wrists, thus increasing inertia and, it was hoped, reducing the tremor. They found the optimum weight had to be judged for each patient individually, maximum benefit being obtained with a weight of between 480 and 600 g. Further increase in weight aggravated the tremor. The results in multiple sclerosis were not spectacular. Of 10 patients, tremor was reduced in 4 but only 2 obtained clinical benefit. Other disabilities, particularly weakness, limited the application of this technique.

The neurosurgical treatment of intention tremor in multiple sclerosis and other diseases was introduced by Irving Cooper[308] and there have been a number of subsequent reports on the effects of stereotaxic thalamotomy. The proportion of patients improved or greatly improved ranges from 25% to 75% or 80%.[309,310,311] Selection of cases is obviously important and Hauptvogel et al[310] advised that tremor should be the predominant disability and that patients in the terminal stages of the disease should not be operated on. In the great majority of reported patients the operation has been unilateral. There are increased risks of bilateral thalamotomy including persistent speech disturbance.[312] In personal experience thalamotomy can occasionally transform the care of patients disabled by violent tremor on attempted movement. A unilateral operation may permit the use of one arm for voluntary movement such as feeding or turning the pages of a book, previously impossible. The outcome is, however, impossible to predict. Kelly[313] states that in all 14 personal cases submitted to thalamotomy the operation was followed within 3 weeks by severe relapse but this is certainly not inevitable. A recent report is, however, not optimistic, benefit being largely outweighed by adverse effects.[314]

SPASTICITY

Spasticity is difficult to define in precise terms but in general is taken to include the effects, mainly adverse, of pathologically increased stretch reflex activity. In many patients with multiple sclerosis, as in other chronic neurological diseases, effective use of remaining strength often seems to be impeded by increased tone and rigidity of movement of the limbs or by spontaneous clonus. Experimentally, it has been shown that loss of reciprocal innervation of opposing muscle groups is a major cause of disability.[315] Painful or distressing extensor or flexor spasms are common in more advanced disease. The treatment of spasticity in multiple sclerosis does not differ in any important way from that in any other condition in which increased reflex activity is largely or wholly the result of spinal cord disease. In multiple sclerosis the symptoms of spasticity requiring treatment, if such is available, are virtually confined to the lower limbs and a condition resembling the arm, spastic in flexion, of the chronic hemiplegic is hardly ever encountered. Apart from the even more intractable nature of spasticity in the upper limb, the action of certain drugs may be different if the heightened reflex activity is the result of cerebral rather than spinal disease.[316]

Increased stretch reflex activity is thought to result, in the great majority of cases, from increased firing of the γ motoneurons, resulting in enhanced sensitivity to stretch of the muscle spindles. As the γ motoneurons are not directly concerned in maintaining muscular contraction, effected by the α motoneurons, it is theoretically possible to inhibit fusimotor firing without affecting the strength of the muscles.[316] In a few examples excessive activity of the α motoneurons appears to be the immediate cause of spasticity, but even here reduction of spindle sensitivity would dampen reflex action. In both forms it is assumed that inhibitory influences derived from or closely associated with the corticospinal tracts have been intercepted by the action of disease. The object of all forms of treatment is therefore either to reinforce or replace inhibitory effect or to interrupt the reflex arc at some point.

Design of clinical trials

Patients are treated for spasticity either because it is hoped to increase their facility of ambulation or to reduce extensor or flexor spasm when recumbent. Walking speed may be affected by a number of factors and any change observed may be the result of conflicting effects on muscle strength and tone, on the state of alertness or motivation and no doubt on other aspects of the patient's total condition. However, if consistent improvement in walking is achieved, particularly in a properly controlled trial, it is reasonable to claim that the intended goal has been achieved, although perhaps not by the intended means.

There have been numerous attempts at measurement of resistance to passive movement by mechanical means but none has come into common use. Resistance is highly variable, being affected by posture, speed of movement, temperature, anxiety, pain, fatigue and by other less ponderable factors. The mere process of attaching the patient's leg to the apparatus and starting the motor used to move the limb may be expected to affect the result. Most investigators, therefore, rely on a simple clinical grading system: 0 — no increased resistance; 1 — just detectable, perhaps as a sudden catch; 2 — moderate resistance; 3 — resistance overcome by the examiner only with difficulty; and 4 — resistance impossible to overcome with legitimate force. A single observer using this method in standard conditions can obtain reliable results but obviously subjective grades, apart from the extremes, cannot be compared between different observers. In the non-ambulant patient the objectives are simpler. Flexor and extensor spasms seriously affect the care and comfort of the immobile spastic patient. If, following treatment, the patient can again sit in a wheelchair, can sleep without disturbance from painful spasms and can be satisfactorily cleaned, the treatment has been successful.

Pharmacological attempts

The pharmacological treatment of spasticity has been disappointing, earlier efforts being firmly rejected by Schwab[317] as 'useless'.

Diazepam appeared to be more promising and was investigated more scientifically. In a double-blind crossover trial[318] the aspects assessed were resistance to passive movement, strength and the patient's opinion on overall benefit, all judged subjectively. The scores were treated statistically and appeared to show benefit in all aspects except strength. The doses of diazepam used in the trial did not exceed 16 mg a day and subsequent experience has shown that to produce a notable effect on spasticity much larger doses are needed. Accompanying drowsiness may diminish spontaneously but is often a limiting factor. The action of diazepam on reflex activity is accompanied by reduction of strength when the drug is given intravenously.

Attention next concentrated on two agents, baclofen and dantrolene sodium. Baclofen is chemically related to GABA, a neurotransmitter with widespread inhibitory effects, at least in the brain, as opposed to the spinal cord. It was introduced for the treatment of spasticity in 1970[319] and was shown to reduce the response to tonic stretch in patients with both complete and incomplete lesions of the spinal cord including multiple sclerosis.[320] It was thought to have a general depressant action on spinal synapses and to exert its main effect on the spinal interneurones. By intravenous injection reduction of spasticity was achieved without inducing weakness.

In a double-blind crossover trial of baclofen versus diazepam, both drugs were shown to be superior to placebo in reducing spasticity but no clear superiority of either drug was found.[321] Function was not assessed. In a similar trial From and Heltberg[322] also found that both drugs reduced spasticity and that patients preferred baclofen, probably because it was less soporific. The patients were severely disabled but of the four patients who could walk at all, this function was adversely affected in three. In later trials more attention has been paid to possible clinical benefit in the ambulant patient and results have been disappointing. No improvement in the activities of daily living may be found[323] or walking ability may be reduced,[324] apparently because of increased weakness of the spastic limbs. It is notoriously difficult to measure the strength of spastic muscles and it is possible that the loss of walking ability is due, at least in part, to the lower limbs no longer being reflexly held in extension, but failure of the legs to support the patient severely limits the use of baclofen in ambulant cases. The other side effects frequently encountered are drowsiness and nausea. There is no doubt, however, that baclofen reduces stretch reflex activity and its main use is in the reduction of distressing clonus and involuntary spasms in non-ambulant patients, such benefits being reported in virtually every trial.

Dantrolene sodium does not affect central reflex mechanisms but has a peripheral action. This is an inhibitory effect on the mechanical force of the muscle fibre through an action on the movement of intracellular calcium.[325] If this is so, the effect must be relatively selective as the means by which dantrolene reduces reflex activity is exerted through the muscle spindle, presumably through a direct action on the intrafusal muscle fibres.[326] As might be expected, however, muscle strength is also reduced when the drug is given intravenously.

The results of clinical trials have been similar to those achieved with baclofen. The effect in spasticity has been confirmed[327] but is not superior to that of diazepam,[328] although causing less drowsiness. Benefit was again confined to reduction in clonus, stiffness and spasms, unfortunately combined with increased weakness and impaired walking speed. Dantrolene sodium has the additional disadvantage of sometimes causing jaundice.

A more recently introduced, centrally acting 'muscle relaxant', tizanidine, has also been the subject of clinical trials in multiple sclerosis and other forms of myelopathy.[329] The effect in reducing resistance to passive movement has been found to be similar to that obtained with baclofen or diazepam and superior to placebo. In a recent comparison of tizanidine with baclofen in a double-blind crossover trial,[330] no significant difference in efficacy was found, although is not clear whether the patients were ambulant or incapacitated. Muscle weakness was more prominent with baclofen and somnolence worse with tizanidine. In a similar trial in severely disabled patients the effect of the two drugs on clonus and spasm were closely similar.[331]

The GABA agonist progabide has been subjected to a double-blind, placebo-controlled crossover trial in patients with multiple sclerosis.[332] A marked effect on spasticity was observed in many patients, although in four, the effect of placebo was more impressive. No improvement in functional tests or in frequency of spasms was obtained. Weakness was not induced but there were many minor side effects. More importantly, progabide is hepato-toxic, 23% of patients developing abnormal serum enzyme levels.

A promising development is the use of intrathecal baclofen.[333-336] This has been found to be remarkably effective in all forms of spasticity, particularly in the reduction of spasms. Unfortunately it must be given either continuously or in frequent doses, necessitating a tube permanently inserted into the lumbar subarachnoid space, joined to a subcutaneously implanted chamber into which injections can be made. The development of a programmable pump that regulates the flow from the chamber to the subarachnoid space is a notable advance.[337] Side effects from the drug appear to be minimal, apart from accidental overdosage which can be reversed by 2 mg of physostigmine intravenously,[337] and treatment has been continued for as long as 2 years. The dose required has varied from 26–780 μg/24h and requires careful initial titration. The benefits in severely disabled patients include relief of pain and discomfort and much greater ease of nursing but there is obviously risk of meningeal infection. Epidural baclofen, which lessens this risk and involves fewer injections, has so far been less successful in multiple sclerosis.[338]

Although the theoretically possible selective inhibition of fusimotor activity with sparing of voluntary power may have been partially achieved by the pharmacological agents at present available, the relief of spasticity combined with improved function in the ambulant patient has not been attained. It is possible that the theory is incorrect. In the severely disabled patient available drugs will lessen discomfort and pain but cannot be relied upon to prevent or alleviate paraplegia in flexion, the end result in many patients with multiple sclerosis.

Surgery

Surgical interruption of the stretch reflex arcs has never been widely used in multiple sclerosis for a number of reasons. The disease is, in general, progressive and there are fears of causing relapse. A proportion of those who suffer most severely from the effects of spasticity are also disabled in other ways, sometimes including mental in-

capacity, so that major surgery on the spinal roots or spinal cord is difficult to justify. Nevertheless the patient with severe disability from flexion contraction or contractures of the lower limbs presents a formidable problem. The prevention of increased flexor tone by the use of Egger's operation has been recommended in ambulant patients,[339] but has never been generally adopted. In essence the procedure involves severing the hamstring tendons and attaching them to the femur, thus converting their action from flexion of the knee to that of extension of the hip. From personal experience this has not been universally successful.

From many similar regimes that of Reyes et al[340] may be selected as providing a judicious measure of activity. The difficulty of distinguishing flexor spasm from contracture can be overcome by examination under general anaesthesia at the time of the operation that has already been decided on. Adductor tenotomy greatly assists nursing problems and care of the sphincters. Flexion is managed by hamstring release but it is not necessary to section the ilio-psoas. In these disabled patients there is nothing to be gained by releasing the Achilles tendon. More heroic surgery is surely inappropriate and ultimately harmful to severely disabled patients.

Intrathecal phenol

This technique was introduced by Maher[341] for the treatment of pain due to carcinoma and was later adapted for use in spasticity. The original concept seems to have been the relief of painful spasm by a selective action on 'pain fibres' but the evident action is the abolition of spasm by interruption of the reflex arc by fibre destruction in the posterior or anterior roots. The technique has been described in detail by a number of authors[342-344] but enthusiasm has waned. Even with the most sophisticated methods of establishing correct needle placement and the direction of the destructive agent to the appropriate roots, the treatment is not suitable, as was at first hoped, for the treatment of the ambulant spastic patient. Sensory loss and even focal weakness might be acceptable risks but there is also danger of damaging sacral roots with resulting retention of urine.

In the bedridden patient the technique is still

valuable in the relief of muscle spasm although, of course, contracture cannot be influenced. In such patients bladder function is nearly always already severely disturbed and there is no prospect of useful movement of the legs. No elaborate technique is required. Lumbar puncture should be performed at the L2–3 space or even at L1–2. Pillows should be placed under shoulders and buttocks so that the lumbar spine is convex downwards to assist the heavy phenol in glycerine or myodil to pool in the vicinity of the lumbar roots it is hoped to treat. Lumbar puncture is often extremely difficult in these patients as the spasm may induce lordosis. Two millilitres of 5% or even 10% phenol in glycerine or myodil is then injected, the viscosity of the solution ensuring that injection is slow. The patient maintains the posture for 20 minutes. There may be a complaint of paraesthesiae but their localisation has not proved to be a reliable guide to the reflex effect. In successful attempts all tone is rapidly lost in the leg placed inferiorly. The procedure can be repeated within a few days, directed at the other leg.

Although permanent destruction of axons results, the clinical effect lasts for no more than six months but can be repeated. Unfortunately, when flexion of the legs is overcome spasm of the spinal musculature may increase and is not amenable to phenol treatment. Patients are naturally often apprehensive but are usually pleased with the relief from pain and spasm and with the possibility of again sitting out of bed.

Other chemical methods of interrupting the reflex arc on either the efferent or afferent side have not been widely used in patients with multiple sclerosis. Such methods include peripheral nerve block with phenol solutions[345] or injection of the motor point with alcohol.[346]

Spasticity, and in particular, flexor spasm, is aggravated by many commonly encountered sources of increased sensory input; bedsores, even small sores on the heel; bladder distension or infection and a distended rectum. The practical implications are important. Even small and painless skin lesions should receive serious attention and the care of the bladder is of wider significance than control of urinary symptoms.

Fatigue

Fatigue, out of proportion to disability or depression, is a common complaint in multiple sclerosis. Amantadine had been tried in the treatment of multiple sclerosis[347] because of its antiviral action, but without benefit. Murray[348] observed relief of fatigue in some patients and the possible effect of amantadine in a dose of 100 mg twice daily on this symptom has been examined in controlled trials.[42] Assessment naturally presented difficulties. Fatigue itself was measured on an improvised scale but attention was also paid to the degree to which fatigue interfered with activity and to the effect of treatment on other troublesome symptoms. No effect on disability was found. Fatigue was improved to a small but significant degree. This was attributed to the effect of amantadine on release of noradrenaline.

Rosenberg & Appenzeller[349] carried out a small double-blind crossover trial of 200 mg of amantadine versus placebo. Of the 10 patients, 6 claimed some relief of fatigue from amantadine, 1 from placebo and 3 from neither. In all patients, serum levels of beta-endorphin-beta-lipoprotein increased on treatment with the active agent, more so in those who responded. Lactate levels were higher and pyruvate lower in non-responders. The relation of these findings to the therapeutic response was not clear. No objective clinical changes were detected.

PHYSIOTHERAPY

Every account of the rehabilitation of patients with multiple sclerosis includes physiotherapy and every physician uses it. As Liversedge[59] pointed out, patients have high expectations of the value of physiotherapy and frequently demand it. No critical evaluation of the merits of physiotherapy in multiple sclerosis appears to have been published. This is scarcely surprising as the difficulties of assessing even a standardised method of treatment are sufficiently daunting and it would perhaps be impossible to devise a method of examining the results of necessarily individualised physiotherapy. Personal experience and common sense indicate that physiotherapy is of value in rehabilitation during recovery from relapse affecting locomotion, although probably not contributing to the degree of recovery finally attained. Another indication is physiotherapy as part of an attempted rescue programme for the patient overwhelmed by mounting disabilities, urinary infection, decubitus ulcers and loss of mobility.

In these examples physiotherapy is given as an inpatient and can be carefully tailored to the patient's needs and endurance. Physiotherapy as an outpatient for those with chronic multiple sclerosis has little to offer. Except in very favourable circumstances, the journey to the department, the waiting, the necessarily brief treatment and infrequent attendance can do no good and often result in exhaustion. Patients with painful spastic legs often obtain temporary symptomatic relief from physiotherapy involving simple supervised exercise, passive movements and even massage, but only if given at home without the attendant fatigue of travel to a department.

Russell[350] advocated a regime of regulated exercise interspersed with periods of rest. He believed that this was more than symptomatic treatment and favourably influenced the course of the disease through an effect on the blood–brain barrier. The regime undoubtedly increased the feeling of wellbeing but did not prevent relapse or the progression of the disease.

PSYCHOLOGICAL MANAGEMENT

Multiple sclerosis is well known as a disease that leads to the wheelchair and is consequently regarded with apprehension or even dread. To learn or to be told that this is the cause of symptoms previously dismissed as 'neuritis' or 'a virus' can scarcely be other than a highly significant and perhaps shocking event. What then should patients be told and when? It is surely undesirable that the diagnosis should be discovered by accident such as overhearing the doctors' discussion on a ward round or reading the notes upside down.[351] It is the author's belief that when the diagnosis is clinically definite the patient should be told, but that in a first attack, however typical, it is usually wise to prevaricate. At a meeting of representatives of European Multiple Sclerosis Societies this view was greeted with astonished exclamations at such an example of Anglo-Saxon stoicism or phlegme britannique. The risk of suicide on learning the diagnosis was heavily emphasised. In published accounts, admittedly from communities with at least an Anglo-Saxon cultural background, it has been found that a definite statement of the diagnosis is often greeted with relief.[351,352] This is certainly a common clinical experience but the ground must be carefully laid with close collaboration between specialist, general practitioner and the patient's near relatives. With such preparation and with sufficient time for explanation both then and later, the author has never known a patient commit suicide. A much more usual response is a resolve to combat what is now known to be a disease with a definite name, combined with relief at the dismissal of often unexpressed fears of madness, brain tumours or the accusation of 'making it all up'.

The approach described above is not appropriate for all patients, who must be treated as individuals. When asked, naturally in retrospect, patients overwhelmingly demand early full information, even when the diagnosis can only be suspected.[353, 354] This approach may well be correct, but patients must be treated as individuals and firm rules are out of place. Certainly those faced with immediate decisions with far-reaching consequences, such as marriage, pregnancy, the adoption of a child or large financial commitments, may well require some explanation at a stage where the disease is no more than possible. I have, however twice encountered a crippling hysterical reaction to the pronouncement of an incorrect diagnosis of early multiple sclerosis, of course made elsewhere.

The individual response to the diagnosis of multiple sclerosis is, as might be expected, highly variable, ranging from trying to dismiss all thought of the disease to the fervid pursuit of any hint of cure. What most patients need and what should be available to all is the opportunity to talk to someone well informed on multiple sclerosis who is prepared to listen. For some, the extension to group counselling may have more to offer[355] but others would find it distasteful. Many articulate patients have expressed their sense of alienation on being actually or potentially disabled. Group counselling or, at a less intense level, membership of a branch of the Multiple Sclerosis Society will prevent isolation but contact with, and natural acceptance by, 'normal' people is more important and more difficult to attain.

The patient with multiple sclerosis may be comfortably and lovingly supported by a devoted family or may be subjected to the harsh stresses of loss of job and income, loss of independence, a vanishing sex life, desertion by spouse and children or even actual cruelty in the home. One disabled patient's 8-year-old son would only pass him the urinal on payment of a small sum. Counselling and professional support are inevitably inadequate. Depression is common among partially disabled but intellectually unimpaired patients.

Particular care may be required when dementia occurs in otherwise relatively active patients. Difficulties at home and at work may arise from lack of emotional control or from thoughtless dispersion of the family assets. Relatives easily become irritated by forgetfulness or unreasonable behaviour and it is often necessary to undertake the difficult task of explaining that these may be a consequence of the disease.

Unconventional treatments

As the scientific approach has so far failed to develop effective treatment for multiple sclerosis a profusion of unconventional methods is to be expected. It is difficult to write of these in detail as no results are published in the scientific press. Snake venom was never popular in Britain and its vogue in the USA is passing. Methods recently encountered include removal of amalgam tooth fillings because of fears of mercury poisoning; nystatin on the grounds that the disease is caused by thrush; severe dietary restriction because of 'universal allergy', and the usual crop of 'vaccines', vitamins and minerals. It is certainly irritating to see some such method uncritically and ignorantly hailed in the press as a breakthrough, on the basis of one or two 'successful' cases. Patients should be dissuaded from spending money they can ill afford or from undergoing potentially harmful treatment with no serious prospect of benefit. Indignation should be reserved for the comparatively rare examples of deliberate exploitation for profit.

REFERENCES

1. Scheinberg L C, Van den Noort S 1986 Multiple sclerosis treatments. Neurology 36: 703–704
2. Schumacher G A, Beebe G, Kibler R F et al 1965 Problems of experimental trials of therapy in multiple sclerosis. Annals of the New York Academy of Sciences 122: 552–568
3. Brown J R, Beebe G W, Kurtzke J F, Loewenson R B, Silberberg D H, Tourtellotte W W 1979 The design of clinical studies to assess therapeutic efficacy in multiple sclerosis. Neurology 29, 9(2): 1–23
4. Weiner H L, Ellison G W 1984 A working protocol to be used as a guideline for trials in multiple sclerosis. Archives of Neurology 40: 704–710
5. Thygesen P 1953 The course of disseminated sclerosis: a close-up of 105 attacks. Rosenkilde and Bagger, Copenhagen
6. Kurtzke J F 1956 Course of exacerbations of multiple sclerosis in hospitalised patients. Archives of Neurology and Psychiatry 76: 175–183
7. Barnes M P, Bateman D E, Cleland P G et al 1985 Intravenous methylprednisolone for multiple sclerosis in relapse. Journal of Neurology, Neurosurgery and Psychiatry 48: 157–159
8. Milligan N M, Newcombe R, Compston D A S 1987 A double-blind controlled trial of high dose methylprednisolone in patients with multiple sclerosis.

Journal of Neurology, Neurosurgery and Psychiatry 50: 511–516
9. McAlpine D (Ed) 1972 In: Multiple sclerosis: a reappraisal 2nd edn. Churchill Livingstone, Edinburgh, p 197
10. Patzold U, Pocklington P R 1982 Course of multiple sclerosis. First results of a prospective study carried out on 102 patients from 1976–80. Acta Neurologica Scandinavica 65: 248–266
11. Weinshenker B G, Ebers G C 1989 Systemic interferon alfa in multiple sclerosis. Archives of Neurology 46: 251–252
12. Poser C M, Paty D W, Scheinberg L et al 1983 New diagnostic criteria for multiple sclerosis: guidelines for research protocols. Annals of Neurology 13: 227–231
13. Rudick R A, Schiffer R B, Schwetz K M, Herndon R M 1986 Multiple sclerosis. The problem of incorrect diagnosis. Archives of Neurology 43: 578–583
14. Compston A 1987 Selection of patients for clinical trials. Neuroepidemiology 6: 34–39
15. Weiss W, Dambrosia J M 1983 Common problems in designing therapeutic trials in multiple sclerosis. Archives of Neurology 40: 678–680
16. Ellison G W, Mickey M R, Myers L W 1988 Alternatives to randomised clinical trials. Neurology 38 (suppl 2): 73–75
17. Maida E, Höcher P, Mann E 1986 Long-term lymphocytapheresis therapy in multiple sclerosis. European Neurology 25: 225–232

18. Fratiglioni L, Siracusa G F, Amato M P, Sita D, Amaducci L 1988 Effectiveness of azathioprine in multiple sclerosis. Italian Journal of Neurological Sciences 9: 261–264
19. Kurtzke J F 1955 A new scale for evaluating disability in multiple sclerosis. Neurology 5: 580–583
20. Kurtzke J F 1965 Further notes on disability evaluation in multiple sclerosis with scale modifications. Neurology 15: 654–661
21. Kurtzke J F 1983 Rating neurologic impairment in multiple sclerosis: an expanded disability status scale (EDSS). Neurology 33: 1444–1453
22. Bauer H J, Krtsch U, Schipper R, Eckhardt I, Minzloff H, Nater B 1984 Disability rating with the IFMSS scales. Acta Neurologica Scandinavica (suppl) 101: 145–152
23. Willoughby E W, Paty D W 1988 Scales for rating impairment in multiple sclerosis: a critique. Neurology 38: 1793–1798
24. Kurtzke J F 1989 The disability status scale for multiple sclerosis: *apologia pro DSS sua*. Neurology 39: 291–302
25. Gordon P A, Caroll D J, Etches W S et al 1985 A double-blind controlled pilot study of plasma exchange versus sham apheresis in chronic progressive multiple sclerosis. Canadian Journal of Neurological Sciences 12: 39–44
26. Kurtzke J F 1987 Problems and pitfalls in treatment trials of multiple sclerosis. Neuroepidemiology 6: 17–33
27. British and Dutch Multiple Sclerosis Azathioprine Trial Group 1988 Double-masked trial of azathioprine in multiple sclerosis. Lancet 2: 179–183
28. Kuzma J W, Namerow N S, Tourtellotte W W et al 1969 An assessment of the reliability of three methods used in evaluating the status of multiple sclerosis patients. Journal of Chronic Diseases 21: 803–814
29. Amato M P, Groppi C, Siracusa G F, Fratiglioni L 1987 Inter and intra-observer reliability in Kurtzke scoring systems in multiple sclerosis. Italian Journal of Neurological Sciences (suppl) 6: 129–132
30. Amato M P, Fratiglioni L, Groppi C, Siracusa G, Amaducci L 1988 Interrater reliability in assessing functional systems and disability on the Kurtzke scale in multiple sclerosis. Archives of Neurology 45: 746–748
31. Khatri B O, McQuillen M P, Harrington G J, Schmoll D, Hoffman R G 1985 Chronic progressive multiple sclerosis: double-blind controlled study of plasmapheresis in patients taking immunosuppressive drugs. Neurology 35: 312–319
32. Rose A S, Kuzma J W, Kurtzke J F, Namerow N S, Sibley W A, Tourtellotte W W 1970 Co-operative study in the evaluation of therapy in multiple sclerosis: ACTH versus placebo. Neurology 5(2): 1–59
33. Tourtellotte W W, Haerer A F, Simpson J F, Kuzma J W, Sikovski J 1965 Quantitative neurological testing I: A battery of tests designed to evaluate in part the neurological function of patients with multiple sclerosis and its use in a therapeutic trial. Annals of the New York Academy of Sciences 122: 480–505
34. Hauser S L, Dawson D M, Lehrich J R et al 1985 Intensive immunosuppression in progressive multiple sclerosis. New England Journal of Medicine 308: 173–180
35. Mickey M R, Ellison G W, Myers L W 1984 An illness severity score for multiple sclerosis. Neurology 34: 1343–1347
36. Sipe J C, Knobler R L, Braheny S L, Rice G P A, Panitch H S, Oldstone M B A 1984 A neurologic rating scale (NRS) in multiple sclerosis. Neurology 34: 1368–1371
37. Alexander L, Berkeley A W, Alexamder A M 1958 Prognosis and treatment of multiple sclerosis: quantitative nosometric study. Journal of the American Medical Association 166: 1943–1949
38. Feinstein A R, Josephy B R, Wells C K 1986 Scientific and clinical problems in indexes of functional disability. Annals of Internal Medicine 105: 413–420
39. Cook S D, Devereux C, Troiano R et al 1986 Effect of total lymphoid irradiation in chronic progressive multiple sclerosis. Lancet 1: 1405–1409
40. IFMSS 1984 Minimal record of disability. Acta Neurologica Scandinavica (suppl) 101: 193–217
41. Robinson I 1987 Analysing the structure of 23 clinical trials in multiple sclerosis. Neuroepidemiology 6: 46–76
42. Canadian MS Research Group 1987 A randomised controlled trial of amantadine in fatigue associated with multiple sclerosis. Canadian Journal of Neurological Sciences 14: 273–278
43. Matthews W B, Small D G 1979 Serial recording of visual and somatosensory evoked potentials in multiple sclerosis. Journal of the Neurological Sciences 40: 11–21
44. Walsh J C, Garrick R, Cameron J, McCleod J G 1982 Evoked potential changes in clinically definite multiple sclerosis: a two year follow up. Journal of Neurology, Neurosurgery and Psychiatry 45: 494–500
45. Confavreux Ch, Mauguière F, Courjon J, Aimard G, Devic M 1981 Evolution des potentials évoqués visuels dans la sclérose en plaques. Revue Neurologique 137: 121–132
46. Dau P C, Petajan J H, Johnson K P, Panitch H S, Bornstein M B 1980 Plasmapheresis in multiple sclerosis: preliminary findings. Neurology 30: 1023–1028
47. Knobler R L, Panitch H S, Braheny S L et al 1984 Systemic alpha-interferon therapy of multiple sclerosis. Neurology 34: 1273–1279
48. Basten A, McLeod J G, Pollard J D et al 1980 Transfer factor in long-term treatment of multiple sclerosis. Lancet 2: 931–934
49. Wiles C M, Clark C R A, Irwin H P, Edgar E F, Swan A V 1986 Hyperbaric oxygen in multiple sclerosis: a double-blind trial. British Medical Journal 292: 367–371
50. Nuwer E R, Packwood J W, Myers L W, Ellison G W 1987 Evoked potentials predict the clinical changes in a multiple sclerosis drug study. Neurology 37: 1754–1761
51. Caputo D, Zaffaroni M, Ghezzi A, Cazullo C L 1987 Azathioprine reduces intrathecal IgG synthesis in multiple sclerosis. Acta Neurologica Scandinavica 75: 84–86
52. Moody D J, Kagan J, Liao D, Ellison G W, Myers L W 1987 Administration of monthly-pulse cyclophosphamide in multiple sclerosis patients. Effects of long-term treatment on immunological parameters. Journal of Neuroimmunology 14: 161–173
53. Hafler D A, Fallis R J, Dawson D M, Schlossman S F, Reinherz E L, Weiner H L 1986 Immunological responses of progressive multiple sclerosis patients treated with an anti-T-cell monoclonal antibody, anti-T-12. Neurology 36: 777–784
54. Trotter J L, Gebel H M, Ferguson T B, Garvey W F, Rodney G E 1983 Thymectomy induced decrease in Ty

cells and OKT8+ cells in multiple sclerosis. Annals of Neurology 14: 656–661

55. Baumhefner R W, Tourtellotte W W, Syndulko K, Shapshak P, Osborne M, Rubenstein G 1988 Copolymer-1 as therapy for multiple sclerosis: the cons. Neurology 37, 7 (suppl 2): 69–71

56. Troiano R, Hafstein M, Ruderman M, Dowling P, Cook S 1984 Effect of high-dose intravenous steroid administration on contrast enhancing computed tomographic scan lesions in multiple sclerosis. Annals of Neurology 15: 257–263

57. Kesselring J, Miller D H, MacManus D G et al 1989 Quantitative magnetic imaging in multiple sclerosis: the effect of high dose intravenous methylprednisolone. Journal of Neurology, Neurosurgery and Psychiatry 52: 14–17

58. Sibley W A 1970 Drug treatment of multiple sclerosis. In: Handbook of clinical neurology, Vol 9. North-Holland, Amsterdam, pp 383–407

59. Liversedge L A 1977 Treatment and management of multiple sclerosis. British Medical Bulletin 33: 78–83

60. Taylor R C, Webster C J 1987 Methodological problems in evaluating hyperbaric treatment of multiple sclerosis. Neuroepidemiology 6: 77–84

61. Miller H, Newell D J, Ridley A 1961 Multiple sclerosis: treatment of acute exacerbations with corticotrophin (ACTH). Lancet 2: 1120–1122

62. Miller H G 1953 Acute disseminated encephalomyelitis treated with ACTH. British Medical Journal 1: 177–183

63. Miller H G, Gibbons J L 1953 Acute disseminated encephalomyelitis and acute disseminated sclerosis: results of treatment with ACTH. British Medical Journal 2: 1345–1349

64. Alexander L, Berkeley A W, Alexander A W 1961 Multiple sclerosis: prognosis and treatment. Thomas, Springfield

65. Veterans Administration Multiple Sclerosis Study Group 1957 Isoniazid in treatment of multiple sclerosis. Journal of the American Medical Association 163: 168–172

66. Hoogstraten M C, Cats A, Minderhout J M 1987 Bed rest and ACTH in the treatment of exacerbations in multiple sclerosis patients. Acta Neurologica Scandinavica 76: 346–350

67. Rawson M D, Liversedge L A, Goldfarb G 1966 Treatment of acute retrobulbar neuritis with corticotrophin. Lancet 2: 1044–1046

68. Rawson M D, Liversedge L A 1969 Treatment of retrobulbar neuritis with corticotrophin. Lancet 1: 222

69. Bowden A N, Bowden O M A, Friedmann A I, Perkin G D, Rose F C 1974 A trial of corticotrophin gelatine injection in acute optic neuritis. Journal of Neurology, Neurosurgery and Psychiatry 37: 869–873

70. Dowling P C, Bosch V V, Cook S D 1980 Possible beneficial effect of high-dose intravenous steroid therapy in acute demyelinating disease and transverse myelitis. Neurology 30, 7(2): 33–36

71. Buckley C, Kennard C, Swash M 1982 Treatment of acute exacerbations of multiple sclerosis with intravenous methylprednisolone. Journal of Neurology, Neurosurgery and Psychiatry 45: 179–180

72. Newman P K, Saunders M, Tilley P J B 1982 Methylprednisolone therapy in multiple sclerosis. Journal of Neurology, Neurosurgery and Psychiatry 45: 941–942

73. Goas J Y, Marion J L, Missoum A 1983 High dose intravenous methylprednisolone in acute exacerbations of multiple sclerosis. Journal of Neurology, Neurosurgery and Psychiatry 46: 99

74. Durelli L, Cocito D, Riccio A et al 1986 High-dose intravenous methylprednisolone in the treatment of multiple sclerosis. Neurology 36: 238–243

75. Abbruzzese G, Gandolfo C, Loeb C 1983 'Bolus' methylprednisolone versus ACTH in the treatment of multiple sclerosis. Italian Journal of Neurological Science 2: 169–172

76. Thompson A J, Kennard C, Swash M et al 1989 Intravenous methylprednisolone and ACTH in the treatment of acute relapse in MS. Neurology 39: 969–971

77. Bindoff L, Lyons P R, Newman P K, Saunders M 1988 Methylprednisolone in multiple sclerosis: a comparative dose study. Journal of Neurology, Neurosurgery and Psychiatry 51: 1108

78. Lyons P R, Newman P K, Saunders M 1988 Methylprednisolone therapy in multiple sclerosis: a profile of adverse effects. Journal of Neurology, Neurosurgery and Psychiatry 51: 285–287

79. Pryse-Phillips W E M, Chandra R K, Bose B 1984 Anaphylactoid reaction to methylprednisolone pulsed therapy for multiple sclerosis. Neurology 34: 1119–1121

80. Warren K G, Catz I, Jeffrey V M, Caroll D J 1986 Effect of methylprednisolone on CSF IgG parameters, myelin basic protein and anti-myelin basic protein in multiple sclerosis exacerbations. Canadian Journal of Neurological Sciences 13: 23–30

81. Troiano J R, Cokk S D, Dowling P C 1987 Steroid therapy in multiple sclerosis. Point of view. Archives of Neurology 44: 803–807

82. Spoor T C, Rockwell D L 1988 Treatment of optic neuritis with intravenous megadose corticosteroids. A consecutive series. Ophthalmology 95: 131–134

83. Flötotto B, Serde D 1988 A pilot study of high dose dexamethasone in patients with multiple sclerosis. Abstracts of IFMSS meeting, Rome V/15

84. Compston D A S, Milligan N M, Hughes P J et al 1987 A double-blind controlled trial of high dose methylprednisolone in patients with multiple sclerosis: 2. Laboratory results. Journal of Neurology, Neurosurgery and Psychiatry 50: 517–522

85. Smith T, Zeeberg I Sjö O 1986 Evoked potentials in multiple sclerosis before and after high-dose methylprednisolone infusion. European Neurology 25: 67–73

86. Miller H, Newell D J, Ridley A 1961 Multiple sclerosis: trials of maintenance treatment with prednisolone and soluble aspirin. Lancet 1: 127–129

87. Fog T 1964 The long-term treatment of multiple sclerosis with corticoids. Acta Neurologica Scandinavica 41 (suppl 13): 473–482

88. Tourtellotte W W, Haerer A F 1965 Use of an oral corticosteroid in the treatment of multiple sclerosis. Archives of Neurology 12: 536–545

89. Millar J H D, Vas C J, Noronha M J, Liversedge L, Rawson M D 1967 Long-term treatment of multiple sclerosis with corticotrophin. Lancet 2: 429–431

90. Rinne U K, Sonninen V, Tuovinen T 1968 Corticotrophin treatment in multiple sclerosis. Acta Neurologica Scandinavica 44: 207–218

91. Hoogstraten M C, Minderhoud J M 1988 A

double-blind controlled trial of high dose methylprednisolone in patients with multiple sclerosis. Journal of Neurology, Neurosurgery and Psychiatry 51: 597

92. Poser C M, Kleefield J, O'Reilly G V, Jolesz F 1987 Neuroimaging and the lesion of multiple sclerosis. American Journal of Neuroradiology 8: 549–552

93. Matthews W B 1985 In: McAlpine's Multiple Sclerosis. Churchill Livingstone, Edinburgh, p 241

94. Buskirk C V, Poffenbarger A L, Capriles L F, Idea B V 1964 Treatment of multiple sclerosis with intrathecal steroids. Neurology 14: 595–597

95. Baker A G 1967 Intrathecal methylprednisolone for multiple sclerosis: evaluation by a standard neurological rating. Annals of Allergy 25: 665–672

96. Lance J W 1969 Intrathecal depo-medrone for spasticity. Medical Journal of Australia 2: 1030

97. Nelson D A, Vates T S, Thomas R B 1973 Complications from intrathecal steroid therapy in patients with multiple sclerosis. Acta Neurologica Scandinavica 49: 176–188

98. Bernat J L, Sadowsky C H, Vincent F M, Nordgren R E, Margolis G 1976 Sclerosing spinal pachymeningitis: a complication of intrathecal administration of depo-medrol for multiple sclerosis. Journal of Neurology, Neurosurgery and Psychiatry 39: 1124–1128

99. Lisak R P 1986 Overview of the rationale for immunomodulating therapies in multiple sclerosis. Neurology 38, 7 (suppl 2): 5–8

100. Girard P F, Aimard G, Pellet H 1967 Thérapeutique immunodépressive en neurologie. Presse Médicale 75: 967–969

101. Aimard G, Girard P F, Raveaou J 1966 Sclérose en plaques et processus d'autoimmunisation: traitement par les antimitotiques. Lyon Médicale 215: 345–353

102. Millac P, Miller H 1969 Cyclophosphamide in multiple sclerosis. Lancet 1: 783

103. Drachman P A, Paterson P Y, Schmidt R T, Spehlmann R F 1975 Cyclophosphamide in exacerbations of multiple sclerosis: therapeutic trial and a strategy for pilot drug studies. Journal of Neurology, Neurosurgery and Psychiatry 38: 592–597

104. Hommes O R, Prick J J G, Lamers K J B 1975 Treatment of the chronic progressive form of multiple sclerosis with a combination of cyclophosphamide and prednisone. Clinical Neurology and Neurosurgery 78: 59–71

105. Hommes O R, Lamers K J B 1977 Immunosuppressive treatment in chronic progressive multiple sclerosis. In : Delmotte P, Hommes O R, Gonsette R (eds) Immunosuppressive treatment in multiple sclerosis. European Press, Gent, pp 48–64

106. Gonsette R E, Demonty L, Delmotte P 1977 Intensive immunosuppression with cyclophosphamide in multiple sclerosis. Journal of Neurology 214: 173–181

107. Gonsette R E, Demonty L, Delmotte P 1977 Intensive immunosuppression with cyclophosphamide in multiple sclerosis. In: Delmotte P, Hommes O R, Gonsette R (eds) Immunosuppressive treatment in multiple sclerosis. European Press, Gent, pp 116–130

108. Hommes O R, Lamers K J B, Reeker S P 1980 Effect of intensive immunosuppression on the course of chronic progressive multiple sclerosis. Journal of Neurology 223: 177–190

109. Theys P, Gossege-Lissoir F, Ketelaer P, Carton H 1981 Short-term cyclophosphamide treatment in multiple sclerosis. Journal of Neurology 225: 119–133

110. Weiner H L, Hauser S L, Hafler D A, Fallis R J, Lehrich J R, Dawson D M 1984 The use of cyclophosphamide in the treatment of multiple sclerosis. Annals of the New York Academy of Sciences 436: 373–381

111. Trouillas P, Neuschwander Ph, Nighoghossian N, Adeleine P, Tremesi P 1989 Immunosuppression intensive dans la sclérose en plaques progressive. Etude ouverte comparant trois groupes: cyclophosphamide, cyclophosphamide-plasmaphrèses et témoins. Résultats à trois ans. Revue Neurologique 145: 369–377

112. Goodkin D E, Plencner S, Palmer–Saxerud J, Teetzen M, Hertsgaard D 1987 Cyclophosphamide in chronic progressive multiple sclerosis. Archives of Neurology 44: 823–827

113. Myers L W, Fahery J L, Moody D J, Mickey M R, Frane M V, Ellison G W 1987 Cyclophosphamide 'pulses' in chronic progressive multiple sclerosis. Archives of Neurology 44: 828–832

114. Killian J M, Bressler R B, Armstrong R M, Huston D P 1988 Controlled pilot trial of monthly intravenous cyclophosphamide in multiple sclerosis. Archives of Neurology 45: 27–30

115. Carter J L, Hafler D A, Dawson D M, Orav J, Weiner H L 1988 Immunosuppression with high-dose iv cyclophosphamide and ACTH in progressive multiple sclerosis: cumulative 6-year experience in 164 patients. Neurology 38 (suppl 2): 9–14

116. Likosky W H 1988 Experience with cyclophosphamide: the cons. Neurology 38 (suppl 2): 14–18

117. Tucker W G, Kapphahn K H 1969 A preliminary evaluation of azathioprine (Imuran) in the treatment of multiple sclerosis. Henry Ford Hospital Medical Journal 17: 89–92

118. Grüninger W, Mertens H G 1973 Uber die immunosuppressive Langzeitbehandlung der Multiplen Sklerose mit Azathioprine. Tenth International Congress of Neurology. Excerpta Medica, Amsterdam, p 148

119. Springer A, Tschabitscher H 1969 Vorlaufiger Bericht uber Therapie Versuche mit Azathioprine bei Multipler Sklerose. Wiener Zeitschrift für Nervenheilkunde 218 (suppl 2): 226

120. Silberberg D, Lisak R, Zweiman B 1973 Multiple sclerosis unaffected by azathioprine in pilot study. Archives of Neurology 28: 210–212

121. Mertens H G, Dommasch D 1977 Long term study of immunosuppressive therapy in multiple sclerosis: Comparison of periods of the disease before and during treatment. In: Delmotte P, Hommes O R, Gonsette R (eds) Immunosuppressive treatment in multiple sclerosis. European Press, Gent, pp 198–210

122. Rosen J A 1979 Prolonged azathioprine treatment of non-remitting multiple sclerosis. Journal of Neurology, Neurosurgery and Psychiatry 42: 338–344

123. Aimard G, Confavreux C, Troullias P, Devic M 1978 L'azathioprine dans le traitement de la sclérose en plaques: une expérience de 10 ans à propos de 77 malades. Revue Neurologique 134: 215–222

124. Aimard G, Confavreux C, Ventre J J, Guillot M, Devic M 1983 Étude de 213 cas de sclérose en plaques traités par l'azathioprine de 1967 à 1982. Revue Neurologique 139: 509–513

125. Sabouraud O, Oger J, Darcel F, Madigaud M, Merienne M 1984 Immunosuppression au long cours dans la sclérose en plaques: evaluation des traitements commencés avant 1972. Revue Neurologique 140: 125–130

126. Lhermitte F, Marteau R, Toullet E, de Saxce H, Loridau M 1984 Traitement prolongé de la sclérose en plaques par l'azathioprine à doses moyennes. Bilan de quinze années d'expérience. Revue Neurologique 140: 553–558

127. Swinburn W R, Liversedge L A 1973 Long-term treatment of multiple sclerosis with azathioprine. Journal of Neurology, Neurosurgery and Psychiatry 36: 124–126

128. Patzold U, Pocklington P 1980 Azathioprine in multiple sclerosis: a three year controlled study of its effectiveness. Journal of Neurology 223: 97–117

129. Patzold U, Hecker H, Pocklington P 1982 Azathioprine in treatment of multiple sclerosis: final results of a $4\frac{1}{2}$ year controlled study of its effectiveness. Journal of the Neurological Sciences 54: 377–394

130. Milanese C, La Mantia L, Salmaggi A et al 1988 Double blind controlled randomised study on azathioprine efficacy in multiple sclerosis. Preliminary results. Italian Journal of Neurological Sciences 9: 53–58

131. Ellison G W, Myers L W, Mickey M R et al 1984 Therapeutic trials in multiple sclerosis: azathioprine. Annals of the New York Academy of Sciences 436: 361–365

132. Ellison G W, Myers L W, Mickey M R, Graves M C, Tourtellotte W W, Nuwer M R 1988 Clinical experience with azathioprine: the pros. Neurology 38, 7 (suppl 2): 20–23

133. Kappos L, Patzold U, Dommasch et al 1988 Cyclosporin versus azathioprine in the long-term management of multiple sclerosis: results of the German multicentre study. Annals of Neurology 23: 56–63

134. Rudge P, Koetsier J C, Mertin J et al 1989 Randomised double blind controlled trial of cyclosporin in multiple sclerosis. Journal of Neurology, Neurosurgery and Psychiatry 52: 559–565

135. Weiner H L, Paty D W 1989 Diagnostic and therapeutic trials in multiple sclerosis: a new look. Neurology 39: 972–976

136. Hafler D A, Weiner H L 1988 Immunosuppression with monoclonal antibodies in multiple sclerosis. Neurology 38 (suppl 2): 42–44

137. Seland T P, McPherson P A, Grace M, Lamoureux G, Blain J G 1974 Evaluation of antithymocyte globulin in acute relapses of multiple sclerosis. Neurology 24: 34–40

138. Kastrukoff L F, McLean D R, McPherson T A 1978 Multiple sclerosis treated with antithymocyte globulin: a five year follow up. Canadian Journal of Neurological Sciences 5: 175–178

139. Walker J E, Hoehn M M, Kashiwagi N 1976 A trial of antilymphocytic globulin in the treatment of chronic progressive multiple sclerosis. Journal of the Neurological Sciences 29: 303–309

140. Lhermitte F, Marteau R, de Saxce H 1979 Traitement des formes graves de la sclérose en plaques par le sérum antilymphocytaire: résultats d'une étude pilote de 50 malades suivis 4 ans. Revue Neurologique 135: 389–400

141. Lhermitte F, Marteau R, de Saxce H 1987 Traitement des formes évolutives et graves de sclérose en plaques par l'association sérum antilymphocytaire, azathioprine, prednisone. Revue Neurologique 143: 98–107

142. Frick E, Angstwurm H, Spath G 1971 Immunosuppressive Therapie der multiplen Sklerose. Münchener Medizinische Wochenschrift 113: 221–231

143. Brendel W, Seifert J, Lob G 1972 Effect of 'maximum' immune suppression with thoracic duct drainage, ALG, azathioprine and cortisone in some neurological disorders. Proceedings of the Royal Society of Medicine 65: 531–535

144. Ring J, Seifert J, Lob G et al 1974 Intensive immunosuppression in the treatment of multiple sclerosis. Lancet 2: 1093–1096

145. Lance E M, Kremer M, Abbosh J 1975 Intensive immunosuppression in patients with disseminated sclerosis. Clinical and Experimental Immunology 21: 1–12

146. Lance E M 1975 Intensive immunosuppression in patients with multiple sclerosis: clinical response. In: Davison A N, Humphrey J H, Liversedge L A, McDonald W I, Porterfield J S (eds) Multiple sclerosis research. HMSO, London, pp 241–254

147. Mertin J, Rudge P, Kremer M 1982 Double-blind controlled trial of immunosuppression in the treatment of multiple sclerosis: final report. Lancet 2: 351–354

148. Cook S D, Devereux C, Troiano R et al 1987 Total lymphoid irradiation in multiple sclerosis: blood lymphocytes and clinical course. Annals of Neurology 22: 634–638

149. Myers L W, Ellison G W, Fahey J L, Tesler A, Gottlich M S 1988 Clinical drawbacks of total lymphoid irradiation: the cons. Neurology 38 (suppl 2): 38–40

150. Capra R, Mattioli F, Vignolo L A, Buffoli A, Micheletti E 1988 Total lymphoid irradiation in chronic progressive multiple sclerosis: preliminary report. Abstracts of IFMSS meeting Rome V/12

151. Brage D 1980 Observations in 166 patients with multiple sclerosis after thymectomy. In: Bauer H J, Poser S, Ritter G (eds) Progress in multiple sclerosis research. Springer, Berlin, pp 451–453

152. Trotter J L, Clifford D B, Montgomery E B, Ferguson T B 1985 Thymectomy in multiple sclerosis: a 3-year follow up. Neurology 35: 1049–1051

153. Aymard J P, Witz F, Conroy T et al 1985 Leucémie aigue secondaire au traitement de la sclérose en plaques par le chlorambucil. Revue Neurologique 141: 152–154

154. Noseworthy J H, Seland T P, Ebers G C 1984 Therapeutic trials in multiple sclerosis. Canadian Journal of Neurological Sciences 11: 355–362

155. Weiner H L, Dawson D M 1980 Plasmapheresis in multiple sclerosis: preliminary study. Neurology 30: 1029–1031

156. Weiner H L 1985 An assessment of plasma exchange in progressive multiple sclerosis. Neurology 35: 320–322

157. Tindall R S A, Walker J E, Ehle A L, Near L, Rollins J, Becker R N 1982 Plasmapheresis in multiple sclerosis: prospective trial of pheresis and immunosuppression versus immunosuppression alone. Neurology 32: 739–743

158. Trouillas P, Neuschwander Ph, Trémisi J P 1986 Modification rapide par les échanges plasmatiques de la sémiologie de formes progressives de la sclérose en plaques. Revue Neurologique 142: 690–695

159. Stefoski D, Schauf C L, McLeod B C, Haywood C P, Davis F A 1982 Plasmapheresis decreases neuroelectric blocking activity in multiple sclerosis. Neurology 32: 904–906

160. Khatri B O, Koethe S M, McQuillen M P 1984 Plasmapheresis with immunosuppressive drug therapy in progressive multiple sclerosis: a pilot study. Archives of Neurology 41: 734–738

161. Scheinberg L C 1984 Treatment of multiple sclerosis. Archives of Neurology 42: 310

162. Maida E, Höcher P, Mann E 1980 Long-term lymphocytapheresis therapy in multiple sclerosis. Preliminary observations. European Neurology 25: 225–232

163. Hauser S L, Fosburg M, Kevy S V, Weiner H L 1984 Lymphocytapheresis in chronic progressive multiple sclerosis: immunologic and clinical effects. Neurology 34: 922–926

164. Medaer R, Eeckhout C, Gautama K, Vermijlen C 1984 Lymphocytapheresis therapy in multiple sclerosis, a preliminary study. Acta Neurologica Scandinavica 70: 111–115

165. Neighbour P A, Miller A E, Bloom B R 1981 Interferon responses of leukocytes in multiple sclerosis. Neurology 31: 561–566

166. Salonen R, Ilonen J, Reunanen M, Salmi A 1982 Defective production of interferon alpha associated with HLA Dw2 antigen in stable multiple sclerosis. Journal of the Neurological Sciences 55: 197–206

167. Zander H, Abb J, Kandewitz P, Riethmüller G 1982 Natural killing activity and interferon production in multiple sclerosis. Lancet 1: 280

168. Abbott R J, Giles P D, Bolderson I 1986 Absence of immunoreactive interferon alpha in CSF from patients with multiple sclerosis. Journal of Neurology, Neurosurgery and Psychiatry 49: 102–103

169. McFarlin D E 1985 Use of interferon in multiple sclerosis. Annals of Neurology 18: 432–433

170. Panitch H S, Francis G S, Hooper C J, Merigan T C, Johnson K P 1985 Serial immunological studies in multiple sclerosis patients treated systemically with human alpha interferon. Annals of Neurology 18: 434–438

171. Jacobs L, O'Malley J, Freeman A, Ekes R 1981 Intrathecal interferon reduces exacerbations of multiple sclerosis. Science 214: 1026–1028

172. Jacobs L, O'Malley J, Freeman A, Murawski J, Ekes R 1982 Intrathecal interferon in multiple sclerosis. Archives of Neurology 39: 609–615

173. Jacobs L, O'Malley J, Freeman A, Ekes R, Reese P A 1985 Intrathecal interferon in the treatment of multiple sclerosis. Patient follow up. Archives of Neurology 42: 841–847

174. Jacobs L, Salazar A M, Herndon R et al 1986 Multicentre double-blind study of effect of intrathecally administered natural human fibroblast interferon on exacerbations of multiple sclerosis. Lancet 2: 1411–1413

175. Jacobs L, Salazar A M, Herndon R et al 1987 Intrathecally administered natural human fibroblast interferon reduces exacerbations of multiple sclerosis. Results of a multicentre, double-blinded study. Archives of Neurology 44: 589–595

176. Jacobs L 1987 Intrathecal interferon, indomethacin and multiple sclerosis. Lancet 1: 326–327

177. Milanese C, Salmaggi A, La Manta L, Corridori F, Nespolo A 1988 Intrathecal beta-interferon in multiple sclerosis. Lancet 2: 563–564

178. Huber M, Bamborschke S, Assheuer J, Heiss W D 1988 Intravenous natural beta interferon treatment of chronic exacerbating-remitting multiple sclerosis: clinical response and MRI/CSF findings. Journal of Neurology 235: 171–173

179. Knobler R L, Panitch H S, Braheny S L et al 1984 Systemic alpha-interferon therapy of multiple sclerosis. Neurology 34: 1273–1279

180. Camenga D L, Johnson K P, Alter M et al 1986 Systemic recombinant alpha-2 interferon therapy in relapsing multiple sclerosis. Archives of Neurology 43: 1239–1246

181. AUSTIMS research group 1988 Interferon-alpha and transfer factor in the treatment of multiple sclerosis. Abstracts of IFMSS meeting, Rome V/9

182. Panitch H S, Hirsch R L, Schindler J, Johnson K P 1987 Treatment of multiple sclerosis with gamma interferon: exacerbations with activation of the immune system. Neurology 37: 1097–1102

183. Lisak R P 1986 Interferon and multiple sclerosis. Annals of Neurology 20: 273

184. Bever C T, Salazar A M, Neely E et al 1986 Preliminary trial of polyICLC in chronic progressive multiple sclerosis. Neurology 36: 494–498

185. Leading Article 1975 Levamisole. Lancet 1: 151–152

186. Dau P C, Johnson K P, Spitler L E 1976 The effect of levamisole on cellular immunity in multiple sclerosis. Clinical and Experimental Immunology 26: 302–309

187. Cendrowski W, Czlonkowska A 1978 Levamisole in multiple sclerosis with special reference to immunological parameters: a pilot study. Acta Neurologica Scandinavica 57: 354–359

188. Gonsette R E, Demonty L, Delmotte P et al 1982 Modulation of immunity in multiple sclerosis: a double blind levamisole-placebo controlled study in 85 patients. Journal of Neurology 228: 65–72

189. Caltagirone C, Carlesimo A 1986 Methisoprinol in the treatment of multiple sclerosis. Acta Neurologica Scandinavica 74: 293–296

190. Pompidou A, Rancurel G, Delsaux M C, Telvi L, Cour V, Buge A 1986 Amélioration clinique et immunologique des scléroses en plaques à forme rémittante par l'isoprinosine. Presse Médicale 15: 930–931

191. Confavreux Ch, Thivolet Ch, Ventre J J, Aimard G, Devic M 1986 Traitement par l'isoprinosine de la sclérose en plaques. Presse Médicale 15: 2256–2257

192. Collins R C, Espinosa L R, Plank C R, Ebers G C, Rosenberg R A, Zabriskie J B 1978 A double-blind trial of transfer factor in multiple sclerosis patients. Clinical and Experimental Immunology 33: 1–11

193. Fog T, Pedersen L, Raun N S et al 1978 Long-term transfer factor treatment for multiple sclerosis. Lancet 1: 851–853

194. Frith J A, McLeod J G, Basten A et al 1986 Transfer factor as a therapy for multiple sclerosis: a follow-up study. Clinical and Experimental Neurology 22: 149–154

195. Van Haver H, Lissoir F, Droissart C et al 1986 Transfer factor therapy in multiple sclerosis: a three-year prospective double-blind clinical trial. Neurology 36: 1399–1402

196. Wisniewski H M, Keith A B 1977 Chronic relapsing experimental allergic encephalomyelitis: an experimental

model of multiple sclerosis. Annals of Neurology
1: 144–148

197. Lassmann H, Wisniewski H M 1979 Chronic relapsing
experimental allergic encephalomyelitis:
clinicopathological comparison with multiple sclerosis.
Archives of Neurology 36: 490–497

198. Alvord E C, Sham, C-M, Hruby S, Kies M 1965
Encephalitogen-induced inhibition of experimental
allergic encephalomyelitis: prevention, suppression and
therapy. Annals of the New York Academy of Science
122: 333–345

199. Driscoll B F, Kies M W, Alvord E C 1974 Successful
treatment of experimental allergic encephalomyelitis
(EAE) in guinea pigs with homologous myelin basic
protein. Journal of Immunology 112: 392–397

200. Campbell B, Vogel P J, Fisher E, Lorenz R 1973
Myelin basic protein administration in multiple
sclerosis. Archives of Neurology 29: 10–15

201. Gonsette R E, Delmotte P, Demonty L 1977 Failure of
basic protein therapy for multiple sclerosis. Journal of
Neurology 216: 27–31

202. Alvord E C, Shaw, C-M, Hruby S, Kies M W 1979
Has myelin basic protein received a fair trial in the
treatment of multiple sclerosis? Annals of Neurology
6: 461–468

203. Salk J, Romine J S, Westall F C, Wiederholt W C
1980 Myelin basic protein studies in experimental
allergic encephalomyelitis and multiple sclerosis: a
summary with theoretical considerations of multiple
sclerosis aetiology. In: Davison A N, Cuzner M L (eds)
The suppression of experimental allergic
encephalomyelitis and multiple sclerosis. Academic
Press, London, pp 141–156

204. Romine J S, Salk J 1983 In: Hallpike J F, Adams
C W M, Tourtellotte W W (eds) Multiple sclerosis.
Chapman, London, pp 621–630

205. Arnon R, Teitelbaum D 1980 Desensitization of
experimental allergic encephalomyelitis with synthetic
peptide analogues. In: Davison A N, Cuzner M L (eds)
The suppression of experimental allergic
encephalomyelitis and multiple sclerosis. Academic
Press, London, pp 195–218

206. Abramsky O, Teitelbaum D, Arnon R 1977 Effect of a
synthetic polypeptide (COP 1) on patients with
multiple sclerosis and with acute disseminated
encephalomyelitis. Journal of the Neurological Sciences
31: 433–438

207. Bornstein M B, Miller A I, Teitelbaum D, Arnon R,
Sela M 1982 Multiple sclerosis: trial of a synthetic
polypeptide. Annals of Neurology 11: 317–319

208. Bornstein M B, Miller A, Slagle S et al 1987 A pilot
trial of COP 1 in exacerbating-remitting multiple
sclerosis. New England Journal of Medicine
317: 408–414

209. Bates D 1986 Hyperbaric oxygen in multiple sclerosis:
discussion paper. Journal of the Royal Society of
Medicine 79: 535–537

210. Warren J, Sacksteder M R, Thuning C A 1978 Oxygen
immunosuppression: modification of experimental
encephalomyelitis in rodents. Journal of Immunology
121: 315–320

211. James P B 1982 Evidence of subacute fat embolism as
the cause of multiple sclerosis. Lancet 1: 380–385

212. Neubauer R A 1978 Treatment of multiple sclerosis
with monoplace hyperbaric oxygenation. Journal of the
Florida Medical Association 65: 101

213. Neubauer R A 1980 Exposure of multiple sclerosis
patients to hyperbaric oxygen at 2 ATA: a preliminary
report. Journal of the Florida Medical Association
67: 498–504

214. Fischer B H, Marks M, Reich T 1983 Hyperbaric
oxygen treatment of multiple sclerosis. New England
Journal of Medicine 308: 181–186

215. Hawkes C H 1984 Hyperbaric oxygen for patients with
multiple sclerosis. British Medical Journal 289: 111

216. Barnes M P, Bates D, Cartlidge N E F, French J M,
Shaw D A 1985 Hyperbaric oxygen in multiple
sclerosis: short-term results of a placebo-controlled,
double-blind trial. Lancet 1: 297–300

217. Barnes M P, Bates D, Cartlidge N F, French J M,
Shaw D A 1987 Hyperbaric oxygen and multiple
sclerosis: final results of a placebo-controlled
double-blind trial. Journal of Neurology, Neurosurgery
and Psychiatry 50: 1402–1406

218. Neiman J, Nilsson B Y, Barr P O, Perrins D J D 1985
Hyperbaric oxygen in chronic progressive multiple
sclerosis: visual evoked potentials and clinical effects.
Journal of Neurology, Neurosurgery and Psychiatry
48: 497–500

219. Wood J, Stell R, Unsworth I, Lance J W, Skuse N
1985 A double-blind trial of hyperbaric oxygen in the
treatment of multiple sclerosis. Medical Journal of
Australia 143: 238–240

220. Harpur G D, Suke R, Bass B H et al 1986 Hyperbaric
oxygen therapy in chronic stable multiple sclerosis:
double-blind study. Neurology 36: 988–991

221. Lhermitte F, Roullet E, Lyon–Caen O et al 1986
Traitement en double insu de 49 formes chroniques de
sclérose en plaques par l'oxygène hyperbare. Revue
Neurologique 142: 201–206

222. Pelaia P, Rasura M, Sparado M et al 1988 Hyperbaric
oxygen therapy in multiple sclerosis patients: 4 year
follow up. International Multiple Sclerosis Conference
Abstracts V/23. IFMSS, Rome

223. Massey E W, Shelton D L, Pact V et al 1985
Hyperbaric oxygen in multiple sclerosis: double-blind
crossover study of 18 patients. Neurology 35 (suppl
1): 104

224. Murthy K M, Maurice P B, Wilmeth J B 1985
Double-blind randomised study of hyperbaric oxygen
(HBO) versus placebo in multiple sclerosis (MS).
Neurology 35 (suppl 1): 104

225. Slater G E, Anderson D A, Sherman R, Ettinger M G,
Haglin J, Hitchcock C 1985 Hyperbaric oxygen in
multiple sclerosis: a double-blind controlled study.
Neurology 35 (suppl 1): 315

226. Neubauer R A 1985 Hyperbaric oxygen therapy of
multiple sclerosis update — 1985.
Lauderdale-by-the-Sea, Florida

227. James P B 1986 Hyperbaric oxygen in multiple
sclerosis. British Medical Journal 292: 692

228. Neubauer R A 1985 Hyperbaric oxygen for multiple
sclerosis. Lancet 1: 810

229. Cook A W 1976 Electrical stimulation in multiple
sclerosis. Hospital Practice 2: 51–58

230. Cook A W, Weinstein S P 1973 Chronic dorsal column
stimulation in multiple sclerosis. New York State
Journal of Medicine 73: 2868–2872

231. Illis L S, Sedgwick E M, Oygar A E, Awadalla M A
1976 Dorsal column stimulation in the rehabilitation of

patients with multiple sclerosis. Lancet 1: 1383–1386

232. Read D J, Matthews W B, Higson R H 1980 The effect of spinal cord stimulation on function in patients with multiple sclerosis. Brain 103: 803–833

233. Proceedings of the 6th International Symposium on External Control of Human Extremities 1978 Yugoslav Committee for Electronics and Automation, Belgrade

234. Young R F, Goodman S J 1979 Dorsal spinal cord stimulation in the treatment of multiple sclerosis. Neurosurgery 5: 225–230

235. Hawkes C H, Wyke M, Desmond A, Bultitude M I, Kanegaonker G S 1980 Stimulation of dorsal column in multiple sclerosis. British Medical Journal 280: 889–891

236. Illis L S, Sedgwick E M, Tallis R C 1980 Spinal cord stimulation in multiple sclerosis: clinical results. Journal of Neurology, Neurosurgery and Psychiatry 43: 1–14

237. Swank R L 1950 Multiple sclerosis: a correlation of its incidence with dietary fat. American Journal of the Medical Sciences 220: 441–450

238. Swank R L, Lerstad O, Strjaum A, Backer J 1952 Multiple sclerosis in rural Norway: its geographical and occupational incidence in relation to nutrition. New England Journal of Medicine 246: 721–728

239. Putnam T J 1935 Studies in multiple sclerosis IV: Encephalitis and sclerotic plaques produced by venular obstruction. Archives of Neurology and Psychiatry 33: 929–940

240. Sinclair H M 1956 Deficiency of essential fatty acids and atherosclerosis, et cetera. Lancet 1: 381–383

241. Allen I V, McKeown S E 1979 A histological, histochemical and biochemical study of the histologically normal white matter in multiple sclerosis. Journal of the Neurological Sciences 41: 81–91

242. Baker R W R, Thompson R H S, Zilkha K J 1963 Fatty acid composition of brain lecthins in multiple sclerosis. Lancet 1: 26–27

243. Gerstl B, Tavastjerna M G, Hayman R B, Eng L F, Smith J K 1965 Alterations in myelin fatty acids and plasmalogens in multiple sclerosis. Annals of the New York Academy of Sciences 122: 405–416

244. Arnetoli G, Pazzagli A, Amaducci L 1969 Fatty acid and aldehyde changes in choline- and ethanolamine-containing phospholipids in the white matter of multiple sclerosis brains. Journal of Neurochemistry 16: 461–463

245. Alling C, Vanier M-T, Svennerholm L 1971 Lipid alterations in apparently normal white matter in multiple sclerosis. Brain Research 35: 325–336

246. Baker R W R, Thompson R H S, Zilkha K J 1964 Serum fatty acids in multiple sclerosis. Journal of Neurology, Neurosurgery and Psychiatry 27: 408–414

247. Baker R W R, Thompson R H S, Zilkha K J 1966 Changes in the amounts of linoleic acid in the serum of patients with multiple sclerosis. Journal of Neurology, Neurosurgery and Psychiatry 29: 95–98

248. Tichy J, Vymazal J, Michalec C 1969 Serum lipoproteins, cholesterol esters and phospholipids in multiple sclerosis. Acta Neurologica Scandinavica 45: 32–40

249. Love W C, Reynolds M, Cashel A, Callaghan N 1973 Fatty acid patterns of serum lipids in multiple sclerosis and other diseases. Biochemical Society Transactions 1: 141–143

250. Wolfgram F, Myers L, Ellison G, Knipprath W 1975 Serum linoleic acid in multiple sclerosis. Neurology 25: 786–788

251. Fisher M, Johnson M H, Natale A M, Levine O H 1987 Linoleic acid levels in white blood cells, platelets and serum of multiple sclerosis patients. Acta Neurologica Scandinavica 76: 241–245

252. Gul S, Smith A D, Thompson R H S, Wright H P, Zilkha K J 1970 Fatty acid composition of phospholipids from platelets and erythrocytes in multiple sclerosis. Journal of Neurology, Neurosurgery and Psychiatry 33: 506–510

253. Thompson R H S 1966 A biochemical approach to the problem of multiple sclerosis. Proceedings of the Royal Society of Medicine 59: 269–276

254. Belin J, Pettet N, Smith A D, Thompson R H S, Zilkha K J 1971 Linoleate metabolism in multiple sclerosis. Journal of Neurology, Neurosurgery and Psychiatry 34: 25–29

255. Lange M S, Shiner M 1976 Small-bowel abnormalities in multiple sclerosis. Lancet 2: 1319–1322

256. Bateson M C, Hopwood D, MacGillivray J B 1979 Jejunal morphology in multiple sclerosis. Lancet 1: 1108–1110

257. Mertin J, Meade C J 1977 Relevance of fatty acids in multiple sclerosis. British Medical Bulletin 33: 67–71

258. Swank R L 1953 Treatment of multiple sclerosis with low fat diet. Archives of Neurology and Psychiatry 91–103

259. Swank R L 1970 Multiple sclerosis: twenty years on a low fat diet. Archives of Neurology 23: 460–474

260. Swank R L, Pullen M 1972 The multiple sclerosis diet book. Doubleday, New York

261. Millar J H D, Zilkha K J, Langman M J S et al 1973 Double-blind trial of linoleate supplementation of the diet in multiple sclerosis. British Medical Journal 1: 765–768

262. Bates D, Fawcett D R W, Shaw D A, Weightman D 1977 Trial of polyunsaturated fatty acids in non-relapsing multiple sclerosis. British Medical Journal 2: 932–933

263. Paty D W, Cousin H K, Read S, Adlakha K 1978 Linoleic acid in multiple sclerosis: failure to show any therapeutic benefit. Acta Neurologica Scandinavica 58: 53–58

264. Bates D, Fawcett D R W, Shaw D A, Weightman D 1978 Polyunsaturated fatty acids in treatment of acute remitting multiple sclerosis. British Medical Journal 2: 1390–1391

265. Dworkin R H, Bates D, Millar J H D, Paty D W 1984 Linoleic acid and multiple sclerosis: a reanalysis of three double-blind trials. Neurology 34: 1441–1445

266. Bates D, Cartlidge N E F, French J M et al 1989 A double-blind controlled trial of long chain n-3 polyunsaturated fatty acids in the treatment of multiple sclerosis. Journal of Neurology, Neurosurgery and Psychiatry 52: 18–22

267. Shatin R 1964 Multiple sclerosis and geography: new interpretation of epidemiological observations. Neurology 14: 338–344

268. McDougall R 1973 No bed of roses. World Medicine 8: 89–99

269. Matheson N 1974 Multiple sclerosis and diet. Lancet 2: 831

270. Fantelli F J, Mitsumoto H, Sebek B A 1978 Multiple sclerosis and malabsorption. Lancet 1: 1039–1040

271. Cook A W, Gupta J K, Pertschuk, Nidzgorski F 1978 Multiple sclerosis and malabsorption. Lancet 1: 1366

272. Jellinek E H 1974 Multiple sclerosis and diet. Lancet 2: 1006

273. Liversedge L A 1975 In: Davison A N, Humphrey J H, Liversedge L A, McDonald W I, Porterfield J S (eds) Multiple sclerosis research. HMSO, London, pp 236–237

274. Miller H, Simpson C A, Yeates W K 1965 Bladder dysfunction in multiple sclerosis. British Medical Journal 1: 1265–1269

275. Bradley W E, Rockswold G L, Timm G W, Scott F B 1976 Neurology of micturition. Journal of Urology 115: 481–486

276. Blaivas J G 1980 Management of bladder dysfunction in multiple sclerosis. Neurology 30, 7 (2): 12–18

277. Anderson J·T, Bradley W E 1976 Abnormalities of detrusor and sphincter function in multiple sclerosis. British Journal of Urology 46: 193–198

278. Blaivas J G, Labib K B, Michalik S J, Zayed A A H 1980 Cystometric response to propantheline in detrusor hyperreflexia: therapeutic considerations. Journal of Urology 124: 259–262

279. Schoenberg H W, Gutrich J, Banno J 1979 Urodynamic patterns in multiple sclerosis. Journal of Urology 122: 648–650

280. Abrahamson A S 1983 Neurogenic bladder: a guide to evaluation and management. Archives of Physical Medicine and Rehabilitation 64: 6–10

281. Blaivas J G, Holland N J, Giesser B, LaRocca N, Madonna M, Scheinberg L 1984 Multiple sclerosis bladder. Studies on care. Annals of the New York Academy of Sciences 436: 328–345

282. Hebjørn S 1977 Treatment of detrusor hyperreflexia in multiple sclerosis. Urologia Internationalis 32: 209–217

283. Hebjørn S, Walter S 1978 Treatment of female incontinence with emepromium bromide. Urologia Internationalis 33: 120–124

284. Hilton P, Hertogs K, Stanton S L 1983 The use of desmopressin (DDAVP) for nocturia in women with multiple sclerosis. Journal of Neurology, Neurosurgery and Psychiatry 46: 854–855

285. Lapides J, Diokno A C, Silber S J, Lowe B S 1972 Clean, intermittent self-catheterisation in the treatment of urinary tract disease. Journal of Urology 197: 184–187

286. Lapides J, Diokno A C, Lowe B S, Kalish M D 1974 Follow up on unsterile intermittent self-catheterisation. Journal of Urology 111: 184–187

287. Warren J W, Muncie H L, Bergquist E J, Hoopes J M 1981 Sequelae and management of urinary infection in patients requiring chronic catheterisation. Journal of Urology 125: 1–8

288. Jakobsen B E, Pedersen E, Grynderup V 1973 Bladder neck resection in multiple sclerosis. Urologia Internationalis 28: 109–120

289. Desmond A D, Shuttleworth K E D 1977 The results of urinary diversion in multiple sclerosis. British Journal of Urology 49: 495–502

290. Toczek S K, McCullough D C, Gargour G W, Kachman R, Baker R, Luessenko A J 1975 Selective sacral rootlet rhizotomy for hypertonic neurogenic bladder. Journal of Neurosurgery 42: 567–574

291. Torrens M J, Griffith H B 1974 The control of the uninhibited bladder by selective sacral neurectomy. British Journal of Urology 46: 639–644

292. Bradley W E, Timm G W, Chou S N 1971 A decade of experience with electronic stimulation of the micturition reflex. Urologica Internationalis 26: 283–303

293. Nathan P 1977 Emptying the paralysed bladder. Lancet 1: 377

294. Medaer L, Kovacs L 1978 Vibration-assisted bladder emptying in multiple sclerosis. Lancet 1: 768–769

295. Lilius H G, Valtonene E J, Wikstrom J 1976 Sexual problems in patients suffering from multiple sclerosis. Journal of Chronic Diseases 29: 643–647

296. Vas C J 1969 Sexual impotence and some autonomic disturbances in men with multiple sclerosis. Acta Neurologica Scandinavica 45: 166–182

297. Kirkeby H J, Poulsen E U, Petersen T, Dørup J 1988 Erectile impotence in multiple sclerosis. Neurology 38: 1366–1371

298. Scott F B, Byrd G J, Karacan I, Olsson P, Beutler L E, Attia S L 1979 Erectile impotence treated with an implantable, inflatable prosthesis. Journal of the American Medical Association 241: 2609–2612

299. Massey E W, Pleet A B 1979 Penile prosthesis for impotence in multiple sclerosis. Annals of Neurology 6: 451–453

300. Sidi A A, Cameron J S, Duffy L M, Lange P H 1986 Intracavernous drug-induced erections in the management of male erectile dysfunction: experience with 100 patients. Journal of Urology 135: 704–706

301. Sabra A F, Hallett M, Sudarski L, Mullaly W 1982 Treatment of action tremor in multiple sclerosis with isoniazid. Neurology 32: 161–174

302. Hallett M, Lindsey J W, Adelstein B D, Riley P O 1985 Controlled trial of isoniazid therapy for severe postural cerebellar tremor in multiple sclerosis. Neurology 35: 1374–1377

303. Morrow J, McDowell H, Ritchie C, Patterson V 1985 Isoniazid and action tremor in multiple sclerosis. Journal of Neurology, Neurosurgery and Psychiatry 48: 282–283

304. Francis D A, Grundy D, Heron J R 1986 The response to isoniazid of action tremor in multiple sclerosis and its assessment using polarised light. Journal of Neurology, Neurosurgery and Psychiatry 49: 87–89

305. Bozek C B, Kastrukoff L F, Wright J M, Perry T L, Larsen T A 1987 A controlled trial of isoniazid therapy for action tremor in multiple sclerosis. Journal of Neurology 234: 36–39

306. Sechi G P, Rosati G, Zuddas M et al 1988 Effects of carbamazepine on cerebellar tremor in multiple sclerosis. Abstracts of IFMSS meeting, Rome V/26

307. Hewer R L, Cooper R, Morgan M H 1972 An investigation into the value of treating intention tremor by weighting the affected limb. Brain 95: 579–590

308. Cooper I S 1960 Neurosurgical alleviation of intention tremor of multiple sclerosis and cerebellar disease. New England Journal of Medicine 263: 441–444

309. Broager B, Fog T 1962 Thalamotomy for the relief of intention tremor in multiple sclerosis. Acta Neurologica Scnadinavica 38 (suppl 3): 153–156

310. Hauptvogel H, Poser S, Orthner H, Roeder F 1975 Indikationen zur stereotaktischen Operation bei Patienten mit multiplen Sklerose. Journal of Neurology 210: 239–251

311. Samra K, Waltz J M, Riklan M, Koslow M, Cooper

I S 1970 Relief of intention tremor by thalamic surgery. Journal of Neurology, Neurosurgery and Psychiatry 33: 7–15

312. Laitinen L, Arsalo A, Hänninen A 1974 Combination of thalamotomy and longitudinal myelotomy in the treatment of multiple sclerosis. Acta Neurochirurgica suppl 21: 89–91

313. Kelly R E In: Vinken P J, Bruyn G W, Klawans H L, Koetsier J C (eds) Handbook of clinical neurology, Vol 47. Elsevier, Amsterdam, p 64

314. Speelman J D, van Manen J 1984 Stereotactic thalamotomy for the relief of intention tremor of multiple sclerosis. Journal of Neurology, Neurosurgery and Psychiatry 47: 596–599

315. Dimitrijevic M R, Nathan P W 1967 Studies of spasticity in man I: Some features of spasticity. Brain 90: 1–30

316. Matthews W B 1965 The action of chlorproethazine on spasticity. Brain 88: 1057–1064

317. Schwab R S 1964 Muscle relaxants. Practitioner 192: 104–108

318. Wilson L A, McKechnie A 1966 Oral diazepam in the treatment of spasticity in paraplegia: a double-blind trial and subsequent impressions. Scottish Medical Journal 11: 46–51

319. Jones R F, Burke D, Marosszeky J E, Gillies J D 1970 A new agent for the control of spasticity. Journal of Neurology, Neurosurgery and Psychiatry 33: 464–468

320. Burke D, Andrews C J, Knowles L 1971 The action of a GABA derivative in human spasticity. Journal of the Neurological Sciences 14: 199–208

321. Cartlidge N E F, Hudgson P, Weightman D 1974 A comparison of baclofen and diazepam in the treatment of spasticity. Journal of the Neurological Sciences 23: 17–24

322. From A, Heltberg A 1975 A double-blind trial with baclofen (Lioresal®) and diazepam in spasticity due to multiple sclerosis. Acta Neurologica Scandinavica 51: 158–166

323. Feldman R G, Kelly-Hayes M, Conomy J P, Foley J M 1978 Baclofen for spasticity in multiple sclerosis: double-blind crossover and three year study. Neurology 28: 1094–1098

324. Sawa G M, Paty D W 1979 The use of baclofen in treatment of spasticity in multiple sclerosis. Journal of the Neurological Sciences 6: 351–356

325. Hainaut K, Desmedt J E 1974 Effect of dantrolene sodium on calcium movements in single muscle fibres. Nature 252: 728–729

326. Mai J, Pedersen E 1979 Mode of action of dantrolene sodium in spasticity. Acta Neurologica Scandinavica 58: 309–316

327. Ladd H, Oist C, Jonsson B 1974 The effect of Dantrium® on spasticity in multiple sclerosis. Acta Neurologica Scandinavica 50: 397–408

328. Schmidt R T, Lee R H, Spehlemann R 1976 Comparison of dantrolene sodium and diazepam in the treatment of spasticity. Journal of Neurology, Neurosurgery and Psychiatry 39: 350–356

329. Rinne U K 1980 Tizanidine treatment of spasticity in multiple sclerosis and chronic myelopathy. Current Therapeutic Research 28: 827–836

330. Stein R, Nordal H J, Offedal S I, Slettebø M 1987 The treatment of spasticity in multiple sclerosis: a double-blind clinical trial of a new anti-spastic drug tizanidine compared with baclofen. Acta Neurologica Scandinavica 75: 190–194

331. Bass B, Weinshenker B, Rice G P A et al 1988 Tizanidine versus baclofen in the treatment of spasticity in patients with multiple sclerosis. Canadian Journal of Neurological Sciences 15: 15–19

332. Rudick R A, Breton D, Krall R L 1987 The GABA-agonist progabide for spasticity in multiple sclerosis. Archives of Neurology 44: 1033–1036

333. Penn R D, Kroin J S 1985 Continuous intrathecal baclofen for severe spasticity. Lancet 2: 125–127

334. Hankey G J, Stewart-Wynne E G, Perlman D 1986 Intrathecal baclofen for severe spasticity. Medical Journal of Australia 145: 465–466

335. Müller H, Zierski J, Dralle D, Börner U, Hoffman O 1987 The effect of intrathecal baclofen on electrical muscle activity in spasticity. Journal of Neurology 234: 348–352

336. Hankey G J, Stewart-Wynne G, Perlman D 1986 Intrathecal baclofen for severe spasticity. Medical Journal of Australia 147: 261

337. Ochs G, Struppler A, Meyerson B A et al 1989 Intrathecal baclofen for long-term treatment of spasticity: a multicentre study. Journal of Neurology, Neurosurgery and Psychiatry 52: 933–939

338. Jones R F, Anthony M, Torda T A, Poulos C 1988 Epidural baclofen for intractable spasticity. Lancet 1: 527

339. Platt G, Russell W R, Willison R G 1958 Flexion spasms and contractures in spinal cord disease. Lancet 1: 757–760

340. Reyes R L, Boothe R, Scorel F 1978 Management of leg contractures in multiple sclerosis. Current Therapeutic Research 23: 673–677

341. Maher R M 1955 Relief of pain in incurable cancer. Lancet 1: 18–20

342. Nathan P W 1959 Intrathecal phenol to relieve spasticity in paraplegia. Lancet 2: 1099–1102

343. Kelly R E, Gautier-Smith P C 1959 Intrathecal phenol in the treatment of reflex spasms and spasticity. Lancet 2: 1102–1105

344. Liversedge L A, Maher R M 1960 Use of phenol in relief of spasticity. British Medical Journal 2: 31

345. Khalili A A, Harmel M H, Forster S, Benton J G 1964 Management of spasticity by selective peripheral nerve block with dilute phenol solutions in clinical rehabilitation. Archives of Physical Medicine 45: 513–519

346. Tardieu G, Hariga J 1964 Traitement des raideurs musculaires d'origine cérébrale par infiltration d'alcool dilue: résultats e 500 injections. Archives Francaises de Pédiatrie 21: 25–41

347. Ellison G W, Mickey M R, Myers L W, Rose A S 1980 A pilot study of amantadine treatment of multiple sclerosis. In: Bauer H J, Poser S, Ritter G (eds) Progress in multiple sclerosis research. Springer, Berlin, pp 407–408

348. Murray T J 1985 Amantadine therapy for fatigue in multiple sclerosis. Canadian Journal of Neurological Sciences 12: 251–254

349. Rosenberg G A, Appenzeller O 1988 Amantadine, fatigue and multiple sclerosis. Archives of Neurology 45: 1104–1105

350. Russell W R 1976 Multiple sclerosis: control of the disease. Pergamon Press, Oxford

351. Burnfield A, Burnfield P 1978 Common psychological problems in multiple sclerosis. British Medical Journal 1: 1193–1194

352. Power P W, Sax D S 1978 The communication of information to the neurological patient: some implications for family coping. Journal of Chronic Diseases 31: 57–63

353. Scheinberg L, Kalb R C, La Rocca N G, Giesser B S, Slater R J, Poser C M 1984 The doctor-patient relationship in multiple sclerosis. In: Poser C M (ed) The diagnosis of multiple sclerosis. Thieme-Stratton, New York, pp 205–215

354. Gorman E, Rudd A, Ebers G C 1984 Giving the diagnosis. In: Poser C M (ed) The diagnosis of multiple sclerosis. Thieme-Stratton, New York, pp 216–222

355. Hartings M F, Parmou M M, Davis F A 1976 Group counselling of multiple sclerosis patients in a program of comprehensive care. Journal of Chronic Diseases 29: 65–73

Genetics and immunology

D. A. S. Compston

Pathology
and its implications

Ingrid Allen

10. Genetic susceptibility to multiple sclerosis

As a disease, multiple sclerosis is not evenly distributed with respect either to region, race, family or individual. As a biological process affecting the nervous system, there are parts which are commonly involved whereas others are spared and the lesions characteristically occur at random intervals. The factors which determine these epidemiological and biological patterns have only been defined to a very limited extent but the distribution of multiple sclerosis has provided many clues to its aetiology and pathogenesis. It was the observation by Charcot over 100 years ago that related individuals may both occasionally develop multiple sclerosis that stimulated studies documenting the frequency of multiplex families; anecdotal accounts were gradually replaced by epidemiologically more robust studies including the careful documentation of concordance rates for multiple sclerosis in twins.

The suggestion that the disease is more common in some parts of the world than others and that prevalence rates differ in ethnically related peoples depending on their location reinforced the idea, first proposed by Pierre Marie in the 1890s, that multiple sclerosis is triggered by infection; from that time a series of putative 'causes' has been proposed, generally reflecting current trends in infectious disease. Thus, in the 1890s bacteria were thought to cause multiple sclerosis whereas in the 1920s the spirochaete was the favoured candidate; the subsequent shift to a viral aetiology has been better sustained and in the last few years there has been a predictable interest in human retroviruses together with a re-run of the spirochaetal hypothesis. Biologists have not been slow to speculate about the mechanisms which could account for the anatomical distribution and temporal pattern of the disease; neuropathological observations and analyses of cerebrospinal fluid have for many years orientated these thoughts along immunological lines and a vast literature now exists documenting observations made in patients with multiple sclerosis and in animal models. Difficulties arise in assembling these into a coherent hypothesis for the pathogenesis of the disease, not least because many of the findings are conflicting or controversial, and it is often difficult to distinguish causative from epiphenomenal observations. This section of the book has two main parts: the first deals with the evidence for genetic susceptibility to multiple sclerosis and the second outlines an interpretation, not free from personal prejudice, on the sequence of events that leads to myelin damage.

GENETIC EPIDEMIOLOGY

The geographical distribution of multiple sclerosis

It may seem curious to open an account of genetic susceptibility to multiple sclerosis with comments on its geographical distribution. An earlier section (Chap. 1) has outlined the methods required to map accurately the frequency of the disease using statistics for prevalence, incidence or mortality and various pitfalls have been highlighted. Multiple sclerosis is common in northern Europe, north America and Australia but rare in the Orient, Asia, the Indian subcontinent, Africa and South America. It has been suggested that the distribution of the disease, varying with latitude, reflects the involvement of an environmental factor in the aetiology. It is however necessary to look critically at these observations since some observers take the view that the putative environmental factor is sufficient to explain the distribution of the disease to the exclusion of all other especially genetic aetiological forces.[1] Three examples have been selected to illustrate both the findings and the difficulties that arise in their interpretation. It is of course not necessary to take either view in isolation; as Davenport commented in 1922: 'there are internal conditions that inhibit and those that facilitate the development of the disease or the factors on which it depends'. This integrated hypothesis is further developed in the sections that follow.

In 1967 Dean[2] provided annual incidence, prevalence and mortality statistics for multiple sclerosis in white South African-born individuals and immigrants to South Africa; the age corrected frequency of the disease was highest in immigrants from Europe, lowest in Afrikaaners and intermediate in South African English both with respect to prevalence and incidence. The very influential finding was that the prevalence in Europeans migrating into South Africa at less than 14 years was $12.8/10^5$ compared with a rate of $50.8/10^5$ for immigrants overall and $66.1/10^5$ in 15–19 year-olds, leading to the reasonable conclusion that the absence of an environmental effect in South Africa protects these juvenile immigrants from developing the disease. These rates depended on 6 and 12 identified cases respectively in the two most informative groups; inaccurate ascertainment or diagnosis affecting only a few individuals would have significantly altered the conclusions of this study and at least a 10% error rate for classification is to be expected even in areas surveyed using more direct methods.[3] In fact, multiple sclerosis has since also been reported as occurring both in coloured South Africans[4] and in a black individual,[5] and an 8-fold increase in incidence has been reported for Afrikaaners.[6] Nevertheless, in a recent survey from Cape Town, the prevalence of multiple sclerosis was 57.5, 14.1, 10.9, and $3.0/10^5$ in immigrants, South African born English, Afrikaaners and pigmented people, respectively[7] suggesting that the pattern results from an interplay between racial differences in susceptibility and an unidentified environmental factor.

The effect of migration from a low to high risk

area has also been studied and the findings seem to implicate an environmental effect. The incidence for multiple sclerosis in the first generation children of West Indian immigrants to the United Kingdom approximates to that seen in other populations native to the United Kingdom and is markedly different from the rate observed in the parental generation both in the West Indies and northern Europe. But this conclusion is based on identifying only 16 cases in Londoners of West Indian origin over a 9-year period;[8] and particular difficulties will have arisen in determining the appropriate denominator for calculating these rates.

The most persuasive epidemiological findings relating to environmental causes of multiple sclerosis are provided by the demonstration of geographical trends in a small area where the disease has been surveyed serially using standardised methods in an ethnically stable population. In continental Australia a gradient, with increasing incidence, prevalence and mortality from multiple sclerosis through Queensland, western Australia, New South Wales and Tasmania was demonstrated in 1961[9] and recently confirmed.[10] As expected, there was a temporal trend resulting from differences in diagnostic criteria, clinical vigilance, improved survival and, in the case of New South Wales, differential immigration of young adults, a relatively high risk group. Since the people inhabiting these parts are all of northern European origin one reasonable conclusion is that environmental factors alone have determined these epidemiological patterns. Furthermore, a preliminary immmunogenetic analysis does not suggest that differential migration or other stratifications of the population at risk can account for this pattern.[11] In contrast to these studies, other observations indicate that the distribution of multiple sclerosis is largely determined by genetic factors.

Racial susceptibility to multiple sclerosis

The incidence and prevalence of multiple sclerosis have been higher in north-east Scotland and the Orkney Islands over a prolonged period than in all other parts of the world and there are regional trends in the distribution of the disease elsewhere in the United Kingdom;[12] difficulties arise in trying to interpret these patterns since the estimates are not all methodologically comparable. Three recent surveys confirm that at least in the southern part of the United Kingdom, the prevalence of multiple sclerosis is now more than $100/10^5$.[13-15] Nevertheless, there is a linear relationship between regional variations in the prevalence and the normal but geographically variable frequency of HLA DR2 — a serologicaelly-defined marker of susceptibility to the disease in most northern European populations,[12] the details of which are discussed below. It had previously been suggested that the prevalence of multiple sclerosis varies with the distribution in Scotland of Nordic but not of Celtic people.[16] Using the unusual approach of scanning the telephone directory for names beginning with Mac or Mc, the distribution of multiple sclerosis has recently been correlated with migration patterns to the south island of New Zealand.[17] Lastly, Ebers[18] has supplemented Davenport's earlier survey,[19] demonstrating that the distribution of multiple sclerosis in the United States of America matches the pattern of immigration from Scandinavia. Poser[20] has summarised this evidence and proposed that multiple sclerosis occurs most frequently where Vandals, Goths and Viking invaders settled from Scandinavia and Germany, and where further migrations occurred of these and local peoples with whom the Viking genes had been liberally shared. If this not altogether far-fetched idea is correct, it would be necessary to explain why there appears to be no documentary evidence for multiple sclerosis having occurred prior to the early part of the nineteenth century,[21] unless this susceptible population only encountered the appropriate environmental triggers in the last two centuries. Although none of these findings are definitive, taken together they make as good a case for genetic factors in the geographical distribution of multiple sclerosis as does the epidemiological evidence favouring an environmental effect.

The concept that genes having a high frequency in Nordic peoples and distributed throughout Europe, the New World and Australasia have determined the epidemiological patterns of multiple sclerosis, can be supplemented by evidence that other populations appear resistant to the disease irrespective of their geographical location. For these purposes it is necessary to ignore details of regional variation in prevalence or the possible significance of migration and to examine how common the disease is in racial groups irrespective of their location. No other race seems quite so vulnerable to multiple sclerosis as northern European caucasoids and there is evidence for especially high Fennoscandian susceptibility;[22] the genes conferring susceptibility may have been further concentrated in the normal population of the Orkney and Shetland Islands.[23] Conversely there are several examples of racial resistance to multiple sclerosis.

The facts relating to South Africa have already been discussed, pointing out that this resistance to multiple sclerosis is relatively preserved in American black West Indians, even though the disease is more commonly seen in the first generation offspring of West Indian immigrants to the United Kingdom.[8] Over and above the biases introduced by problems of case ascertainment and clinical vigilance, multiple sclerosis has been of legendary rarity in black Africans; clinicians experienced in the diagnosis have repeatedly observed that whilst Europeans resident in the African continent develop, or in some cases bring with them, multiple sclerosis this is almost never recognised in the native population.[20] Cases are now being reported and it seems likely that this represents a change in pattern rather than improved recognition. However, in areas where populations which are at high and low risk of multiple sclerosis are mixed, the disease does occur more commonly in black individuals and this is especially evident in the United States where the frequency of multiple sclerosis increases with known racial admixture of caucasian and black genes.[20,24]

Multiple sclerosis is seldom if ever diagnosed in American Indians, Lapps, Hutterites, Eskimos and in Hungarian gypsies,[20,25-27] groups in which comparisons have been made with peoples of ethnically different origin residing in the same geographical regions, but this list is not intended to be exhaustive and no doubt many other small communities exist in which multiple sclerosis would be rare if surveyed.

There is reasonably good evidence that orientals have much lower susceptibility to multiple sclerosis than caucasoids. Thus, the prevalence of the disease has been estimated at between 0.88–4/10[5] in Chinese and Japanese populations from Hong Kong, Taiwan, Korea, and Japan[28–30] and even though in many instances these are first estimates which may rise with time, rates obtained in Europe using comparable methods are many times higher. Japanese migrants to north America have a higher prevalence than other orientals,[31] but whether this reflects enhanced clinical vigilance in their identification or a genuine shift in incidence is uncertain. Multiple sclerosis occurs both in Ashkenazi and non-Ashkenazi Jews; Israel is one of the geographical regions where sufficient outward and inward migration has occurred to allow comparison of the relative contribution of environmental and genetic factors by comparing the frequency of multiple sclerosis in Jewish populations throughout the world. From an overall comparison it is clear that Jews are susceptible to multiple sclerosis even though variations in prevalence may have arisen depending on geographical location.[32]

Multiple sclerosis occurs in Arabs in a form that is clinically indistinquishable from other patients with the disease, but the prevalence is low. Studies from Jordan,[33] Iraq[34] and Kuwait[35] indicate that the disease has a prevalence of about 5/10[5], but comparisons of the same ethnic groups in areas where the indigenous population has a higher frequency of multiple sclerosis have not been performed, so that the contribution of genetic resistance to this low prevalence has yet to be established. Nevertheless, the probability is that Arabs are relatively resistant to multiple sclerosis. The disease occurs in Indians but the available evidence and the observations of local observers suggest that this may be more common in individuals from the north of India who are of Indo-European origin and in Parsis than in the southern Indian Tamils and Dravidians;[36,37] the existing prevalence studies suggest that, as a region, the Indian subcontinent represents a low prevalence zone but again the distinction of environmental from genetic influences on this pattern have yet to be established.

Although the available evidence indicates that multiple sclerosis is predominantly a disease of caucasians which has probably emerged in the last 200 years in response to an environmental trigger, it will be clear from this discussion that documenting the prevalence of the disease in one population in one place does not provide sufficient evidence on which to make firm judgements about racial susceptibility. What is needed is to study the same ethnic group in high and low prevalence zones and to assess the effect of migration.

Sex differences in susceptibility to multiple sclerosis

Differences in susceptibility to multiple sclerosis also exist within single ethnically homogenous populations. Apart from studies which have surveyed highly-selected populations of patients, multiple sclerosis is almost always found to be more common in females than males. The reported figures vary but a ratio of 2:1 F:M is usually found whatever the ethnic origin of the population being described.[38,39] There is a relationship between age of onset and sex; in childhood multiple sclerosis, the excess of females is no less marked[40] whereas it would be the experience of many clinicians that multiple sclerosis presenting in the 5th and 6th decades, in which the course is typically progressive from onset and the prognosis relatively poor, usually affects males. It is unusual for a genetic trait to be expressed more commonly in females: sex-linked disorders and some others perhaps arising from mitochondrial inheritance more commonly affect males, even though symptomatic female carriers are well described. It seems unlikely that there is primarily a genetic explanation for this finding; although it is possible that penetrance of a genetic trait is modified differently in males and females. Many other putatively auto-immune diseases are more common in females and although the reasons are not well understood, one interpretation is that this arises from interactions between endocrine factors and the immune system.

Familial multiple sclerosis

The second aspect of susceptibility to multiple sclerosis within one ethnic group is the tendency for the disease to occur in families. This has been the most influential observation in thinking about the genetics of multiple sclerosis and one which may yet prove the most reliable for determining the number and location of the genes which confer susceptibility to the disease. Following the original 19th century reports of familial multiple sclerosis, cases were reported sporadically in the literature so that by 1950 there were 188 examples described in 85 families.[41] It soon became clear that bias in the selection of informative families had to be eliminated by taking an epidemiological approach to the problem of genetic susceptibility. Pedigree analysis led to general speculation about the nature of susceptibility to the disease but rather than force an interpretation that clearly could not accommodate much conflicting information, the majority of investigators took the view that nurture was more important than nature in the aetiology of multiple sclerosis.

To some extent interpretation is still a matter of opinion but at least the facts which have to be accommodated are now clear. The basic observations are that multiple sclerosis does occur more commonly in relatives of affected patients than in the rest of the population. Usually only two individuals are affected and pedigrees with more cases are unusual; in fact serious consideration should be given to the possibility that the diagnosis is incorrect if multiple sclerosis is diagnosed in several relatives. The commonest relationship between affected individuals is sibship. Although it is convenient for the purposes of appreciating the size of the risk and for counselling to express the occurrence of familial multiple sclerosis as the number of index cases who have an affected relative — i.e. the prevalence of multiplex families — the observations are better expressed as the recurrence risk for individual categories of relative. This avoids difficulties arising from variation of family structure within populations and at the same time gives an indication of the chance that a particular relative will develop the disease. To take these two approaches separately, approximately 15% of patients are known to have an affected relative[42,43] whereas the highest recurrence risk is observed in siblings (5%). A definitive study has been carried out in British Columbia;[44] in this population-based survey 19.9% of index cases had an affected relative — this is a high but perhaps more reliable figure than some of the non-population based estimates, although it includes cases of 'possible MS'

which are usually excluded from other surveys. In this series, recurrence risks differed slightly depending on the sex of the relative and affected individual but overall, the highest risk was observed in siblings (4%), then parents (3%), children (2.5%), uncles, aunts and cousins (2%) and nephews and nieces (1.5%). These rates are age-adjusted and take into account the fact that clinical status cannot be defined accurately in many relatives by nature of their current age. If only the cases with definite or clinically definite multiple sclerosis are considered and the figures not adjusted for age, the data available from epidemiologically less reliable surveys,[45] give overall recurrence risks of 1.2%, 0.6% and 0.5% for siblings, parents and offspring respectively. The size of the problem can be appreciated by considering that the life-time risk of developing multiple sclerosis for any individual growing up in northern Europe is approximately 1:800 or 0.00125% and this may reduce to 1:20 for the female sibling of an affected woman.

However, others have claimed that the excess of females consistently observed in sporadic multiple sclerosis is not so obvious in the familial cases, especially those that have more than two affected individuals.[46] By this account, there is no increase in the recurrence risk within individual categories for male and female relatives and the sex ratio of unaffected offspring in patients with the disease does not differ from the normal population.[47] There is an increase in the number of like-sexed pairs of affected siblings or more distantly related doublets but not parent/child combinations. This finding is consistent with an interaction between gender and the genes that confer susceptibility to multiple sclerosis or their expression. In fact there are slightly more like- than unlike-sexed sibling pairs in the normal population and there will be a tendency for like-sexed siblings to share a closer environment than other partners. Sex concordance in siblings can be used in the assessment of any familial disease to identify interactions between environmental and genetic effects.[48]

These findings have practical importance in the management of individual cases. Young patients often ask for advice about pregnancy; several issues arise in this context, including the risk of increased disease activity and difficulties in coping with both young children and neurological disability (see pp. 109) but the issue of recurrence is often uppermost in patients' thoughts. The simple distinction needs to be made between the risk of having any affected relative (about 15%) and the risk to a particular individual. In general, a recurrence risk for children of 1–4% is regarded as acceptable by most patients, bearing in mind that almost a third will know from their own experience that the disease is not necessarily disabling and many others may have had the disease for a sufficiently short time not to have appreciated the day-to-day significance of a chronic neurological disorder. The difference in the risk for parents and offspring is surprising if genetic factors are primarily responsible for familial multiple sclerosis, but the observed rates in offspring are likely to be confounded by variable age at onset of the disease or its clinical expression, suggesting that the age-corrected risk (4%) may be the more accurate.

The fact that every category of relative has a recurrence risk of well under 10% more or less completely excludes the possibility that susceptibility arises from the effect of a single gene whatever its mode of inheritance; any other interpretation would require invoking a very considerable reduction in penetrance. However, the consistently higher recurrence risk in siblings than other relatives strongly suggests a recessive mode of inheritance for all or some of the genes that confer susceptibility to the disease.[45] Those who favour the view that the major aetiological factor in the development of multiple sclerosis is environmental legitimately point out that a shared environment could as easily account for the slight increase in cases amongst siblings. It is therefore necessary to consider the evidence available from twin studies in order further to judge the merits and demerits of the genetic case for familial multiple sclerosis.

Twin studies in patients with multiple sclerosis

There have been several studies of twins in which one of each pair is already known to have multiple sclerosis. Several of these studies have been criticised on the basis that the sample has been collected with a bias towards monozygotic pairs

who are concordant. The value of twin studies is that higher concordance in monozygotic than dizygotic pairs implies a genetic contribution to the aetiology — the greater the difference the more the contribution. The reason is simple: monozygotic twins are genetically identical; dizygotic twins are no more alike than any other pair of siblings. However, dizygotic twins are more likely than other siblings to have had a shared environmental exposure including simultaneous infection by the organisms that cause childhood exanthematous diseases, and this is particularly true for identical twins. Conversely, monozygotic twins rapidly cease to be genetically identical in some important respects; although the germ line is the same, somatic mutations occur during life involving genes which regulate and restrict immune responses, such as the T cell receptors, so that immunological behaviour is not necessarily the same in twins who are phenotypically identical. Because of the differences in methodology, the studies will briefly be described.

In 1951 Thums[49] identified 96 MS patients who had a living twin and he was able to study 13 monozygotic and 30 dizygotic pairs. One pair of monozygotic twins was concordant; all the dizygotic pairs were discordant. Methods for establishing zygosity and the precision with which multiple sclerosis was diagnosed were not discussed.

McKay & Myrianthopoulous[50] collected twin pairs by appeal through the news media and obtained a sample biased in favour of monozygotic pairs, like-sexed dizygotic twins and females, problems for which they tried to correct when presenting an 8-year follow-up of their study.[51] They found no difference in the concordance rate for multiple sclerosis in monozygotic (23% in 9 pairs) and dizygotic (21% in 29 pairs). 22% of cases had other affected relatives and these high-risk families were particularly common when monozygotic twins were concordant for multiple sclerosis. Of such families, 67% had additional cases, compared with 10% of families with monozygotic twins discordant for multiple sclerosis.

Cendrowski[52] found no concordance for multiple sclerosis in 3 dizygotic twin pairs identified in an epidemiological survey of 300 patients. He reviewed 13 previous studies and found that 35/234 (15%) dizygotic pairs were concordant for multiple sclerosis. In an earlier study he had found significantly higher concordance for multiple sclerosis in monozygotic twins (24/90; 27%) than in dizygotic pairs (11/85; 13%) but the methods of ascertainment were not population-based.

Williams et al[53] collected 12 monozygotic and 12 dizygotic twin pairs in which at least one individual had definite multiple sclerosis. The concordance rates for multiple sclerosis were 50% and 17% respectively. Although the method of ascertainment has been criticised, this study was the first to use laboratory markers as an index of subclinical disease in the seemingly unaffected partner of index cases. The presence of oligoclonal bands would not be regarded as diagnostic of multiple sclerosis, but it is nevertheless of importance that 4 monozygotic and 8 dizygotic unaffected twin partners had qualitative abnormalities of cerebrospinal fluid.[54] The authors also introduced an important age correction for their study showing that 2/3 monozygotic but none of the dizygotic pairs aged 50 years or more were concordant.

Heltberg & Holm[55] took advantage of the Danish registers of twins and of patients with multiple sclerosis to identify 47 twin pairs in which an affected individual with multiple sclerosis and the living co-twin were personally examined; 4/19 monozygotic and 1/28 dizygotic pairs were concordant. A more recent study from Scandinavia sought to establish the prevalence of multiple sclerosis using sickness insurance and hospital discharge registers; 11 monozygotic pairs were identified, one of which was concordant, whereas all 10 dizygotic pairs were discordant for the disease.[56]

Bobowick and colleagues[57] estimated the frequency of multiple sclerosis in 16 000 male twin pairs registered through military service and identified 16 affected individuals from 15 pairs; 9 sibships were examined and concordance was established in 1 monozygotic but none of the dizygotic pairs. The purpose of this survey was to identify epidemiological risk factors and a higher prevalence of trauma, infection, surgery, allergy and animal exposure was present in the affected than unaffected individuals.

Alperovitch[58] studied 54/116 twin pairs identified in a cohort of 7942 patients; only 1/14 monozygotic and 1/40 dizygotic pairs were concordant using clinical criteria.

Undoubtedly the most careful study was carried out in Canada and reported in 1986:[59] 27 monozygotic and 43 dizygotic pairs were identified from 5463 patients attending 10 multiple sclerosis clinics, thus approximating to a population-based study. The concordance rates were 26% and 2.3%, respectively, compared with a rate in 4582 siblings identified from 2 of these centres of 1.9%. These patients have since been investigated by magnetic resonance, revealing a high prevalence of imaging abnormalities in the clinically unaffected co-twins.

Therefore, although a clear difference has been demonstrated in concordance between the monozygotic and dizygotic pairs, even allowing for problems with ascertainment bias, certain questions remain unanswered; these include the absolute differences in concordance rate needed in order to derive an overall assessment of heritability, and perhaps most importantly whether there is a difference between the concordance rate in dizygotic twins and all other siblings; if this were conclusively demonstrated, the implication would be that environmental factors operate to increase the risk of multiple sclerosis in multiplex families; if not, genetic factors are likely to be the main determinant of familial multiple sclerosis.

MARKERS OF SUSCEPTIBILITY TO MULTIPLE SCLEROSIS

The problem of identifying genes which increase susceptibility to multiple sclerosis has been considered at various times during the last few decades in order to provide laboratory support for the evidence obtained using classical genetic methods. Although clues to the location of these genes have been provided, subsequent work has not substantiated some of the preliminary associations, such as that with blood groups. This situation changed in 1972 with the report of a relationship between the major histocompatibility antigen HLA A3 and multiple sclerosis.[60] A great deal of subsequent work has so far failed to provide a comprehensive explanation for susceptibility to the disease, but the importance of the histocompatibility system in altering thresholds for the development of multiple sclerosis is now accepted and this has more general implications for the pathogenesis of the disease.

The findings to be described, both with respect to genetic susceptibility and immunological abnormalities in patients with multiple sclerosis, require some understanding of the mechanism of immune response (see also Ch. 11).

The major histocompatibility complex (MHC)

Contact between cells involved in immune response is determined by cell surface proteins which are the products of linked histocompatibility genes. In man, these are encoded on the short arm of the 6th chromosome. There are 3 types of gene: class 1 (HLA — A, B and C); class 2 (HLA — DR, DQ and DP) and class 3 (some, but not all of the complement component genes). The structure and organisation of the HLA system has been worked out using three types of analysis serological cellular and molecular; classifications have changed rapidly and correlations between new findings and old observations have not always been made, adding difficulties to an inherently confusing topic. Much of the early work was done using serological techniques; antibodies that recognised class 1 or 2 products were used to detect these antigens on cell surfaces, usually by lysing the cell in the presence of complement. Cellular typing techniques were developed simultaneously which depended on the ability of cells from one individual to proliferate on contact with different class 2 antigens; several refinements of this principle were adopted in determining the full range of these class 2 antigens, but difficulties arose in correlating the antigens defined by the serological and cellular techniques.

Most recently, molecular techniques have been used to define the structure and organisation of the HLA system by DNA restriction fragment length polymorphism (RFLP) analysis, gene cloning and sequencing. DNA is extracted from whole blood, cut with a panel of restriction enzymes which snip the genomic DNA at preferential sites — usually affecting introns, i.e. those parts of the genome which are not expressed as gene products — after which the pieces are separated by electrophoresis. Individual fragments of interest can be highlighted by hybridisation to a radio-labelled sequence which is complementary to the genomic fragment; in gene jargon this is called a probe. There is normal variation in the distribution of these restriction sites which is inherited in a predictable manner and so can be used to type individuals within a family. Because DNA is cut at different places depending on the distribution of the restriction sites, the length of individual fragments, and hence their position on electrophoretic gels, also differs between individuals. In most instances these variations occur in parts of the genome which do not code for important gene products and so they cannot be detected by phenotypic characteristics, but this does not detract from their usefulness as genetic markers. Needless to say, this field is moving fast and application of the techniques to multiple sclerosis has lagged behind the basic developments.

The structure of MHC molecules

Class 1 molecules consist of two associated chains inserted into the membrane of all nucleated cells.[61] The structure of one chain, beta 2 microglobulin, does not vary between individuals and is encoded outside the HLA system on chromosome 15. The other is the product of an HLA A, B or C locus gene; it has a portion within the cell, one that straddles the membrane and three extracellular parts. As might be expected, the two most exposed domains vary most in their structure, accounting for the polymorphisms that exist both at a genotypic and phenotypic level. Over fifty class 1 specificities have been defined serologically, one of which (HLA A3) gave rise to the original HLA association with multiple sclerosis.[60] Molecular analysis has not provided any new information on this weak association and in common with most other putatively auto-immune diseases, the stronger associations are with class 2 antigens. But the class 1 region should not altogether be ignored; some of the associations seen in patients with myasthenia are stronger with class 1 than 2 antigens and several new class 1 loci have been identified. Thus, whilst it has long been known that there are loci within the class 1 region that do not give rise to gene products (so called pseudogenes), three new class 1 genes that do encode detectable protein products have been described and the possibility arises that these will be informative with respect to disease susceptibility.[62]

The class 2 genes are more complicated. They also consist of paired alpha and beta chains both encoded within the HLA system and having cytoplasmic, transmembrane and extracellular domains, but unlike the class 1 products, each is variable in its structure.[63] Molecular analysis has identified complexities at two levels: firstly, more than one alpha or beta chain may exist for each locus and secondly, there are several genes which do not appear to encode protein products (or at any rate these have yet to be identified). Thus, for practical purposes, susceptibility has to be considered in terms of the genes which encode DR (one alpha and three beta), DP (two alpha and two beta) and DQ (one alpha and one beta), whereas the DO beta, DZ alpha, DX alpha, DX beta, and other pseudogenes of DR beta, DP alpha, and DP beta can thankfully be ignored. The situation is further simplified since most of the variation in structure which gives rise to the serologically-defined polymorphisms occurs because of amino acid substitutions in the outermost extracellular domain of DR beta, DQ beta, DP beta can thankfully be ignored. The situation is further simplified since most of the variation in structure which gives rise to the serologically-defined polymorphisms occurs because of amino acid substitutions in the outermost extracellular domain of DR beta, DQ beta, DP beta and DQ alpha so it is not surprising that DNA RFLP correlations exist with most but not all of the serologically-defined specificities. Difficulties arise in discriminating between some serotypes using RFLP methods but fortunately, these turn out not to be those of special interest in the context of multiple sclerosis. For example molecular analysis distinguishes 19 RFLP patterns within the DR beta 1 gene which correspond to 6 DR serotypes. DR beta 2 (characterised by 1.3, 1.6 and 12.5 kilobase fragments after digestion with the restriction enzyme Taq 1) associates with DR2; DR beta 2sh associates with the serological split of DR2, called DR2S.[64] Thus, the three main types of analysis have identified a range of polymorphisms, the definition of which is constantly being updated; the polymorphisms detected by serological, cellular and molecular methods are usually comparable since the same gene or its product is being recognised and precise comparisons can often be made between studies carried out by different investigators; however, some disease associations involve the use of local reagents which have not been widely evaluated, or depend on the identification of rare alleles recognised by only one of these techniques.

Population differences in the distribution of MHC gene products

Certain serological polymorphisms encoded by neighbouring loci tend to occur together more often than expected by chance — a phenomenon known as linkage disequilibrium which may depend upon evolutionary pressures for these antigens to remain associated because of complementary biological functions. In addition, HLA antigens are not evenly distributed amongst populations. Therefore there is an uneven distribution of haplotypes between populations and these stratifications can also be used to categorise individuals within geographically defined groups. HLA A1, B8 and DR3 is the most frequent haplotype in northern Europeans whereas A24 Dw52 and DR2 is more common in Japanese. There is a gradient from northern to southern Europe for the haplotype A3, B7 and DR2 which shows a higher frequency in Scandinavian, English, German and Swiss than in Celtic, Dutch, French, Italian, Spanish and Austrian populations.[65] These clines are of interest since they may provide clues to racial differences in disease susceptibility.

Linkage disequilibrium is also seen for genotypes detected by RFLP analysis. Thus, the serological specificities DR2 and DQw1 are in linkage disequilibrium; they correspond broadly to the antigen Dw2 defined by cellular typing techniques. As mentioned above the DR2 associated DNA RFLP is DR beta 2 and the DQw1 associated RFLPs are DQ beta 1b and DQ alpha 1b and these also are in linkage disequilibrium.[64] For this particular group of antigens the number of splits of the serologically-defined antigens revealed by molecular analysis is relatively small, unlike some other combinations; for example, DR6 is associated with 7 RFLPs. However, previous analysis has shown that DR2 can be separated into at least 5 subtypes by cellular typing using mixed lymphocyte cultures or related techniques and these do not each seem to represent different genotypes. Given the complexity of antigenic recognition that underlies proliferation in mixed lymphocyte cultures it is not surprising that functional tests of this kind, which presumably approximate better to what happens in vivo, provide more complex typing patterns than classification by genotype or phenotype. However, the cross-reactivity between antigens familiar to serologists is matched to some extent by shared molecular sequences, although in the case of DR2 the 1.3, 1.6 and 12.5 kilobase fragments which define DR beta 2 are not shared with other genotypes. DQ beta RFLPs cover the DQw2 and 3 serotypes but also define the serological splits evident from linkage disequilibrium with DR and Dw types; variation in the DQ alpha gene determines DQw1. Combining RFLP information from DR beta, DQ alpha and DQ beta analysis allows definition of most of the serological allotypes and their splits.

Associations between multiple sclerosis and MHC antigens

Population studies using serological markers

It is against this background that HLA associations with multiple sclerosis should be considered. The most consistent observation has been that multiple sclerosis is associated with HLA A3, B7, Dw2, DR2 and DQw1 in northern Europeans. The presence of any one of these antigens increases the risk that an individual will develop the disease by a factor of between 2.9 and 5.5. Associations with this group of antigens are also seen in northern European migrants to Australasia and North America and there is a relationship between one or other of these antigens and the disease in some other populations that have been studied including Greeks, Iranians, coloured South Africans and black Americans, even though the strength of the association weakens through southern Europe and the Mediterranean.[66] Allowing for population inter-

breeding, these observations are broadly consistent with the interpretation that the genes conferring susceptibility to multiple sclerosis — epitomised by HLA DR2 — are over-represented in northern Europeans and that this accounts for the high prevalence of multiple sclerosis both in this region and in areas populated by northern Europeans.

This simple hypothesis requires some modification. The prevalence of multiple sclerosis has been consistently higher in the Orkney Islands and north-east Scotland than anywhere else in the world[67] but there is no association with HLA A3, B7 or DR2. The reason is not that these antigens are any less frequent in patients with multiple sclerosis than affected individuals, but because DR2 has a very high normal frequency in north-east Scotland.[23,68] In fact, provisional estimates indicate that the distribution of multiple sclerosis in the United Kingdom correlates well with variations in the normal frequency of HLA DR2[12] (see above). But several findings clearly indicate that the presence of DR2, defined serologically, is not a sufficient explanation for lowering the threshold for susceptibility to multiple sclerosis. First, multiple sclerosis is rare in several populations where the normal frequency of DR2 is high: examples include Japanese, black Africans, American Indians and Hungarian gypsies.[69,70] Secondly, in some populations, multiple sclerosis shows no HLA association or it is linked to antigens other than DR2; thus in Sardinian patients,[71] where multiple sclerosis has a higher prevalence than many neighbouring parts of the Mediterranean, and in Jordanian Arabs[33] there is an association with DR4 even though DR2 has an increased frequency in Mediterranean Arabs,[35] and no very clear pattern emerges from studies of Indians,[72,73] Jews[74,75] and orientals[76,77] irrespective of their geographical location.

In view of this confusing pattern, immunogeneticists have turned to the more recently defined class 2 phenotypes in the hope that a clearer picture would emerge. In contrast to the distribution of DR2 in patients with multiple sclerosis and controls in north-east Scotland, there is a weak association with DQw1, defined serologically, suggesting that DQw1 may be a closer marker of susceptibility to the disease than DR2.[68] Conversely, there is a stronger association between multiple sclerosis and DR2 than DQw1 in south east Wales,[78] and in Mediterranean Arabs.[79] In a more recent study of caucasian patients from New Zealand,[80] DR2 was more strongly associated with multiple sclerosis than DQw1 which, as in the United Kingdom, had a higher normal frequency than DR2; also, although the frequency of DQw1 was similar in normal Maoris — in whom multiple sclerosis rarely occurs — and caucasians, DR2 was less commonly detected in the former group. Further evidence that DQw1 is also not the elusive multiple sclerosis susceptibility gene, is provided from the Sardinian study which showed an association with DQw3 but the relative risk was no higher than for DR4.[71]

Family studies

The alternative approach to demonstrating disease associations in groups of unrelated individuals is to study families in which more than one case of multiple sclerosis has occurred, assessing whether the disease segregates in association with a particular HLA marker. Difficulties arise in reconciling evidence on the relationship between the major histocompatibility complex and multiple sclerosis available from family and population studies. Unusual single pedigrees or series involving a very few informative families provide some evidence for HLA linkage to disease susceptibility. Hartung et al[81] described 3 families, one with 4 affected siblings; another had 3 definitely and one probably affected siblings and an unidentified neurological disease in 2 earlier generations; the last family had 3 affected siblings, 2 others with an undiagnosed neurological disorder, and 1 affected and a suspected case amongst the children of the index case. All affected individuals in these families who were studied typed positively for HLA DR2 and DQw1.

Even if results are pooled from many individually small family studies, evidence for linkage is too weak to maintain the strong associations seen in population studies. In all families published down to 1982, but not derived from a systematic sample,[82] observed rates of haplotype sharing were 85/103 (83%) in siblings, 11/11 in parent/offspring pairs, and 4/9 in cousins. These figures are not significantly different from the expected rates of 75%, 100%, 25% and 12.5% respectively. In families in which more than 2 individuals were affected (the minority), a common haplotype was shared by all cases in 15 (68%) compared with an expected rate of 35%. Previous analyses using published sources led to the conclusion that there is evidence for HLA-linked susceptibility to multiple sclerosis involving a gene situated 5–20 recombination units from the HLA-D locus;[83] others have extended this type of analysis to correct for estimated age of disease onset and genetic heterogeneity, concluding that there is tight linkage between susceptibility to multiple sclerosis and the HLA complex in families where HLA DR2 is associated with multiple sclerosis, whereas there is no evidence for linkage in the remaining families.[84] More recently it has been shown in families with only one affected person that DR2 and the extended haplotype on which it is located is over-represented in affected individuals by comparison with the paired parental haplotype not transmitted to that child suggesting that DR2 is itself a risk factor for multiple sclerosis and not merely a marker of increased susceptibility in the population.[85] Conversely the epidemiologically more secure strategy of working from a population base provides conflicting evidence for linkage; in a study involving 40 sibling pairs derived from 611 patients there was no difference in observed and expected rates of haplotype sharing[86] but HLA typing in familial cases of multiple sclerosis derived from a population base has also shown statistically significant segregation in association with the HLA DR2/DQw1/C2C/C4A3, C4B1 haplotype.[87]

Molecular genetic associations with multiple sclerosis

Given this tantalising but confusing picture it is understandable that attention should turn to molecular analysis in the expectation that a genotypic association would be identified that accounted for the different associations seen within and between populations. The picture that might have emerged is illustrated by findings in juvenile onset diabetes demonstrating that susceptibility occurs preferentially in individuals who do not have the amino acid aspartate at position 57 in the

DR beta chain.[88] This resistance to diabetes is seen irrespective of HLA phenotype although it is well established that juvenile diabetes is associated both with HLA DR3 and 4. It immediately raises questions about the fine structure of DR molecules and how this may alter depending on small variations in sequence at critical points in the molecule affecting its tertiary structure and function. The story for multiple sclerosis is less dramatic.

Using a cDNA DQ beta gene probe and the Eco RI restriction enzyme, Cohen et al[89] identified a RFLP which was found in DR2 positive normal individuals and French patients with multiple sclerosis but not those with diabetes. Whilst not providing a substantial new insight into the mechanism of susceptibility to multiple sclerosis, this study did highlight the fact that genotyping and phenotyping provide different segregation patterns in the context of multiple sclerosis. Marcadet et al[90] classified individuals with multiple sclerosis on the basis of typing patterns produced using a restriction enzyme, which cleaves DNA at a different site, and another DQ beta gene probe; one RFLP typing pattern associated with all DR1 and some DR2, DRw6 positive individuals (defined serologically) and the other matched the remaining DR2 and DRw6 positive cases; this geno type was positively associated with multiple sclerosis, the frequencies between cases and controls being 97% and 63% respectively. Subsequently, Olerup et al[91] carried out genomic HLA typing by RFLP analysis using DR beta and DQ beta cDNA probes. In a small series they found that the frequency of a DR beta fragment identified by digestion with Pvu II (designated P-DR beta II) and a DQ beta fragment identified by digestion with Bam HI (designated DQ beta II) carried a similar relative risk to each other and to DR2 defined serologically. The DR and DQ beta II fragments were shown to be in linkage disequilibrium both in patients with multiple sclerosis and controls. This study of Scandinavian patients does not therefore provide evidence for a stronger association with any genotypic or phenotypic DQ allele than with DR2 and similar findings have been reported from Australia.[92] Marrosu et al[72] found no disturbance in the distribution of fragments identified with a DR beta gene probe after digestion with Bam HI and Taq I, or with a DQ

beta probe using the restriction enzymes Bam HI, Taq 1, Hind III and Bg1 II in Sardinian patients with multiple sclerosis and controls.

There have been very few studies of class 2 antigen frequencies defined by primed lymphocyte cellular typing — the DP alleles — but Moen and colleagues described an association with DPw4 in French cases[93] and subsequently Odum et al[94] have reported a higher frequency of DPw4 (93%) in patients with multiple sclerosis from Sardinia than controls (72%), using both primed lymphocyte and restriction fragment length polymorphism typing. In this group, the relative risk for developing multiple sclerosis in the presence of DP4 was about the same as for DR2 but these two class 2 antigens were not in linkage disequilibrium and were therefore independently associated with susceptibility. Nevertheless, their combined presence conferred a higher risk than either antigen alone, implying synergy in their effects on susceptibility.

Evidence for a DQ genotypic association supplementing the previously reported DQ serological association has been provided by Heard et al[95] using a strategy in which DNA was first pooled from MS patients or controls, with and without DR2 and thereby making up 4 groups: this approach demonstrated that following digestion with the enzyme Msp 1 and using a full length DQ alpha probe, a 3.25 kilobase fragment was present in the pool of patients with DR2 which was absent in the corresponding group of controls. Hybridisation with a DR beta probe after digestion with a different enzyme also demonstrated a fragment which discriminated between DR2 positive cases and controls but all other enzyme/probe/DNA pool combinations were uninformative. This finding suggested that the fragment was not itself associated with DR2 and this was confirmed by studying individual patients drawn from the Grampian region of Scotland and northern Ireland. Using 3 fragments of known specificity, characterising respectively Dw2, DQw1 and DQw1.2, it was shown in the Scottish patients that both patients and controls typing serologically for DR2 were of the Dw2, DQw1.2 subtype but the 3.25 kb cluster, identified by a DQ alpha probe after Msp 1 digestion, discriminated DR2 positive cases and controls in Scotland and northern Ireland.

This fragment occurred rarely in the presence of DR2 but was associated with DRw8 and DR7; indeed it may be allelic to DQw1 which is associated with multiple sclerosis, at least in Scotland. This raises the possibility that this DQ alpha fragment may be inherited on the other haplotype from DR2/DQw1 thus representing a second susceptibility gene for multiple sclerosis.

If these findings are confirmed, it will be of considerable interest to determine whether a similar relationship exists in other geographical regions since the emergence of subsidiary genetic associations, in areas of high prevalence where susceptibility factors conferring an increased biological risk are over-represented in the normal population, is a prediction of the polygenic model of inheritance as applied to multiple sclerosis and other diseases. Under this hypothesis, risk factors — be they genetic or environmental — are presumed to make differing contributions to the development of disease and not to be evenly distributed. If one factor confers a high risk and is common in the population, prevalence of the disease will rise since the chance of the remaining events also occurring in individuals is relatively increased. However, the important risk factor may itself show an inappropriately weak association with the disease or none at all, since it is present in such a high proportion of the at-risk population. In these circumstances, other factors which make a relatively small contribution to overall susceptibility will tend to emerge in population-based disease association studies. Conversely, where all risk factors are infrequent in the population at risk, those which make the greatest contribution to disease susceptibility will be seen to be associated with the disease and more detailed studies will be needed to demonstrate the subsidiary associations.[79] Thus in Scotland, but not in areas of lower prevalence, no association is seen with DR2 but a weak association emerges with DQw1 and, with the recent evidence, the allelic fragment defined by the DQ beta probe after enzyme digestion with Msp 1. Thus, rather than being interpreted as conflicting evidence on susceptibility to multiple sclerosis, the associations with genes and gene products encoded within and outside the major histocompatibility complex, varying within and between populations or geographical regions, provide evidence in support of this hypothesis.

Other phenotypic and molecular associations with multiple sclerosis

Other polymorphic systems have also been studied in the attempt to identify genes, not necessarily linked to HLA, which confer susceptibility to multiple sclerosis, but to date no more definite relationship has been established than with the HLA DR/DQ region of the major histocompatibility complex. Various complement component polymorphisms are encoded within the major histocompatibility complex and at first it looked as if these might be acting as independent susceptibility gene products; originally the cluster of BfS alleles attracted attention in part through their linkage to DR2/Dw2/DQw1 in caucasians and subsequently through the claim that BfF alleles protect individuals from developing multiple sclerosis but not isolated episodes of demyelination.[96] Subsequently, no disturbance in the distribution of Bf alleles has been demonstrated in populations of patients with demyelination selected for extremes of severity.[69] Nevertheless, it remains likely that whatever mechanism underlies genetic susceptibility to multiple sclerosis, an increased risk is conferred by the presence of genes encoding the products which make up the extended haplotype A3/B7/DR2/DQw1/C4A4 and BfS.[87]

Two other polymorphic systems need to be considered as candidate loci for susceptibility to multiple sclerosis. Immunoglobulins consist of paired heavy and light chains. The heavy chains are made up of sections that vary in their structure, giving rise to the separate classes and subclasses of antibody together with their diversity of specificity. Other parts that are constant within and between individuals have slight structural alterations which account for the Gm allotypes. These serve as useful genetic markers but do not seem to confer differences in function. These Gm types and a further set of genes which determine the switch from synthesis of one antibody class to another during immune response are encoded on chromosome 14. The classification of Gm phenotype incorporates identification both of the variable region subclass (IgG 1, 2, 3, etc.) and the Gm allotype. Initially groups of Gm allotypes which appeared to increase or reduce the risk of multiple sclerosis were described[97–99] but the strength and specificity of these associations are not yet established. The finding reported most consistently has been an increase in G1m1, 17 and G3m21 but perhaps the most interesting finding is an interaction between HLA class 1 and 2 alleles and Gm allotype in determining susceptibility and resistance to multiple sclerosis.[100,101] Restriction fragment length polymorphisms have been used to extend the range of Gm allotypes. Gaiser et al[102] digested DNA with BstII and found a 5.9 kb band to be less common, and a 4.1 kb band more frequent in patients with multiple sclerosis from France and North America than controls. These bands correlated with the presence of the G3m21 and G3m5, 10, 11, 13 haplotypes respectively; the strength of these molecular associations was similar but their specificity different from the phenotypic studies. As with the study of Bf associations, inconsistency of results may have arisen from sampling errors but geographical and racial differences in the distribution of these antigens may also be important.

Knowledge has accumulated rapidly in the last few years on the genetic organisation of the receptor on T cells which accounts in part for diversity of cellular immune responses. Four separate T cell receptor chains have been identified which seem to associate in pairs — alpha with beta, gamma with delta — and each pairwise combination identifies T cells at different stages in development.[103] The fine structure of these chains is variable and arises from recombinations of the basic genetic units occurring during development as the molecules are assembled. An important consequence of this reassembly is that monozygotic twins are not identical with respect to structures which play a vital role in the development of immune response.

Attempts to demonstrate associations between T cell receptor gene rearrangements and susceptibility to multiple sclerosis have not been particularly informative; Heard et al[95] failed to demonstrate differences in polymorphisms between cases and controls with gene probes for the T cell receptor alpha and beta chains using pooled

DNA and others have also failed in this respect using a variety of enzymes and cDNA probes against the T cell receptor alpha and beta chains. For example, Oksenberg et al[104] defined several restriction fragment length polymorphisms using a beta chain probe and enzyme digestion with Kpn I and Bgl II, and an alpha chain gene probe with Taq I; dominant inheritance was established in family studies and all sections of the two chains were detected by these reagents but there were no differences in the frequency of these fragments in patients with multiple sclerosis or myasthenia gravis compared with a panel of normal controls. But more encouraging results have recently been reported; first, using a panel of cDNA probes directed against variable parts of the T cell receptor beta chain, Beall and colleagues have shown a disturbance in the distribution of restriction fragment length polymorphism haplotypes by comparison both with random and DR2 positive normal controls.[105] Secondly, Seboun et al have demonstrated an abnormal pattern of T cell receptor alpha chain gene rearrangements in patients with multiple sclerosis using a different combination of restriction enzymes and molecular probes.[106]

The mechanism of genetic susceptibility to multiple sclerosis

Despite this imperfect understanding of the genetic basis of susceptibility to multiple sclerosis, attempts have been made from an early stage to interpret the associations in terms of immunological phenomena. The approach has been to compare a given abnormality previously shown to be characteristic of the disease in cases and controls, grouped according to whether or not individuals possess the marker under consideration. No consistent pattern of altered immune reactivity has emerged from these studies. In a comparison of serological and historical evidence for viral exposure in 177 cases and 164 controls,[107] differences in age of infection and/or antibody titre to rubella, measles, mumps and parainfluenza 1 were identified, especially in comparisons of DR2 positive cases and controls. HLA DR3 positive patients had increased titres of varicella zoster and adenovirus antibodies; this antigen has previously been associated with a history of upper respiratory tract infections in childhood.[108]

In a subsequent study, non-specific tests of immune function were correlated with serological evidence for exposure to 15 infectious agents in cases and controls, including those having close contact with the patients themselves. Antibody titres against none of the infective agents selected for study correlated with changes in circulating CD8 cells, but periodic reductions in this lymphocyte subpopulation did correlate with the presence of HLA DR2.[109] Perhaps the best explanation for these observations is that they provide very indirect evidence for an interplay between environmental and genetic factors in determining the immunological milieu of patients with multiple sclerosis. A similar approach has been taken using molecular markers. Jacobsen et al[110] identified an HLA DR2/Dw2 associated RFLP segregating with expression of one of two distinct DR beta polypeptide chains (DR beta 2) and correlating with HLA class 2 restriction of T4 positive measles virus-specific cytotoxic T cell clones.

Alterations in the concentration of complement components occur in the cerebrospinal fluid of patients with multiple sclerosis, some of which have been correlated with the presence of major histocompatibility alleles; these include associations between low levels of C2, C3, total haemolytic activity and factor B in a subgroup of patients with multiple sclerosis, abnormalities that were linked to HLA B18 and BfF1.[111]

Susceptibility to multiple sclerosis and the clinical course

It has always proved attractive to consider that the extreme variation in the clinical course of multiple sclerosis depends on heterogeneity in the pathogenesis which in turn may result from differences in genetic susceptibility. The question is often asked whether multiple sclerosis, as presently defined, is more than one disease. Several authors have claimed that more severe multiple sclerosis occurs in individuals who are HLA DR2 positive and this has been extended to the suggestion that one form of the disease is characterised by oligoclonal bands or increased intrathecal IgG

synthesis, severity, early onset and the presence of DR2/Dw2.[112] Conversely, it has been claimed that a milder form of the disease occurs in DR3 positive cases[113] but this finding has been refuted by others.[114] There are sporadic reports — none confirmed — claiming that less severe disease is seen in individuals with A25/B18,[115] that HLA A3 is associated with an increased relapse rate which is modified by treatment with azathioprine[116] and that HLA DR3 cases are less responsive to this drug than DR2 positive cases.[113] But most investigators have been unable to confirm reports of an association between HLA antigens and severity or category of disease.[69,117]

Olerup and colleagues[118] have applied molecular techniques to this problem and found a pattern of restriction fragment length polymorphisms, following digestion with Taq 1 and hybridisation with a DQ beta gene probe, that characterised patients in whom multiple sclerosis had been progressive from onset. This pattern was not detected in cases with relapsing disease and occurred rarely in normal controls. More recently, Heard et al[95] found a normal distribution of the DQ alpha polymorphism in patients with multiple sclerosis with respect to disease severity. The hypothesis that multiple sclerosis is more than one disease and that genetic factors are instrumental in determining the course may turn out to be correct but the complex interplay between genetic, environmental and other factors involved in disease activity and clinical disability makes it likely that more powerful methods of analysis will be needed other than simply correlating outcome with the presence or absence of a single genetic marker.

CONCLUDING REMARKS

Studies on the genetics of multiple sclerosis, using classical techniques, have ranged from determining patterns of racial susceptibility, recurrence risks in relatives of affected individuals, concordance rates in twins and the distribution of the disease. With the availability of serological and molecular techniques for studying genetic polymorphisms, the emphasis has been on identifying genes and their products which confer susceptibility. The opportunity now exists to define the number and location of these genes using a combined clinical and molecular genetic approach. The incomplete and heterogenous associations demonstrated so far probably reflect the multifactorial and polygenic nature of multiple sclerosis. The power of molecular genetics is such that once the genes have been mapped, the mechanism whereby they confer susceptibility will become clear; these genes may be involved in determining the structure and function of myelinated axons in the central nervous system, the complex interactions of immune response and unexpected facets of this difficult disease.

REFERENCES

1. Kurtzke J F 1987 Multiple sclerosis in twins. New England Journal of Medicine 317: 51
2. Dean G 1967 Annual incidence, prevalence and mortality of multiple sclerosis in white South African born and in white immigrants to South Africa. British Medical Journal 2: 724–730
3. Hennessy A, Swingler R J, Compston D A S 1989 The incidence and mortality of multiple sclerosis in south east Wales. Journal of Neurology, Neurosurgery and Psychiatry 52: 1085–1089
4. Ames F R, Lou W S 1977 Multiple sclerosis in coloured South Africans. Journal of Neurology, Neurosurgery and Psychiatry 40: 729–735
5. Bhigjee A I 1987 Multiple sclerosis in a black patient. A case report. South African Medical Journal 72: 873–875
6. Rossman K D, Jacobs H A, Van der Merwe 1985 A new multiple sclerosis epidemic? South African Medical Journal 68: 162–163
7. Kies B (personal communication)
8. Elian M, Dean G 1987 Multiple sclerosis among the United Kingdom born children of immigrants from the West Indies. Journal of Neurology, Neurosurgery and Psychiatry 50: 327–332
9. McCall M G, Breareton T Le G, Dawson A, Millingen K, Sutherland J M, Acheson E D 1968 Frequency of multiple sclerosis in three Australian cities — Perth, Newcastle and Hobart. Journal of Neurology, Neurosurgery and Psychiatry 31: 1–9
10. Hammond S R, McLeod J G, Millingen K S et al 1988 The epidemiology of multiple sclerosis in three Australian cities: Perth, Newcastle and Hobart. Brain 111: 1–25
11. Hammond S R 1989 The epidemiology of multiple sclerosis in Australia. PhD Thesis, University of Sydney, pp 335–368
12. Swingler R J, Compston D A S 1986 The distribution of multiple sclerosis in the United Kingdom. Journal of Neurology, Neurosurgery and Psychiatry 49: 1115–1124
13. Swingler R J, Compston D A S 1988 The prevalence of multiple sclerosis in south east Wales. Journal of Neurology, Neurosurgery and Psychiatry 51: 1520–1524
14. Williams E S, McKeron R O 1986 Prevalence of multiple sclerosis in a south London borough. British Medical Journal 293: 237–239
15. Roberts M, Martin J P, McLellan D L 1989 Multiple sclerosis in the Southampton and S W Hampshire Health Authority. Journal of Neurology, Neurosurgery and Psychiatry 52: 1206–
16. Sutherland J M 1956 Observations on the prevalence of multiple sclerosis in northern Scotland 79: 635–654
17. Skegg D C G, Corwin P A, Craven R S, Malloch J A,

18. Pollock M 1987 Occurrence of multiple sclerosis in the north and south of New Zealand. Journal of Neurology, Neurosurgery and Psychiatry 50: 134–139
18. Ebers G C, Bulman D 1986 The geography of MS reflects genetic susceptibility. Neurology 36 (suppl 1) 108
19. Davenport C B 1922 Multiple sclerosis from the standpoint of geographic distribution and race. Archives of Neurology and Psychiatry 8: 51–58
20. Poser C M 1990 Multiple sclerosis in tropical and subtropical countries. In: Roman G, Toro G (eds) Tropical Neurology. CRC press, Florida
21. Compston D A S 1988 The 150th anniversary of the first depiction of the lesions of multiple sclerosis. Journal of Neurology, Neurosurgery and Psychiatry 51: 1249–1252
22. Kurtzke J F 1974 Further features of the Fennoscandian focus of multiple sclerosis. Acta Neurologica Scandinavica 50: 478–502
23. Compston D A S 1981 Multiple sclerosis in the Orkneys. Lancet 2: 98
24. Reed T 1969 Racial admixture in US blacks. Science 165: 762–768
25. Gronning M, Mellgren S 1985 MS in the two northern-most counties of Norway. Acta Neurologica Scandinavica 72: 321–327
26. Hader W J 1982 Prevalence of multiple sclerosis in Saskatoon. Canadian Medical Journal 127: 295–297
27. Pálffy G Y 1982 MS in Hungary including the gypsy population. In: Kuroiwa Y, Kurland L T (eds) Multiple sclerosis east and west. Karger, Basel, pp 149–158
28. Yu Y L, Woo E, Hawkins B R et al 1989 Multiple sclerosis amongst Chinese in Hong Kong. Brain 112: 1445–1467
29. Hung T P, Landsborough D, Shi M S 1976 Multiple sclerosis amongst Chinese in Taiwan. Journal of the Neurological Sciences 27: 459–484
30. Kuroiwa Y, Shibasaki H, Ikeda M 1983 Prevalence of multiple sclerosis and its north to south gradient in Japan. Neuroepidemiology 2: 62–69
31. Detels R, Visscher B, Malmgren R M et al 1977 Evidence for lower susceptibility to multiple sclerosis in Japanese-Americans. American Journal of Epidemiology 105: 303–310
32. Leibowitz U, Kahana E, Alter M 1973 The changing frequency of multiple sclerosis in Israel. Archives of Neurology 29: 107–110
33. Kurdi A, Ayesh I, Abdallat A et al 1977 Different B lymphocyte alloantigens associated with multiple sclerosis in Arabs and North Europeans. Lancet 1: 1123–1125
34. Hamdi T 1975 MS in Iraq. A clinical and geomedical survey. Journal of Postgraduate Medicine 21: 1–9
35. Al-Din A S N 1986 Multiple sclerosis in Kuwait;

clinical and epidemiological study. Journal of Neurology, Neurosurgery and Psychiatry 49: 928–931

36. Bharucha N E, Bharucha E P, Wadia N H et al 1988 Prevalence of multiple sclerosis in the Parsis of Bombay. Neurology 38: 727–729

37. Jain S, Maheshwari M C 1985 Multiple sclerosis; Indian experience in the last 30 years. Neuroepidemiology 4: 96–107

38. Weinshenker B G, Bass B, Rice D P A et al 1989 The natural history of multiple sclerosis; a geographically based study. 1: Clinical course and disability. Brain 112: 133–146

39. Confavreux C, Aimard D, Devic M 1980 Course and prognosis of multiple sclerosis assessed by the computerised data processing of 349 patients. Brain 103: 281–300

40. Duquette P, Murray T J, Pleines J et al 1987 Multiple sclerosis in childhood; clinical profile in 125 patients. Journal of Paediatrics 111: 359–363

41. Pratt R T C, Compston N D, McAlpine D 1951 The familial incidence of multiple sclerosis and its significance. Brain 74: 191–232

42. Ebers G C 1983 Genetic factors in multiple sclerosis. Neurologic Clinics 1: 645–654

43. Roberts D F, Bates D 1982 The genetic contribution to multiple sclerosis; evidence from north east England. Journal of the Neurological Sciences 54: 287–293

44. Sadovnick A D, Baird P A, Ward R H 1988 Multiple sclerosis; updated risks for relatives. American Journal of Medical Genetics 29: 533–541

45. Spielman R S, Nathanson N 1982 The genetics of susceptibility to multiple sclerosis. Epidemiologic Reviews 4: 46–65

46. Weitkemp L R 1983 Multiple sclerosis susceptibility. Interaction between sex and HLA. Archives of Neurology 40: 399–401

47. Alperovitch A, Feingold N 1981 Sex ratio in offspring of patients with multiple sclerosis. New England Journal of Medicine 305: 1157

48. Grufferman S, Barton J W, Eby N L 1987 Increased sex concordance of sibling pairs with Behçet's disease, Hodgkins disease, multiple sclerosis and sarcoidosis. American Journal of Epidemiology 126: 365–369

49. Thums K 1951 Einelige Zwillinge mit koncordanter multiplen Sklerose. Weiner Zeitschrift für Nervenheilkunde 4: 173–203

50. McKay R F, Myrianthopoulous N C 1958 Multiple sclerosis in twins and their relatives. Archives of Neurology 80: 667–674

51. McKay R F, Myrianthopoulous N C 1966 Multiple sclerosis in twins and their relatives. Final report. Archives of Neurology 15: 449–462

52. Cendrowski W S 1968 Multiple sclerosis; discordance of three dizygotic twin pairs. Journal of Medical Genetics 5: 266–268

53. Williams A, Eldridge R, McFarland H et al 1980 Multiple sclerosis in twins. Neurology 30: 1139–1147

54. Xu X–H, McFarlin D E 1984 Oligoclonal bands in CSF; twins with MS. Neurology 34: 769–774

55. Heltberg A, Holm N V 1982 Concordance in twins and recurrence in sibships in multiple sclerosis. Lancet 1: 1068

56. Kinnunen E, Koskenvuo M, Kaprio J, Aho K 1987 Multiple sclerosis in a nationwide series of twins. Neurology 37: 1627–1629

57. Bobowick A R, Kurtzke J F, Brody J A et al 1978 Twin study of multiple sclerosis; an epidemiologic enquiry. Neurology 28: 978–987

58. Alperovitch A 1989 Multiple sclerosis in twins — a French study. In: 5th ECTRIMS congress proceedings. Elsevier, Amsterdam (in press)

59. Ebers G C, Bulman D E, Sadovnick A D et al 1986 A population based study of multiple sclerosis in twins. New England Journal of Medicine 315: 1638–1642

60. Jersild C, Svejgaard A, Fog T 1972 HL-A antigens and multiple sclerosis. Lancet 1: 1240–1241

61. Strachan T 1987 Molecular genetics and polymorphism of class 1 HLA antigens. British Medical Bulletin 43: 1–14

62. Holmes N 1989 New HLA class 1 molecules. Immunology Today 10: 52–53

63. Strominger J L 1987 Structure of class 1 and class 2 HLA antigens. British Medical Bulletin 43: 81–93

64. Bidwell J 1988 DNA-RFLP analysis and genotyping of HLA-DR and DQ antigens. Immunology Today 9: 18–23

65. Bodmer J G, Kennedy L J, Lindsay J, Wasik A M 1987 Applications of serology and the ethnic distribution of 3 locus HLA haplotypes. British Medical Bulletin 43: 94–121

66. Compston D A S 1986 Genetic factors in the aetiology of multiple sclerosis. In: McDonald W I, Silberberg D (eds) Multiple Sclerosis: BIMR Neurology 6. Butterworths, London, pp 56–73

67. Cook S D, Cromarty M B, Tapp W et al 1985 Declining incidence of multiple sclerosis in the Orkney Islands. Neurology 35: 545–551

68. Francis D A, Batchelor J R, McDonald W I et al 1987 Multiple sclerosis in north east Scotland; an association with HL-A-DQw1. Brain 110: 181–196

69. Troup G M, Schanfield M S, Singaraju C H et al 1982 The study of HLA alloantigens of the Navajo Indians of North America. Tissue antigens 20: 339–351

70. Gyódi E, Tauszik T, Petranyi G et al 1981 The HLA antigen distribution in the gypsy population in Hungary. Tissue Antigens 18: 1–12

71. Marrosu M G, Muntoni F, Murru M R et al 1988 Sardinian multiple sclerosis is associated with HLA-DR4. Neurology 38: 1749–1753

72. Wadia N H, Trikanad V S, Krishnaswamy P R 1981 HLA antigens in multiple sclerosis amongst Indians. Journal of Neurology, Neurosurgery and Psychiatry 44: 849–851

73. Trikinnad V S, Wadia N H, Krishnaswamy P R 1982 Multiple sclerosis and HLA B12 in Parsi and non-Parsi Indians. A clarification. Tissue Antigens 19: 155–157

74. Brautbar C, Cowen I, Kahana E et al 1977 Histocompatibility determinants in Israeli Jewish patients with multiple sclerosis. Tissue Antigens 10: 291–302

75. Brautbar C, Amar A, Cowen I et al 1982 Histocompatability (HLA) antigens and multiple sclerosis in Israelis. Israeli Journal of Medical Science 18: 631–634

76. Naito S, Tabira T, Kuroiwa Y 1982 HLA studies of multiple sclerosis in Japan. In: Kuroiwa Y, Kurland L T (eds) Multiple sclerosis east and west. Karger, Basel, pp 215–222

77. Hawkins B R, Yu Y L, Woo E, Huang C Y 1988 No apparent association between HLA and multiple

sclerosis in southern Chinese. Journal of Neurology, Neurosurgery and Psychiatry 51: 443–445

78. Swingler R J, Kirk P F, Darke C, Compston D A S 1987 HLA and multiple sclerosis in south east Wales. Journal of Neurology, Neurosurgery and Psychiatry 50: 1153–1155

79. Al–Din A S N, Al–Saffa R M, Siboo R, Behbehani K 1986 Association between HLA-region epitopes and multiple sclerosis in Arabs. Tissue Antigens 27: 196–200

80. Miller D H, Hornabrook R W, Dagger J, Fong R 1989 Class II HLA antigens in multiple sclerosis. Journal of Neurology, Neurosurgery and Psychiatry 52: 575–577

81. Hartung H–P, Will R G, Francis D et al 1988 Familial multiple sclerosis. Journal of the Neurological Sciences 83: 259–268

82. Compston D A S, Howard S V 1982 HLA typing in multiple sclerosis. Lancet 2: 661

83. Stewart G J, McLeod J G, Basten A, Bashir H V 1981 HLA family studies in multiple sclerosis; a common gene dominantly expressed. Human Immunology 3: 13–29

84. Haile R W, Iselius L, Hodge S E 1981 et al Segregation and linkage analysis of 40 multiplex multiple sclerosis families. Human Heredity 31: 252–258

85. Hauser S L, Fleishnick E, Weiner H L et al 1989 Extended major histocompatability complex haplotypes in patients with multiple sclerosis. Neurology 39: 275–277

86. Ebers G C, Paty D W, Stiller C R 1982 et al HLA typing in multiple sclerosis sibling pairs. Lancet 2: 88–90

87. Francis D A, McDonald W I, Batchelor J R 1987 HLA determinants in familial multiple sclerosis: a study from the Grampian region of Scotland. Tissue Antigens 29: 7–12

88. Todd J A, Bell J I, McDevitt H O 1987 HLA-DQ beta gene contributes to susceptibility and resistance to insulin dependent diabetes mellitus. Nature 329: 599–604

89. Cohen D, Cohen O, Marcadet A et al 1984 Class 2 HLA-DC beta chain DNA restriction fragments differentiate among HLA-DR2 individuals in insulin dependent diabetes and multiple sclerosis. Proceedings of the National Academy of Sciences of the USA 81: 1774–1778

90. Marcadet A, Massart C, Semana G et al 1985 Association of Class 2 HLA DQ beta chain DNA restriction fragments with multiple sclerosis. Immunogenetics 22: 93–96

91. Olerup O, Carlsson B, Wallin J et al 1987 Genomic HLA typing by RFLP analysis using DR beta and DQ beta cDNA probes reveals normal DR-DQ linkages in patients with multiple sclerosis. Tissue Antigens 30: 135–138

92. Reid M A, Buhler M, Stewart G J, Sergeantson S W 1986 HLA Class 2 RFLPs in multiple sclerosis. Abstract, 6th International Congress of Immunology, Toronto, Canada

93. Moen T, Stein R, Bratlie A, Bondervik E 1984 Distribution of HLA-SE antigens in multiple sclerosis. Tissue Antigens 24: 126–127

94. Odum N, Hyldig–Nielsen G J, Morling N et al 1988 HLA-DP antigens are involved in the susceptibility to multiple sclerosis. Tissue Antigens 31: 235–237

95. Heard R N S, Cullen C, Middleton D et al 1989 An allelic cluster of DQ alpha restriction fragments is associated with multiple sclerosis; evidence that a second haplotype may influence disease susceptibility. Human Immunology 25: 111–123

96. Fielder A H, Batchelor J R, Vakarelis B N, Compston DAS, McDonald WI 1981 Optic neuritis in multiple sclerosis; do factor B alleles influence progression of disease? Lancet 2: 1246–1248

97. Pandey J R, Goust J–M, Salier J–P 1981 Immunoglobulin G heavy chain (Gm) allotypes in multiple sclerosis. Journal of Clinical Investigation 67: 1797–1800

98. Propert D N, Bernard C C A, Simons M J 1982 Gm allotypes and multiple sclerosis. Journal of Immunogenetics 9: 359–361

99. Blanc M, Clanet M, Berr C et al 1986 Immunoglobulin allotypes and susceptibility to multiple sclerosis. Journal of the Neurological Sciences 75: 1–5

100. Salier J–P, Sesbouiié R, Martin–Mondière C et al 1986 Combined influences of Gm and HLA phenotypes upon multiple sclerosis susceptibility and severity. Journal of Clinical Investigation 78: 533–538

101. Francis D A, Brazier D M, Batchelor J R et al 1986 Gm allotypes in multiple sclerosis influence susceptibility in HLA-DQw1 positive patients from the north east of Scotland. Clinical Immunology and Immunopathology 41: 406–409

102. Gaiser C N, Johnson M J, De Lange G et al 1987 Susceptibility to multiple sclerosis associated with an immunoglobulin gamma 3 restriction fraction length polymorphism. Journal of Clinical Investigation 79: 309–313

103. Wraith D C, McDevitt H O, Steinman L, Acha–Orbea-Germline repertoire of T cell receptor beta chain genes intervention in autoimmune disease. Cell (in press)

104. Oksenberg J R, Gaiser C N, Cavalli–Svorza L L, Steinman L 1988 Polymorphic markers of human T cell receptor alpha and beta genes. Family studies and comparison of frequencies in healthy individuals and patients with multiple sclerosis and myasthenia gravis. Human Immunology 22: 111–121

105. Beall S S, Concannon P, Charmley P et al 1989 The germline repertoire of T cell receptor beta chain genes in patients with chronic progressive multiple sclerosis. Journal of Neuroimmunology 21: 59–66

106. Seboun E, Robinson M A, Doolittle T H et al 1989 A susceptibility locus for multiple sclerosis is linked to the T cell receptor β chain locus. Cell 57: 1095–1100

107. Compston D A S, Vakerelis B M, Paul E, McDonald W I, Batchelor J R, Mims CA 1986 Viral infection in patients with multiple sclerosis and HLA-DR matched controls. Brain 109: 325–344

108. Lamoureux G, Lapierre Y, Ducharme G 1983 Past infectious events and disease evolution in multiple sclerosis. Journal of Neurology 230: 81–90

109. Hughes P J, Kirk P F, Dyas J, Munro J A, Welsh K I, Compston D A S 1987 Factors influencing circulating OKT8 cell phenotypes in patients with multiple sclerosis. Journal of Neurology, Neurosurgery and Psychiatry 50: 1156–1159

110. Jacobsen S, Sorrentino R, Nepom G T, McFarlin D E, Strominger J L 1986 DNA restriction fragment length polymorphism of HLA-DR2; correlation with HLA-DR2 associated functions. Journal of Neuroimmunology 12: 195–203

111. Trouillas P, Berthoux F, Betuel H, Boisson D, Aimard G, Devic M 1976 Hypocomplementaemic MS. Heterozygous C2 deficiency link to HLA A10 B18. Lancet ii: 1023

112. Engell T, Raus N E, Thomsen M, Platz P 1982 HLA and heterogeneity of multiple sclerosis. Neurology 32: 1043–1046

113. Madigand D M, Oger J J–F, Fauchet R, Sabouraud O, Genetet B 1982 HLA profiles in multiple sclerosis suggest two forms of disease and the existence of protective haplotypes. Journal of the Neurological Sciences 53: 519–529

114. Poser S, Ritter G, Bauer H J et al 1981 HLA antigens and the prognosis of multiple sclerosis. Journal of Neurology 225: 219–221

115. Meyer–Rienecker H J, Wegener S, Hitzschke B, Richter K V 1982 Multiple sclerosis — relation between HLA haplotype A25, B18 and disease progression. Acta Neurologica Scandinavica 66: 709–712

116. Mertin J, Rudge P, Kremer M et al 1982 Double blind controlled trial of immunosuppression in the treatment of multiple sclerosis; final report. Lancet 2: 351–354

117. British and Dutch Multiple Sclerosis Azathioprine Trial Group 1988. Histocompatability antigens in multiple sclerosis patients participating in a multicentre trial of azathioprine. Journal of Neurology, Neurosurgery and Psychiatry 51: 412–415

118. Olerup O, Fredrikson S, Olsson T, Kam–Hansen S 1987 HLA class 2 genes in chronic progressive and in relapsing/remitting multiple sclerosis. Lancet 2: 327

11. Immunological aspects of multiple sclerosis

Observations made several decades ago on samples of cerebrospinal fluid first implicated immunological mechanisms in the pathogenesis of multiple sclerosis.[1] Since that time, knowledge on the complex organisation of the immune system has rapidly increased, providing more and more opportunities for documenting immunological phenomena in this disease. However, investigation of the immune system in patients with multiple sclerosis has necessarily been indirect since access to affected tissue is limited. Those who wish to investigate the pathogenesis by studying the disease itself have routinely to be content with samples of peripheral blood or cerebrospinal fluid and rarely have access to affected tissue during life; even autopsy material is scarce and may only depict the end-stage of a disease process which is dynamic and evolves with time.

Attention has therefore turned to experimental models of demyelination for understanding the human disease. This provides investigators with the advantage of being able to manipulate experimental conditions in the laboratory and so theoretically to dissect out each stage in the sequence of events leading to demyelination. The problem is that the most extensively studied animal model of multiple sclerosis — acute experimental allergic encephalomyelitis — is not characterised by widespread demyelination; even though a great deal has been learned about this disease over several decades, the question remains open as to its relevance for the study of human demyelinating disease.

More recently it has become possible to study aspects of multiple sclerosis by recreating conditions in vitro, albeit in a simplified and artificial way, which may mimic immunological events occurring in the central nervous system. It is now possible to grow relatively pure cultures of most individual cell types which contribute to the structure and function of myelinated axons and to study their interactions with cellular and humoral components of the immune system. This approach offers the possibility of building step by step an in vitro model of the complex sequence of events which leads to myelin injury in vivo.

Using these three approaches — analysis of clinical samples, animal models and tissue culture — in combination, immunologists have been able to go some way towards explaining the mechanism of tissue damage in multiple sclerosis. One problem is in defining the essential features of the disease. Clinically, the production of transient symptoms, the development of fixed signs, the pattern of relapses and slow progression all require explanation. At a pathological level, mechanisms must be provided for the development of reversible myelin injury, persistent demyelination and perivascular lymphocytic infiltration. Fundamental dilemmas such as whether the disease is primarily a disorder of the blood–brain barrier, which normally excludes immune mediators from the central nervous system, with secondary bystander demyelination, or an autoimmune process directed at one or other of the structural components of myelin have to be resolved.

Since so many questions remain unanswered, scepticism is understandably expressed about the immunological nature of the disease. The argument usually arises from adopting too narrow a concept of immunology in which the distinction between primary and epiphenomenal aspects is overstated and spurious distinctions are made between the various cellular and soluble factors

321

involved in the induction, mediation and repair of inflammation. A key question is whether a given observation is abnormal and potentially pathogenic or merely part of normal immunological homeostasis. For example the presence of a particular set of genes is not abnormal but may predispose an individual to demyelinating disease given other circumstances; oscillations in populations of lymphocytes which normally regulate immune responses may be appropriate but nevertheless induces instability in the cellular interactions that constantly go on in a changing immunological environment. Immunologists have to decide at what stage the immune system has lost control or specificity and become involved in a pathological process. Much therefore hinges on the proper use and selection of controls. Given all these uncertainties it is inevitable that any one reviewer is bound to pick amongst the evidence and take what suits his own hypothesis, leaving the rest as unreliable or unconfirmed observations. There is also the inevitable tendency to build elaborate hypotheses based on one aspect of what is clearly a very complex process. What follows is a version of the immunology of demyelinating disease which switches from man to mouse to molecule in an attempt to present a coherent but somewhat personal view of what might be going on.

THE MECHANISM OF IMMUNE RESPONSE

Immune response involves a sequence in which antigen is first detected, processed and then presented to effector components of the system: certain antigens must be tolerated since they are either innocuous or not foreign, and there must be a method for terminating responses which are complete or temporarily in abeyance. In essence, the processing, presentation and executive arms of immune response are carried out by specialised cellular subpopulations; communication between these cells is mediated by soluble factors as well as cell — cell contact, and the whole system is genetically restricted. Lymphocyte education takes place in the thymus during a critical period in development as a result of which there is positive and negative selection for cells responding to an enormous range of antigens; thereafter, major

histocompatibility complex restriction on immune response and tolerance to autoantigens are established.[2]

Immune responses occurring within the central nervous system are of special interest since it is normally protected from immune mediators by the blood–brain–nerve barrier; however, circulating immunocompetent cells routinely patrol the central nervous system and others, also systemically derived, are permanently resident. The list of participants in the immune response which could therefore be studied is enormous and includes genes, T cells and their numerous subpopulations, B cells, antibodies and their various classes, soluble mediators, including cytokines, macrophages and their mediators and complement — not to mention substances produced endogenously in response to viral infection such as the interferons.

Antigen presentation

Once the physical barriers that protect animals and man from environmental agents have been breached, defence depends on the ability of specialised cells to ingest and destroy potential pathogens. This can happen more easily if the agents become attached to antibody and complement but ultimately the pathogens need to be recognised and dealt with by phagocytic or cytotoxic cells. The initial step by which complex antigen is recognised involves antigen presenting cells. Macrophages are able to process antigen, in addition to having a primary role as phagocytes, but this is also carried out by follicular dendritic cells which trap antigen and induce predominantly B cell responses, and by interdigitating cells which may be more intimately involved in T cell antigen presentation.[3] Both cell types are to be found throughout the body but when antigen is trapped, they migrate to lymph nodes for the initiation of immune responses. The interaction between lymphocytes and antigen-presenting cells leads both to antibody synthesis through the action of T cell dependent B cell responses and the production of effector T cells. Thus within lymph nodes there are germinal centres containing dendritic cells and B cells which stimulate plasma cells to synthesise antibody. Elsewhere there is proliferation of the effector T cell repertoire which includes clonal expansion of helper, cytotoxic and suppressor subpopulations. Antigen presentation does not occur exclusively within lymph nodes; in the central nervous system, type 1 astrocytes can be induced to express class 2 major histocompatibility antigens; they can then present antigen to activated T cells[4] and provide all the requirements for a local immune response surrounding areas of damage to the blood-brain barrier (see below).

Induction of the immune response

One important feature of these events is that antigen can only be presented in association with major histocompatibility complex molecules; indeed this is their major biological function and in simple terms offers a mechanistic explanation for associations between the HLA system and disease. The tertiary structure of these molecules has recently been shown to contain a cleft in the polymorphic portion in which sit denatured fragments of processed antigen.[5] Cellular interactions only occur if antigen is presented with a class 2 molecule of the same allelic specificity as that expressed on the surface of the responding T cell.[6] In addition to the processed antigen and the associated class 2 molecule, two other structures are involved in the docking of cells involved in regulating the immune response. One is the group of accessory molecules including CD4 and CD8 which are present on the responding T cell.[7] CD4 anchors antigen-presenting cells to T cells and serves as a useful surface marker for this class of lymphocyte, i.e. the T helper/inducer cell. The quartet of molecules required for cellular interaction is made up by the T cell receptor itself which accepts the antigen in question if the arrangement of accessory and class 2 molecules is appropriate.

The T cell receptor consists of several glycoprotein chains at least two of which are encoded by genes which undergo rearrangement during development accounting for the diversity of T cell responses.[8] Any one T cell uses two from an available pool of four chains but usually alpha pairs with beta and gamma with delta; the latter are found on thymic cells[9] whereas mature circulating cells express alpha/beta T cell receptors. In addition, the T cell receptor is associated with the invariable CD3 antigen consisting of three chains; this is ubiquitous and so can be used as a marker by which all T cells are recognised.[10] Mature T cells leaving the thymus also express either the CD4 or CD8 antigen. Although the CD4 marker allows them provisionally to be classified as helper/inducer cells, it is unfortunately now clear that CD4 positive cells have several functions, some of which involve immune suppression and the CD8 population is equally heterogenous.

One type of CD4 cell will enhance specific and polyclonal B cell responses directly or through the release of interleukins; the other mediates B cell suppression, T cell cytotoxicity and delayed type hypersensitivity responses.[11] The density of yet another surface marker, the CD45 antigen recognisable by a variety of monoclonal antibodies, can now be used to distinguish these two types of helper cell.[12]

Effector mechanisms of the immune system

After antigen presentation and induction of the immune response, action is required. This may consist of T cell cytotoxicity or the production of antibody, or both, but also involves suppression of the immune response. The effector mechanisms are also restricted by major histocompatibility complex antigens and molecules which anchor cytotoxic and target cells. In the case of T cell cytotoxicity these molecules are the class 1 histocompatibility antigens and the CD8 accessory molecule.[13] The mechanism of killing involves the release of soluble perforins which have structural and functional similarities with the membrane attack complexes of complement and belong to a family of pore-forming proteins which perforate the membrane of target cells leading to metabolic changes and osmotic disruption of the cell and its contents.[14] Cytotoxic cells are fortunately not susceptible to their own perforins. The release of perforins is enhanced by those interleukins which are known to mediate the interaction of cytotoxic cells and their targets, especially IL-2. Other molecules which kill target cells include tumour necrosis factors, serine esterase and proteoglycans.[14]

Antibody responses differ, depending on the state of vigilance amongst B cells, i.e. the primary and secondary response. Primary response involves T cell dependent stimulation which results in the production both of plasma cells, which secrete antibody, and memory cells; when antigen is encountered for the second time, responses are quicker and achieve a higher antibody titre. The role of B cells in mounting these responses may not be entirely passive and there is evidence that the antibody present by definition on the surface of all B cells may initially bind the offending antigen and present this to the T cells which in turn help that same B cell clone to expand.[15]

Just as specificity is an integral part of immunity, so also suppression is necessary if the system is to be efficient. Originally, it was thought that this function was achieved by a discrete population of T cells with their own lineage; suppression was assigned to the CD8 subpopulation[16] but it has since proved difficult to identify the cells which are primarily responsible for this immunological phenomenon. More recently, the suggestion has been made that suppression is mediated both by CD4 and CD8 cells and that the phenomenon involves responses to unique sequences or idiotypes presented by the arrangement of T cell receptor, major histocompatibility complex product and foreign antigen; these self-reactive effector cells damp down the responding T cell population; thus T helper and T suppressor cells can be regarded as different sides of the same coin.[17]

It will be clear from this account that many of the cellular interactions involved in the immune response can be replaced or are entirely mediated by other soluble factors, collectively known as interleukins. Interleukin 1 is produced by macrophages and a variety of other cells and stimulates one population of CD4 T helper cells to produce interleukins 4, 5 and 6 (formerly known as beta interferon) which in turn stimulate B cells and between them regulate the sequential synthesis of the different antibody classes.[18] Interleukin 1 has no effect on those CD4 positive cells which stimulate T cell cytotoxic responses, effects which are mediated by interleukin 2.[19] Responding cells express receptors for these interleukins; thus both the lineage and functional activity of lymphocyte subpopulations can be inferred at any one time from studies of their surface markers.

ENVIRONMENTAL TRIGGERS

All hypotheses for the mechanism of autoimmune disease take as their starting point the notion that extrinsic factors trigger the disease process in individuals rendered susceptible through their genetic background. In the case of multiple sclerosis many candidates, most of them viruses, have been proposed. Initially, the evidence was based on population serology demonstrating that randomly tested patients with multiple sclerosis had higher antibody titres to viruses that cause childhood exanthematous viral infections than controls and this evidence was specifically taken to implicate measles in the aetiology of multiple sclerosis.[20] Since more direct evidence for an abnormal host response to measles has not been forthcoming, the concept emerged that measles merely epitomised a general disturbance of immunological behaviour in patients with multiple sclerosis;[21] later the suggestion was made, again using measles as an example, that individuals developed multiple sclerosis because they were exposed to a common viral illness relatively late in childhood during a brief window of susceptibility.[22] Others took the view that measles antibody titres were high because of cross-reactivity with a closely related paramyxovirus and for a while the favoured candidate was canine distemper virus;[23] although lacking laboratory support, this idea was felt to be consistent with epidemiological observations on exposure to domestic animals[24] and changes in incidence of multiple sclerosis in several small islands in the North Atlantic.[25] Meanwhile, sporadic reports of viral isolation from tissue obtained from patients with multiple sclerosis have continued to appear, providing a steady trickle of new candidates for the cause of the disease.

A variety of techniques has been used in these studies, some of which are extremely sensitive and may merely have detected the presence of persistent viruses living symbiotically with the host. The distinction between agents that initiate the disease process and those that precipitate new events in patients with pre-existing disease has not always been made clear in these reports. Four recent studies will be used to illustrate these points.

In 1965 Sibley & Foley[26] reported that up to

50% of relapses are preceded by a clinically significant infection; in 1985 Sibley et al[27] showed prospectively that 27% of relapses followed a recognisable infection even though infections were reported less often in patients with multiple sclerosis than controls; overall a relapse was three times more likely to occur at the time of an infection, irrespective of disease severity. Nearly 9% of all episodes which were deemed to be viral infections were followed by a relapse.

Approximately 10 years ago Russell and colleagues reported the isolation of a virus from the bone marrow of several patients with multiple sclerosis[28] and later identified the organism as SV5. Subsequently it became clear that this paramyxovirus could be recovered from the bone marrow of other individuals and population serology showed a high prevalence of exposure in the community;[29] however the organism was not known to be associated with any human disease. Subsequently the substantial claim was made that a high proportion of the oligoclonal bands demonstrated by electrophoresis in over 90% of patients with multiple sclerosis could be absorbed with SV5 antigen but not other paromyxoviruses;[30] in addition it was reported that this reactivity to SV5 antigen was peculiar to patients with multiple sclerosis and the electrophoretic patterns were unaffected by absorption with SV5 antigen in those individuals without multiple sclerosis who nevertheless appeared to have SV5 antibodies in their spinal fluid. However, the absorption procedure was evidently not confined to the oligoclonal bands, raising questions about technical aspects of the study: to date, there has been no positive confirmation of the findings and others have failed to demonstrate SV5 antibody in association with the oligoclonal bands appearing in the spinal fluid of patients with multiple sclerosis.[31]

Attention has since turned to the relationship between retrovirus infection and multiple sclerosis. Serological tests demonstrated antibodies to human T cell lymphotropic viruses (HTLV) I, II and III (HIV 1) in up to 70% of patients and molecularly cloned probes revealed the existence of HTLV I related nucleotide sequences in cells from the cerebrospinal fluid of some affected individuals.[32] It was initially suggested that these observations resulted from cross-reactivity with an as yet unidentified retrovirus. These findings provoked widespread interest, but many counter claims were soon made based on repeating the serological studies in a variety of groups of cases and controls.[33-35] The same authors have more recently reported the identification of HTLV I DNA sequences recognising the *gag* and *env* portions of the genome in peripheral blood mononuclear cells from 6 patients with multiple sclerosis compared with 1/20 controls;[36] as before they found serological evidence for retrovirus exposure. The recent work has been achieved using the polymerase chain reaction which detects tiny amounts of DNA in the infected cell and amplifies this up to levels at which molecular cloning and sequencing can be performed. The technique is sufficiently sensitive to detect DNA sequences which are harmlessly integrated within the host genome and by the very nature of its sensitivity it is particularly vulnerable to contamination.[37] One further study in part confirms the claim that a retrovirus may be involved in the pathogenesis of multiple sclerosis: Greenberg et al[38] have demonstrated DNA sequences of the *pol* and *env* parts of the HTLV I genome in patients with multiple sclerosis but not controls; however, they failed to confirm the disease specificity of the *gag* sequences detected by Reddy et al.[36]

For many years ideas about the viral basis for multiple sclerosis have depended on comparisons with diseases in which viruses can mimic some or many of the clinical and pathological characteristics of human demyelinating diseases. This approach can now be extended to· the study of retrovirus infection and the nervous system, since it is clear that tropical spastic paraplegia (otherwise known as Jamaican neuropathy or HTLV associated myelopathy) is associated with and probably caused by infection with HTLV I.[39] Twenty five years after the clinical and pathological features of this inflammatory demyelinating disease confined to selected fibre pathways within the spinal cord was first described,[40] population serology has demonstrated a strong association between this disease and antibodies to HTLV I in the Carribean, Europe, Africa and Japan.[41] This association is substantiated by the finding that oligoclonal bands in the spinal fluid of patients with TSP are specific for HTLV I and recently

HTLV I has itself been demonstrated in the peripheral blood mononuclear cells of patients with tropical spastic paraplegia by polymerase chain reactions using probes for various components of the HTLV genome.[42] Even if the evidence is poor with respect to multiple sclerosis, the lesson here is that retroviruses can cause chronic demyelinating disease which is confined to selected parts of the central nervous system.

SYSTEMIC IMMUNOLOGICAL ABNORMALITIES IN MULTIPLE SCLEROSIS

Peripheral blood phenotype

Enumerating lymphocytes in the blood and cerebrospinal fluid and documenting their function has been used extensively as a means for understanding the immune basis of multiple sclerosis. The assumption underlying these investigations has been that variations from normal may help in understanding the immunopathogenesis of the disease. The basic idea is sound and proved extremely informative early in the AIDS epidemic but comparable studies in patients with multiple sclerosis need to be very carefully controlled. The opportunity for making observations has been enormous but the knowledge accrued rather disappointing. The general sequence has been for basic immunologists to provide panels of monoclonal antibodies which are thought to define subpopulations of lymphocytes having increasingly discrete functions; it is then relatively easy to enumerate cells in single samples from a small cohort of cases and controls from which rather extravagant generalisations have been made. Subsequently the function of the cell population recognised by the monoclonals has more often than not been brought into question but by then another antibody is usually being tested. Nevertheless, some conclusions can be reached based on serial studies, adequately controlled and carried out using well-validated methods and reagents. Lymphocyte populations are given cluster (CD) numbers but within each CD group, several reagents can be used to define the population of interest. The CD4 group is usually detected by Leu 3a, 3b or OKT 4 and the CD8 group by OKT 8, OKT 5 or Leu 2a. Many of the other clusters

so far defined have not been studied extensively in the context of multiple sclerosis.

Originally, several groups reported a reduction in percentage of OKT 8 cells in patients with multiple sclerosis, especially during periods of disease activity, based on serial measurements in carefully monitored cases with relapsing or progressive disease.[43–47] The subsequent failure to confirm this observation justifiably brought into question the role of lymphocyte phenotyping[48,49] but the consensus would seem to be that, allowing for variations in technique, reagents and methods for expressing results, CD8 cells are reduced in number in patients with chronic progressive disease.[50,51] However monoclonal antibodies can be used singly or in combination to identify less heterogenous lymphocyte populations including those characterised by the presence of activation markers expressed transiently during T cell maturation. Within the CD8 subset, suppressor and cytotoxic cells can be distinguished by several antibodies and activated cells can be enumerated apart from those in the resting state.

One subpopulation of CD4 cells — the suppressor inducer (OKT4/2H4 positive) lymphocyte — which stimulates the CD8 suppressor subset, is reduced in the circulation in patients with chronic progressive multiple sclerosis,[52] even though the parent CD4 population has not attracted much attention from lymphocyte subpopulators. This finding is of course consistent with the notion that suppressor activity. is deficient in patients with multiple sclerosis, at least during the progressive phase. In a study involving patients with multiple sclerosis, healthy relatives and unrelated controls, Hughes et al[53] showed, as expected, that there was a strong correlation between Leu 2a phenotype and the percentage of OKT 8 cells, but also that each correlated with the sub-population of Leu 2a/15 (functional suppressor) cells. Moreover, the reduction in CD8 cells observed in patients with multiple sclerosis could be accounted for by alterations in the number of these functional suppressor lymphocytes.

There is an increase in T cells expressing early and late activation markers in patients with multiple sclerosis;[54–59] these antigens are present on activated CD4 and CD8 cells, whereas the expression of others is not confined to T lymphocytes at all. Hughes and colleagues[53] found no difference in the percentage of activated CD8 cells between groups and no pattern to the fluctuations observed in this subpopulation during serial studies of affected individuals or their relatives. Activated T cells express interleukin 2 receptors (Tac positive) and other early antigens (4/F2, insulin and transferrin receptors) within 48 hours; DR antigen is expressed within a few days whereas Ta1, Ts2/77 and MLR 1, 2, 3 or 4 appear later. There are reports of an increase in the proportion of cells expressing the Tac or interleukin 2 receptor in patients with multiple sclerosis,[56-59] but this does not correlate with disease activity and the findings are inconsistent; in two recent surveys, Crockard et al[60] found no increase in the proportion of cells expressing IL-2 receptors in 50 patients with multiple sclerosis irrespective of disease activity, whereas Konttinen et al[61] identified more lymphocytes carrying DR antigen, IL-2 receptors and the glycoprotein pg 40/80 in patients during remission than in normal controls. Others also have failed to confirm the original observation of increased IL-2 receptor expression.[54,55,61] Some other activation markers can also be detected more frequently on cells from patients with multiple sclerosis than controls, but none distinguishes CD8 from CD4 cells.[54,56]

Peripheral blood lymphocyte function

An alternative approach has been to study the function of lymphocyte populations without reference to their surface phenotype. The problem with this approach is that function has to be defined in the context of a specific challenge — for example the acetyl choline receptor in the case of myasthenia gravis — in the absence of which non-specific stimulation using plant lectins, which differentially stimulate one population of cells or another, or myelin antigens which are of doubtful significance for the pathogenesis of multiple sclerosis have been used. Concanavalin A preferentially stimulates T suppressor cells whereas pokeweed mitogen is a T cell dependent B cell activator. There is rather a poor correlation between functional and phenotypic results carried out in the same individuals or comparable groups,

presumably because complex interactions involving several subsets are involved in responsiveness to antigen or plant lectins. This lack of correlation is not peculiar to studies on multiple sclerosis to the extent that it is now fashionable in immunological circles not to believe in the existence of suppressor cells even though suppression as a phenomenon is integral to immune regulation. As discussed above, this view arises not from conceptual difficulties with the nature of immune suppression but from difficulty in assigning suppressor activity to a particular category of lymphocyte, defined by phenotype or function.

Peripheral blood mononuclear cell responses to concanavalin A and pokeweed mitogen are each abnormal in patients with multiple sclerosis. This can be detected either by assaying cell division or the production of immunoglobulin from the supernatant of cells in culture. IgG synthesis by unstimulated peripheral blood B lymphocytes is increased in multiple sclerosis patients, especially during relapse[62] and this response is enhanced by PWM stimulation.[63] More complicated culture systems have been used to sort out which lymphocyte subset is contributing to this result, by carrying out sequential assays in which con A is first used to expand the available pool of T suppressor cells; these are then inhibited from further cell division but remain functionally intact and can be added to mononuclear cells from the same patient which are stimulated either to respond again to con A or to secrete IgG in response to pokeweed. The results are consistent with the interpretation that suppressor function is impaired in multiple sclerosis, especially during the chronic progressive phase.[64-67] However, mixing cells from healthy controls and patients with multiple sclerosis, in vitro, suggests that B cell responses are abnormal in patients with multiple sclerosis over and above this impairment of T suppression.[68,69]

The next step has therefore been to decide whether the complicated, time-consuming and expensive tests of lymphocyte function can be replaced by simpler phenotypic studies which are more economical on time and resources. The answer is that they do not provide the same information and so are not interchangeable. Abnormalities of pokeweed-stimulated IgG secretion and the number of OKT 8 positive cells or T cells expressing receptors for IgG immune complexes were originally correlated in groups of patients with multiple sclerosis in relapse.[70] Using a two stage concanavalin A-mixed lymphocyte reactivity culture, Tjernlund et al[71] reported that the OKT 4/8 ratio and spontaneous or pokeweed-stimulated IgG synthesis were increased with reduced stimulation indices in chronic progressive patients, but not those in remission. Phenotype and function correlated poorly in the individual. Ojer et al[72] showed that CD8 cell percentages (demonstrated by Leu 2a and OKT 8) and concanavalin A-concanavalin A proliferative responses were comparable in normal individuals but not in cases of multiple sclerosis. This topic has been studied most intensively by Antel and colleagues,[63,64,73,74] who attribute the alterations in suppressor function to a combined alteration in the number and function of CD8 cells. Their most recent published work[75] shows that CD8 cell lines grown from patients with multiple sclerosis during periods of disease stability have significantly higher, and near normal, activity in a concanavalin A-concanavalin A suppressor assay compared with cell lines grown up from patients with progressive disease. Conversely, cytotoxic activity does not differ in these same cell lines, suggesting that it is the suppressor population of the CD8 cell group which is defective in the context of multiple sclerosis.

In another recent look at this question, Hughes & Compston[55] showed that spontaneous and PWM-stimulated IgG synthesis were significantly increased in patients with multiple sclerosis compared with controls. IgG synthesis after sequential concanavalin A-pokeweed stimulation was, as expected, reduced compared with PWM stimulation alone, both in cases and controls, but the results were not statistically significant. The differences were more apparent when cases with chronic progressive multiple sclerosis were compared with healthy or other neurological disease controls. The percentage of CD8 cells was lower in patients with multiple sclerosis than controls, but suppressor function and CD8 phenotype did not correlate in individual patients or controls. Others have however shown a correlation between the number of OKT4/2H4 cells and suppressor function assessed

in an autologous mixed lymphocyte reactivity assay.[76]

Why has there been this preoccupation with documenting changes in the circulation in the context of a disease that is confined to the central nervous system? One reason is that the blood can easily be sampled but the main stimulus has been to find an explanation for the blood–brain barrier damage that now seems to be the first readily recognisable step in the sequence of events that leads to myelin injury and its clinical expression. An attractive hypothesis is that the defect in suppressor function lowers the threshold for T cell activation and since activated T cells have the ability to penetrate the blood–brain barrier, this would disrupt immunological equilibrium within the 'not-so' privileged central nervous system.

THE BLOOD–BRAIN BARRIER

Cells and macromolecules which circulate through the cerebral vasculature are normally excluded from contact with the brain parenchyma by the blood–brain barrier; as in other vascular tissues, this is made up by a network of endothelial cells but these are surrounded by a basement membrane associated with pericytes. The abluminal surface is covered by a network formed from the foot processes of type 1 astrocytes.[77] These specialised glial cells induce the endothelial cells to form tight junctions; together, this anatomical structure achieves the complex function of excluding the transfer of large molecules from the circulation, whilst remaining permeable to water and lipid. Specific mechanisms exist for transporting some essential nutrients, including glucose and other metabolically active substances, across cerebral vessels. Regional variation in structure partly accounts for selective permeability, but this depends more on a variety of physiological mechanisms acting in health and disease, including macromolecular vesicular transport and endocytosis. Over and above these mechanisms, there is now evidence that T cells activated against a variety of neural and irrelevant antigens can penetrate the normal blood–brain barrier.[78,79] Hafler & Weiner,[80] in a therapeutic trial of monoclonal antibodies directed against the CD3 T cell marker, found that labelled cells remained viable in vivo and moved rapidly through the blood–brain barrier into the nervous system, where they constituted 70% of all cells recovered from cerebrospinal fluid within 72 hours of the infusion. Not only does this study demonstrate that the cerebral capillaries are permeable in multiple sclerosis, but it also supports the idea that systemic immunotherapy will influence the central nervous system.

In the context of immunological disease of the central nervous system, the passage of immune mediators also seems to take place by increased vesicular transport and partial relaxation of endothelial tight junctions.[81] This has lead to the idea that blood–brain barrier damage is a necessary and sufficient cause for inducing experimental and human demyelinating disease. Sadly, this has encouraged some individuals to promote the idea that multiple sclerosis is caused by non-specific vascular damage occurring as a result of sludging[82] or fat deposition[83] in the capillaries — hypotheses which have sometimes been associated with prolonged and expensive therapeutic diversions. Demyelination can be induced in intact experimental animals merely by increasing T cell mediated permeability of the blood–brain barrier, but more than lymphocytic infiltration is necessary for the experimental induction of demyelination within the central nervous system. Clinical signs appear shortly after the onset of blood–brain barrier damage in experimental allergic encephalomyelitis, but do not develop if vascular injury is prevented using the alpha-1 adrenoceptor antagonist prazosin;[84] and conversely, a form of experimental allergic encephalomyelitis can be induced by inoculation with a preparation of brain-derived endothelial cell membranes.[85]

The opportunity to dissect the sequence of events that leads to tissue damage using animal models is illustrated by experiments in which the protocol for inducing experimental allergic encephalomyelitis is used in susceptible animals which have been made macrophage deficient,[86] or depleted of complement by pre-treatment with cobra venom factor[87] which induces uncontrolled activation of C3. In these situations blood–brain barrier damage and T cell infiltration of the nervous system develop as expected, but clinical signs either do not occur or are significantly modified. This indicates that T cell infiltration of the nervous system is not directly responsible for impaired function of myelinated axons. Further evidence for the dissociation between blood–brain barrier damage and myelin injury is provided by the finding that animals in which host T cell responses are inhibited by induction of leucopenia can nevertheless show severe blood–brain barrier damage and tissue oedema with clinical signs of experimental allergic encephalomyelitis but no perivascular cellular infiltrate.[88] In subsequent experiments, Sedgwick[89] has shown that CD8 cells are not required for the induction or, more interestingly, the long-term resistance to re-induction of experimental allergic encephalomyelitis seen in animals which have recovered from an initial episode. More recently it has been shown that the resistance is mediated by a population of CD4 suppressor lymphocytes.[90]

The next problem is therefore to determine what happens once T cells have passed through the blood-brain barrier. Cells recovered from the abluminal surface of the cerebral capillaries or the brain parenchyma show major histocompatibility complex class 2 antigen restriction in their ability to induce experimental allergic encephalomyelitis,[91] suggesting that interactions with cells resident within the central nervous system and able to express class 2 antigen may be involved in these local immune responses. Some pericytes, perivascular monocytes and microglia express low levels of these antigens in vivo;[92] class 2 antigen expression can be induced on type 1 astrocytes[4,93] and it has therefore been suggested that their interaction with infiltrating T cells may compromise blood–brain barrier function further increasing vascular permeability.[77]

Studies carried out in patients with multiple sclerosis support the idea that blood–brain barrier damage is not sufficient for the induction of myelin injury. The evidence includes the poor anatomical correlation between areas of perivascular infiltration and demyelination in multiple sclerosis, and the observation that retinal vascular sheathing is present in a high proportion of patients with optic neuritis, whether as an isolated phenomenon or a manifestation of multiple sclerosis.[94] Histological examination of these sheaths confirms that the appearances are due to the presence of perivascular infiltration by mononuclear cells occurring at a site where there are no myelinated axons.[95] More recent observations have used the techniques of magnetic resonance imaging to demonstrate the early and reversible nature of blood–brain barrier damage using gadolinium DPTA[96]

Taken with the somewhat conflicting evidence for an increase in T cell activation in the circulation of patients with multiple sclerosis and the demonstration of class 2 antigen expression on microglia and endothelial cells in tissue from patients with multiple sclerosis,[97–99] this evidence is consistent with the hypothesis that blood–brain barrier damage is necessary early in the development of focal demyelination but only in the sense that it permits entry of cellular and soluble mediators with pathogenic potential into the central nervous system.

CEREBROSPINAL FLUID IN PATIENTS WITH MULTIPLE SCLEROSIS

Analysis of cerebrospinal fluid provides the most direct opportunity for studying in life events taking place within the central nervous system which underlie the symptoms and signs by which the disease is recognised and defined. Repeated access provides some information on the dynamics of immunological activity within the central nervous system, but sampling the spinal fluid can never reveal whether these changes are the cause or consequence of myelin injury. Qualitative and quantitative abnormalities of spinal fluid have been in use for several decades as a means of supplementing the clinical evidence for diagnosis, and for assessing the effects of treatment. The spinal fluid therefore provides practical information and can be used to understand the pathogenesis of multiple sclerosis. The emphasis of these studies has been on the presence and nature of inflammatory cells and antibodies, but some other components of spinal fluid have also attracted attention.

Inflammatory cells in the cerebrospinal fluid

About 65% of patients with multiple sclerosis have an excess of inflammatory cells in the cerebrospinal fluid. Opinions differ on whether this is more likely to occur during periods of disease activity; the distinction is difficult since lumbar puncture tends more often to be carried out during relapse, but conversely, it is now clear that the disease process, likely to be reflected by changes in the cerebrospinal fluid, correlates poorly with clinical activity. This increase is due mainly to the presence of T cells, but plasma cells, macrophages and occasional polymorphonuclear leucocytes are also to be found. The total count is therefore usually between 5–50/mm^3 and although other diagnoses should be considered when there are more than 100 cells or large numbers of polymorphs, these abnormalities are occasionally seen in otherwise typical cases of multiple sclerosis. The use of monoclonal antibodies for discriminating lymphocyte subpopulations initially indicated that the pleocytosis is due to a selective increase in the number of CD4 cells;[100] more recent investigations have shown that this is typical of any other disorder in which there is acute inflammation within the central nervous system.[101]

The cells recovered from the spinal fluid are activated, showing increased DNA synthesis during relapse;[102] attempts to define more precisely the specificity of activation markers on cerebrospinal fluid cells include the demonstration of increased DR/Ia[103] and IL-2 receptors,[59] but neither observation has consistently been reported. Weber et al[104] have characterised the function of cells appearing in the cerebrospinal fluid and find that although CD8 cytotoxic cells are present, the main cell type is a precursor cytotoxic cell of CD4/helper phenotype. Rotteveel and colleagues[105] studied T cell receptor gene rearrangements in 30 T cell lines cloned from each of two patients with multiple sclerosis; their failure to demonstrate a shared pattern in these clones indicates that the T cell response in the cerebrospinal fluid is polyclonal and not restricted to a common or shared antigen. Conversely, Hafler et al[106] reported that a high proportion of clones derived from the cerebrospinal fluid of one patient with multiple sclerosis had a shared T cell receptor beta gene rearrangement. However, the specific responsiveness of T cells present in the spinal fluid has remained elusive; in a separate report, Hafler et al[107] found no increase in the proliferative response to myelin basic protein or proteolipid protein in a large number of T cells cloned from the cerebrospinal fluid of patients with multiple sclerosis.

It has been known for many years that plasma and B cells present in cerebrospinal fluid can synthesise immunoglobulin;[108] there is no difference in the proportion that can synthesise IgG, IgM and IgA, although the balance differs between patients[109] and although antibody synthesis occurs mainly within the nervous system, the same pattern of secretion is exhibited by peripheral blood samples from individual patients.

Immunoglobulin in the cerebrospinal fluid

The protein content of cerebrospinal fluid is considerably less than the serum concentration in normal individuals. Both in health and disease, this protein consists mainly of albumin, but the most characteristic abnormality is a selective increase in immunoglobulin due to local synthesis, together with leak of serum proteins through a damaged blood–brain barrier. Proteins can be detected in cerebrospinal fluid using quantitative or qualitative techniques. The quantity of IgG in cerebrospinal fluid is expressed using different formulae which vary in the sensitivity with which they discriminate patients with multiple sclerosis from those with other neurological diseases,[110] but all adjust for passive transfer of proteins across a damaged blood–brain barrier. Oligoclonal bands are detected by electrophoretic techniques in which cerebrospinal fluid is applied to various gels and the proteins migrate through an electric field at a constant pH after which they are stained, usually with Coomassie blue. In patients with multiple sclerosis, approximately 10 bands appear in the gamma region — collectively known as the oligoclonal pattern which is present in over 90% of patients;[111] this finding is not specific to multiple sclerosis and occurs in a wide variety of other neurological diseases, not all of which are the result of an immunological or infective process. Greater sensitivity can be introduced by adding a pH gradient to the electrophoretic field followed by silver staining; this technique, known as isoelectric focusing, increases the number of bands visible in samples from patients with oligoclonal

bands; in most cases these bands are not detected in serum. Once present, they persist and do not as a rule fluctuate in intensity or number depending on disease activity. Rather more variation is, however, seen in the concentration of immunoglobulin present in the spinal fluid.

Apart from their role in diagnosis, oligoclonal bands have been used to predict prognosis, particularly in patients with isolated episodes of demyelination. Several investigators have demonstrated a higher rate of conversion to multiple sclerosis in individuals with optic neuritis showing oligoclonal bands at presentation than those with normal cerebrospinal fluid[112–114] and Moulin et al[115] have extended this type of analysis to include isolated demyelination also affecting the cerebrum, brainstem, cerebellum or spinal cord. Conversely, detecting a single electrophoretic band is of considerably less value in diagnosis; Bass et al[116] found that only a quarter of these cases were eventually diagnosed as having multiple sclerosis, the remainder having an alternative diagnosis.

Immunoglobulin consists of paired heavy and light chains; Ig class is determined by the heavy chains (IgA, D, E, G and M) and there are subclasses within each of these categories (e.g. IgG1, IgG2, IgG3 and IgG4). Additional alterations in amino acid structure, the Gm allotypes, are found for each immunoglobulin subclass. There is also variation in the light chains — these consisting either of kappa or lambda forms. Free kappa and lambda chains are often detected in spinal fluid from patients with multiple sclerosis. Bracco et al[117] detected only kappa chains in 3, lambda in 10 and both in 15/32 cases, whereas no free chains were present in the remaining 4. In a quantitative assessment, Fagnart and colleagues[118] demonstrated free kappa chains in 81% of samples from patients with multiple sclerosis compared with 60% in infections of the central nervous system and 19% in patients with other neurological disorders. This difference was even more marked when corrections were made for passive transfer of free light chains from serum and this approach also revealed a high frequency of free lambda chains in patients with multiple sclerosis. Since free light chains correlate well with the presence of oligoclonal bands and IgG index, their detection supplements, but does not replace more conventional immunological assays applicable to spinal fluid.

The specificity of antibodies synthesised intrathecally in patients with multiple sclerosis has not been resolved, even though some of the bands may be directed against viral proteins or brain antigens.[119,120] Myelin basic protein is released from brain whatever the mechanism of injury, and can be detected as antigen or antibody in cerebrospinal fluid from patients with isolated forms of demyelination and multiple sclerosis in relapse;[121] in patients with progressive disease, the amount of free antigen decreases and the concentration of antibody increases by comparison with cases in relapse.[122]

HUMORAL MECHANISMS OF MYELIN INJURY

There is evidence that humoral mechanisms are involved in myelin injury, their mediators being introduced into the nervous system or synthesised locally following T cell damage to the blood–brain barrier. Although the experimental findings are incomplete and assumptions have to be made, one hypothesis is that demyelination is mediated by antibody, complement and macrophages which act synergistically to produce potentially reversible myelin injury. In constructing this hypothesis, it is necessary to switch from observations made in samples from patients with multiple sclerosis to animal models of demyelination or oligodendrocytes grown in tissue culture; extrapolating from one system and species to another may of course turn out not to be appropriate.

The lesions of multiple sclerosis contain B lymphocytes and plasma cells in addition to the populations of T cells already described; these synthesise immunoglobulin which can be detected immunocytochemically[123] and in the spinal fluid as a result both of spillage from the brain parenchyma and local production by those plasma cells which enter the subarachnoid space.[108]

Until recently, there has been no obvious role for this intrathecal antibody in the pathogenesis of demyelination. Now, however, it is clear that the well-established T cell mediated model of acute inflammatory experimental allergic encephalomyelitis, in which there is only scanty

demyelination, can be modified to produce widespread loss of myelin by synergistic use of myelin basic protein sensitised T cells, together with a monoclonal antibody directed against myelin oligodendrocyte glycoprotein.[124] In this model, demyelination seems to depend on complement activation occurring at the surface of oligodendrocytes and from non-specific phagocytosis by macrophages attracted by their receptors for the Fc portion of antibody.

The role of complement in mediating myelin injury is currently of considerable interest. Oligodendrocytes synthesise the myelin sheath that enfolds short sections of neighbouring axons within the central nervous system. The otherwise bare axonal segment found between the territory of each oligodendrocyte — the node of Ranvier — is covered by the foot processes of type 2 astrocytes. The type 2 astrocyte and oligodendrocytes are derived from a common precursor cell, the 0-2A progenitor.[125] Techniques for studying oligodendrocyte development in vitro can also be used indirectly to investigate the myelin injury that occurs in human and experimental demyelinating disease. A very simple experiment, but one which has proved informative, is to incubate rat cultured oligodendrocytes, in vitro, with constituents of normal serum mimicking what might happen if the blood brain–barrier were to be broken down.[126] Within a few minutes, the cells lose their processes and the membrane becomes permeable; soon after, the cells are lysed. This serum effect is restricted to oligodendrocytes and does not affect type 2 astrocytes or neurones, although 0-2A progenitors are partly susceptible.[127] Oligodendrocytes which have grown in culture for 6 days show maximum sensitivity to homologous serum. The factor in serum which is responsible for this cytotoxicity is complement, activation occurring through the classical pathway and in the absence of antibody. Normally, the classical pathway is activated only when antibody becomes membrane-bound and this leads to fixation of C1, after which sequential activation of the complement cascade occurs, leading both to the formation of short-lived activation products which are chemotactic and activate macrophages, and to membrane-attack complexes of complement which insert into the cell membrane and act initially as a calcium ionophore, later causing disruption of the cell and its contents.[128]

Oligodendrocyte lysis in vitro depends on the formation of membrane attack complexes and occurs in the absence of macrophages, although these cells are of importance in vivo (see below). The evidence for involvement of the membrane attack complex is that serum obtained from animals depleted of complement by cobra venom factor is inactive, as is serum specifically depleted of the terminal complement component, C9. The final piece of evidence is that C9 can be detected immunocytochemically on the surface of cells exposed to fresh autologous serum.

Complement activation at the surface of oligodendrocytes is followed by a rapid rise in intracellular calcium which precedes cell death. However, if the availability of complement is reduced by using diluted serum, the rise in intracellular calcium is controlled and starts to fall within approximately 5 minutes. This calcium transient is associated with a remarkable change in the appearance of the cell;[129,130] two minutes after exposure to maximum sub-lethal complement attack, the oligodendrocyte surface shows multiple vesicular extrusions on which membrane attack complexes are concentrated. Within 6 minutes, the cells resume their pre-exposure appearance, having removed the vesicles. These contain a high density of membrane-attack complexes, demonstrable both by electron microscopy and by immunological methods, and contain oligodendrocyte surface antigens. Following recovery, the cell is morphologically intact and able to continue synthesising structural components appropriate for its stage of development. It does, however, have a limited capacity for recovery and is unable to withstand repeated cycles of exposure to sub-lethal concentrations of complement.

The recovery mechanism is dependent on the change in intracellular calcium and agents which interfere with calcium activated intracellular proteins such as calmodulin inhibit the vesicular repair mechanism and promote cell lysis. The calcium transient depends on the formation of membrane-attack complexes and entry of calcium from outside the cell, in addition to some release from intracellular stores. It is greater, but not of longer duration, when antibody and complement are used synergistically to injure oligodendrocytes and under these circumstances may reach the level at which irreversible cell injury occurs. More importantly,

there are differences in the peak level of intracellular calcium reached depending on which antibody is used; responses are higher using antimyelin oligodendrocyte glycoprotein than other antimyelin antibodies.[129] This is of particular importance, since myelin oligodendrocyte glycoprotein is orientated on the external surface of the oligodendrocyte cell body and its myelin processes, whereas other antigens such as myelin basic protein are internalised and so not available for interaction with components of the immune system. It is of interest that the density of myelin oligodendrocyte glycoprotein increases on the surface of developing oligodendrocytes at the same time as sensitivity to homologous serum reaches its peak. Although complement activation by oligodendrocytes is sufficient in vitro to injure reversibly myelinating cells, albeit reversibly, local availability of antibody — as occurs in multiple sclerosis — may be sufficient to cause permanent cell damage, mediated by a rise in intracellular calcium. Changes in intracellular calcium can be expected to have a variety of other effects on the oligodendrocyte/myelin complex depending on their location, changes in calcium ion concentration will affect conduction through myelinated pathways and stimulate calcium-activated proteases which cause myelin autolysis.[131]

There is evidence that these experimental findings are revelant for the pathogenesis of human demyelinating disease and that intrathecal complement activation in patients with multiple sclerosis. C9 and the neo-antigen formed when the membrane attack complex is finally assembled have been demonstrated immunocytochemically in the adventitia surrounding the endothelial cells which line small blood vessels in plaques, irrespective of their histological age.[132] This finding is not specific to multiple sclerosis and is also observed in conditions characterised by intrathecal antibody synthesis, such as subacute sclerosing panencephalitis. Although the assays are not in routine use, and may have no role in the management of individual patients, studies of spinal fluid also provide evidence for complement activation occurring within the central nervous system in patients with multiple sclerosis. Concentrations of C2 and C3 do not differ in patients with multiple sclerosis depending on disease activity, but C4 has been shown to be reduced compared with controls.[133] The short-lived activation products C3a and C4a can be detected in the spinal fluid of patients with multiple sclerosis, but not in controls.[134] There is a significant reduction in the concentration of C9, implying complement activation, and consumption[135,136] which correlates inversely with increased IgG synthesis. The concentration of C9 increases at the time of improved clinical status resulting from treatment with high dose intravenous methylprednisolone.

Evidence that complement activation occurring in patients with multiple sclerosis involves the formation of membrane attack complexes is provided by the detection of the membrane attack complex neo-antigen, which only forms when the terminal complex is fully assembled through the sequential addition of C5b C9.[137] Following demonstration of the recovery mechanism of oligodendrocytes and the identification of vesicles in the supernatant of cells grown in tissue culture, identical particulate material has been found in the cerebrospinal fluid of patients with multiple sclerosis, but not in individuals with mechanical nerve root irritation or intracranial mass lesions.[130] These vesicles bind C8, C9 and the neo-antigen of membrane attack complexes, but not C3 and are shown by electron microscopy to have a high concentration of membrane pores; galactocerebroside but not myelin basic protein is present on their surface.

THE ROLE OF MICROGLIA AND MACROPHAGES IN MULTIPLE SCLEROSIS

Histological evidence suggests that macrophages are ultimately responsible for contacting and stripping away myelin from axons.[138,139] Vesicular disruption of myelin occurs in proximity to macrophages and the myelin lamellae are removed by a process which involves the attachment of myelin to coated pits, after which the sheets are incorporated into macrophages as elongated vesicles. The presence of coated pits suggests that this process is receptor-mediated and macrophages seen to contact oligodendrocytes and the myelin sheath are coated with antibody. The source of these macrophages is controversial. The intact central nervous system is traditionally regarded as not containing cells which are primarily immunocompetent, but during development, circulating macrophages enter the nervous system, seemingly through an intact blood–brain barrier in response to neuronal death, and establish themselves as resident microglial cells.[140] Thereafter, it can be difficult to distinguish one cell type from the other and no substantial differences may exist. Circulating activated macrophages can also cross the blood–brain barrier and so contribute to the local inflammatory process.

Therefore, the implication is that the mature central nervous system contains large numbers of cells which are capable of secreting and responding to a wide range of inflammatory mediators: in addition, they have the ability to phagocytose intact cells and debris.[134] The list of soluble factors which interact with macrophages is enormous. Interferon gamma, produced in response to viral infection, is a potent activator of macrophages and stimulates the release of interleukins, tumour necrosis factors, toxic oxygen species and some early complement components;[134] it also activates macrophage-mediated cytotoxicity. Many of these cytokines and inflammatory mediators form part of powerful positive feed forward loops; thus complement activation leads to the production of activation products which are chemotactic for and activate macrophages, which in turn produce more early complement components. Conversely, the production by macrophages of other molecules such as prostaglandins, which are immunosuppressive, is reduced by interferon gamma. Several of these macrophage products, including tumour necrosis factor, leukotrienes and oxygen radicals have been shown to damage myelin in vitro either by a direct effect or through oligodendrocyte injury.[141,142]

Complement activation, intrathecal antibody synthesis and other pro-inflammatory cytokines provide the local conditions needed for macrophage activation. What remains uncertain is whether macrophages activated damage to myelin and oligodendrocytes or merely act as scavengers of tissue that is already irreversibly injured through humoral mechanisms of immunity.

CONCLUDING REMARKS

The hypothesis that emerges from a consideration

of the evidence available from human samples and experimental studies is that in genetically susceptible individuals, activated T cells and macrophages, responding to environmental triggers, increase their normal surveillance of the nervous system and interact with type 1 astrocytes further to disrupt the blood–brain barrier and cause a leak of immune mediators into the nervous system. Oligodendrocytes are unduly sensitive to contact with complement, especially when antibody directed against a variety of surface components of the oligodendrocyte or its myelin processes is also present. The interaction of these soluble mediators

increases membrane permeability and leads to a rise in intracellular calcium, the degree and duration of which determines whether or not reversible injury ensues. As complement activation proceeds, macrophages are recruited and they contribute to cell injury through release of cytokines and phagocytosis of the myelin lamellae. The sequence of events that leads to tissue injury needs to be understood so that a mechanistic approach is taken in selecting new treatments and the resource of patients available for the clinical trials, on which definitive strategies for treatment will be based, is not squandered.

REFERENCES

1. Kabat E A, Moore D H, Landow H 1942 An electrophoretic study of the protein components in cerebrospinal fluid and their relationship to the serum protein. Journal of Clinical Investigation 21: 571–577
2. Von Boehmer H, Teh H S, Kisielow P 1989 The thymus selects the useful, neglects the useless and destroys the harmful. Immunology Today 10: 57–61
3. Unanue E R 1984 Antigen presenting function of the macrophage. Annals and Reviews in Immunology 2: 395–428
4. Fontana A, Fierz W, Wekerle H 1984 Astrocytes present myelin basic protein to encephalitogenic T cell lines. Nature 307: 276–278
5. Brown J H, Jardetzky T, Saper M A et al 1988 A hypothetical model of the foreign antigen binding site of Class 2 histocompatibility molecules. Nature 332: 845–850
6. Zinkernagel R M, Doherty C 1974 Restriction of in vitro T cell mediated cytotoxicity in lymphocytic choriomeningitis within a syngeneic or semiallogeneic system. Nature 248: 701–702
7. Shaw S 1989 Not all in a name. Nature 338: 539–540
8. Marrack P, Kappler J 1988 The T cell repertoire for antigen and MHC. Immunology Today 9: 308–315
9. Janeway C A, Jones B, Hayday A 1988 Specificity and functional T cells bearing gamma/delta receptors. Immunology Today 9: 73–76
10. Anderson P, Morimoto C, Breitmeyer J B, Schlossman S F 1988 Regulatory interactions between members of the immunoglobulin superfamily. Immunology Today 9: 199–203
11. Bottomly K 1988 A functional dichotomy in CD4 + T lymphocytes. Immunology Today 9: 268–274
12. Streuli M, Matsuyama T, Morimoto C et al 1987 Identification of the sequence required for expression of the 2H4 epitope on the human leukocyte common antigen. Journal of Experimental Medicine 166: 1567–1572
13. McMichael A J, Ting A, Zweerink H J, Askonas B A 1977 HLA restriction of cell mediated lysis of influenza virus infected human cells. Nature 270: 524–526
14. Liu C-C 1988 Multiple mechanisms of lymphocyte mediated killing. Immunology Today 9: 140–144
15. Abbas A K 1988 A reassessment of mechanisms of antigen-specific T-cell-dependent B-cell activation. Immunology Today 9: 89–94
16. Reinherz E L, Schlossman S F 1980 Regulation of the immune response-inducer and suppressor T lymphocyte subsets in human beings. New England Journal of Medicine 303: 370–373
17. Batchelor J R, Lombardi G, Lechler R I 1989 Speculations on the specificity of suppression. Immunology Today 10: 37–40
18. O'Garra A 1989 Interleukins in the immune system 2. Lancet 1: 1003–1005
19. O'Garra A 1989 Interleukins in the immune system 1. Lancet 1: 943–946
20. Adams J M, Imagawa D T 1962 Measles antibodies in multiple sclerosis. Proceedings of the Society for Experimental Biology and Medicine 111: 562–566
21. Patterson P Y, Whitacre C C 1981 The enigma of oligoclonal immunoglobin G in cerebrospinal fluid from multiple sclerosis patients. Immunology Today 1: 111–117
22. Alter M 1977 Is multiple sclerosis an age-dependent host response to measles? Lancet 1: 456–457
23. Haile R, Smith P, Read D et al 1982 A study of measles virus and canine distemper virus antibodies, and of childhood infections in multiple sclerosis patients and controls. Journal of the Neurological Sciences 56: 1–10
24. Cook S D, Dowling P C 1980 Multiple sclerosis and viruses; an overview. Neurology 30 (suppl): 80–91
25. Kurtzke J F, Hyllested K 1986 Multiple sclerosis in the Faroe Islands. Clinical update, transmission and the nature of MS. Neurology 36: 307–328
26. Sibley W A, Foley J M 1965 Infection and immunisation in multiple sclerosis. Annals of the New York Acadamy of Sciences 122: 457–468
27. Sibley W A, Bamford C R, Clark K 1985 Clinical viral infections and multiple sclerosis. Lancet i: 1313–1315
28. Mitchell D N, Porterfield J S, Micheletti R et al 1978 Isolation of an infectious agent from bone marrows of patients with multiple sclerosis. Lancet ii: 387–391
29. Goswami K K A, Lange L S, Mitchell D N et al 1984. Does Simian virus 5 infect humans? Journal of General Virology 65: 1295–1303
30. Goswami K K A, Randall R E, Lange L S, Russell

W C 1987 Antibodies against the paramyxovirus SV5 in the cerebrospinal fluid of some multiple sclerosis patients. Nature 327: 244–247

31. Vandvik B, Norrby E 1989 Paramyxovirus SV5 and multiple sclerosis. Nature 338: 769–771

32. Koprowski H, DeFreitas E C, Harper M E et al 1985 Multiple sclerosis and human T-cell lymphotroplic retroviruses. Nature 318: 154–160

33. Swingler R J, Hughes P J, Munro J A, Compston D A S 1987 Human T-cell lymphotroplic viruses in patients with multiple sclerosis. Journal of Neurology 234: 448

34. Rice G P A, Armstrong H A, Bullman D E et al 1986 Absence of HTLV I and III in sera of Canadian patients with multiple sclerosis and chronic myelopathy. Annals of Neurology 20: 533–534

35. Karpas A, Kampf U, Sidden A et al 1986 Lack of evidence for involvement of known retroviruses in multiple sclerosis. Nature 322: 177–178

36. Reddy E P, Sandberg–Wollheim M, Mettus R V et al 1989 Amplification and molecular cloning of HTLV I sequences from DNA of multiple sclerosis patients. Science 243: 529–533

37. Waksman B H 1989 Multiple sclerosis: relationship to a retrovirus? Nature 337: 599

38. Greenberg S J, Ehrlich G D, Abbott M A et al 1989 Detection of sequences homologous to human retroviral DNA in multiple sclerosis by gene amplification. Proceedings of the National Academy of Sciences of the USA 86: 2878–2882

39. Gessain A, Barin F, Vernant J C et al 1985 Antibodies to human T lymphotropic virus type I in patients with tropical spastic paraparesis. Lancet 2: 407–409

40. Montgomery R D, Cruickshank E K, Robertson W B, McMenemey W H 1964 Clinical and pathological observations on Jamaican neuropathy. Brain 87: 425–462

41. Newton M, Cruickshank K, Miller D H et al 1987 Antibody to human lymphotropic virus type I in West Indian born UK residents with spastic paraparesis. Lancet 1: 415–416

42. Bangham C R M, Duenke S, Phillips R E, Bell J E 1988 Enzymic amplification of exogenous and endogenous retroviral sequences from DNA of patients with tropical spastic paraparesis. EMBO Journal 7: 4179–4184

43. Compston D A S 1983 Lymphocyte sub-populations in patients with multiple sclerosis. Journal of Neurology, Neurosurgery and Psychiatry 46: 105–114

44. Hauser S L, Reinherz E L, Hoban C J et al 1983 Immunoregulatory T-cell and lymphocytotoxic antibodies in active multiple sclerosis; weekly analysis over a six month period. Annals of Neurology 13: 418–425

45. Bach M–A, Martin C, Cesaro P et al 1985 T-cell subsets in multiple sclerosis — a longitudinal study of exacerbating remitting cases. Journal of Neuroimmunology 7: 331–343

46. Compston D A S, Hughes P J 1984 Peripheral blood lymphocyte sub-populations and multiple sclerosis. Journal of Neuroimmunology 6: 105–114

47. Reder A T, Antel J P, Oger J J–G et al 1984 Low T8 antigen density on lymphocytes in active multiple sclerosis. Annals of Neurology 16: 242–249

48. Rice G P A, Finney D, Braheny S L et al 1984 Disease activity markers in multiple sclerosis. Another look at suppressor cells defined by monoclonal antibodies OKT4, OKT5 and OKT8. Journal of Neuroimmunology 6: 75–84

49. Mingioli E S, McFarlin D 1984 Leucocyte surface antigens in patients with multiple sclerosis. Journal of Neuroimmunology 6: 131–139

50. Paty D W, Kastrukoff L, Morgan N, Hiob L 1983 Suppressor T lymphocytes in multiple sclerosis; analysis of patients with acute relapsing and chronic progressive disease. Annals of Neurology 14: 445–449

51. Hughes P J, Kirk P F, Compston D A S 1986 Suppressor T cells in family members of patients with multiple sclerosis. Brain 109: 969–985

52. Morimoto C, Hafler D A, Weiner H L et al 1987 Selective loss of the suppressor-inducer T-cell subset in progressive multiple sclerosis. New England Journal of Medicine 316: 67–72

53. Hughes P J, Kirk P F, Compston D A S 1989 Dual labelling of circulating CD8 cells in patients with multiple sclerosis. Journal of Neurology, Neurosurgery and Psychiatry 52: 118–121

54. Golaz J, Steck A, Moretta L 1983 Activated T lymphocytes in patients with multiple sclerosis. Neurology 33: 1371–1373

55. Hughes P J, Compston D A S 1988 Peripheral blood lymphocyte phenotype and function in multiple sclerosis. Journal of Neurology, Neurosurgery and Psychiatry 51: 1187–1192

56. Hafler D A, Hemler M E, Christenson L et al 1985 Investigation of in vivo activated T-cells in multiple sclerosis and inflammatory central nervous system diseases. Clinical Immunology and Immunopathology 37: 163–171

57. Selmaj K, Plater–Zyber K C, Rockett K A et al 1986 Multiple sclerosis; increased expression of interleukin 2 receptors on lymphocytes. Neurology 36: 1392–1395

58. Bellamy A S, Calder V L, Feldmann M, Davison A N 1985 The distribution of interleukin 2 receptor bearing lymphocytes in multiple sclerosis; evidence for a key role of activated lymphocytes. Clinical and Experimental Immunology 61: 248–256

59. Tournier–Lasserve E, Lyon–Caen O, Roullet E, Bach M–A 1987 IL-2 receptor and HLA Class 2 antigens on cerebrospinal fluid cells of patients with multiple sclerosis and other neurological diseases. Clinical and Experimental Immunology 67: 581–586

60. Crockard A D, McNeill T A, McKirgan J, Hawkins S A 1988 Determination of activated lymphocytes in peripheral blood of patients with multiple sclerosis. Journal of Neurology, Neurosurgery and Psychiatry 51: 139–141

61. Konttinen Y T, Bergroth V, Kinnunen E et al 1987 Activated T lymphocytes in patients with multiple sclerosis in clinical remission. Journal of the Neurological Sciences 81: 133–139

62. Goust J M, Hoffman P M, Pyrjma J et al 1980 Defective immunoregulation in multiple sclerosis. Annals of Neurology 8: 526–523

63. Antel J P, Rosenkoetter M, Reder A et al 1984 Multiple sclerosis; relation to in vitro IgG secretion to T suppressor cell number and function. Neurology 34: 1155–1160

64. Antel J P, Arnason B G W, Medof M E 1979 Suppressor cell function in multiple sclerosis.

Correlation with clinical disease activity. Annals of Neurology 5: 338–342

65. Gonzalez R L, Dau P C, Spitler L E 1979 Altered regulation of mitogen responsiveness by suppressor cells in multiple sclerosis. Clinical and Experimental Immunology 36: 78–84

66. Wallen W C, Houff S A, Iivanainen M, Calebrese V P, Devrier G H 1981 Suppressor cell activity in multiple sclerosis. Neurology 31: 668–674

67. Haahr S, Muller–Larsen A, Pedersen E 1983 Immunological parameters in multiple sclerosis patients with special reference to the Herpes virus group. Clinical and Experimental Immunology 51: 197–206

68. Kelly R E, Ellison G W, Myers L W et al 1981 Abnormal regulation of in vitro IgG production in multiple sclerosis. Annals of Neurology 9: 267–272

69. Goust J–M, Hogan E L, Arnaud P 1982 Abnormal regulation of IgG production in multiple sclerosis. Neurology 32: 228–234

70. Huddlestone J R, Oldstone M V A 1982 Suppressor T-cells are activated in vivo in patients with multiple sclerosis coinciding with remission from acute attack. Journal of Immunology 129: 915–917

71. Tjernlund U, Cesaro P, Tournier E et al 1984 T-cell subsets in multiple sclerosis; a comparative study between cell surface antigens and function. Clinical Immunology and Immunopathology 32: 185–197

72. Ojer J, Kastrukoff L, O'Gorman M, Paty D W 1986 Progressive multiple sclerosis; abnormal immune functions in vitro and abberent correlation with enumeration of lymphocyte sub-populations. Journal of Neuroimmunology 12: 37–48

73. Antel J P, Bania M B, Reder A, Cashman N 1986 Activated suppressor cell dysfunction in progressive multiple sclerosis. Journal of Immunology 137: 137–141

74. Antel J P, Nicholas M K, Bania M B et al 1986 Comparison of T8+ cell mediated suppressor and cytotoxic function in multiple sclerosis. Journal of Neuroimmunology 12: 215–224

75. Antel J, Brown M, Nicholas M K et al 1988 Activated suppressor cell function in multiple sclerosis — clinical correlations. Journal of Neuroimmunology 17: 323–330

76. Chofflon M, Weiner H L, Morimoto C, Hafler D A 1988 Loss of functional suppression is linked to decreases in circulating suppressor inducer (CD4+ 2H4+) T-cells in multiple sclerosis. Annals of Neurology 24: 185–191

77. Bradbury M W (ed) 1983 In: Concept of the blood brain barrier. John Wiley and Sons, London

78. Wekerle H, Linington C, Lassmann H, Meyerman R 1986 Cellular immune reactivity within the CNS. Trends in Neuroscience 9: 271–277

79. Simmons R D, Buzbee T M, Linthicum D S et al 1987 Simultaneous visualisation of vascular permeability change and leucocyte egress in the central nervous system during autoimmune encephalomyelitis. Acta Neuropathologica 74: 191–193

80. Hafler D A, Weiner H L 1987 In vivo labelling of blood T cells; rapid trafficking to cerebrospinal fluid in multiple sclerosis. Annals of Neurology 22: 89–93

81. Hirano A, Dembitzer H M, Becker N H Levine S, Zimmerman H M et al 1970 Fine structural alterations of the blood brain barrier in experimental allergic encephalomyelitis. Journal of Neuropathology and Experimental Neurology 29: 432–440

82. Simpson L O 1989 Immunological treatment for multiple sclerosis. Lancet 1: 1272–1273

83. James P B 1989 Immunological treatment for multiple sclerosis. Lancet 1: 1273

84. Goldmutz E A, Brosnan C F, Norton W T 1986 Prazosin treatment suppresses increased vascular permeability in both acute and passive transferred EAE in the Lewis rat. Journal of Immunology 137: 3444–3450

85. Tsukada N, Koh C S, Yanagisawa N et al 1987 A new model for multiple sclerosis; chronic experimental allergic encephalomyelitis induced by immunisation with cerebral endothelial cell membrane. Acta Neuropathologica 73: 259–266

86. Brosnan C F, Bornstein M B, Bloom B R 1981 The effects of macrophage depletion on the clinical and pathologic expression of experimental allergic encephalomyelitis. Journal of Immunology 126: 614–620

87. Linington C, Morgan B P, Scolding N J et al 1989 The role of complement in the pathogenesis of experimental allergic encephalomyelitis. Brain 112: 895–911

88. Sedgwick J, Brostoff S, Mason D 1987 Experimental allergic encephalitis in the absence of a classical delayed type hypersensitivity. Severe paralytic disease correlates with the presence of interleukin 2 receptor positive cells infiltrating the central nervous system. Journal of Experimental Medicine 165: 1058–1075

89. Sedgwick J D 1988 Long-term depletion of CD8+ T-cells in vivo in the rat; no observed role for CD8+ (cytotoxic/suppressor) cells in the immunoregulation of experimental allergic encephalomyelitis. European Journal of Immunology 18: 495–502

90. Ellerman K E, Powers J M, Brostoff S W 1988 A suppressor T-lymphocyte cell line for autoimmune encephalomyelitis. Nature 331: 265–267

91. Brostoff S, Mason D W 1986 The role of lymphocyte subpopulations in the transfer of rat EAE. Journal of Neuroimmunology 10: 331–339

92. Vass K, Lassmann H, Wekerle H, Wisniewski H M 1986 The distribution of Ia antigen in the lesions of rat experimental allergic encephalitis. Acta Neuropathologica 70: 149–160

93. Matsumoto Y, Fujiwara M 1986 In situ detection of Class 1 and 2 major histocompatibility complex antigens in the rat central nervous system during experimental allergic encephalitis — an immunohistochemical study. Journal of Neuroimmunology 12: 265–277

94. Lightman S, McDonald W I, Bird A C et al 1987 Retinal venous sheathing in optic neuritis. Its significance for the pathogenesis of multiple sclerosis. Brain 110: 405–414

95. Shaw P J, Smith N M, Ince P G, Bates D 1987 Chronic periphlebitis retinae in multiple sclerosis. A histopathological study. Journal of Neurological Sciences 77: 147–152

96. Miller D H, Rudge P, Johnson G et al 1988 Serial gadolinium enhanced magnetic resonance imaging in multiple sclerosis. Brain 111: 927–939

97. Hayes M, Roodroofe M N, Cuzner M L 1987 Microglia of the major cell type expressing MHC Class 2 in human white matter. Journal of the Neurological Sciences 80: 25–37

98. Hayashi T, Morimoto C, Burks J S et al 1988 Dual label immunocytochemistry of the active multiple

sclerosis lesions; major histocompatibility complex and activation antigens. Annals of Neurology 24: 523–531

99. Traugott U, Scheinberg L C, Raine C S 1985 The presence of Ia positive endothelial cells and astrocytes in multiple sclerosis and its relevance to antigen presentation. Journal of Neuroimmunology 8: 1–14

100. Hafler D A, Fox D A, Manning M E et al 1985 In vivo activated T lymphocytes in the peripheral blood and cerebrospinal fluid of patients with multiple sclerosis. New England Journal of Medicine 312: 1405–1411

101. Kuroda Y, Shibaski H 1987 CSF mononuclear cell subsets in active MS; lack of disease-specific alteration. Neurology 37: 497–499

102. Noronha A B C, Richman D P, Arnason B G W 1980 Detection of in vivo stimulated cerebrospinal fluid lymphocytes by flow cytometry in patients with multiple sclerosis. New England Journal of Medicine 303: 713–717

103. Fredrikson S, Karlsson–Parra A, Olsson T, Link H 1987 HLA-DR antigen expression on T cells from cerebrospinal fluid in multiple sclerosis and aseptic meningoencephalitis. Clinical and Experimental Immunology 68: 298–304

104. Weber W E J, Buurman W A, Vandermeeren M M P P et al 1987 Fine analysis of cytolytic and natural killer T lymphocytes in the CSF in multiple sclerosis and other neurological diseases. Neurology 37: 419–425

105. Rotteveel F T M, Kokkelink I, van Walbeek H K et al 1987 Analysis of T cell receptor-gene rearrangement in T cells from the cerebrospinal fluid of patients with multiple sclerosis. Journal of Neuroimmunology 15: 243–249

106. Hafler D A, Duby A D, Lee S J et al 1988 Oligoclonal T lymphocytes in the cerebrospinal fluid of patients with multiple sclerosis. Journal of Experimental Medicine 167: 1313–1322

107. Hafler D A, Benjamin D S, Burks J, Weiner H L 1987 Myelin basic protein and proteolipid protein reactivity of brain and cerebrospinal fluid-derived T cell clones in multiple sclerosis and post infectious encephalomyelitis. Journal of Immunology 139: 68–72

108. Cohen S R, Bannister R 1967 Immunoglobulin synthesis within the central nervous system in disseminated sclerosis. Lancet i: 366–367

109. Henriksson A, Kam–Hansen S, Link H 1985 IgM, IgA and IgG producing cells in cerebrospinal fluid and peripheral blood in multiple sclerosis. Clinical and Experimental Immunology 62: 176–184

110. Schuller E A C, Benabdallah S, Sagar H J et al 1987 IgG synthesis within the central nervous system. Comparison of 3 formulas. Archives of Neurology 44: 600–604

111. Thompson E J, Kaufmann P, Shortman R C et al 1979 Oligoclonal immunoglobulins and plasma cells in spinal fluid of patients with multiple sclerosis. British Medical Journal 1: 16–17

112. Sandberg–Wollheim M 1975 Optic neuritis; studies on the cerebrospinal fluid in relation to clinical course in 61 patients. Acta Neurologica Scandinavica 52: 167–178

113. Nikoskelainen E, Frey H, Salmi I 1981 Prognosis of optic neuritis with special reference to cerebrospinal fluid, immunoglobulin and measles virus antibodies. Annals of Neurology 9: 545–550

114. Stendahl–Brodin L, Link H 1983 Optic neuritis; oligoclonal bands increase the risk of multiple sclerosis. Acta Neurologica Scandinavica 67: 301–304

115. Moulin D, Paty D W, Ebers G C 1983 The predicted value of cerebrospinal fluid electrophoresis in possible multiple sclerosis. Brain 106: 809–816

116. Bass B H, Armstrong H, Weinshenker B et al 1988 Interpretation of single band patterns in CSF protein electrophoresis. Canadian Journal of the Neurological Sciences 15: 20–22

117. Bracco F, Gallo P, Menna R et al 1987 Free light chains in the CSF in multiple sclerosis. Journal of Neurology 234: 303–307

118. Fagnart O C, Sindic C J M, Laterre C 1988 Free kappa and lambda light chain levels in the cerebrospinal fluid of patients with multiple sclerosis and other neurological diseases. Journal of Neuroimmunology 19: 119–132

119. Schadlich H–J, Karber H, Felgenhauer K 1987 The prevalence of locally-synthesised virus antibodies in various forms of multiple sclerosis. Journal of the Neurological Sciences 80: 343–349

120. Brankin B, Allen I V, Hawkins S A, Wisdom G B 1988 Screening of multiple sclerosis cerebrospinal fluid for autoantibodies. Journal of the Neurological Sciences 84: 29–40

121. Martin–Mondière C, Jacque C, Delassalle A et al 1987 Cerebrospinal myelin basic protein in multiple sclerosis 44: 276–278

122. Warren K G, Katz I 1987 A correlation between cerebrospinal fluid, myelin basic protein and antimyelin basic protein in multiple sclerosis patients. Annals of Neurology 21: 183–189

123. Esiri M N 1980 Multiple sclerosis; a quantitative and qualitative study of immunoglobulin containing cells in the central nervous system. Neuropathology and Applied Neurobiology 6: 9–21

124. Linington C, Bradl M, Lassmann H et al 1988 Augmentation of demyelination in rat acute allergic encephalomyelitis by circulating mouse monoclonal antibodies directed against a myelin oligodendrocyte glycoprotein. American Journal of Pathology 130: 443–454

125. Raff M C, Miller R H, Noble M 1983 A glial cell precursor that develops in vitro into an astrocyte or an oligodendrocyte depending on culture medium. Nature 303: 390–396

126. Scolding N J, Morgan B P, Houston A et al 1989 Normal rat serum cytotoxicity against syngeneic oligodendrocytes. Complement activation and attack in the absence of antimyelin antibodies. Journal of the Neurological Sciences 89: 289–300

127. Scolding N J, Morgan B P, Campbell A K, Compston D A S 1990 Complement mediated serum cytotoxicity against oligodendrocytes; a comparison with other cells of the oligodendrocyte-type 2 lineage. Journal of the Neurological Sciences (in press)

128. Morgan B P 1989 Complement mediated attack on nucleated cells: resistance, recovery and non-lethal effects. Biochemical Journal 264: 1–14

129. Scolding N J, Houston W A J, Morgan B P et al 1989 Reversible injury of cultured rat oligodendrocytes by complement. Immunology 67: 441–446

130. Scolding N J, Morgan B P, Houston W A J et al 1989 Vesicular removal by oligodendrocytes of membrane attack complexes formed by activated complement.

Nature 339: 620–622

131. Chantry A, Earl C, Groome N, Glynn P 1988
Metalloprotease cleavage of 18.2–14.1 kilodalton basic
protein dissociating from rodent myelin membrane
generates 10.0 and 5.9 kilodalton terminal fragments.
Journal of Neurochemistry 1988 50: 688–694

132. Compston D A S, Morgan B P, Campbell A K et al
1989 Immunocytochemical localisation of the terminal
complement complex in multiple sclerosis.
Neuropathology and Applied Neurobiology 15: 307–316

133. Jans H, Heltberg A, Zeeberg I et al 1984 Immune
complexes and the complement factor C4 and C3 in
cerebrospinal fluid and serum from patients with
chronic progressive multiple sclerosis. Acta Neurologica
Scandinavica 69: 34–38

134. Hartung H–P, Heininger K 1989 Non-specific
mechanisms of inflammation and tissue damage in MS.
Annals of the Institute Pasteur 140: 226–233

135. Morgan B P, Campbell A K, Compston D A S 1984
Terminal component of complement (C9) in
cerebrospinal fluid of patients with multiple sclerosis.
Lancet 2: 251–254

136. Compston D A S, Morgan B P, Oleesky D et al 1986
Cerebrospinal fluid C9 in demyelinating disease.
Neurology 36: 1503–1506

137. Sanders M E, Koski C L, Robbins D et al 1986
Activated terminal complement in cerebrospinal fluid
in Guillain–Barré syndrome and multiple sclerosis.
Journal of Immunology 136: 4456–4459

138. Prineas J W 1985 The neuropathology of multiple
sclerosis. In: Koetsier J (ed) Handbook of clinical
neurology — demyelinating diseases, Vol 3 (47).
Elsevier, Amsterdam, pp 213–257

139. Esiri M M 1987 Macrophage populations associated
with multiple sclerosis plaques. Neuropathology and
Applied Neurobiology 13: 451–465

140. Perry V H, Gordon S 1988 Macrophages and microglia
in the nervous system. Trends in Neurosciences
11: 273–277

141. Camma W, Blume B R, Norton W T, Gordon S 1978
Degradation of basic protein in myelin by neutral
proteases secreted by stimulated macrophages; a
possible mechanism for inflammatory demyelination.
Proceedings of the National Academy of Sciences of
the USA 75: 1554–1558

142. Selmaj K W, Raine C S 1988 Tumour necrosis factor
mediates myelin and oligodendrocyte damage in vitro.
Annals of Neurology 23: 339–346

12. Pathology of multiple sclerosis

THE PATHOLOGICAL CONCEPT OF DEMYELINATING DISEASE

The early descriptions of the pathology of multiple sclerosis by Cruveilhier,[1] Carswell,[2] Charcot,[3] and Dawson[4] established the concept of demyelinating disease, the pathological hallmark of which is periaxial demyelination, i.e. myelin destruction with relative axonal preservation (Fig. 12.1). Pathologists have therefore designated a variety of conditions 'demyelinating', based on this common pathological feature and these are usually classified into two main groups:

Acute disseminated perivenous encephalomyelitis (acute perivascular myelinoclasis)

Classic (parainfectious; postimmunisation; idiopathic)
Hyperacute (acute haemorrhagic leucoencephalitis)

Multiple sclerosis (disseminated sclerosis)

Classic (Charcot type)
Acute (Marburg type)
Diffuse cerebral sclerosis (Schilder type)
Concentric sclerosis (Balò type)
Neuromyelitis optica (Dévic type)

The validity of grouping conditions both acute and chronic, and with varying clinical and anatomical features, must be questioned. The classification, however, is based on histological description and not on aetiology; moreover, there are sufficient common features to justify such an interim grouping until the pathogenesis of these diseases is firmly established. The emphasis on myelin destruction as the unifying histological feature in demyelinating disease is justified by the prominence of oligodendrocyte and myelin loss at autopsy. It must be conceded, however, that most pathological studies have concentrated on these demyelinating lesions to the detriment of other more subtle and diffuse abnormalities, which may nevertheless be significant pointers to basic pathogenesis. Multiple sclerosis is the most common of the demyelinating diseases; other diseases originally included in the group but in which pathogenesis is now established (e.g. central pontine myelinolysis), are now considered as distinct entities. Genetic disorders of myelin and conditions in which neuronolytic demyelination occurs, are excluded by definition.

PATHOLOGY

Most cases of multiple sclerosis coming to autopsy are of the classical (Charcot) type with an initial history of remission and relapse, but ultimately showing continuous deterioration.[5] Four additional, much rarer, forms are recognised, i.e. Dévic's neuromyelitis optica,[6] Marburg's acute type,[7] Schilder's variety with massive confluent demyelination in the cerebral hemispheres,[8] and Balò's type,[9] in which the demyelination appears to be concentric.

The chronic and severe nature of the neurological deficit in most cases is indicated in autopsy series by the high incidence of secondary infections of the renal and respiratory tracts and of limb contractures and pressure sores (Table 12.1). However a change in the pattern of these nonspecific secondary complications is now apparent, presumably largely due to improvements in general care and in antibiotic therapy. Fewer

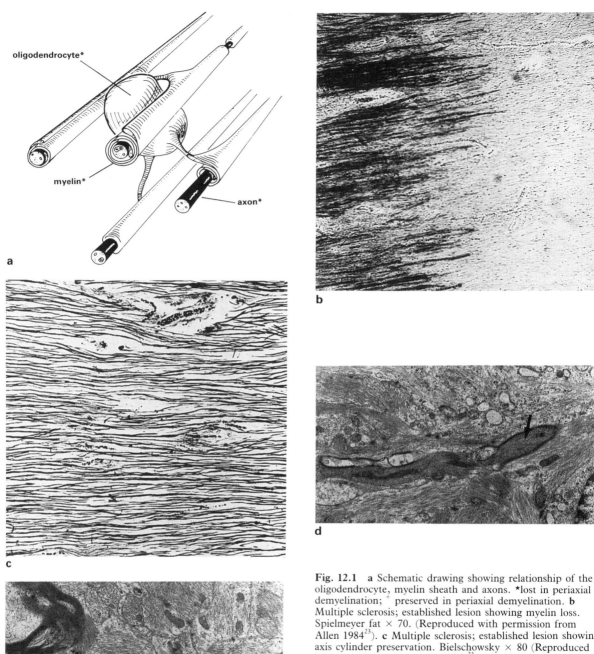

Fig. 12.1 **a** Schematic drawing showing relationship of the oligodendrocyte, myelin sheath and axons. *lost in periaxial demyelination; + preserved in periaxial demyelination. **b** Multiple sclerosis; established lesion showing myelin loss. Spielmeyer fat × 70. (Reproduced with permission from Allen 1984[23]). **c** Multiple sclerosis; established lesion showing axis cylinder preservation. Bielschowsky × 80 (Reproduced with permission from Allen 1984[23]). **d** Periaxial demyelination in multiple sclerosis; a thinly myelinated nerve fibre (arrow) shows irregular blebbing and displacement of myelin as it traverses an astrocytic scar. Electron micrograph × 6250. **e** Loss of a myelin internodal segment in multiple sclerosis can leave paranodal axolemmal specialisations in place (between arrows). Filament-rich astrocytic processes surround the axon. Electron micrograph × 6800. (Reproduced with permission from Allen 1984[23].)

Table 12.1 Significant complications in multiple sclerosis

Complication	Number of cases
Bronchopneumonia	55
Cystitis and pyelonephritis	53
Renal and/or vesical calculi	10
Pelvic abscess and localised peritonitis	9
Venous thrombosis: leg veins	5
periprostatic	3
adrenal vein	1
renal vein	1
cerebral vein	1
Pulmonary emboli	6
Adrenal haemorrhage	1
Stercoral ulceration	1
Volvulus	2
Bacterial endocarditis	1
Hypothermia	1
Epilepsy	1
Burns	1
Suicide	3

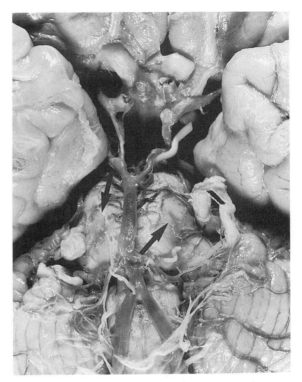

Fig. 12.2 Plaques seen externally on the surface of the pons (arrows) after stripping of the leptomeninges.

patients die with extensive pressure sores or septicaemia complicating renal sepsis, and not all patients die as a direct result of their disease; in a series of 120 cases, collected over many years, approximately 25% of patients died from apparently unrelated conditions.[10]

The essential lesion — anatomy and evolution

Anatomy of plaque distribution

In classical multiple sclerosis, in which the patient has been severely affected and has had many years of illness, the brain at autopsy may appear slightly atrophic with widening of cerebral sulci and some ventricular dilation, and the spinal cord may also show some atrophy. The characteristic specific pathological abnormality is the presence of scattered demarcated lesions in which periaxial demyelination can be demonstrated histologically. Irregular, grey, firm depressed plaques can often be seen externally in the optic nerves, on the surface of the pons, (Fig. 12.2), medulla and spinal cord, and on the superior surface of the corpus callosum. These may be up to 5 mm in diameter

and are best seen if the arachnoid is stripped from the underlying surface.

In the unfixed, sectioned brain, old lesions are grey, often somewhat translucent and firm (hence the use of the term 'sclerosis'), and recent lesions are soft and appear pink: after fixation, the distinguishing hardness of the old lesion is lost and the recent lesions are difficult to see.

The pattern of plaque distribution varies considerably from case to case and within any one case plaques may vary considerably in size and age. A clear impression of the most common distribution of lesions within the brain is best obtained by the study of a series of cases, altering in each the plane of cerebral section. Thus, with coronal sectioning, a wide scatter of lesions is seen in both cerebral hemispheres, often with a degree of symmetry (Fig. 12.3); predominant involvement of one hemisphere is rare. The relationship of plaques to the ventricular system is striking, particularly to the lateral angles of the lateral ventricles and to

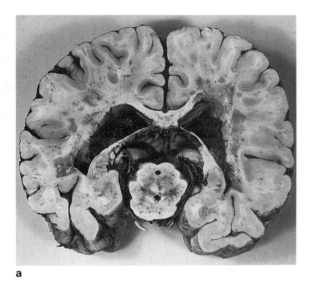
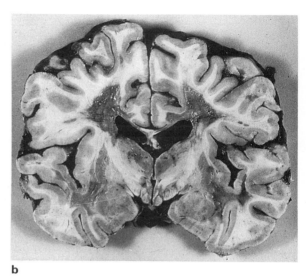

a

b

Fig. 12.3 Classical chronic multiple sclerosis. **a** Numerous scattered plaques in deep white matter and brain stem. **b** Symmetrical periventricular demyelination. (Reproduced with permission from Allen 1984[23]).

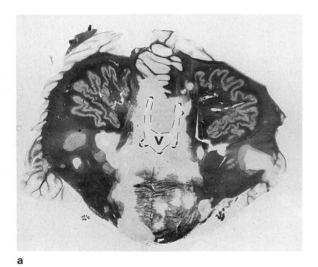

a

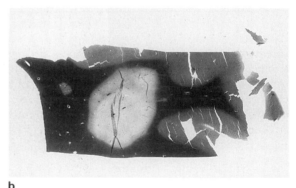

b

Fig. 12.4 **a** Brainstem plaques with confluent demyelination around the IVth ventricle (**V**). **b**. Subcortical plaque with sparing of the immediate subcortical myelin. Weigert-Pal × 1.

the floor of the aqueduct and the fourth ventricle (Fig. 12.4a). Other scattered plaques are seen throughout the white matter, many extending close to the cortex but sparing the immediate subcortical myelin (Fig. 12.4b). The involvement of grey matter is frequently underestimated[11] unless extensive histological investigation is carried out. Brownell and Hughes,[12] in a study of the cerebrum in multiple sclerosis, found that 74% of

plaques involved the white matter, 17% were sited at the junction of grey and white matter, 5% were entirely cortical and 4% were restricted to the central grey matter. Of all cerebral plaques, 22% were frontal, 15% parietal, 12% temporal and only 1% occipital. The periventricular plaques look relatively small in the coronal plane, but on sagittal section are often seen to extend from the limits of the anterior and inferior horns of the lateral ven-

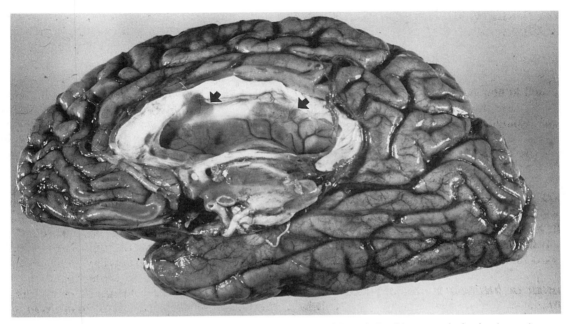

Fig. 12.5 Classical chronic multiple sclerosis. Note plaques with striking relationship to terminal veins (arrows).

tricle to the tip of the posterior horn. Also in the sagittal plane, the striking relationship of demyelination to terminal veins is most easily seen (Fig. 12.5) and in this site small perivenular, spherical plaques may be identified.

The optic nerve, brainstem and spinal cord are usually extensively involved (Figs. 12.6 and 12.7), and in some patients these sites are severely affected while the cerebrum contains only a few plaques. In a study of 36 optic nerves from 18 patients,[13] demyelination was found in 35, thus confirming the vulnerability of the optic nerve in multiple sclerosis. Plaques in the brain stem may be difficult to see with the naked eye, but they are often numerous and involve the periaqueductal grey and white matter and also important midline

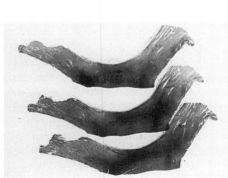

a

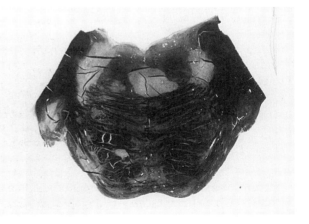

b

Fig. 12.6 a Demyelination in optic nerves adjacent to the optic chiasm. Spielmeyer × 2.5. (Reproduced with permission from Allen 1984[23].) **b** Plaques in the pons. Weigert-Pal × 2.5.

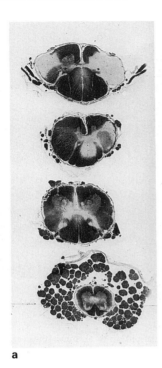

a

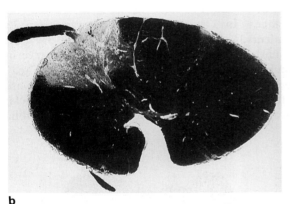

b

Fig. 12.7 a Classical chronic multiple sclerosis with extensive spinal cord involvement. Note symmetrical lesions in the lateral columns of the cervical cord. These must be distinguished from secondary long tract degeneration due to plaques in the brainstem. Weigert-Pal × 3. **b** Fan-shaped plaque in the cervical cord, closely related to the denticulate ligament. Spielmeyer fat × 6.

structures such as the medial longitudinal fasciculus.[14] Cranial nerves may be involved at their junction with central nervous tissue in the brainstem, and plaques within the cerebellum are common and are usually easily seen. The spinal cord

shows a marked predilection for involvement with plaques in the dorsum septum, subpial regions and adjacent to the anterior fissure. Oppenheimer[15] in a study of the spinal cord in 18 cases of multiple sclerosis found that the cervical cord is involved much more commonly than lower levels. He also noted the predominance of fan-shaped cervical cord lesions with a broad base, adjacent to the lateral pial surface of the cord and closely associated with the denticulate ligament (Fig. 12.7b).

Evolution of the plaque

Very few detailed descriptions of the earliest phases of demyelination in multiple sclerosis exist because of the lack of suitable pathological material. Even those patients designated 'acute' usually have been ill for some months before death, and the pathological lesions are already well established. Cerebral biopsy is rarely necessary for diagnosis and is not justified for research purposes; although some biopsy descriptions exist, these have usually been taken in cases of several weeks duration to exclude other pathological conditions. There is therefore controversy and speculation as to the primary histological abnormality; pathologists have been forced to tackle the problem either by study of the plaque edge or of the supposedly unaffected white matter. Each of these approaches produces scientific difficulties. The plaque edge is the interface between damaged and non-damaged tissue, and the observed abnormalities must result both from the disease itself and from tissue response. The apparently normal white matter, particularly in the established case, undoubtedly shows abnormalities of a secondary nature and it is difficult to distinguish these from primary pathology. It is not surprising, therefore, that observers differ in description of the early lesion and emphasise different features.

At least three contrasting views are held. According to these, the early lesion is characterised by: (i) physical disintegration of myelin without increased cellularity (Fig. 12.8); (ii) increased cellularity in which microglial hyperplasia is prominent (Fig. 12.9); (iii) perivascular inflammation in which lymphocytes are present (Fig. 12.10). Zimmerman & Netsky,[16] Seitel-

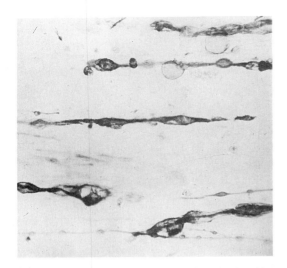

Fig. 12.8 Early demyelination in multiple sclerosis with disintegration of myelin sheath. At this phase the fragments of myelin retain their histochemical staining properties. Myelin × 270. (Reproduced with permission from Allen 1984[23].)

berger,[17] Greenfield and Norman[18] and Lumsden[11] all consider myelin disintegration, occurring in the absence of hypercellularity, as the initial change. Seitelberger states 'myelin sheaths are irregularly swollen, pale-staining and beaded and there is associated microglial phagocytosis of myelin'. Seitelberger also emphasises the inflammatory component in the plaque, but considers that in the early stages demyelination may be observed without an immune cellular response. By contrast, Dawson,[4] and Adams and Kubik[14] argue that hypercellularity with myelin pallor and microglial infiltration is the earliest abnormality, while Adams[19] suggests that perivascular lymphocytic cuffs in near-normal myelin may represent the initial lesion. Most workers are agreed that oligodendrocytes can still be recognised in the very early lesions though they are not necessarily normal. Raine, Scheineberg and Waltz[20] suggest that not only are oligodendrocytes surviving at this very early stage but they may proliferate. Brown[21] has described increased pinocytosis in cerebral vessels

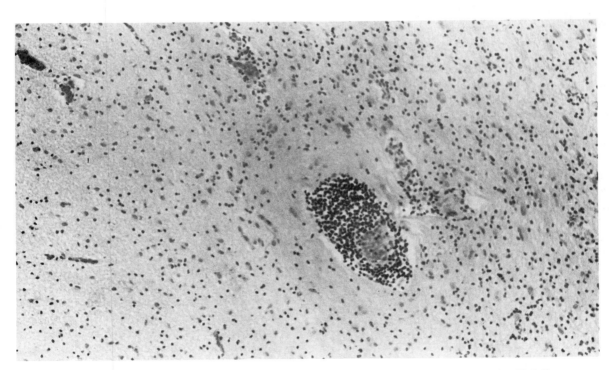

Fig. 12.9 Acute plaque in multiple sclerosis, showing perivascular inflammation and increased cellularity. H & E × 100.

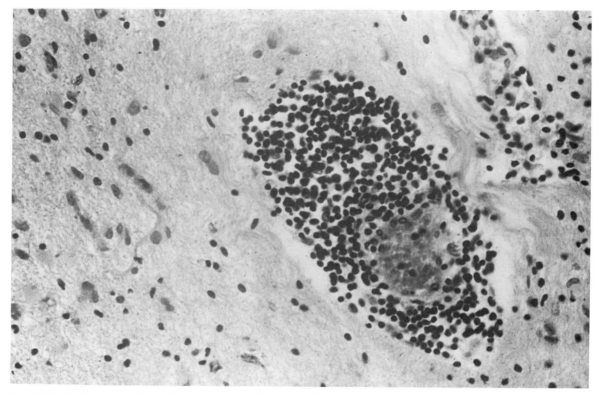

Fig. 12.10 Perivascular inflammation (enlarged from Fig. 12.9) shows predominant lymphocytic response in an area of acute demyelination. H & E × 250.

in biopsy tissue from early MS; this abnormality may have significance for some MRI changes.

Although a number of ultrastructural patterns of myelin disruption have been reported in and around developing, established, and old plaques in multiple sclerosis (see list below), it is not yet certain which of these indicate the operation of primary or secondary mechanisms and which are artefactual. Moreover, many of these recognisable patterns are likely to be stages in continuous processes which may involve more than one pattern at the same or different times (e.g. see 10 below).

1. Increased inter-lamellar spacing in myelin[22–24] (Fig. 12.11a)
2. Vesicular dissolution of myelin[24–27] (Fig. 12.11b)
3. Splitting and vacuolation of sheaths[28,29] (Fig. 12.11b)
4. Dilatation of periaxonal space and partial

detachment from included axon[20,30–32] (Fig. 12.12)
5. Sheath fragmentation, ball and ovoid formation[22,11,29] (Fig. 12.13)
6. Granular-lamellar degeneration within sheath[11,22,28,29] (Fig. 12.14)
7. Filamentous accumulations in sheath[29] (Fig. 12.14)
8. Irregularly thin myelin sheaths[22,28,29] (Fig. 12.15)
9. Macrophage-associated myelin thinning, with or without accompanying micropinocytosis vermiformis[23,24,29,30,33] (Fig. 12.16)
10. Myelin phagocytosis which may follow endocytotic thinning, lamellar widening, or vesicular dissolution and which may involve active peeling of layers of myelin by the processes of invading macrophages or of resident astrocytes[23,24,29,33–35] (Figs. 12.17 and 12.18).

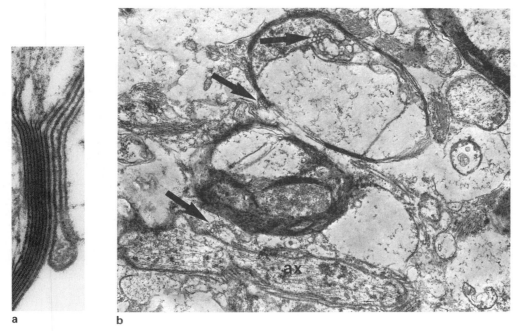

Fig. 12.11 a Lamellar separation of successive outer myelin lamellae. Electron micrograph ×120 000. **b** Vesicular-tubular myelin dissolution (arrows) and an almost naked axon (**ax**) in the partially demyelinated margin of an active plaque in acute multiple sclerosis. Electron micrograph × 14 700.

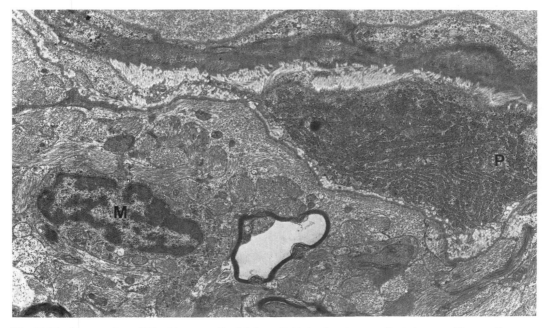

Fig. 12.12 A macrophage (**M**) without myelin debris or lipid, is close to a myelinated axon with a swollen sheath. There is a plasma cell (**P**) in the perivascular Virchow-Robin space nearby. Electron micrograph × 4600.

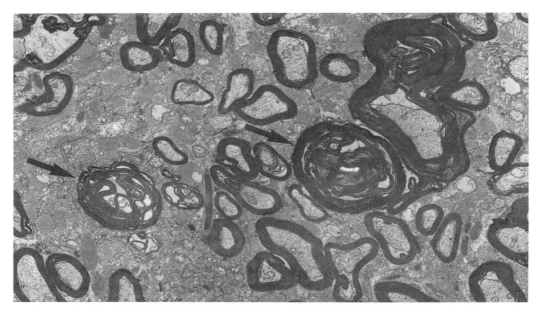

Fig. 12.13   Large masses of myelin (arrows), may in some cases represent myelin shed from large sheaths during the process of partial demyelination. Electron micrograph × 4000.

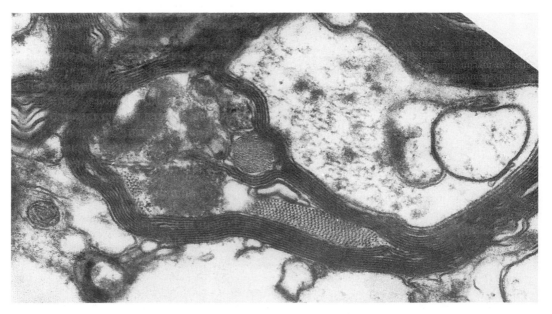

Fig. 12.14   Amorphous and filamentous material has accumulated within the myelin lamellae (major dense line) and distends the sheath. Electron micrograph × 44 000.

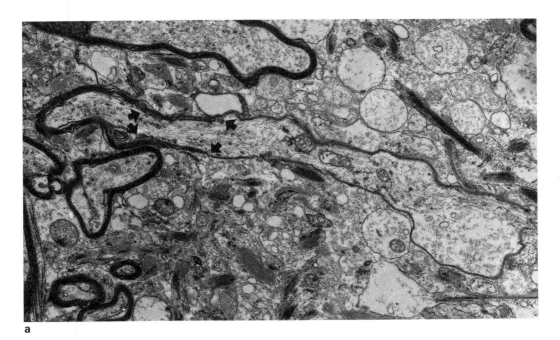

a

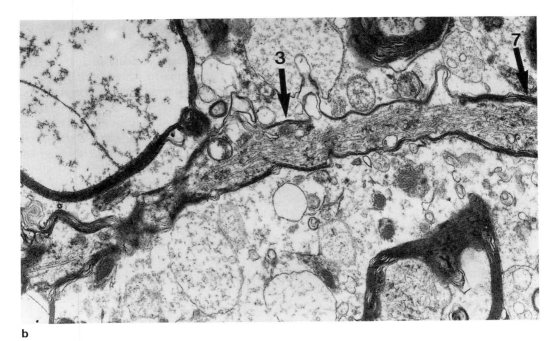

b

Fig. 12.15 **a** Abrupt tapering of a myelin sheath which appears to continue as a very thin myelin cover. The unusual presence of paranodal loops and specialisations (between arrows) as part of a continuous myelin covering suggests that the outermost nodal loops may have grown out (from left to right) to re-cover a demyelinated internode. Electron micrograph × 9100. **b** An internodal myelin sheath which is thinner in the centre of the field (3 lamellae) than at either extremity (7 lamellae). Irregular blebbing in the thinned region may indicate a localised demyelinating process. Electron micrograph × 13 100.

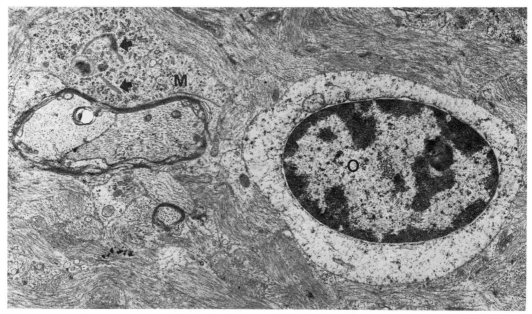

Fig. 12.16 A macrophage process (**M**) containing lyre bodies (arrows) makes intimate contact with a thinly myelinated nerve fibre which has a swollen oligodendroglial inner tongue. Interpretation of the adjacent swollen and pale oligodendrocyte (**O**) is difficult in autopsy tissue. However since not all oligodendrocytes appear so, it may have some pathological significance. Electron micrograph × 9100.

Interpretation of patterns of demyelination as indicating particular mechanisms of demyelination is only possible if due regard is paid to the context of any observed change. Thus, a pattern found only rarely in the depths of chronic plaques and never in the active acute plaque is unlikely to be an indicator of a primary mechanism in the formation of the early lesion.

The established early lesion

Despite the controversy regarding the initial lesion, there is general agreement as to the histological appearances of the established early lesion. Such plaques are generally hypercellular due to the mixed macrophage/astrocytic response (Fig. 12.19); myelin sheaths show physical disintegration with 'myelin ball' formation and this is accompanied by chemical breakdown of myelin (*vide infra*). Axons are generally preserved (Fig. 12.20) and in grey matter there is striking preservation of nerve cell bodies. A variable degree of perivascular inflammation is apparent; most of the cells look lymphocytic, but specialised histochemistry and electron microscopy indicates that there is a mixed cellular population in which lymphocytes, plasma cells and macrophages are all present (Fig. 12.21). Prineas[24] suggests that the hypercellularity is mainly the result of infiltrating microglia, some of which are in contact with intact myelin sheaths. Other sheaths, however, appear thinned and fragments of recognisable myelin are seen within macrophages, in some cases forming distinctive 'lyre bodies' (Figs. 12.17a and 12.22). Although the perivascular inflammatory response may be considerable, and immuno-competent cells can be identified in the Virchrow-Robin space (Fig. 12.21), only a few such cells are seen within the brain parenchyma and these are mainly plasma cells.

Electron microscopy of the acute lesion has confirmed the cellular constitution of the plaque but has not resolved the problem of the initial pathological reaction. The fundamental question as to whether myelin can disintegrate without cellular activity, or whether macrophages or other cells are essential for initial damage has not been resolved. Guo and Gao[27], and Lassmann[26] describe

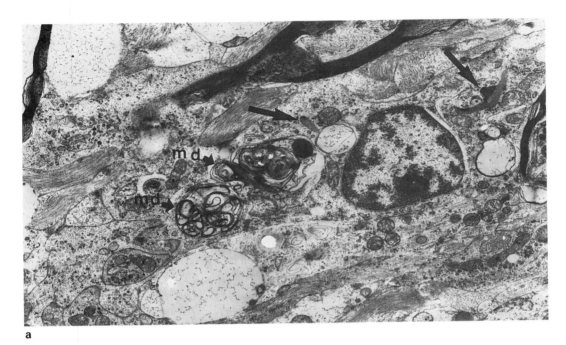

a

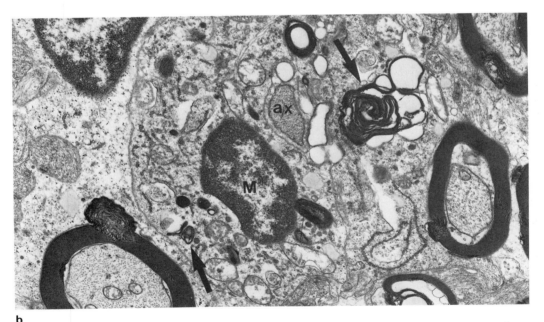

b

Fig. 12.17 a A macrophage with typical extensive processes contacts myelin sheaths. Its cytoplasm contains both recognisable, native-period, myelin debris (**md**) and partly degraded, 'lyre' bodies (arrows). Electron micrograph × 8800. **b** Macrophage-associated demyelination. A naked axon (**ax**) is enveloped by a macrophage (**M**) which contains fragments of undegraded myelin debris (arrows), indicative of very recent uptake. Electron micrograph × 12 800.

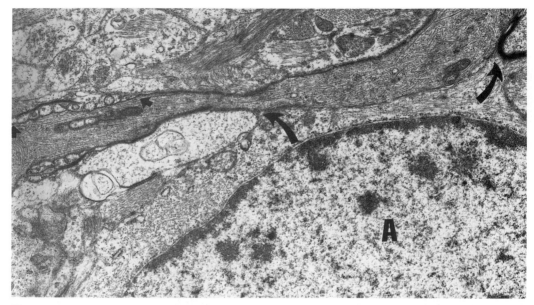

Fig. 12.18 A Filament-rich astrocyte (**A**) is separated from an axon by only myelin lamella (between curved arrows). The nine surviving nodal loops (between small arrows) of the adjacent node of Ranvier indicate the sheath's former thickness. Electron micrograph × 9600.

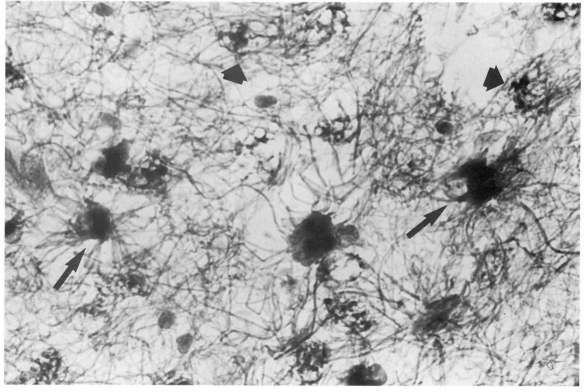

Fig. 12.19 Area of active demyelination in a classical case of multiple sclerosis stained for acid phosphatase; Astrocytes (arrows) and macrophages (arrowheads) are present. Acid phosphate × 500.

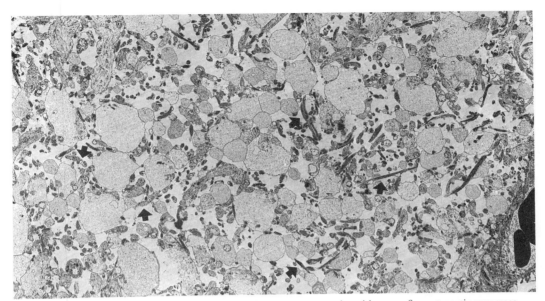

Fig. 12.20 Axonal preservation in an established plaque; axons co-exist with many fine astrocytic processes (arrows), in an oedematous plaque. Electron micrograph × 2400.

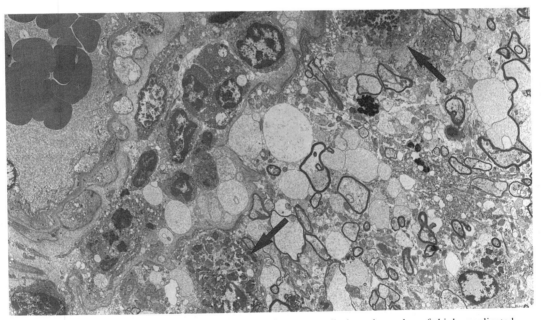

Fig. 12.21 Perivascular inflammatory cuff in a region of severe myelin loss. A number of thinly myelinated fibres are present amongst naked axons and occasional macrophages (arrows). Electron micrograph × 2300.

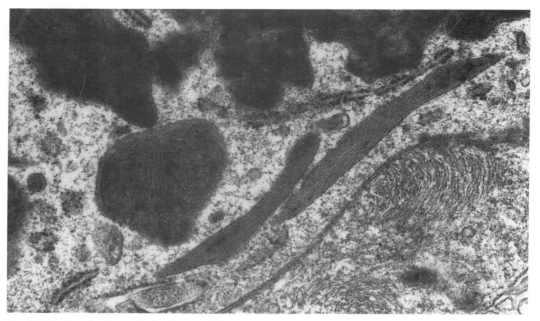

Fig. 12.22   Lyre bodies and other forms of phagolysosomes containing degraded myelin in the cytoplasm of a macrophage. Electron micrograph × 38 300.

extensive extracellular vesicular dissolution as the major pattern of myelin disruption (Fig. 12.11b). Kirk[25] had earlier described a focus of vesicular demyelination in an acute plaque (Fig. 12.11b), in a case of MS sampled at early autopsy. Prineas[24] in discussing the significance of these reports, pointed out that myelin vesiculation around chronic established lesions had been most pronounced in cases where autopsy had been delayed, which suggests that such changes had occurred postmortem. Against this however, is the fact that vesicular dissolution is a prominent feature of experimental inflammatory demyelinating disease and can be readily demonstrated in perfusion-fixed animal tissues.[36] Nevertheless Prineas,[24] reviewing the findings of Prineas & Raine[33] and Brown[21] in their studies of small numbers of cases of acute MS fixed at early autopsy or biopsy, concluded that myelin breakdown appeared to be effected chiefly by infiltrating macrophages which phagocytosed compact myelin.

It must be emphasised that the initial destruction of myelin is probably rapid and is likely to trigger a series of cellular and chemical reactions (e.g. lysosomal enzyme and complement acti-

vation) which may produce further secondary demyelination. Thus interpretation of histology in terms of initial events may not be possible even in acute cases. The occurrence of early remyelination may further confuse the issue.

The active, non-acute lesion

It is difficult to define accurately the active lesion in terms of age: the time taken for acute lesions to become inactive is unknown and probably varies according to the initial size of the plaque and its anatomical situation. Some lesions remain active for many months and during that time are capable of enlarging. The pathologist has to use arbitary descriptive features to characterise such lesions which have a variable overall cellularity, but which show astrocytic and macrophage hyperplasia and contain myelin lipid degradation products (Fig. 12.23). Perivascular inflammation is usually present but often slight, although lipid-containing macrophages and lipofuscin deposits may be seen in the Virchrow–Robin space. The central regions of such plaques may be hypocellular and gliosed and have some of the features of old, inactive

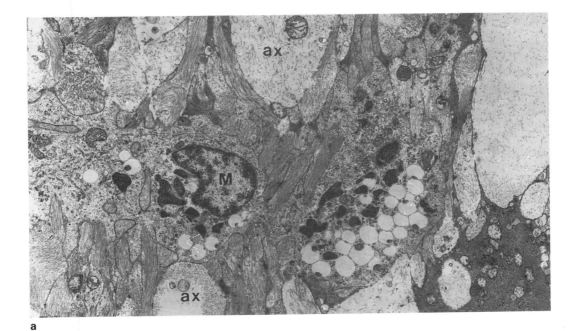

a

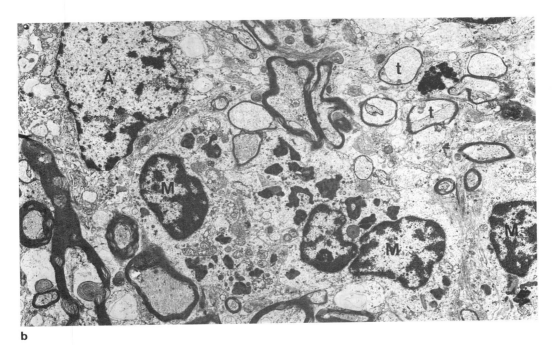

b

Fig. 12.23 a Macrophages (**M**) containing degraded myelin and lipid droplets remain within a dense astroglial scar. Note the swollen naked axons (**ax**). Electron micrograph × 6300. **b** Grouped, thinly myelinated axons (**t**) in a gliosed area with little sign of ongoing demyelination suggest that remyelination has occurred. The numerous macrophages (**M**) contain lyre bodies and other dense, partly degraded myelin phagolysosomes but neither fresh myelin debris nor lipid droplets are present. Thickly myelinated (probably normal) fibres and a large reactive astrocyte (**A**) are also present. Electron micrograph × 6300.

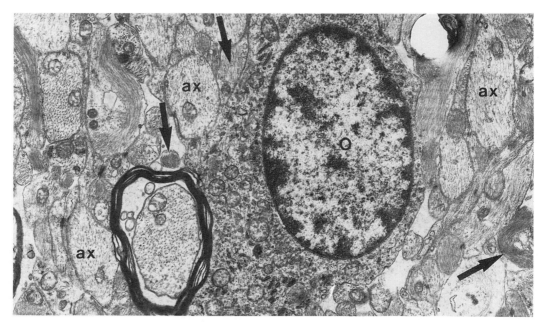

Fig. 12.24 An isolated oligodendrocyte (**O**) and myelin sheath present amongst naked axons (**ax**) and astrocytic processes (arrows). Electron micrograph × 8500.

plaques; however, occasional surviving oligo-dendrocytes may be seen (Fig. 12.24). Active plaques have a hypercellular edge which may extend from 1–3 cm into surrounding tissue; within this zone macrophages and hypertrophied astrocytes are seen and some authors claim that oligodendrocyte hyperplasia is apparent.[37,38] In the periplaque area both normal and disintegrating myelin sheaths may be seen, and Prineas[24] has suggested that the mechanism of demyelination in the plaque edge may differ from that of the early lesion.

The inactive lesion

These lesions, of which the large periventricular plaques are often the most characteristic, are hypocellular, demyelinated and gliosed and show massive oligodendrocytic loss. Electron microscopy confirms the presence of naked axons and astrocytic processes and Raine[39] has described modified contacts between astrocytes and axons. Increased diameter of demyelinated axons in inactive plaques in the spinal cord has been described by Shintaku, Hirano and Llena,[40] though the

phenomenon is not confined to such plaques (Fig. 12.23a). These workers suggest that this abnormality may be a manifestation of increased water content in the axoplasm, secondary to increased permeability of the demyelinated axolemma. Small venules in these inactive lesions are not inflamed but have thickened hyalinised walls. Myelin breakdown products are absent from the inactive plaque.

Remyelination

While the ability of the interfasicular oligodendrocyte to regenerate is uncertain, few would now agree with the view expressed by Greenfield[41] that 'it seems certain that in the CNS, myelin, once lost is not replaced'. Remyelination has been observed in many experimental animal models and in the human, remyelination, albeit imperfect, is possible. This potential for recovery is supported by immunohistochemical evidence of a precursor cell, shared with the type II astrocyte and capable of division and differentiation.[42] Nevertheless, in multiple sclerosis this remyelination process (Figs. 12.21, 12.23b, 12.25) is far

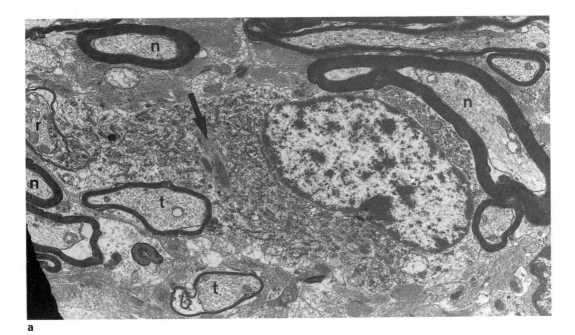

a

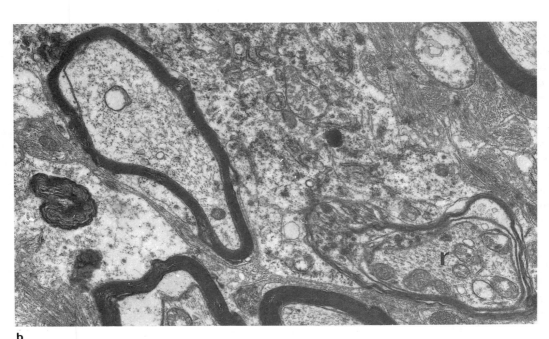

b

Fig. 12.25 **a** Thinly myelinated (**t**) and normal (**n**) fibres co-exist in a dense astrocytic scar. Another fibre (**r**) is loosely invested by part-compacted myelin which is in continuity with the microtubule-rich cytoplasm of a hypertrophic light oligodendrocyte. The glial filaments (arrow) are contained in an astrocyte process which passes over the oligodendrocyte. Electron micrograph × 5600. **b** Detail of fibre (**r**) The lack of myelin compaction, the association with a microtubule-rich oligodendrocyte and the absence of macrophages suggest that this is remyelinating activity. Electron micrograph × 20 000.

from complete and factors which limit the process are not understood. Massive early remyelination in acute multiple sclerosis has been described.[43] In chronic cases the shadow plaques, in which loss of myelin is not total, are thought to be undergoing demyelination and remyelination (as indicated by uniformly thin internodes) simultaneously.[28,30,44,45]

Remyelination with peripheral type myelin, due to Schwann cell invasion, has also been demonstrated in multiple sclerosis.[46–49] This type of remyelination is usually seen in the brainstem or spinal cord where the proximity of Schwann cells in nerve roots may be the decisive factor. As in experimental models, an inverse relationship of astrocytic proliferation and Schwann cell remyelination has been noted.[50] It has also been suggested that Japanese patients show more extensive peripheral type remyelination than do white races.[51]

Diffuse abnormalities within the central nervous system in multiple sclerosis

In the established case of multiple sclerosis, widespread but relatively mild histological abnormalities may be found in white matter which appears normal to the naked eye, a fact which has profound implications for biochemical and other studies. In a combined histological, histochemical and biochemical study of such tissue, 72% of samples were found to be histologically abnormal.[52] Abnormalities included small foci of demyelination, diffuse gliosis (Fig. 12.26), perivascular inflammation and deposition of lipofuscin, iron and calcium, (Fig. 12.27). Collagenisation of small blood vessels (Fig. 12.28) and diffuse corpora amylacea formation were also noted (Fig. 12.29). It can be argued that many of these changes are secondary to plaque formation. In a further study, however, of a series of selected mild or predominantly spinal cases,[53] similar abnormalities were found, suggesting that a more diffuse lesion, of which astrocytes form a prominent component, can occur in the absence of significant plaque formation. It is possibly relevant to this argument that abnormally thin myelin and an increase in astrocyte lysosomes has been reported in biopsies from cerebral white matter

outside plaques.[54] The meninges also may be involved in the diffuse process and macrophages, lymphocytes and plasma cells can be identified in the subarachnoid space.[55]

Retinal pathology

The clinical association of multiple sclerosis with retinal periphlebitis and uveitis is discussed in detail in Chapter 4 and several pathological studies have been undertaken.[56,57] Perivascular inflammation, particularly perivenular inflammation, is the most common abnormality (Fig. 12.30): the inflammatory response is mixed and lymphocytes and plasma cells can be identified. Other lesions include retinitis, uveitis and retinal vein sclerosis. Association with optic nerve lesions is 100%.

Peripheral nerve pathology

The relationship of multiple sclerosis to peripheral neuropathy is discussed in Chapter 9. Much of the pathological literature on this subject relates to reports of single cases or small series in which both multiple sclerosis and peripheral neuropathy have been present. Thus the association of hypertrophic neuropathy[49,58] and inflammatory demyelinating polyradiculitis[59,60] with multiple sclerosis has been described. However, few systematic pathological studies of peripheral nerves in a large series of multiple sclerosis cases have been undertaken, but Argyrakis[61] describes a wide spectrum of pathological changes in peripheral and cranial nerves, in early autopsies of well-documented multiple sclerosis patients. Increased endothelial pinocytosis, oedematous expansion of the endoneurial space, mononuclear cell infiltration and demyelination were all found. The process was milder than that in the central nervous system and was not plaque-like. Axonal degeneration was also seen, but was often independent of the demyelination. Some of these abnormalities may be secondary to inflammation and tract degeneration within the central nervous system, but Poser[62] and others have argued that a common immunopathology may underlie both central and peripheral lesions.

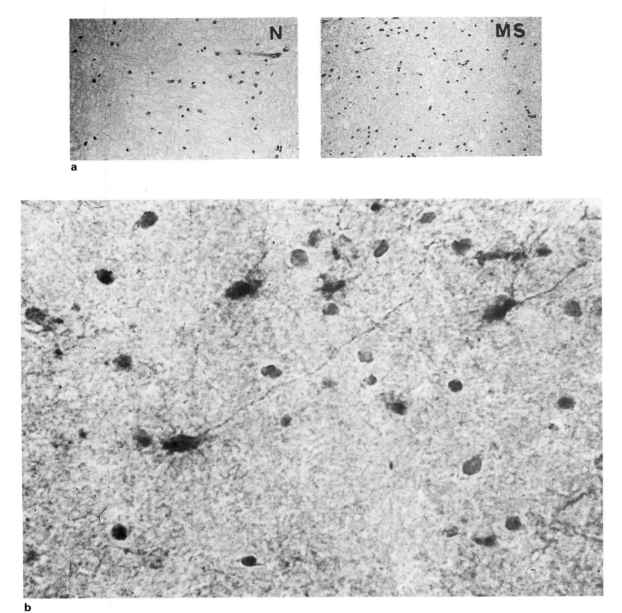

Fig. 12.26 a Macroscopically-normal white matter in multiple sclerosis (**MS**) brain shows increased cellularity in comparison with normal (**N**) brain. H & E × 100. **b** Reactive astrocytes in the macroscopically normal white matter stained for acid phosphatase × 250.

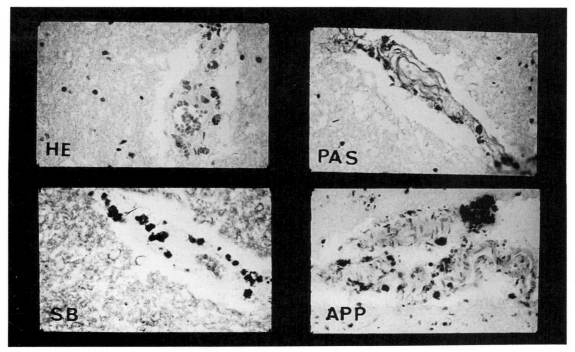

Fig. 12.27 Perivascular abnormalities in the macroscopically normal white matter in multiple sclerosis include lipofuscin deposition. This pigment probably originates from macrophages and is demonstrated in H & E (**HE**), Sudan black (**SB**) and by the periodic acid Schiff (**PAS**), and acid phosphatase (**APP**) reactions × 100.

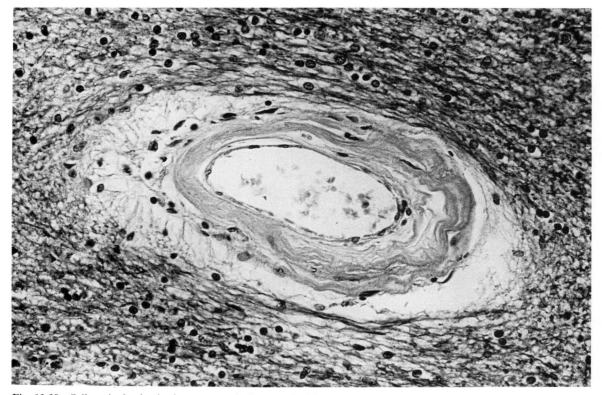

Fig. 12.28 Collagenised veins in the macroscopically normal white matter in multiple sclerosis. H & E/Luxol fast blue × 250.

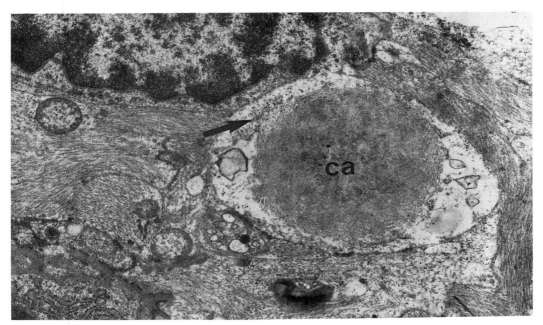

Fig. 12.29 Corpora amylacea (**ca**) formation within a degenerate cell process which contains a few remnant intermediate filaments (arrow). Electron micrograph × 12 600.

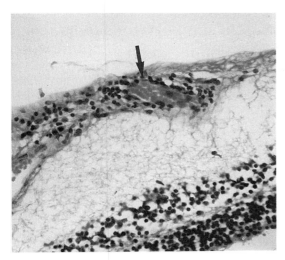

Fig. 12.30 Retinal periphlebitis in a case of classical multiple sclerosis (arrow). Separation of retinal layers is a postmortem artefact. H & E × 160.

Histochemistry of multiple sclerosis

In understanding the histochemical changes which accompany and follow demyelination in the central nervous system in multiple sclerosis, some under-

standing of the structure and chemistry of myelin is essential. Myelin has a complicated molecular structure (Figs. 12.31a and b) which accounts not only for its inherent physical and physiological properties but also for its histochemical reactivity. Chemical changes resulting from periaxial demyelination (Fig. 12.31c) are similar to those which occur in Wallerian degeneration, liberating proteins and lipids which are digested by lysosomal enzymes, mainly within macrophages but also to some extent within astrocytes.

Lipids

For many years, lipid histochemistry was extensively investigated with the idea that the inherent constitution of myelin in multiple sclerosis might be abnormal. It is now generally accepted, however, that lipid abnormalities in the macroscopically normal white matter are the result either of Wallerian degeneration or of unsuspected demyelination and there is no evidence of an inherent metabolic defect. Lipid histochemistry in multiple sclerosis therefore reflects the normal, enzyme-effected, biochemical degradation of myelin.

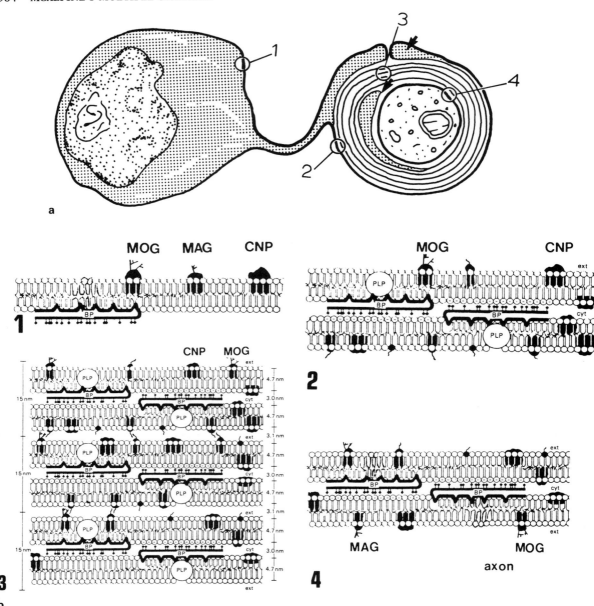

Fig. 12.31 a Schematic drawing (not to scale) of the relationship between an oligodendrocyte and the internodal myelin of a nerve fibre. Despite being continuous from cell to compact sheath, the membrane is not uniform in either chemical composition or molecular architecture. (The proposed structure and composition of the four zones indicated are described in part **b** of this figure.) Note also that oligodendroglial cytoplasm extends right through the sheath and is identifiable on this diagram as the outer and inner loops (arrows); in paranodal myelin it becomes even more plentiful in the form of the nodal loops (not shown). **b** Schematic representation (not to scale) of the molecular architecture of the central myelin sheath, prepared by Dr Brenda Brankin based on Rumsby 1978,[63] Schwob et al 1985[64] and Brunner et al 1989.[65] The occurrence and disposition of proteins in the different zones of the oligodendrocyte-myelin unit is shown. **1** The oligodendrocyte membrane associated zone. **2** The myelin surface associated zone. Highest amounts of **MOG** are found in this zone. **3** The compact myelin zone; the controversy as to whether **MAG** is present in compact myelin has not yet been resolved. **4** The myelin/axon interface zone; highest amounts of the cell adhesion molecule **MAG** are found in this zone.

MOG = myelin oligodendroglial glycoprotein; **MAG** = myelin-associated glycoprotein; **BP** = basic protein; **PLP** = proteolipid protein; **CNP** = 2'3'-cyclic nucleotide 3'-phosphodiesterase.

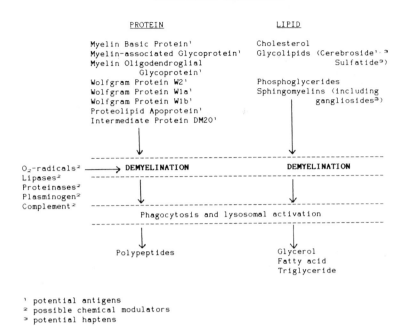

NORMAL MYELIN CONSTITUENTS

PROTEIN

Myelin Basic Protein¹
Myelin-associated Glycoprotein¹
Myelin Oligodendroglial
          Glycoprotein¹
Wolfgram Protein W2¹
Wolfgram Protein W1a¹
Wolfgram Protein W1b¹
Proteolipid Apoprotein¹
Intermediate Protein DM20¹

LIPID

Cholesterol
Glycolipids (Cerebroside¹·³
              Sulfatide³)

Phosphoglycerides
Sphingomyelins (including
              gangliosides³)

O₂-radicals² ────→ DEMYELINATION   DEMYELINATION
Lipases²
Proteinases²
Plasminogen²
Complement²

          Phagocytosis and lysosomal activation

          Polypeptides   Glycerol
                                          Fatty acid
                                          Triglyceride

¹ potential antigens
² possible chemical modulators
³ potential haptens

Fig. 12.31   c Histochemistry of myelin and demyelination.

These changes occur slowly within the central nervous system and probably have little relevance to initial mechanisms of demyelination.

Myelin proteins

Recently, greater pathogenetic significance has been placed on proteins and glycoproteins because of the known antigenic and encephalitogenic potential of these components. Early descriptions[66] of the immunohistochemistry of myelin basic protein (MBP) and myelin-associated glycoprotein (MAG) indicated a decreased staining for MAG involving the plaque and also extending far beyond. By contrast, MBP loss was restricted to areas of macrophage infiltration in which degenerating myelin sheaths often showed increased MBP staining. These observations led to the hypothesis that MAG could be an initiating antigen in multiple sclerosis which is therefore lost before the subsequent physical disruption of myelin. Later reports, however, indicated that not all acute plaques are surrounded by a zone of poor MAG

staining and this abnormality, while unexplained, cannot be considered an essential feature of the plaque.[67]

Irrespective of primary immunopathogenetic significance, macrophages containing MBP-positive and MAG-positive fragments of myelin have been identified, and this phenomenon has been associated with the presence of MHC class II antigens in these cells.[68] This upregulation of microglia and infiltrating macrophages may reflect antigen presentation in demyelinating lesions, but its significance for the basic pathology of multiple sclerosis is unknown.

Lysosomal enzymes

Lysosomal enzyme abnormalities in the plaque and periplaque are well substantiated and few workers doubt that this is a secondary phenomenon,[69] though there is some unconfirmed evidence of an inherent abnormality of lysosomal function.[70] A gradient of lysosomal enzyme activity can be demonstrated with highest levels in

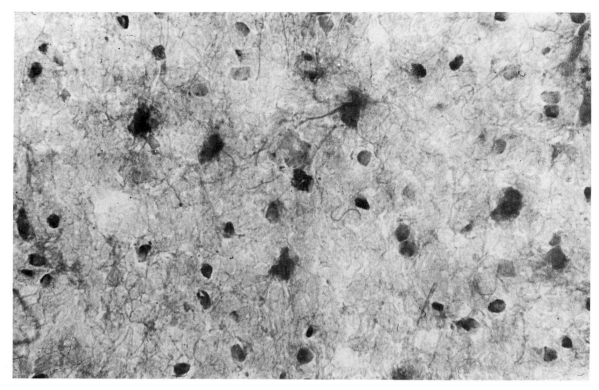

Fig. 12.32 Lysosomal enzyme activity in astrocytes in a chronic plaque. Acid phosphatase × 250.

plaque, intermediate levels in periplaque, and lower but still abnormal levels in macroscopically normal white matter.[71] Levels of lysosomal enzymes are equally high in acute and chronic plaques, and although inflammatory cells are an important source of these enzymes, astrocytes also make a significant contribution[72] (Fig. 12.32). The increases in enzyme activity in the macroscopically normal white matter can be largely correlated with gliosis, but abnormalities in β-glucosaminidase exist in white matter which is not obviously gliosed, as judged by standard microscopy. Elevated lysosomal enzyme levels could clearly be of importance in the process of demyelination and in the rendering of non-demyelinated tissue susceptible to a demyelinating influence.

Immunohistochemistry

The clinical immunology of multiple sclerosis has been extensively studied and is reviewed in Chapter 11. Parallel with these investigations, immunohistochemical studies relevant to immune function have been carried out in the central nervous system. Although patterns of abnormality have been established, results are inconsistent, difficult to interpret and at best can be considered preliminary. Undoubtedly, the immune response in multiple sclerosis is complex and is influenced by many factors, with the added complication that in the central nervous system, neurotransmitters and brain-derived cytokines have an immunomodulatory effect.[73] It seems clear that tissue-directed immunohistochemistry will not be sufficient to elucidate the sequence of immune events, particularly as cellular markers may not be entirely specific and immune cells may lose specific markers on entering the central nervous system. As will be seen from the following discussion, however, such studies may act as pointers to aetiopathogenesis and assist in formulating a broad pathogenetic concept in which both exogenous factors and host response have significance.

Light and electron microscopical studies in which lymphocytes and plasma cells have been demonstrated in the perivascular region and in myelinated tissue[74–76] have been extended by the use of specific immunohistochemistry. Immunoglobulin-containing cells have been demonstrated within the central nervous system,[77,78] although in a combined histological and biochemical study,[79] plaque levels of immunoglobulin could not be correlated positively with the inflammatory cell response. The general lymphocytic response has been studied using T and B cell markers,[80,81] and T cell subsets have been studied in relationship to plaque anatomy and antigen-presenting cells.[82,83] One set of results[82] indicates the importance of helper-inducer cells in lesion progression, while in the other[82] cytotoxic-suppressor cells were found in greater numbers in the CNS parenchyma. There are several explanations for the apparent discrepancy,[83] not least being the difficulty of comparable case selection and agreed criteria for tissue categorisation. More recent studies for T cell subsets have not clarified these issues, though it is suggested that within active lesions, suppressor-cytotoxic cells predominate[84] and that there is a paucity of suppressor-inducer cells.[85]

Expression of MHC class II gene products (Ia antigen) has been extensively investigated in MS. Ia positivity has been demonstrated on macrophages, endothelial cells and astrocytes and its relevance to antigen presentation discussed.[86–90]

In MS, Ia-positive astrocytes and macrophages are predominantly associated with active lesions,[89,91] although Ia-positive macrophages have also been found in normal-appearing white matter.[92] A low percentage of Ia-positive endothelial cells has also been found, randomly distributed throughout both white and grey matter. Thus, within the plaque the potential for antigen presentation exists and Ia-positive macrophages (and other cells) could thereby participate in a postulated immunopathogenic progression of the lesion.

Interferons have also been studied in the central nervous system in multiple sclerosis and while all types of interferon have been demonstrated in active chronic lesions, IFN-gamma is found mainly on astrocytes and IFN-alpha on macrophages.[93] In patients with intercurrent infection, IFN-gamma and Ia positive astrocytes are detectable throughout wide areas of normal-appearing white matter,[94] thus suggesting a mechanism for systemic infection-related relapse in multiple sclerosis.

The involvement of complement in demyelination has long been considered a possibility and complement studies have been undertaken in cerebrospinal fluid and in brain tissue. Granular deposits of C9 and the terminal complex (TCC) have been demonstrated immunocytochemically in association with capillary endothelial cells, predominantly within plaques and adjacent white matter.[95] Complement activation therefore may be an early event in the demyelinating process.

In summarising the immunohistochemistry of the central nervous system in multiple sclerosis, it is clearly premature to produce an overall scheme which synthesises cellular and chemical events. There is undoubted evidence that many of the abnormalities are secondary in nature and are not specific.[96,97] Nevertheless, this view does not detract from the importance of immunohistochemistry in understanding the progression of multiple sclerosis and in the development of scientifically-based therapeutic strategies.

Subtypes of multiple sclerosis

Acute multiple sclerosis — Marburg type

Marburg[7] in 1906 described three cases in which multiple, recently-demyelinated lesions were found at autopsy in the central nervous system with a preceding, relatively acute illness. This form of multiple sclerosis is monophasic, but a similar acute fulminant phase of the disease may occur as a terminal event in more chronic cases, and this observation strengthens the argument[98] that the differences between acute and classic multiple sclerosis are quantitative. This variety is probably not as rare as has been suggested and usually occurs in relatively young patients. At autopsy, myelin destruction may be very extensive and axonal loss severe, but plaques can be recognised. Areas of demyelination are surrounded by a wide oedematous zone (Fig. 12.33) and often in

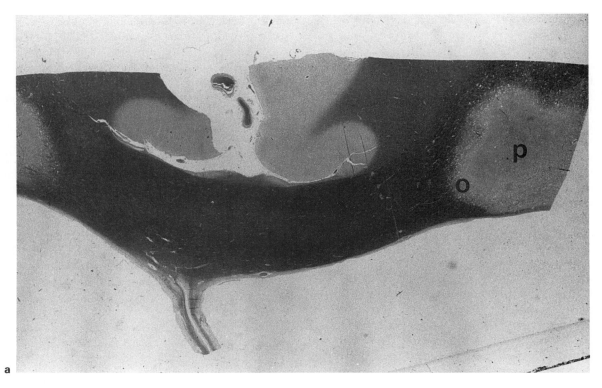

a

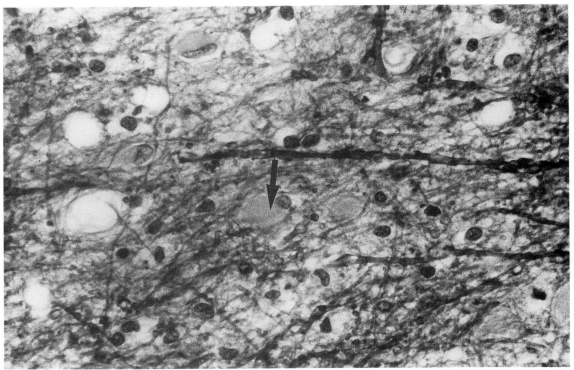

b

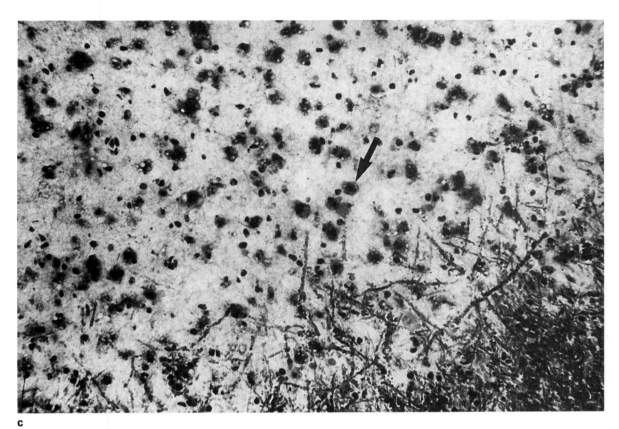

c

Fig. 12.33 **a** Acute multiple sclerosis. Plaque-like area of demyelination (**p**) is surrounded by a zone of oedema (**o**). H & E/Luxol fast blue × 5. **b** Acute multiple sclerosis; area of active demyelination showing marked astrocytic response (arrow). H & E/Luxol fast blue × 250. **c** Acute multiple sclerosis: area of active demyelination showing infiltration of lipid-filled macrophages (arrows) close to plaque edge. Spielmeyer/Sudan black × 250.

this area there is secondary disintegration of myelin with Wallerian degeneration. Usually patients have been treated with anti-inflammatory drugs and perivascular inflammation at autopsy may be slight.

Schilder type multiple sclerosis

The subject of Schilder's disease (diffuse cerebral sclerosis) has caused great confusion in the past. Schilder's original description[8] concerns a previously healthy child who developed severe, relatively acute demyelinating disease. In subsequent publications he added a further two cases, though later reviews suggest that these are probably examples of leucodystrophy and subacute sclerosing panencephalitis respectively.[99]

Leucodystrophies and other forms of genetic disorders of myelin are now not included in this category of demyelinating disease, but the relatively acute form of demyelination seen in previously healthy children remains recognisable and is designated Schilder type multiple sclerosis. At autopsy, these cases show widespread confluent demyelination, usually involving both cerebral hemispheres, brainstem and cerebellum (Fig. 12.34). In the cerebral hemispheres the lesions are not usually symmetrical, are sharply outlined and do not involve the subcortical rim of white matter. Axonal preservation is only partial and there is widespread Wallerian degeneration. At a late stage, cavitation of the lesions may occur. Transitional cases which contain numerous scattered discrete plaques in addition to diffuse

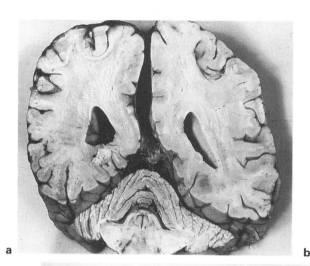

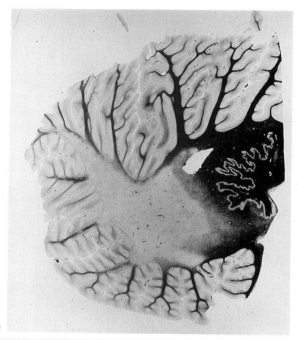

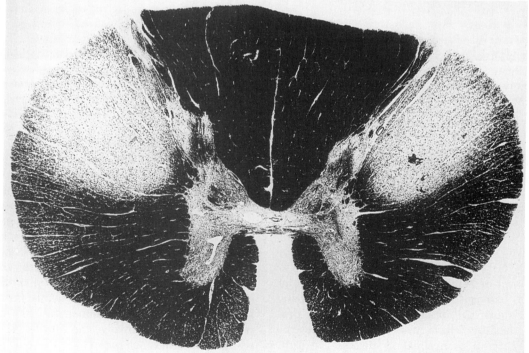

Fig. 12.34 Schilder's disease following a febrile illness in a child of 9. **a** Diffuse demyelination in the cerebral hemispheres. **b** Demyelination in the cerebellar white matter. Weigert-Pal × 3 (Reproduced with permission from Allen 1984.[23]) **c** Secondary long tract (Wallerian) in the spinal cord. Weigert-Pal × 15 (Reproduced with permission from Allen 1984.[23])

demyelination are recognised and their occurrence supports the argument that Schilder's disease is indeed a form of multiple sclerosis. Poser's[100] series of 105 cases of Schilder type multiple sclerosis contained 72 with classical plaques. The age range in this group was similar to that of classical multiple sclerosis and the clinical course was variable.

Concentric sclerosis — Balò type multiple sclerosis

This is a rare form of multiple sclerosis which few have had the opportunity to study extensively. Courville[101] in a series of 20 cases, found that although the age range was 10–51, 14 cases were aged between 20 and 33. In all but 5, survival was under one year and the shortest history was two weeks. At autopsy, large plaques are seen in the white matter and are frequently symmetrical in the cerebral hemispheres and cerebellum. Myelin staining of these lesions (Fig. 12.35) reveals the concentric pattern of demyelination, alternating with zones of myelin preservation. Other, more irregular, complex patterns of demyelination may be seen, with interweaving and circular formations. The basis of this pattern of demyelination is incompletely understood. Demyelinated zones are hypercellular and contain macrophages; the areas of myelin preservation may be at least in part remyelinated. Cases have been described in older patients in whom the illness was more chronic and was characterised pathologically by demyelinated gliosed zones in which axons were preserved. In one case report[102] concentric sclerosis was associated with neuromyelitis optica.

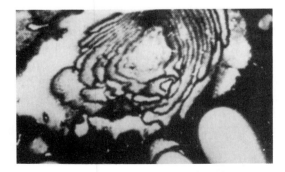

Fig. 12.35 Balò type multiple sclerosis. Concentric demyelination in deep white matter. Woelcke × 50.

Neuromyelitis optica — Dévic type multiple sclerosis

The frequent and severe involvement of optic nerves and spinal cord in multiple sclerosis means that clinically, the combined symptomatology of partial or complete blindness and paraplegia is not unusual. In most cases, however, there is evidence of more generalised involvement and the term neuromyelitis optica is reserved for those in which visual and spinal cord signs develop about the same time and dominate the clinical illness. Onset is usually acute and 50% of patients die within months; surviving patients may show partial or total recovery. There has been much controversy as to whether the syndrome has a single pathological basis and is related to classical multiple sclerosis. It is now clear, however, that several diseases may produce the syndrome,[103] but the term 'neuromyelitis optica' is not used for systemic conditions such as syphilis and systemic lupus erythematosus;[104] rather, it is reserved for cases in which no generalised disease process can be identified. In this latter group, the exact relationship to classical multiple sclerosis is still debatable. Some have argued that the pathology is distinctive,[105] but careful clinicopathological studies indicate that a variety of recognised demyelinating diseases may produce the syndrome.[18,103] Appropriate, associated histological abnormalities have been found in cases in which neuromyelitis optica was present with classical, acute, Schilder's type and Balò type multiple sclerosis and with diffuse encephalomyelitis.

At autopsy, all cases show partial or total demyelination of the optic nerves and spinal cord (Fig. 12.36). If the condition has been chronic, the cord is often thinned and the affected segment of the cord (most frequently the upper thoracic) shows marked gliosis and meningeal thickening. Remyelination by Schwann cells is often seen in the posterior root entry zone. The development of oedema in the acute phase of demyelination may be particularly important for necrosis in the spinal cord, restricted as it is by pia, and in the optic nerves, similarly encircled and encased in the optic foramina. In very severe cases, therefore, general tissue necrosis may occur and this may explain the finding of antibody to glial fibrillary acidic protein in cerebrospinal fluid in these cases.[106]

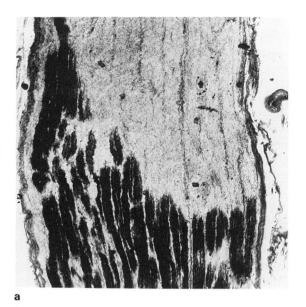

a

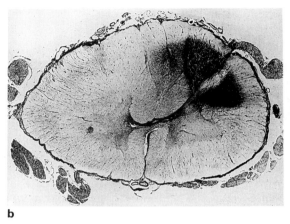

b

Fig. 12.36 Dévic type multiple sclerosis. **a** Demyelination of optic nerve. Spielmeyer × 65. (Reproduced with permission from Allen 1984[23].) **b** Severe demyelination of the cervical cord. Spielmeyer × 10.

Hughes (1978)[107] has collected a series of cases of acute necrotic myelopathy and has reviewed a further 20 well-documented cases. These may well be examples of demyelinating disease and this view is supported by a previous history of optic neuritis in one case and of associated plaque formation in the brain of a second case.

SUMMARY AND SIGNIFICANCE OF THE PATHOLOGICAL LESIONS IN MULTIPLE SCLEROSIS

Anatomical and histological findings

To the non-histologist, detailed descriptions of the plaque in multiple sclerosis and of mechanisms of demyelination must be confusing. While acknowledging the dangers of oversimplification, an attempt has been made to summarise salient features (Fig. 12.37, Table 12.2) and to indicate possible primary or secondary significance.

A constant and well-documented feature of multiple sclerosis is the anatomical distribution of the lesions, and many studies have confirmed the susceptibility of myelin in the periventricular region and in the optic nerves and spinal cord, yet the

significance of plaque distribution is unknown. The susceptibility of the periventricular white matter has been explained on the basis of a circulating toxin or an antibody effect. Not all periventricular white matter is equally vulnerable, however, and a recent study[108] suggests that the periventricular plaque results from the formation of a lesion around a subependymal vein, which later coalesces with adjacent lesions. These workers argue that, as there is no origin of plaques from ependyma, it is unlikely that CSF plays a part in their initial development. Chronic lesions often show an overlying granular ependymitis and this inflamed ependyma could secondarily allow molecular exchange between plaque and CSF.

The relationship of plaques to veins and venules is a continuing theme in the literature and is supported by the careful anatomical studies of Fog,[109] who observed that most plaques had a close anatomical relationship with one, two or more central veins. Although it is now accepted that there is no evidence of vascular thrombosis as the basis of plaque formation, it has been suggested that local susceptibility may be particularly great in regions situated in the boundary zones between the territories of supply of major cerebral

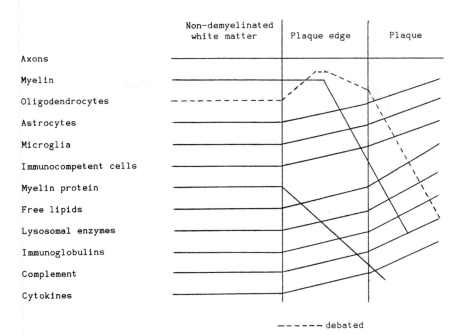

	Non-demyelinated white matter	Plaque edge	Plaque
Axons			
Myelin			
Oligodendrocytes			
Astrocytes			
Microglia			
Immunocompetent cells			
Myelin protein			
Free lipids			
Lysosomal enzymes			
Immunoglobulins			
Complement			
Cytokines			

– – – – – – debated

Fig. 12.37 Schematic view of the plaque and periplaque in multiple sclerosis. The changes in oligodendrocytes are controversial.

Table 12.2 Pathological reactions in multiple sclerosis

Structure	Pathological reaction	Primary (P) or secondary (S)
Astrocyte	Hypertrophy, hyperplasia, potential antigen presentation	?
Macrophages	Hyperplasia, phagocytosis, potential antigen presentation	S
Immune competent cells	Infiltration	?
Oligodendrocyte	Necrosis	?
Myelin sheath	Necrosis or disorganisation	P
	Incomplete healing	S
Neuronal perikaryon	Unaffected	–
Axons	Unaffected initially. Some late degeneration	S
Blood–brain barrier	Increased permeability	?
Endothelial cell	Increased pinocytosis, potential antigen presentation	?
Blood vessel wall	Hyalinisation	S
Meninges	Mild inflammation	S

arteries.[12] Fan-shaped lesions in the spinal cord have been described by Oppenheimer,[15] who suggests that mechanical stress, induced by repeated minor injury during neck flexion, may predispose the cervical cord to plaque formation.

In summary, it must be emphasised that all white matter is susceptible in multiple sclerosis, but for unknown reasons certain anatomical sites are more constantly damaged. The relationship of plaques to veins seems to be significant and the possibility that endothelium is primarily involved in the multiple sclerosis lesion is supported by the occurrence of increased pinocytosis in the acute lesion and by similar perivenular inflammatory lesions in the retina, a non-myelinated structure in the human. Despite very extensive study of early lesions in multiple sclerosis, there is no consensus view as to the earliest phase of myelin damage and its relationship to the inflammatory response. It seems likely, however, that subsequent events are complicated by secondary release of enzymes, complement and cytokines, and in the established lesion several patterns of tissue destruction may be seen. The perivascular position of many plaques has led to speculation that the myelinotoxic factors, known to be present in the serum of multiple sclerosis patients,[110] could be responsible for demyelinating activity, but there is no proof of this. Although there is evidence of the possible importance of immune-competent and antigen-presenting cells in demyelination in multiple sclerosis, there can be no firm conclusion that the disease is 'autoimmune'. Tissue immunohistochemistry has not established a uniform pattern of cellular reaction and the exact relationship of immune-competent cells to the elevated immunoglobulin in the cerebrospinal fluid is unknown.

The fact that diffuse astrocytosis is observed in the macroscopically-normal white matter, even in those cases which are predominantly spinal, could be interpreted as supportive evidence for primary involvement of astrocytes in the pathological response, though it must be conceded that such an effect may be non-specific. The involvement of retinal veins in multiple sclerosis suggests that myelin may not be the primary target and future studies should concentrate on early endothelial reactions using structural, biochemical and immune techniques.

Mechanisms of lesion growth

The eventual shape and size of chronic plaques probably depends on several factors, two of which may be coalescence of adjacent lesions and finger-like extensions (Dawson's fingers) from the plaque edge. Although the coalescence of adjacent, expanding plaques can easily be understood, the mechanisms responsible for growth by extension at the periphery remain uncertain. Among several factors which could be involved at this site are the increased levels of lysosomal enzymes and the degree and extent of inflammation. For example, lysosomal enzyme levels are known to be elevated in the periplaque, rendering it potentially more vulnerable to further attack. Moreover, the cellular inflammatory response is more prominent towards the edge of old plaques, the centre of which may be hypocellular and appear inactive. Thus, the presence of perivascular inflammation at the plaque edge may mean that a continuous inflammatory process takes place, inducing further demyelination. Brosnan et al[111] have suggested that the common mechanism of lymphokine activation of macrophages will lead to release of products such as neutral proteases and these, in the presence of plasma proteins (plasminogen and complement), could cause myelinolysis. Selmaj & Raine[32] have proposed that the cytokines alpha tumour necrosis factor (αTNF) and lymphotoxin (βTNF), secreted respectively by activated macrophages and activated T lymphocytes, could be involved in the progression of the multiple sclerosis lesion through their effects on ionic channels in oligodendrocytes, myelin and axons. They reported that recombinant human TNF, when applied to myelinated cultures of mouse spinal cord causes a sequence of changes comprising oligodendroglial necrosis, irreversible myelin swelling of characteristic morphology, and eventual demyelination.

Overall significance of the neuropathology of multiple sclerosis

Many years of study have established accurate

descriptions of the neuropathological abnormalities in multiple sclerosis with good overall correlation with the clinical findings. It is apparent, however, that many unresolved problems remain and no aetiological hypothesis can be formulated without comparing multiple sclerosis with other demyelinating diseases and with experimental models of demyelination. These comparisons are covered in Chapter 3.

Acknowledgements

I am pleased to acknowledge the considerable help given by the following: Mr Roy Creighton for photographic expertise; Mr George Glover and staff for technical assistance; Mrs Esther McNamee for secretarial support and Mr Robert McConnell for help in preparation of the final draft.

REFERENCES

1. Cruveilhier J 1829–42 Anatomie pathologique du corps humain, Vol 2, Livraison 52, Plate 2. Baillière, Paris
2. Carswell R 1838 Atrophy. In: Pathological anatomy. Illustration of elementary forms of disease, Plate IV. Longman, Orme, Brown, Green and Longman, London
3. Charcot J M 1877 Lectures on the diseases of the nervous system (trans G Sigerson). The New Sydenham Society, London. First series, lecture 6 (delivered 1868)
4. Dawson J W 1916 The histology of disseminated sclerosis. Transactions of the Royal Society of Edinburgh 50: 517–740
5. McDonald W I 1982 Clinical problems of multiple sclerosis. In: Sears T A (ed) Neuronal-glial cell interrelationships. Dahlem Konferenzen 1982. Springer, Berlin, pp 11–24
6. Dévic M E 1894 Myélite subaigüe compliquée de névrite optique. Bulletin Medical (Paris) 8: 1033
7. Marburg O 1906 Die sogenannte 'akute multiple sklerose.' Jahrbuch für Psychiatrie und Neurologie 27: 211–312
8. Schilder P 1912 Zur Kenntnis der sogenannte diffusen sklerosen. Zeitschrift für die gesamte. Neurologie und Psychiatrie 10: 1–60
9. Balò J 1928 Encephalitis periaxialis concentrica. Archives of Neurology and Psychiatry 19: 242–264
10. Allen I V, Millar J H D, Hutchinson M J 1978 General disease in 120 necropsy-proven cases of multiple sclerosis. Neuropathology and Applied Neurobiology 4: 279–284
11. Lumsden C E 1970 The neuropathology of multiple sclerosis. In: Vinken P J, Bruyn G W (eds) Handbook of clinical neurology, Vol 9. North Holland, Amsterdam, pp 296–298
12. Brownell B, Hughes J T 1962 The distribution of plaques in the cerebrum in multiple sclerosis. Journal of Neurology, Neurosurgery and Psychiatry 25: 315–320
13. Ulrich J, Waltraut G-L 1963 The optic nerve in multiple sclerosis. Neuro-opthalmology, Vol 3, part 3. Aeolus Press, Amsterdam, pp 149–159
14. Adams R D, Kubik C S 1952 The morbid anatomy of the demyelinative disease. American Journal of Medicine 12: 510–546
15. Oppenheimer D R 1978 The cervical cord in multiple sclerosis. Neuropathology and Applied Neurobiology 4: 151–162
16. Zimmerman H M, Netsky M G 1950 The pathology of multiple sclerosis. Association for Research into Nervous Diseases Proceedings 28: 271–312
17. Seitelberger F 1960 Histochemistry of demyelinating diseases proper, including allergic encephalomyelitis and Pelizaeus–Merzbacher's disease. In: Cummings J N (ed) Modern scientific aspects of neurology. Edward Arnold, London, pp 146–187
18. Greenfield J G, Norman R M 1963 Demyelinating diseases. In: Blackwood W, McMenemey W H, Meyer A, Norman R M, Russell D S (eds) Greenfield's neuropathology, 2nd edn. Edward Arnold, London, pp 475–519
19. Adams C W M 1977 Pathology of multiple sclerosis: progression of the lesion. British Medical Bulletin 33: 15–20
20. Raine C S, Scheinberg L, Waltz J M 1981 Multiple sclerosis. Oligodendrocyte survival and proliferation in an active established lesion. Laboratory Investigation 45: 534–546
21. Brown W J 1978 The capillaries in acute and subacute multiple sclerosis plaques: a morphometric analysis. Neurology 28: 84–92
22. Gonatas N K 1970 Ultrastructural observation in a case of multiple sclerosis (abs). Journal of Neuropathology and Experimental Neurology 29: 149
23. Allen I V 1984 Demyelinating diseases. In: Adams J H, Corsellis J A N, Duchen L W (eds) Greenfield's neuropathology, 4th edn. Edward Arnold, London, pp 338–384
24. Prineas J W 1985 The neuropathology of multiple sclerosis. In: Koetsier J C (ed) Handbook of clinical neurology 3(47): 213–257
25. Kirk J 1979 The fine structure of the CNS in multiple sclerosis. II. Vesicular demyelination in an acute case. Neuropathology and Applied Neurobiology 5: 289–294
26. Lassmann H 1983 Comparative neuropathology of chronic experimental allergic encephalomyelitis and multiple sclerosis. Springer, Berlin
27. Guo Yu–Pu, Gao Shu-Fang 1983 Concentric sclerosis. In: Tyrer J H, Eadie M J (eds) Clinical and Experimental Neurology. Proceedings, Australian Association of Neurologists, Sydney 19: 67–76
28. Suzuki K et al 1969 Ultrastructural studies of multiple sclerosis. Laboratory Investigation 20: 444–454
29. Prineas J 1975 Pathology of the early lesion in multiple sclerosis. Human Pathology 6: 531–554
30. Prineas J W, Connell F 1978 The fine structure of chronically active multiple sclerosis plaques. Neurology 28: 68–75

31. Prineas J W, Graham J S 1981 Multiple sclerosis: capping of surface immunoglobulin G on macrophages engaged in myelin breakdown. Annals of Neurology 10: 149–158

32. Selmaj K W, Raine C S 1988 Tumor necrosis factor mediates myelin and oligodendrocyte damage in vitro. Annals of Neurology 23: 339–346

33. Prineas J W, Raine C S 1976 Electron microscopy and immunoperoxidase studies of early multiple sclerosis lesions. Neurology 26: 29–32

34. Lampert 1978 Autoimmune and virus-induced demyelinating diseases. American Journal of Pathology 91: 175–208

35. Raine C S 1984 Biology of disease, analysis of autoimmune demyelination: its impact upon multiple sclerosis. Laboratory Investigation 50: 608–635

36. Dal Canto M C, Wisniewski H M, Johnson A B et al 1975 Vesicular disruption of myelin in autoimmune demyelination. Journal of the Neurological Sciences 24: 313–319

37. Friede R L 1961 Enzyme histochemical studies in multiple sclerosis. Archives of Neurology 5: 433–443

38. Ibrahim M Z M, Adams C W M 1965 The relation between enzyme activity and neuroglia in early plaques of multiple sclerosis. Journal of Pathology and Bacteriology 90: 239–243

39. Raine C S 1978 Membrane specialisations between demyelinated axons and astroglia in chronic EAE lesions and multiple sclerosis plaques. Nature (London) 275: 326–327

40. Shintaku M, Hirano A, Llena J F (1988) Increased diameter of demyelinated axons in chronic multiple sclerosis of the spinal cord. Neuropathology and Applied Neurobiology 14: 505–510

41. Greenfield J G 1958 Demyelinating diseases. In: Greenfield J G et al (eds) Neuropathology. Edward Arnold, London, pp 441–474

42. Raff M C, Miller R H, Noble M 1983 A glial progenitor cell that develops in vitro into an astrocyte or an oligodendrocyte, depending on culture medium. Nature 303: 390–396

43. Prineas J W et al 1987 Massive early remyelination in acute multiple sclerosis (abs). Neurology 37 (suppl 1): 109

44. Andrews J M 1972 The ultrastructural neuropathology of multiple sclerosis. In: Wolfgram F, Ellison G W et al (eds) Multiple sclerosis. Immunology, virology and ultrastructure. New York, pp 23–52

45. Prineas J W, Connell F 1979 Remyelination in multiple sclerosis. Annals of Neurology 5: 22–31

46. Feigin I, Popoff N 1966 Regeneration of myelin in multiple sclerosis: the role of mesenchymal cells in such regeneration and in myelin formation in the peripheral nervous system. Neurology 16: 364–372

47. Ghatax N R, Hirano A et al 1973 Remyelination in multiple sclerosis with peripheral type myelin. Archives of Neurology 29: 262–267

48. Ogata J, Feigin I 1975 Schwann cells and regenerated peripheral myelin in multiple sclerosis: an ultrastructural study. Neurology 25: 713–716

49. Schoene W C, Carpenter S, Behan P O, Geschwind N 1977 'Onion bulb' formations in the central and peripheral nervous system in association with multiple sclerosis and hypertrophic polyneuropathy. Brain 100: 755–773

50. Itoyama Y, Ohnishi A, Tateishi J, Kuroiwa Y, Webster H deF 1985 Spinal cord multiple sclerosis lesions in Japanese patients: Schwann cell remyelination occurs in areas that lack glial fibrillary acidic protein (GFAP). Acta Neuropathologica Berlin 65: 217–223

51. Itoyama Y, Webster H deF, Richardson E P Jr, Trapp B D 1983 Schwann cell remyelination of demyelinated axons in spinal cord multiple sclerosis. Annals of Neurology 14: 339–346

52. Allen I V, McKeown S R 1979 A histological, histochemical and biochemical study of the macroscopically normal white matter in multiple sclerosis. Journal of the Neurological Sciences 41: 81–91

53. Allen I V, Glover G, Anderson R 1981 Abnormalities in the macroscopically normal white matter in cases of mild or spinal multiple sclerosis. Acta Neuropathologica (suppl 7): 176–178

54. Arstila A U, Riekkinen P, Rinne U K, Laitinen L 1973 Studies on the pathogenesis of multiple sclerosis — participation of lysosomes on demyelination in the central nervous system white matter outside plaques. European Neurology 9: 1–20

55. Adams C W M 1983 The general pathology of multiple sclerosis: morphological and chemical aspects of the lesions. In: Hallpike J F, Adams C W M, Tourtellotte W W (eds) Multiple sclerosis. Pathology, diagnosis and management. Williams and Wilkins, Baltimore, pp 203–240

56. Arnold A C, Pepose J S, Hepler R S 1984 Retinal periphlebitis and retinitis in multiple sclerosis. Opthalmology 91: 255–262

57. Shaw P J, Smith N M, Ince P G, Bates D 1987 Chronic periphlebitis retinae in multiple sclerosis. A histological study. Journal of the Neurological Sciences 77: 147–152

58. Rosenberg N L, Bourdette D 1983 Hypertrophic neuropathy and multiple sclerosis. Neurology 33: 1361–1364

59. Lassman H, Budka H, Schnaberth G 1981 Inflammatory demyelinating polyradiculitis in a patient with multiple sclerosis. Archives of Neurology 38: 99–102

60. Best P V 1985 Acute polyradiculoneuritis associated with demyelinated plaques in the central nervous system: report of a case. Acta Neuropathologica 67: 230–234

61. Argyrakis A. 1988 PNS alterations in MS (abs). Clinical Neuropathology 7: 143

62. Poser C M 1987 The peripheral nervous system in multiple sclerosis. A review and pathogenetic hypothesis. Journal of the Neurological Sciences 79: 83–90

63. Rumbsy M G 1978 Organization and structure in central nerve myelin. Biochemical Society Transactions 6: 448–462

64. Schwob V S et al 1985 Electron microscopic immunocytochemical localisation of myelin proteolipid protein and myelin basic protein to oligodendrocytes in rat brain during myelination. Journal of Neurochemistry 45: 559–571

65. Brunner C, Lassman H, Waehneldt T, Matthieu J, Linington C 1989 Differential ultrastructural localization of myelin basic protein, myelin/oligodendroglial glycoprotein, and 21',3'-cyclic nucleotide 3'-phosphodiesterase in the CNS of adult

rats. Journal of Neurochemistry 52: 296–304
66. Itoyama Y, Sternberger N H, Webster H deF, Quarles R H, Cohen S R, Richardson E P 1980 Immunocytochemical observations on the distribution of myelin-associated glycoprotein and myelin basic protein in multiple sclerosis lesions. Annals of Neurology 17: 167–177
67. Prineas J W, Kwon E E, Sternberger N H, Lennon V A 1984 The distribution of myelin-associated glycoprotein and myelin basic protein in actively demyelinating multiple sclerosis lesions. Journal of Neuroimmunology 6: 251–264
68. Hayes G M, Woodroofe M N, Cuzner M L 1987 The identification of myelin basic protein by class II microglia in white matter from multiple sclerosis brain. Journal of Neuroimmunology 16: 75
69. Cuzner M L, Davison A N 1979 The scientific basis of multiple sclerosis. Molecular Aspects of Medicine 2: 147–248
70. McKeown S R, Allen I V, 1979 The fragility of cerebral lysosomes in multiple sclerosis. Neuropathology and Applied Neurobiology 5: 405–415
71. McKeown S R, Allen I V 1978 The cellular origin of lysosomal enzymes in the plaque in MS: a combined histological and biochemical study. Neuropathology and Applied Neurobiology 4: 471–481
72. Allen I V, Glover G, McKeown S R, McCormick D 1979 The cellular origin of lysosomal enzymes in the plaque in multiple sclerosis. II. A histochemical study with combined demonstration of myelin and acid phosphatase. Neuropathology and Applied Neurobiology 5: 197–210
73. Merrill J 1988 The natural immune system in autoimmune and neurological disease. In: Reynolds C W, Wiltrout R H (eds) Functions of the natural immune system. Plenum, New York, pp 411–431
74. Guseo A, Jellinger K 1975 The significance of perivascular infiltrations in multiple sclerosis. Journal of Neurology 211: 51–60
75. Tanaka R, Iwasaki Y, Koprowski H 1975 Ultrastructural studies of perivascular cuffing cells in multiple sclerosis brain. American Journal of Pathology 81: 467–474
76. Prineas J W, Wright R G 1978 Macrophages, lymphocytes, and plasma cells in the perivascular compartment in chronic multiple sclerosis. Laboratory Investigation 38: 409–421
77. Mussini J-M, Hauw J J, Escourolle R 1977 Immunofluorescence studies of intracytoplasmic immunoglobulin binding lymphoid cells (CILC) in the central nervous system. Report of 32 cases including 19 multiple sclerosis. Acta Neuropathologica 40: 227–232
78. Esiri M M 1980 Multiple sclerosis: a quantitative and qualitative study of immunoglobulin-containing cells in the central nervous system. Neuropathology and Applied Neurobiology 6: 9–21
79. Cuzner M L, Allen I V, Glynn P, Newcombe J 1981 Antigenic specificity of intrathecally synthesised immunoglobulins in multiple sclerosis. Neuropathology and Applied Neurobiology 7: 503
80. Nyland H, Mork S, Matre R 1982 In-situ characterization of mononuclear cell infiltrates in lesions of multiple sclerosis. Neuropathology and Applied Neurobiology 8: 403–411
81. Kreth H W, Dunker R, Rodt H, Meyerman R 1982 Immunohistochemical identification of T-lymphocytes in the central nervous system of patients with multiple sclerosis and subacute sclerosing panencephalitis. Journal of Neuroimmunology 2: 177–183
82. Traugott U, Reinherz E L, Raine C S 1983 Multiple sclerosis. Distribution of T cells, T cell subsets and Ia-positive macrophages in lesions of different ages. Journal of Neuroimmunology 4: 201–221
83. Booss J, Esiri M M, Tourtellotte W W, Mason D Y 1983 Immunohistological analysis of T lymphocyte subsets in the central nervous system in chronic progressive multiple sclerosis. Journal of the Neurological Sciences 62: 219–232
84. Hayashi T, Morimoto C, Burke J S et al 1987 Double-label immunochemical analysis of T-cell activation markers and MHC expression in active multiple sclerosis lesions (abs). Journal of Neuroimmunology 16: 74
85. Sobel R A, Castro E E, Hafler D A, Morimoto C, Schlossman S F, Weiner H L 1987 Immunohistochemical analysis of suppressor-inducer and helper-inducer T cells in multiple sclerosis brain tissue. Journal of Neuroimmunology 16: 163–164
86. Traugott U, Scheinberg L C, Raine C S 1985 On the presence of Ia-positive endothelial cells and astrocytes in multiple sclerosis lesions and its relevance to antigen presentation. Journal of Neuroimmunology 8: 1–14
87. Traugott U, Raine C S 1985 Multiple sclerosis. Evidence for antigen presentation in situ by endothelial cells and astrocytes. Journal of the Neurological Sciences 69: 365–370
88. Woodroofe M N, Bellamy A S, Feldmann M, Davison A N, Cuzner M L 1986 Immunocytochemical characterisation of the immune reaction in the central nervous system in multiple sclerosis. Possible role for microglia in lesion growth. Journal of the Neurological Sciences 74: 135–152
89. Traugott U 1987 Multiple sclerosis: relevance of class I and class II MHC-expressing cells to lesion development. Journal of Neuroimmunology 16: 283–302
90. Esiri M M, Reading M C 1987 Macrophage populations associated with multiple sclerosis plaques. Neuropathology and Applied Neurobiology 13: 451–465
91. Hauser S L, Bhan A K, Gilles F H 1983 Immunohistochemical staining of human brain with monoclonal antibodies that identify lymphocytes, monocytes and Ia antigen. Journal of Neuroimmunology 5: 197–205
92. Hayes G M, Woodroofe M N, Cuzner M L 1987 Microglia are the major cell type expressing MHC class II in human white matter. Journal of the Neurological Sciences 80: 25–37
93. Traugott U, Lebon P 1987 Demonstration of alpha, beta and gamma interferon in active chronic multiple sclerosis lesions (abs). Journal of Neuroimmunology 16: 172
94. Traugott U, Lebon P 1987 Multiple sclerosis: association between intercurrent infections and diffuse astrocyte immunopathology. Neurology 38: 236
95. Compston D A S, Morgan B P, Campbell A K et al 1989 Immunocytochemical localisation of the terminal complement complex in multiple sclerosis. Neuropathology and Applied Neurobiology (in press)
96. Sobel R A, Ames B A 1988 Major histocompatibility complex molecule expression in the human central

nervous system: immunohistochemical analysis of 40 patients. Journal of Neuropathology and Experimental Neurology 47: 19–28

97. Esiri M M, Reading M C, Squier M V, Hughes J T 1989 Immunocytochemical characterisation of the macrophage and lymphocyte infiltrate in the brain in 6 cases of human encephalitis of varied aetiology. Neuropathology and Applied Neurobiology (in press)

98. Peters G 1968 Multiple sclerosis. In: Minckler J (ed) Pathology of the nervous system, Vol 1. McGraw-Hill, New York, pp 821–843

99. Lumsden C E 1951 Fundamental problems in the pathology of multiple sclerosis and allied demyelinating diseases. British Medical Journal 1: 1035–1043

100. Poser C M 1957 Diffuse-disseminated sclerosis in the adult. Journal of Neuropathology and Experimental Neurology 16: 61–78

101. Courville C B 1970 Concentric sclerosis. In: Vinken P J, Bruyn G W (eds) Handbook of clinical neurology, Vol 9. North Holland, Amsterdam, pp 437–451

102. Currie S, Roberts A H, Urich H 1970 The nosological position of concentric lacunar leucoencephalopathy. Journal of Neurology, Neurosurgery and Psychiatry 33: 131–137

103. Cloys D E, Netsky M G 1970 Neuromyelitis optica. In: Vinken P J, Bruyn G W (eds) Handbook of Clinical neurology, Vol 9. North Holland, Amsterdam, pp 426–435

104. Allen I V, Millar J H D, Kirk J, Shillington R 1979 Systemic lupus erythematosus clinically resembling multiple sclerosis and with unusual pathological and ultrastructural features. Journal of Neurology, Neurosurgery and Psychiatry 42: 392–401

105. Hassin G B 1937 Neuroptic myelitis versus multiple sclerosis. A pathologic study. Archives of Neurology and Psychiatry 37: 1083–1099

106. Chou C H J, Chou F C H, Tourtellotte W W, Kibler R F 1984 Dèvic's syndrome: antibody to glial fibrillary acidic protein in cerebrospinal fluid. Neurology 34: 86–88

107. Hughes J T (ed) 1978 Pathology of the spinal cord. Lloyd–Luke, London, pp 152–156

108. Adams C W M, Abdulla Y H, Torres E M, Poston R N 1987 Periventricular lesions in multiple sclerosis: their perivenous origin and relationship to granular ependymitis. Neuropathology and Applied Neurobiology 13: 141–152

109. Fog T 1965 Multiple sclerosis. Acta Neurologica Scandinavica (suppl 15): 5–161

110. Grunke-Iqbal I, Bornstein M B 1979 Multiple sclerosis: immunochemical studies on the demyelinating serum factor. Brain Research 160: 489–503

111. Brosnan C F, Cammer W et al 1988 Myelin antigens and demyelination. In: Crescenzi G S (ed) A multidisciplinary approach to myelin diseases. Plenum, pp 207–218

13. Aetiological hypotheses for multiple sclerosis — evidence from human and experimental diseases

Numerous hypotheses as to the cause of multiple sclerosis have been advanced over the years, often influenced by current scientific fashion. As yet, no published hypothesis explains satisfactorily all the 'hard facts' of the disease, though no doubt claims to the contrary can be made. It is probable that several factors are involved in the pathogenesis and although there is genetic predisposition, probably of a polygenic nature (see Ch. 10), epidemiological evidence suggests that exogenous factors are also involved (see Ch. 1).

In recent years interest has been concentrated on the genetic control and function of the immune system, particularly in its interactions with infectious agents, though the effect of toxins, trauma and vascular factors have also been considered.[1,2] Major current working hypotheses are summarised in Table 13.1, and much of the evidence in support of these, e.g. genetic predisposition, deregulation of the immune system, and putative autoantigens, has been discussed in earlier chapters. However, some additional evidence from the pathology and virology of multiple sclerosis, and from other human and experimental demyelinating diseases will be evaluated in this chapter.

Table 13.1 Aetiological hypotheses and supportive evidence in multiple sclerosis

Hypothesis	Supportive evidence
Autoimmune	Increased incidence of other autoimmune diseases[0] Genetic predisposition[+] Deregulation of immune system[+] Identifiable autoantigens[0] Autoimmune-induced human and experimental models[+]
Infective	Viral antibodies[+] Isolates from tissues[0] Virus-like particles in tissues[0] Viral persistence — antigen[+] — genome[+] Virally-associated immune dysfunction[+] Virally-induced experimental models[+]
Combined infective allergic	Evidence from other human demyelinating diseases[+] Virally-induced experimental models in which autoimmune reactions occur[+]
Other (including toxic, dietary and vascular)	[0]

[0]Evidence negative or incomplete.
[+]Some positive evidence available.

Additional evidence for an autoimmune aetiology

Studies on other autoimmune diseases in multiple sclerosis

Well-characterised autoimmune diseases, e.g. myasthenia gravis, apart from fulfilling the necessary criteria for such a designation, are known to be associated in affected patients with other autoimmune conditions and with altered patterns of malignancy. By analogy, it has been suggested that the association of multiple sclerosis with autoimmune diseases such as Hashimoto's thyroiditis, might support the idea that multiple sclerosis itself is an autoimmune disorder. Lumsden[3] in a series of 60 necropsy-proven cases (apparently uncontrolled), noted a high incidence of thyroid adenoma and thyroid involution. However, Allen and co-workers,[4] in a series of 120 necropsy-proven cases, with matched controls, did not confirm an increased incidence of thyroid disease, but noted however that the most severe cases of thyroid atrophy occurred in the multiple sclerosis series. It could be argued that both these necropsy studies were too small to be statistically significant, but a large clinical study of 828 cases of definite multiple sclerosis[5] found an incidence of autoimmune disease no higher than that estimated for the general population (see Ch. 4). The same author found a significantly higher prevalence of generally low titres of one or more autoantibodies in the multiple sclerosis group, and interpreted the result as non-specific B-cell overactivity. Similarly increased levels of autoantibodies, directed against antigenic determinants in pituitary growth hormone-producing cells and in structures containing vasopressin/oxytocin have been found in patients with multiple sclerosis,[6] but the specificity of these antibodies is unknown. A further study of 188 patients with multiple sclerosis[7] found a three-fold increased frequency of autoimmune thyroid disease, but no increase in other autoimmune diseases. Other reports include that of multiple sclerosis and lupus erythematosus in the same family,[8] multiple sclerosis associated with myasthenia gravis[9,10] and with bullous pemphigoid.[11] Overall there is no firm association of autoimmune diseases with multiple sclerosis, though genetic background may occasionally predispose to one or more of these conditions in patients with multiple sclerosis.

Studies on non-central nervous system malignancy in multiple sclerosis

The occasional coexistence of cerebral tumours and multiple sclerosis is well documented and is discussed in Chapter 4. The incidence and pattern of non-central nervous system malignancy in multiple sclerosis has been the subject of several studies. Zimmerman & Netsky[12] suggested that the overall incidence of malignancy in multiple sclerosis was unduly high, but Lumsden,[3] Allen et al[4] and Wender et al[13] all failed to confirm this finding. As with autoimmune diseases, therefore, the studies of malignancy to date do not suggest an immune disorder predisposing to increased or altered patterns of malignancy.

Relationship of genetic background, immune abnormalities and autoantigens in multiple sclerosis

The genetic background to multiple sclerosis and immune abnormalities associated with the disease have been discussed in detail previously (Chs. 10, 11). However, in assessing the case for an autoimmune pathogenesis, these factors have to be considered in relationship to each other and to the neuropathological abnormalities in multiple sclerosis and in various animal models. The best documented genetic abnormality is the association with antigens encoded within the major histocompatibility complex (MHC) and, as with diseases such as rheumatoid arthritis and insulin-dependent diabetes mellitus, the association is strongest with the MHC class II gene products. However, many inconsistencies have been found and clearly the whole genetic picture is not yet available. Several genes may be involved,[14] including not only those controlling antigen presentation to T-lymphocytes (MHC class II genes), but also those controlling T-cell receptors. Allelic polymorphisms of MHC class II genes are directly involved in regulating patterns of immune responsiveness and even a few amino acid substitutions in MHC class II molecules may increase significantly susceptibility to autoimmune diseases.[15] Such genetic evidence as does exist in multiple sclerosis suggests that similar factors may operate and may instigate an autoimmune response irrespective of other pathogenetic factors. Genetic background is of equal importance in animal models of demyelination with an autoimmune or combined infective/autoimmune pathogenesis (see below).

It is speculative and indeed premature at this stage to link genetic predisposition in multiple sclerosis with reported T-cell abnormalities and in particular with reduction in suppressor-inducer T-cells. Clearly, if such a genetic link did exist, then B-cell overactivity (both in relationship to exogenous and autoantigens), and cytokine release could all be explained as secondary effects. Much further work needs to be done both in humans and in experimental models to test such an hypothesis.

Autoimmune-induced human and experimental models of demyelination

The potential for an autollergic response to central nervous system tissue in man is supported by the fatal cases of demyelinating encephalitis following antirabies treatment by injections of emulsions of nervous tissue.[16–18] Similar lesions resulted from the injection of calf's brain extract for Parkinson's disease.[19] The lesions are generally of the perivascular type and mainly involve the spinal cord, although in some cases the demyelination is more confluent and the brain and optic nerves are involved. In all of these cases the antigen was administered repeatedly and there was no evidence of a relapsing-remitting condition. Lumsden[20] produced similar patterns of demyelination by repeated cyanide intoxication.

The injection of brain extracts to induce demyelination experimentally was first used in monkeys.[21] Since these initial experiments, the model, known as experimental allergic encephalitis, has been refined and a wide variety of pathological features produced by variations in injection schedules and by the use of various adjuvants and encephalitogenic antigens. Species and strain of animal also influence the pathological outcome.[22] Passive transfer by injection of lymphocytes from an affected to a normal animal is possible,[23] suggesting the importance of a cell-mediated response in pathogenesis.

In the hyperacute form of experimental allergic encephalitis the neuropathology is similar to acute haemorrhagic leucoencephalitis in man (see below) and is characterised by perivascular haemorrhage, fibrin deposition, focal necrosis and acute inflammation.[24] In a less severe but still acute form, the lesions resemble those of acute perivenous leucoencephalitis in man, with perivascular demyelination and cuffs of lymphocytes and macrophages (Fig. 13.1). Despite the dissimilarity of acute forms of experimental allergic encephalitis and multiple sclerosis, the development of the chronic relapsing model has shown that immunological and structural abnormalities similar to those seen in multiple sclerosis can be produced in susceptible strains of animals.[25–27] Circumscribed demyelinated lesions are found in cerebral white matter, in the periventricular region and in the optic nerves and spinal cord. Coalescence of perivascular plaques is a prominent feature (Fig. 13.2), but there may also be radial extension of plaques. Perivascular cuffing by lymphocytes is accompanied by oligodendrocyte loss, demyelination, macrophage reaction and gliosis. B-lymphocytes predominate in the perivascular location, whereas T-cells are found within the parenchyma.[28] Plasma

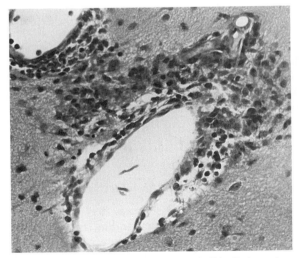

Figure 13.1 Experimental allergic encephalitis. Perivascular inflammation. (H&E × 250).

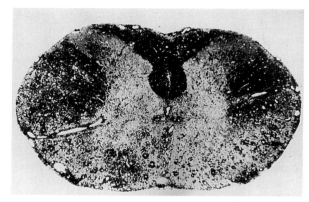

Figure 13.2   Chronic relapsing experimental allergic encephalitis. Spinal cord demyelination. (Woelcke × 100).

cells are present within the lesions and there is associated intrathecal IgG synthesis. It has been shown that genes controlling the induction of MHC class II antigen expression affect disease susceptibility in different rat strains and therefore, as in multiple sclerosis, genetic background is important.[29] There are, however, major differences between the two diseases which prevent experimental allergic encephalitis being used as the ideal model for multiple sclerosis. The induction and progression of experimental allergic encephalitis depends on the combination of a cell-mediated immune response to myelin basic protein and an antibody reaction to lipid markers such as galactocerebroside. There is as yet no convincing evidence of an antimyelin or antioligodendrocytic antibody response in multiple sclerosis, and therefore the significance of myelin as a potential source of autoantigens must be questioned. It may be that non-myelin antigens are primarily involved and destruction of myelin in multiple sclerosis is a secondary 'bystander effect'.

Additional evidence for an infective aetiology

The idea that multiple sclerosis may have an infective aetiology is of long standing and a variety of pathogens, including protozoa, bacteria, spirochaetes and mycoplasma, have been implicated in the past. Studies concerning identification or isolation of these organisms have not been con-

firmed and some of the observations can now be interpreted as artefactual. Most reproducible evidence of infection implicates viruses, and a variety of laboratory methods has been used to test the viral hypothesis, which is also supported by various epidemiological studies.[30,31]

Studies on viral antibodies

The observation, first made by Adams & Imagawa,[32] that patients with multiple sclerosis have high titres of measles antibody in serum and cerebrospinal fluid has been confirmed many times. Further work has shown that in addition to measles, other viral antibody levels, e.g. herpes simplex virus, mumps and rubella[33–35] may be raised and there is evidence of viral antibody synthesis within the central nervous system. The demonstration of antibodies to the retrovirus HTLV I in patients with tropical spastic paraparesis (HTLV I associated myelopathy)[36] has raised the possibility that a retrovirus might be implicated in multiple sclerosis. In a study of serum and cerebrospinal fluid antibody from multiple sclerosis patients[37] an elevation of antibodies against HTLV I was found: however, several studies have failed to confirm this result[38–41]

It has been shown that antiviral activity in multiple sclerosis is not restricted to IgG but can also be demonstrated in IgA[42] and that this response is not significantly affected by immunosuppressant therapy.[43] Supernatant fluids from cultured cerebrospinal fluid cells from multiple sclerosis patients contain viral antibodies, most commonly measles and rubella.[44] The pattern of antiviral response in the cerebrospinal fluid may change in the course of the disease[45] and may differ quantitatively from the various viral proteins as compared with serum.[46]

The significance of these antibody responses and their relationship to the cerebrospinal fluid immunoglobulins and oligoclonal bands is uncertain. Viral antigens will absorb only part of the immunoglobulin and similarly the oligoclonal bands are only partly absorbed.[47] It may well be that a non-specific, increased B-cell response explains the antibody phenomenon,[48] though the possibility of continual stimulation due to viral persistence cannot be excluded.

Studies on viral isolates and virus-like particles

Over the years, there have been several reports of isolation of viruses from multiple sclerosis tissues, including rabies, herpes simplex virus, measles and parainfluenza type I.[49] Most of these concern single cases and no consistent pattern has emerged. Again, many reports of virus-like particles in multiple sclerosis tissue, including brain and bone marrow, have appeared. Most of these are also of single cases in which very few particles have been seen in very small tissue samples. Further study has shown that many of these particles can be explained as artefactual or as normal intracellular organelles.[50,51] Thus it is clear that virus cannot be identified easily in multiple sclerosis by classical techniques, though the advent of newer, much more sensitive techniques keeps the viral hypothesis alive.

Studies on viral antigens and genome in multiple sclerosis

The concepts of viral persistence, latency and reactivation are of possible significance in multiple sclerosis and could explain the viral antibody response and the relapsing-remitting nature of the disease, similar to that of herpetic lesions of the skin. The failure to demonstrate virus morphologically or indeed by many other techniques in multiple sclerosis is not inconsistent with persistence and latency. In the case of the herpes viruses it is well documented that in the latent phase, no particles can be seen in ganglion cells and antigen cannot be detected. With varicella-zoster, the organism cannot be recovered from human ganglia during latency, but viral genome can be demonstrated by in situ hybridisation.[52] It is possible that similar mechanisms could operate in multiple sclerosis and the possibility of persistence in sites other than the nervous system, e.g. the reticuloendothelial system and the uvea, must be considered, as these can be affected in potentially demyelinating infections, e.g. canine distemper.[53]

In the last few years, several studies using immunohistochemical and molecular biological techniques have been undertaken in multiple sclerosis in an attempt to demonstrate viral persistence. Both positive and negative results have

been obtained, which have to be interpreted taking into account technique sensitivity and specificity. Using immunohistochemistry with antibodies to specific viral components, two positive studies have been reported. Cook and co-workers[54] found positivity within plaques using antisera to a feline-derived agent, thought to be a morbillivirus related to measles and distemper. Positive results have also been obtained in plaques using antisera to herpes virus (HSV-2).[55] With the advent of viral molecular techniques, several new studies have been undertaken looking for viral genomic sequences. Genetic information for cytomegalovirus and herpes simplex virus has not been found,[56] though the techniques used were not particularly sensitive. Measles virus has been the subject of several studies. Stevens and co-workers[57] examined four cases of multiple sclerosis by the technique of solution hybridisation with negative results. In a further study of eleven cases,[58] negative results were also obtained. In both studies, the techniques used were relatively insensitive and the brain sampling not extensive. By contrast, measles virus sequences were found in one of four multiple sclerosis brains,[59] though in a later study positive hybridisation was also found in controls.[60] In both of these studies, the method of probe preparation raises the possibility of cross-reaction with human tissues. In a recent study,[61] measles virus genome was demonstrated in two of eight multiple sclerosis cases (Fig. 13.3), but not in any of the 56 controls. The techniques used were sensitive and the brain sampling extensive: confirmation by polymerase chain reaction is required. Sequences related to human T-lymphotrophic virus type I have been described in peripheral blood mononuclear cells of six patients with multiple sclerosis[62] using the techniques of gene amplification molecular cloning and sequence analysis. However, in interpreting these results, the possibility of artefact in the gene amplification phase has to be considered and this result has not been confirmed.

Studies on virally-associated immune dysfunction in multiple sclerosis

Interactions of viruses and the immune system is complex and genetically determined host factors and viral molecular structure are both of import-

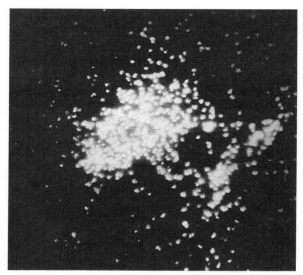

Figure 13.3   Periventricular MS plaque. Measles virus N genomic probe following RNase treatment. (Reflection contrast × 500).

ance. For example, it is known that HLA antigen can control immune response to separate sites on a viral protein antigen either directly through immune response genes or through linkage with other genes[63] and differences exist in the normal immune response to various viruses.[64] Evidence is accumulating that in multiple sclerosis some of the immune abnormalities observed are related to viral infection and possibly to viral persistence; therefore in assessing the viral hypothesis, these observations must be taken into account. As discussed previously (Ch. 11), serial measurements of suppressor T cells in multiple sclerosis patients and in their spouses and siblings have demonstrated that, while the siblings did not show the fluctuations with periodic reductions found in the patients, spouses showed responses similar and simultaneous to those occurring in the patient.[65] These findings indicate the importance of environmental factors, possibly infections, in multiple sclerosis but do not implicate a specific infection. Other reported immunological abnormalities, however, are of a specific nature and are related to possible measles persistence in multiple sclerosis. In a study of the cellular immune response to measles in twins, including pairs discordant and concordant for multiple sclerosis, a

difference in response to measles virus has been demonstrated in those twins with active multiple sclerosis as opposed to their normal twin sibling.[66] Affected twins had a persistently elevated response to measles virus, suggesting the presence of clonally-expanded, measles-specific, T-cell populations. A substantial number of patients with multiple sclerosis have been shown to have a reduced capacity to generate measles virus-specific cytotoxic T-lymphocytes,[67] even though responses to other viruses are normal.[68] Further studies have shown that there is no defect in the T-cell repertoire, nor is there cell sequestration due to cross-reactivity with a myelin antigen. It is more likely that there is an abnormality of induction or maintenance of the measles virus-cytotoxic T-lymphocyte response, or that there is cell sequestration within the central nervous system due to recognition of measles virus antigens.[69] A similar response in subacute sclerosing panencephalitis, a measles infection in which viral persistence in the central nervous system is a key factor in pathogenesis,[70] suggests that perhaps it is more likely that the response in multiple sclerosis is the result of cell sequestration within the central nervous system.

Studies on virally-induced experimental models of demyelination

The ability of viruses to induce demyelination in man (e.g. progressive multifocal leucoencephalopathy due to papovavirus) and in animals is undoubted. Mechanisms of demyelination include (i) viral infection with consequent cytolysis of myelin-bearing oligodendrocytes, (ii) immune-induced cytolysis of myelin-bearing cells by immune reactions directed against viral antigens, (iii) immune complex formation of viral antigen, host antibodies and complement causing secondary damage, (iv) virally-induced antimyelin autoimmunity.[71] Demyelinating viral infections which have been studied in their natural host include the JHM strain of mouse hepatitis virus, Theiler's murine encephalomyelitis, visna in sheep and canine encephalomyelitis.[72] Other experimentally-induced models include pathogens such as vesicular stomatitis, chandipura, measles, herpes simplex, Venezuelan encephalomyelitis and Semliki Forest virus. Using such models, the importance of factors such as age, genetic background and immune status of the host and the strain, and dose and route of inoculation are all seen to be relevant to the induction of demyelination.[73] Clearly, many of the viruses used in these models have no direct relevance to multiple sclerosis and can only be used to study pathogenetic mechanisms.[74] For example, using the Theiler encephalomyelitis model, it has been suggested that the mechanism of demyelination is immune-mediated.[75] The immunopathology, however, differs from that of experimental allergic encephalitis in that serum and cells from infected mice do not injure myelinating cultures or produce in vivo transfer of disease.[76] Recently, it has been suggested that the immune system plays a role in the initiation of virus replication which appears to be a prerequisite for demyelination.[77] In the case of JHM mouse hepatitis strain, subacute demyelination has been produced in 4–5 week old Lewis rats. Lymphocytes from these animals are sensitised to myelin basic protein and will transfer the disease passively to recipients. Thus, it is tempting to speculate that the virus generates an autoimmune response against myelin basic protein, because the initial infection is abortive or chronic in a young unnatural host.[78]

Three models are of more direct relevance to multiple sclerosis in that they all concern pathogens which have been implicated as a possible cause of the disease, i.e. measles, distemper and herpes simplex virus. Various measles models have been used: of particular interest is that of measles intracerebral inoculation in hamsters producing chronic relapsing myelitis,[79] with the onset of the myelitis 5–50 weeks after injection. In canine distemper infection, demyelination has been described both in the naturally occurring and experimental forms[80–82] (Fig. 13.4). In this model, early demyelination probably results from oligodendrocytic infection, whereas progressive, later lesions are probably immune mediated. By contrast, in the herpes simplex type 2 model in mice, demyelination appears to be related to neuronal infection with axonal transport of virus and subsequent infection of oligodendrocytes.[83–85]

Additional evidence for a combined infective/autoimmune aetiology in multiple sclerosis

Studies in other human demyelinating diseases

The clinical aspects of acute perivenous encephalomyelitis and its possible relationship to multiple sclerosis have been discussed in Chapter 6. However, in assessing the possibility of a combined infective-autoimmune pathogenesis for multiple sclerosis, the pathology of acute perivenous demyelination needs to be assessed because of its known association in many cases with viral infections and its similarity in some respects to acute, Marburg-type multiple sclerosis.

At necropsy in the *classical form* the brain and spinal cord may look normal or merely show slight congestion and oedema. Mild discoloration of the white matter may be seen, but no plaque-like lesions are apparent. The most distinctive histological feature is perivenular demyelination (Fig. 13.5) with total myelin disintegration, associated macrophage lipid phagocytosis, but with relative preservation of axis cylinders. A mild inflammatory response (initially neutrophil polymorph, later lymphocytic) is seen in the perivascular zone and in the meninges but this is not a pronounced feature. The cerebral hemispheres are usually symmetrically involved: occasionally, lesions become confluent, particularly in the spinal cord, but the tongue-like extensions seen in multiple sclerosis plaques are

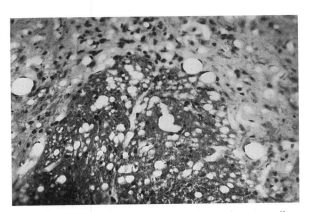

Figure 13.4 Canine distemper. Large plaque virus + small plaque virus, 8 days post inoculation. Demyelination, posterior columns, spinal cord. (H&E/Luxol-fast-blue × 500).

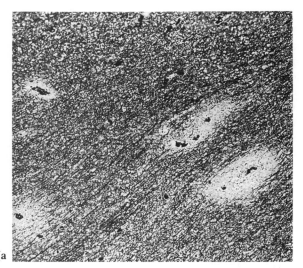

(a

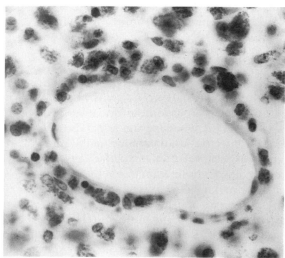

(b

Figure 13.5   Acute perivenous encephalomyelitis.
a) Perivenular demyelination. (Spielmeyer × 40).
b) Perivenular demyelination. Lipid laden macrophages.
(Scharlach R × 250).

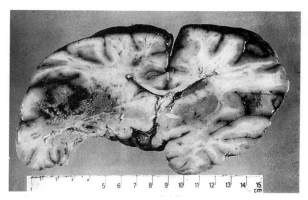

Figure 13.6   Acute haemorrhagic leucoencephalitis.

necropsy the brain is swollen and on section numerous small haemorrhages are seen mainly in the white matter, though the grey matter is also involved (Fig. 13.6). Histologically, the main abnormalities are related to blood vessels, with fibrinoid necrosis of small veins and fibrinous exudation. Oedema is marked and there is usually perivascular demyelination, neutrophil polymorph infiltration and ball and ring haemorrhages, centred on thrombosed capillaries. As tissue destruction proceeds, macrophages and astrocytes become prominent in the cellular response.

Subacute, late and recurrent forms of acute haemorrhagic leucoencephalitis have been described. Malamud[86] published a case of post measles encephalitis in which remissions and relapses occurred, and several further cases with this pattern have been described.[87,88] While it is generally accepted that acute disseminated perivenous encephalomyelitis is a monophasic disease, cases in which there has been recurrence of the syndrome, often related to different antigens, have been described.[89,90] Hart & Earle[91] have described four cases in which typical viral glial nodules (Babès nodes) were found in the brain in addition to perivenous demyelination, suggestive of viral infection.

Factors which can be cited against a classical infectious aetiology in these forms of demyelinating disease include the interval between the initiating and neurological illness, the relatively mild inflammatory response and the failure to recover organisms by classical virological techniques. In

not in evidence. Old lesions are characterised by astrocytic gliosis and an increase in perivascular reticulin. Neurons often appear normal though some may show chromatolysis, possibly related to axis cylinder destruction. The pathology has many features in common with experimental allergic encephalitis and, as in this model, the human disease has an acute counterpart — *acute haemorrhagic leucoencephalitis*. In this hyperacute form, at

these respects, this form of human demyelinating disease is similar to the demyelinating myelopathy induced with measles inoculation in the hamster.[79] The importance of cerebral vascular endothelium in the lesion has been emphasised by various workers,[92] but the exact pathogenesis is uncertain. In a study of seven cases, complicating measles, using in situ hybridisation for viral genome, virus could be demonstrated in many tissues but not in the central nervous system.[93] It is tempting therefore to suggest that virus, if it invades the brain at all, is cleared rapidly from this site and the subsequent demyelination is of immune or inflammatory origin.

Virally-induced experimental models of demyelination in which autoimmune reactions occur

Evidence is strong that in various experimental viral models of demyelination, autoimmune reactions against myelin occur. For example in experimental vaccinia,[94] reactions against whole myelin, myelin basic protein and oligodendrocytes have been described, and against galactocerebroside in Theiler's infection,[95] and glycolipids in Semliki Forest virus infection.[96] Moreover, the combination of viral infection with infection of central nervous system tissue can greatly increase the degree of demyelination in mice.[97] Perhaps the most thoroughly studied model is that of Theiler's murine encephalomyelitis which has several features of significance for multiple sclerosis. In this model, viral infection of oligodendrocytes is a prerequisite for the subsequent development of demyelination, though immune-mediated pathology is thought to contribute to the progression of the lesion.[77] Evidence implicating autoimmune factors has come from successful treatment of animals with immunosuppressive regimes[98] and from specific cell depletion experiments.[99] As with multiple sclerosis, susceptibility to demyelination in the mouse model is related to MHC locus antigens. Helper T-cells have been shown to be the key factor in preventing demyelination in strains of mice which are resistant to the process. Susceptibility to demyelination occurs either in athymic strains of mice or in normal mice by the depletion of CD4+ T-cells.[100]

In conclusion, it is premature to deduce from the experimental evidence available that we have an exact or even a good model of multiple sclerosis. There is much circumstantial evidence, however, implicating the importance of interaction of infectious agents, particularly viruses, with genetically-controlled factors in the immune system, and these may be the key to our understanding of the development of multiple sclerosis.

REFERENCES

1. Poser C M 1986 Pathogenesis of multiple sclerosis. Acta Neuropathologica (Berlin) 71: 1–10
2. Sayetta R B 1986 Theories of the etiology of multiple sclerosis: A critical review. Journal of Clinical Laboratory Immunology 21: 55–70
3. Lumsden C E 1970 In: Vinken P J, Bruyn G W (eds) Handbook of clinical neurology, Vol 9. North Holland Publishing, Amsterdam & American Elsevier, New York, pp 232–233
4. Allen I V, Millar J H D, Hutchinson M J 1978 General disease in 120 necropsy-proven cases of multiple sclerosis. Neuropathology and Applied Neurobiology 4: 279–284
5. De Keyser J 1988 Autoimmunity in multiple sclerosis. Neurology 38: 371–374
6. Møller A, Hansen B L, Hansen G N, Hagen C 1985 Autoantibodies in sera from patients with multiple sclerosis directed against antigenic determinants in pituitary growth hormone-producing cells and in structures containing vasopressin/oxytocin. Journal of Neuroimmunology 8: 177–184
7. Wynn D R, Codd M B, Kurland L T, Rodriguez M 1987 Multiple sclerosis: A population-based investigation of the association with possible autoimmune diseases or diabetes mellitus. Neurology 37 (3): 272
8. Sloan J B, Berk M A, Gebel H M, Fretzin D F 1987 Multiple sclerosis and systemic lupus erythematosus. Archives Internal Medicine 147: 1317–1320
9. Lo R, Feasby T E 1983 Multiple sclerosis and autoimmune diseases. Neurology (NY) 33: 97–98
10. Somer H, Muller K, Kinnunen E 1989 Myasthenia gravis associated with multiple sclerosis. Epidemiological survey and immunological findings. Journal of the Neurological Sciences 89: 37–48
11. Simjee S, Konqui A, Ahmed A R 1985 Multiple sclerosis and bullous pemphigoid. Dermatologica 170: 86–89

12. Zimmerman H M, Netsky G 1950 The pathology of multiple sclerosis. Association for Research in Nervous and Mental Disease Proceedings 28: 271–312

13. Wender M, Lenart-Jankowska D, Kowal P, Pruchnik–Grabowska D 1987 Incidence of malignant neoplasms in patients with multiple sclerosis. Neurologia Neurochir Pol 21 (1): 40–44

14. Heard R N S et al 1989 An allelic cluster of DQα restriction fragments is associated with multiple sclerosis: Evidence that a second haplotype may influence disease susceptibility. Human Immunology 25: in press

15. Gregersen P K 1989 HLA class II polymorphism: Implications for genetic susceptibility to autoimmune disease. Laboratory Investigation 61 (1): 5

16. Bassoe P, Grinker R R 1930 Human rabies and rabies vaccine encephalomyelitis. Archives of Neurology and Psychiatry 23: 1138–1160

17. Lesniowski S 1931 Inflammation de la substance grise du tronc cérébral (polioencephalitis superior et inferior) après vaccination antirabique. Journal of Neurology and Psychiatry 31: 427–440

18. Uchimura I, Shiraki H 1957 A contribution to the classification and the pathogenesis of demyelinating encephalomyelitis, with special reference to the central nervous system lesions caused by preventative inoculation against rabies. Journal of Neuropathology and Experimental Neurology 16: 139–208

19. Jellinger K, Seitelberger F 1958 Akute todliche Entmarkungsencephalitis nach wiederholten Hirntrockenzelleninjektionen. Klinische Wochenschrift 36: 437–441

20. Lumsden C E 1950 Cyanide leucoencephalopathy in rats and observations on the vascular and ferment hypotheses of demyelinating diseases. Journal of Neurology, Neurosurgery and Psychiatry 13: 1–15

21. Rivers T M, Sprunt D H, Berry G P 1933 Observations on attempts to produce acute disseminated encephalomyelitis in monkeys. Journal of Experimental Medicine 58: 39–53

22. Raine C S 1984 Analysis of autoimmune demyelination: its impact upon multiple sclerosis. Laboratory Investigation 50 (6): 608–635

23. Paterson P Y 1960 Transfer of allergic encephalomyelitis in rats by means of lymph node cells. Journal of Experimental Medicine 111: 119–135

24. Wisniewski H M, Lassmann H, Brosnan C F, Mehta P D, Lidsky A A, Madrid R E 1982 Multiple sclerosis: immunological and experimental aspects. In: Matthews W B, Glaser G H (eds) Recent advances in clinical neurology, Vol 3. Churchill Livingstone, Edinburgh, pp 95–124

25. Raine C S 1978 Membrane specialisations between demyelinated axons and astroglia in chronic EAE lesions and multiple sclerosis plaques. Nature (London) 275: 326–327

26. Brown A, McFarlin D E, Raine C S 1982 Chronologic, neuropathology of relapsing experimental allergic encephalomyelitis in the mouse. Laboratory Investigation 46: 171–185

27. Lassmann H, Kitz K, Wisniewski H M 1981 The development of periventricular lesions in chronic relapsing experimental allergic encephalomyelitis in guinea pigs: a light and scanning electron microscopic study. Neuropathology and Applied Neurobiology 7: 1–11

28. Traugott U, Shevach E, Chiba J, Stone S H, Raine C S 1982 Chronic relapsing experimental allergic encephalomyelitis: Identification and dynamics of T- and B-cells within the central nervous system. Cellular Immunology 68: 261–275

29. Male D, Pryce G 1989 Induction of Ia molecules on brain endothelium is related to susceptibility to experimental allergic encephalomyelitis. Journal of Neuroimmunology 21: 87–90

30. MacGregor J D, MacDonald J, Ingram E A, McDonnell M, Marshall B 1981 Epidemic measles in Shetland during 1977 and 1978. British Medical Journal 282: 434–436

31. Cook S D, Cromarty J I, Tapp W, Poskanzer D, Walker J D, Dowling P C 1985 Declining incidence of multiple sclerosis in the Orkney Islands. Neurology 35 (4): 545–551

32. Adams J M, Imagawa D T 1962 Measles antibodies in multiple sclerosis. Proceedings of the Society for Experimental Biology and Medicine 111: 562–566

33. Norrby E, Link H, Olsson J, Panelius M, Salmi A, Vandvik B 1974 Comparison of antibodies against different viruses in cerebrospinal fluid and serum samples from patients with multiple sclerosis. Infection and Immunity 10: 688–694

34. Goswami K K A, Randall R E, Lange L S, Russell W C 1987 Antibodies against the paramyxovirus SV5 in the cerebrospinal fluids of some multiple sclerosis patients. Nature 327: 244–247

35. Brankin B, Wisdom G B, Allen I V, Hawkins S A, Cosby S L 1989 Antibodies to simian virus 5 in patients with multiple sclerosis and other neurological disorders. Journal of the Neurological Sciences 89: 181–187

36. Gessain A et al 1985 Antibodies to human T-lymphotrophic virus type-I in patients with tropical spastic paraparesis. Lancet 2: 407–409

37. Koprowski H et al 1985 Multiple sclerosis and human T-cell lymphotropic retroviruses. Nature 318: 154–160

38. De Rossi A, Gallo P, Tavolato B, Callegaro L, Chieco-Bianchi L 1986 Search for HTLV-I and LAV/HTLV-III antibodies in serum and CSF of multiple sclerosis patients. Acta Neurol Scandinavica 74: 161–164

39. Epstein L et al 1987 Serum antibodies to HTLV-I in human demyelinating disease. Acta Neurol Scandinavica 75: 231–233

40. Kuroda Y, Shibasaki H, Sato H, Okochi K 1987 Incidence of antibody to HTLV-I is not increased in Japanese MS patients. Neurology 37 (1): 156–158

41. Madden D L et al 1988 Serologic studies of MS patients, controls, and patients with other neurologic diseases: Antibodies to HTLV-I, II, III. Neurology 38: 81–84

42. Coyle P K, Brook S 1988 Antigenic specificity and electrophoretic pattern of polymeric and monomeric IgA in multiple sclerosis. Neurology 38 (suppl 1): 197

43. Nath A, Wolinsky J S, Kerman R H 1989 Effect of cyclosporine on rubella virus-specific immune responses in chronic progressive multiple sclerosis. Journal of Neuroimmunology 22: 143–148

44. Salmi A A, Hyypiä T, Ilonen J, Reunanen M, Remes

M 1989 Production of viral antibodies in vitro by CSF cells from mumps, meningitis and multiple sclerosis patients. Journal of the Neurological Sciences 90: 315–324

45. Sandberg-Wollheim M, Vandvik B, Nadj C, Norrby E 1987 The intrathecal immune response in the early stage of multiple sclerosis. Journal of the Neurological Sciences 81: 45–53

46. Walsh M J, Shapshak P, Graves M C, Imagawa D T, Tourtellotte W W 1987 Isoelectric point restriction of cerebrospinal fluid and serum IgG antibodies to measles virus polypeptides in multiple sclerosis. Journal of Neuroimmunology 14: 243–252

47. Roström B 1981 Specificity of antibodies in oligoclonal bands in patients with multiple sclerosis and cerebrovascular disease. Acta Neurologica Scandinavica (suppl) 86

48. Leinikki P et al 1982 Virus antibodies in the cerebrospinal fluid of multiple sclerosis patients detected with Elisa tests. Journal of the Neurological Sciences 57: 249–255

49. ter Meulen V, Stephenson J R 1983 The possible role of viral infections in multiple sclerosis and other related demyelinating diseases. In: Hallpike J F, Adams C W M, Tourtellotte W W (eds) Multiple sclerosis: pathology, diagnosis and management. Chapman and Hall, London, pp 241–275

50. Kirk J, Hutchinson W M 1978 The fine structure of the CNS in multiple sclerosis. I. Interpretation of cytoplasmic papovavirus-like and paramyxovirus-like inclusions. Neuropathology and Applied Neurobiology 4: 343–356

51. Kirk J 1979 Pseudoviral hollow-cored vesicles in multiple sclerosis brain. Acta Neuropathologica 48: 63–66

52. Johnson R T 1984 Relapsing and remitting viral diseases of the nervous system. Trends in Neurosciences 7 (8): 268–269

53. Summers B A, Greisen H A, Appel M J G 1983 Does virus persist in the uvea in multiple sclerosis, as in canine distemper encephalomyelitis? Lancet 2: 372–373

54. Cook R D, Flower R L P, Dutton N S 1986 Light and electron microscopical studies of the immunoperoxidase staining of multiple sclerosis plaques using antisera to a feline-derived agent and to galactocerebroside. Neuropathology and Applied Neurobiology 12: 63–79

55. Martin J R, Holt R K, Webster H de F 1988 Herpes simplex-related antigen in human demyelinative disease and encephalitis. Acta Neuropathologica 76 (4): 325–337

56. Aulakh G S, Albrecht P, Tourtellotte W W 1980 Search for cytomegalovirus and herpes simplex virus genetic information in multiple sclerosis. Neurology 30: 530–532

57. Stevens J G, Bastone V B, Ellison G W, Myers L W 1979 No measles virus genetic information detected in multiple sclerosis-derived brains. Annals of Neurology 8 (6): 625–627

58. Dowling P C et al 1986 Measles virus nucleic acid sequences in human brain. Virus Research 5: 97–107

59. Haase A T, Ventura P, Gibbs C J, Tourtellotte W W 1981 Measles virus nucleotide sequences: detection by hybridization in situ. Science 212: 672–675

60. Haase A T et al 1984 Detection of hybridization of viral infection of the CNS. Annals of the New York Academy of Sciences 436: 103–108

61. Cosby S L et al 1989 Examination of eight cases of multiple sclerosis and 56 neurological and non-neurological controls for genomic sequences of measles virus, canine distemper virus, simian virus 5 and rubella virus. Journal General Virology 70: 2027–2036

62. Premkumar Reddy E, Sandberg-Wollheim M, Mettus R V, Ray P E, DeFreitas E, Koprowski H 1989 Amplification and molecular cloning of HTLV-I: Sequences from DNA of multiple sclerosis patients. Science 243: 529–533

63. Mäkelä M J 1989 Antibody response to different antigenic sites on measles virus surface polypeptides in patients with multiple sclerosis. Journal of the Neurological Sciences 90: 239–246

64. McFarland H F, McFarlin D E 1979 Cellular immune response to measles, mumps, and vaccinia viruses in multiple sclerosis. Annals of Neurology 6: 101–106

65. Hughes P J, Kirk P F, Compston D A S 1986 Suppressor T-cells in family members of patients with multiple sclerosis. Brain 109: 969–985

66. Greenstein J I, McFarland H F, Mingioli E S, McFarlin D E 1984 The lymphoproliferative response to measles virus in twins with multiple sclerosis. Annals of Neurology 15: 79–87

67. Jacobson S, Flerlage M L, McFarland H F 1985 Impaired measles virus-specific cytotoxic T cell responses in multiple sclerosis. Journal of Experimental Medicine 162: 839–850

68. Goodman A D, Jacobson S, McFarland H F 1989 Virus-specific cytotoxic T-lymphocytes in multiple sclerosis: a normal mumps virus response adds support for a distinct impairment in the measles virus response. Journal of Neuroimmunology 22: 201–209

69. Dhib-Jalbut S, McFarlin D E, McFarland H F 1989 Measles virus-polypeptide specificity of the cytotoxic T-lymphocyte response in multiple sclerosis. Journal of Neuroimmunology 21: 205–212

70. Dhib-Jalbut S, Jacobson S, McFarlin D E, McFarland H F 1989 Impaired human leukocyte antigen-restricted measles virus-specific cytotoxic T-cell response in subacute sclerosing panencephalitis. Annals of Neurology 25: 272–280

71. Lampert P W 1978 Autoimmune and virus-induced demyelinating diseases. American Journal of Pathology 91: 176–208

72. Dal Canto M C, Rabinowitz S G 1982 Experimental models of virus-induced demyelination of the central nervous system. Annals of Neurology 11: 109–127

73. Buchmeier M J, Dalziel R G, Koolen M J M 1988 Coronavirus-induced CNS disease: a model for virus-induced demyelination. Journal of Neuroimmunology 20: 111–116

74. Whitaker J N, Kingsburn D W 1984 Viruses and the pathogenesis of multiple sclerosis. Trends in Neurosciences 7 (3): 57–60

75. Dal Canto M C, Lipton H L 1975 Primary demyelination in Theiler's virus infection. Laboratory Investigation 33 (6): 626–637

76. Barbano R L, Dal Canto M C 1984 Serum and cells from Theiler's virus-infected mice fail to injure myelinating cultures or to produce in vivo transfer of disease. Journal of the Neurological Sciences 66: 283–293

77. Blakemore W F, Welsh C J R, Tonks P, Nash A A

1988 Observations on demyelinating lesions induced by Theiler's virus in CBA mice. Acta Neuropathologica 76: 581–589

78. Watanabe R, Wege H, ter Meulen V 1983 Adoptive transfer of EAE-like lesions from rats with coronavirus-induced demyelinating encephalomyelitis. Nature (London) 305: 150–153

79. Carrigan D R, Johnson K P 1980 Chronic relapsing myelitis in hamsters associated with experimental measles virus infection. Proceedings National Academy Science 77: 4297–4300

80. Vandevelde M, Kristensen F, Kristensen B, Steck A J, Kihm U 1982 Immunological and pathological findings in demyelinating encephalitis associated with canine distemper virus infection. Acta Neuropathologica (Berlin) 56: 1–8

81. Vandevelde M, Higgins R J, Kristensen B, Kristensen F, Steck A J, Kihm U 1982 Demyelination in experimental canine distemper virus infection: immunological, pathologic and immunohistological studies. Acta Neuropathologica (Berlin) 56: 285–293

82. Allen I V, Cosby S L, Kirk J, Martin S J, Dinsmore S 1987 Neuropathology and neurovirulence of canine distemper virus plaque isolates in the hamster. Neuropathology and Applied Neurobiology 13: 349–369

83. Martin J R 1982 Spinal cord and optic nerve demyelination in experimental herpes simplex virus type 2 infection. Journal of Neuropathology and Experimental Neurology 41 (3): 253–266

84. Flynn T E, Martin J R 1983 Topography of remyelinated chronic spinal cord lesions in herpes simplex virus type 2 infections of mice. Journal of the Neurological Sciences 61: 327–339

85. Martin J R 1984 Intra-axonal virus in demyelinative lesions of experimental herpes simplex type 2 infection. Journal of Neurological Sciences 63: 63–74

86. Malamud N 1939 Sequelae of postmeasles encephalomyelitis. A clinicopathologic study. Archives of Neurology and Psychiatry 41: 943–954

87. Bérard–Badier M, Gastaut H, Payan H 1961 Comparative clinico-pathological study of one early and two late cases of measles encephalitis (with an electroencephalographic study of one case). In: van Bogaert L, Radermecker J, Hozay J, Lowenthal A (eds) Encephalitides: proceedings of a symposium on the neuropathology, electronencephalography and biochemistry of encephalitides, Antwerp, 1959. Elsevier, London, pp 106–123

88. Oppenheimer D R 1966 A case of so-called demyelination encephalitis. Neuropatologia Polska 4 (suppl): 151–162

89. Alcock N S, Hoffman H L 1962 Recurrent encephalomyelitis in childhood. Archives of Diseases in Childhood 37: 40–44

90. van Bogaert L 1950 Post-infectious encephalomyelitis and multiple sclerosis. Journal of Neuropathology and Experimental Neurology 9: 219–249

91. Hart M N, Earle K M 1975 Haemorrhagic and perivenous encephalitis: a clinical-pathological review of 38 cases. Journal of Neurology, Neurosurgery and Psychiatry 38: 585–591

92. Poser C M, Roman G, Emery E S III 1978 Recurrent disseminated vasculomyelinopathy. Archives of Neurology 35: 166–170

93. Moench T R, Griffin D E, Obriecht C R, Vaisberg A, Johnson R T 1988 Distribution of measles virus antigen and RNA in acute measles with and without neurologic involvement. Journal of Infective Diseases 158: 433–442

94. Steck A J, Tschannen R, Schaefer R 1981 Induction of antimyelin and antioligodendrocyte antibodies by vaccinia virus. Journal of Neuroimmunology 1: 117–124

95. Fujinami R S, Zurbriggen A, Powell H C 1988 Monoclonal antibody defines determinant between Theiler's virus and lipid-like structures. Journal of Neuroimmunology 20: 25–32

96. Khalili-Shirazi A, Gregson N, Webb H E 1986 Immunological relationship between a demyelinating RNA enveloped budding virus (Semliki Forest) and brain glycolipids. Journal of the Neurological Sciences 76: 91–103

97. Salmi A, Wu L–X, Röyttä M, Mäkelä M J 1987 Modulation of experimental allergic encephalomyelitis in mouse by virus infection. Journal of Neuroimmunology 16 (1): 152–153

98. Lipton, Dal Canto M 1979 Infection and Immunity 26: 369–374

99. Welsh C J R, Tonks P, Nash A A, Blakemore W W 1987 The effect of L3T4 T-cell depletion on the pathogenesis of Theiler's murine encephalomyelitis virus infection in CBA mice. Journal General Virology 68: 1659–1667

100. Rosenthal A, Fujinami R S, Lampert P W 1986 Mechanism of Theiler's virus-induced demyelination in nude mice. Laboratory Investigation 54: 515–522

Index